DIABETIC FOOT
Lower Extremity Arterial Disease and Limb Salvage

FIRST EDITION

DIABETIC FOOT
Lower Extremity Arterial Disease and Limb Salvage

FIRST EDITION

EDITOR

— **ANTON N. SIDAWY, MD, MPH, FACS**

Chief, Surgical Services
Veterans Affairs Medical Center
Professor of Surgery
George Washington and Georgetown Universities Medical Centers
Washington, District of Columbia

LIPPINCOTT WILLIAMS & WILKINS
A **Wolters Kluwer** Company

Philadelphia • Baltimore • New York • London
Buenos Aires • Hong Kong • Sydney • Tokyo

Acquisitions Editor: Brian Brown
Managing Editor: Julia Seto
Project Manager: Fran Gunning
Manufacturing Manager: Ben Rivera
Marketing Manager: Adam Glazer
Design Coordinator: Terry Mallon
Production Services: Laserwords Private Limited
Printer: Edwards Brothers

First Edition
© 2006 by Lippincott Williams & Wilkins
530 Walnut Street
Philadelphia, PA 19106
www.LWW.com

Printed in the United States

Library of Congress Cataloging-in-Publication Data
Diabetic foot : lower extremity arterial disease and limb salvage / editor, Anton N. Sidawy.-- 1st ed.
   p. ; cm.
 Includes bibliographical references and index.
 ISBN 0-7817-6068-2
 1. Foot--Blood-vessels--Diseases. 2. Foot--Surgery. 3. Diabetes--Complications.
   4. Limb salvage. I. Sidawy, Anton N.
 [DNLM: 1. Diabetic Foot. WK 835 D53517 2006]
RD563.D493 2006
617.5'85059--dc22

                                                       2005028208

Care has been taken to confirm the accuracy of the information presented and to describe generally accepted practices. However, the authors, editors, and publisher are not responsible for errors or omissions or for any consequences from application of the information in this book and make no warranty, expressed or implied, with respect to the currency, completeness, or accuracy of the contents of the publication. Application of this information in a particular situation remains the professional responsibility of the practitioner.

The authors, editors, and publisher have exerted every effort to ensure that drug selection and dosage set forth in this text are in accordance with current recommendations and practice at the time of publication. However, in view of ongoing research, changes in government regulations, and the constant flow of information relating to drug therapy and drug reactions, the reader is urged to check the package insert for each drug for any change in indications and dosage and for added warnings and precautions. This is particularly important when the recommended agent is a new or infrequently employed drug.

Some drugs and medical devices presented in this publication have Food and Drug Administration (FDA) clearance for limited use in restricted research settings. It is the responsibility of health care providers to ascertain the FDA status of each drug or device planned for use in their clinical practice.

The publisher has made every effort to trace copyright holders for borrowed material. If they have inadvertently overlooked any, they will be pleased to make the necessary arrangements at the first opportunity.

To purchase additional copies of this book, call our customer service department at (800) 638-3030 or fax orders to (301) 223-2320. International customers should call (301) 223-2300. Lippincott Williams & Wilkins customer service representatives are available from 8:30 am to 6:30 pm, EST, Monday through Friday, for telephone access. Visit Lippincott Williams & Wilkins on the Internet: http://www.lww.com.

                                             10 9 8 7 6 5 4 3 2 1

To Mary, Michelle, and Nicholas
Their patience, support, and inspiration made this contribution possible.

Contents

Preface

The incidence and prevalence of diabetes mellitus continue to rise. Over half of all lower extremity amputations are performed in diabetics. The topic of the diabetic foot, including its prevention and management, is of paramount importance to individuals afflicted with this disease. Three factors converge in diabetics to form the "perfect storm" that leaves in its wake a foot badly injured and infected, leading to major amputation if not appropriately managed. These factors are neuropathy that renders the foot insensate, compromised immunity that increases the propensity for infections, and ischemia due to arterial occlusive disease, particularly in the tibioperoneal distribution. Most books dealing with the diabetic foot dedicate only a small part to the discussion and management of lower extremity arterial disease in these patients. In contrast, while planning this book, I wanted to emphasize arterial disease and its management while also addressing other factors that play major roles in lower extremity complications of diabetes.

The chapters in this book could be organized in two major groups: The first dealing with the diabetic foot proper, and the next section covering lower extremity arterial disease and its management in diabetics. However, instead of grouping the chapters as such, I felt that their sequence should follow how physicians encounter patients with this disease and then proceed with its diagnosis and management. The book concludes with the coverage of major leg amputations to emphasize that, in these patients, a major amputation should be a last-resort procedure. The impact of neuropathy and alterations in gait biomechanics on the formation of foot wounds and Charcot foot seen in diabetic patients independent of occlusive arterial disease is detailed so that the importance of prevention can be appreciated. Appropriate wound management and closure techniques are of paramount importance to limb salvage. Medical and surgical control of foot infections is important in preventing major amputations and optimizing length and functionality of foot amputations. Angiogenesis and the concept of angiosomes and their role in healing foot lesions are discussed in detail.

While planning the strategy to improve arterial blood flow using reconstructive surgery or endovascular techniques, it is important to understand the distribution of peripheral arterial disease in these patients. Although the femoral-popliteal segment is the region most commonly affected, infragenicular occlusive disease in the anterior tibial, posterior tibial, and peroneal arteries is the classic distribution in diabetics, and it is the disease most challenging to correct. It is not unusual to encounter diabetic patients with ischemic foot lesions having a palpable popliteal pulse with occlusive disease isolated to the infragenicular arteries of the leg, sparing the arterial system in the foot, which renders it amenable to successful vascular reconstruction. Endovascular techniques and bypasses to distal tibioperoneal and pedal arteries are highly demanding, requiring skill and time to perform. Placement of femoral-to-tibial or popliteal-to-tibial bypass is a meticulous procedure that distinguishes the surgeon. All aspects of pathophysiology, anatomy, diagnosis, and management of infragenicular disease need to be well understood for optimal patient care and are presented in detail in this text. Throughout this book, various terms are used interchangeably to describe the particular distribution of atherosclerotic disease that involves the anterior tibial, posterior tibial, and peroneal arteries sparing the pedal vessels; these terms are also used interchangeably to describe bypasses that treat this disease. These terms include: Tibial, tibioperoneal, distal, crural, infragenicular, and infrapopliteal.

It is my hope that this book will further the understanding of this disease and its management leading to optimal limb salvage and functionality. This objective can only be attained through a multidisciplinary team approach that combines the efforts of not only vascular and reconstructive surgeons but other specialists, as well. I would like to thank wholeheartedly the authors that contributed time and effort to this project; they indeed represent the multidisciplinary approach required for optimal management of this difficult problem.

Anton N. Sidawy, MD, MPH, FACS
Washington, D.C.

Foreword

There may be dramatic challenges facing vascular surgeons today, but none of these challenges is more complex and vexing than those presented by diabetic patients who have progressed to the point of neuropathy, vascular disease, and impaired response to infection. This triad accounts for an inordinate number of amputations in diabetic patients, and yet much of this horrendous toll is preventable by the knowledge so carefully detailed and discussed in this book. It contains just about everything that one needs to know to make a significant difference, for the better, in managing these patients, regardless of whether they present with neurotrophic ulcers, foot sepsis, or chronic critical ischemia. This knowledge is imparted in great detail, and is organized into multiple expertly written chapters, which cover every conceivable aspect of this subject.

Those who wish to aspire to the proud designation of "limb salvage surgeon," and even those who are already devoting much of their surgical efforts in this direction, should have this book. It goes far beyond the scope of even the most comprehensive vascular surgical text. Furthermore, it goes into details well beyond vascular surgery, with chapters written by other specialists on many basic considerations such as the microbiology of foot sepsis, the biomechanical consequences of the associated neuropathy, preventative foot care, the use of orthotics and proper foot wear, and other considerations which should make this book valuable to any physicians and health care professionals involved with diabetic foot problems.

This book will not only serve as a read-through text but as a valuable reference to be consulted whenever these problems confront the reader. Dr. Sidawy and his many carefully selected contributors are to be congratulated on producing a needed and valuable addition to our knowledge base. It is a very important topic, and they have indeed done an excellent job of covering all of its critical aspects.

Robert B. Rutherford, MD, FACS

Contributors

CHRISTOPHER J. ABULARRAGE, MD General Surgery Resident, Department of Surgery, Georgetown University Hospital, Washington, District of Columbia

ERIC D. ADAMS, MD Staff, Vascular Surgeon, Department of Surgery, Section of Vascular Surgery, Walter Reed Army Medical Center, Washington, District of Columbia; Adjunct Assistant Professor, Department of Surgery, Uniformed Services University of the Health Sciences, Bethesda, Maryland

CAMERON M. AKBARI, MD, MBA Senior Attending in Vascular Surgery and Director of Vascular Diagnostic Laboratory, Department of Vascular Surgery, Washington Hospital Center; Assistant Professor, Department of Surgery, Georgetown University School of Medicine, Washington, District of Columbia

SUBODH ARORA, MD Associate Professor of Surgery, Department of Surgery, George Washington University Hospital and Veterans Affairs Medical Center, Washington, District of Columbia

ENRICO ASCHER, MD Director, Department of Vascular Surgery, Maimonides Medical Center, Brooklyn, New York; Professor of Surgery, Mount Sinai School of Medicine, New York, New York

CHRISTOPHER E. ATTINGER, MD Medical Director, The Limb Center, Georgetown University Hospital, Washington, District of Columbia

BERNADETTE AULIVOLA, MD, RVT Attending Vascular Surgeon, Departments of Surgery and Radiology, Loyola University Health System; Assistant Professor, Departments of Surgery and Radiology, Loyola University Chicago-Stritch School of Medicine, Maywood, Illinois

IAN H. BEISER, DPM Assistant Clinical Professor, Department of Surgery, George Washington University, Washington, District of Columbia

CHRISTOPHER T. BUNCH, MD Staff Physician, Department of Surgery, Duluth Clinic/SMDC Health System, Duluth, Minnesota

KEITH D. CALLIGARO, MD Chief, Section of Vascular Surgery, Pennsylvania Hospital; Clinical Professor, Department of Surgery, University of Pennsylvania, Philadelphia, Pennsylvania

BENJAMIN B. CHANG, MD Attending Vascular Surgeon, Division of Vascular Surgery, Albany Medical Center Hospital; Assistant Professor of Surgery, Albany Medical College, Albany, New York

MICHAEL S. CONTE, MD Associate Surgeon, Department of Vascular Surgery, Brigham and Women's Hospital; Associate Professor, Department of Surgery, Harvard Medical School, Boston, Massachusetts

HERBERT DARDIK, MD Chairman, Department of Surgery, Englewood Hospital and Medical Center, Englewood, New Jersey; Clinical Professor, Department of Surgery, Mount Sinai School of Medicine, New York, New York

R. CLEMENT DARLING, III, MD Chief, Division of Vascular Surgery, Albany Medical Center Hospital; Professor, Department of Surgery, Albany Medical College, Albany, New York

KEVIN DOERR, RVT Section of Vascular Surgery, Pennsylvania Hospital, Philadelphia, Pennsylvania

MATTHEW J. DOUGHERTY, MD Section of Vascular Surgery, Pennsylvania Hospital, Philadelphia, Pennsylvania

KAREN KIM EVANS, MD Attending Plastic Surgeon, Veterans Affairs Medical Center, Washington, District of Columbia

CHARLES J. FOX, MD Attending Surgeon, Vascular Surgery Service, Walter Reed Army Medical Center, Washington, District of Columbia; Assistant Professor, Department of Surgery, Uniformed Services University of the Health Sciences, Bethesda, Maryland

ROBERT G. FRYKBERG, DPM, MPH Chief, Podiatric Surgery, Department of Surgery, Carl T. Hayden Veterans Affairs Medical Center, Phoenix; Adjunct Professor of Podiatric Medicine, Arizona Podiatric Medicine Program, Midwestern University, Glendale, Arizona

DAVID L. GILLESPIE, MD Chief and Program Director, Department of Vascular Surgery, Walter Reed Army Medical Center, Washington, District of Columbia; Associate Professor of Surgery, Division of Vascular Surgery, Uniformed Services University of the Health Sciences, Bethesda, Maryland

JOSEPH GIORDANO, MD Professor and Chairman, Department of Surgery, George Washington University Hospital, Washington, District of Columbia

PETER GLOVICZKI, MD Professor and Chair, Department of Vascular Surgery, Mayo Clinic; Professor and Chair, Department of Vascular Surgery, Gonda Vascular Center, Mayo Clinic and Foundation, Rochester, Minnesota

PETER HENDERSON, MD Division of Vascular Surgery, New York-Presbyterian Hospital Weill Medical College of Cornell University, Columbia University College of Physicians and Surgeons, New York, New York

ANIL HINGORANI, MD Division of Vascular Surgery, Maimonides Medical Center, Brooklyn; Associate Professor, Department of Surgery, Mount Sinai School of Medicine, New York, New York

JAMAL J. HOBALLAH, MD, MBA Chairman, Division of Vascular Surgery, University of Iowa Hospitals and Clinics; Professor of Surgery, Department of Surgery, University of Iowa, Iowa City, Iowa

THERESA M. IMPEDUGLIA, MD Assistant Director of Vascular Fellowship Training Program, Director of Surgical Research Laboratory, Department of Surgery, Englewood Hospital and Medical Center, Englewood, New Jersey; Assistant Clinical Professor of Surgery, Department of Surgery, Mount Sinai School of Medicine, New York, New York

MANJU KALRA, MBBS Assistant Professor, Department of Vascular Surgery, Mayo Clinic; Assistant Professor, Department of Vascular Surgery, Gonda Vascular Center, Mayo Clinic and Foundation, Rochester, Minnesota

VIRGINIA L. KAN, MD Associate Chief, Infectious Diseases Section, Department of Medical Service, Veteran Affairs Medical Center; Associate Professor, Department of Medicine, George Washington University School of Medicine, Washington, District of Columbia

K. CRAIG KENT, MD Chief, Division of Vascular Surgery, New York Presbyterian Hospital; Professor of Surgery, Weill Medical College of Cornell University, Columbia College of Physians and Surgeons, New York, New York

GLENN M. LAMURAGLIA, MD Visiting Surgeon, Department of Vascular and Endovascular Surgery, Massachusetts General Hospital, Boston, Massachusetts; Associate Professor of Surgery, Harvard Medical School, Cambridge, Massachusetts

JOHN C. LANTIS, II, MD Director of Clinical Research, Department of Surgery, St. Luke's-Roosevelt Hospital; Assistant Professor, Department of Surgery, Columbia University, New York, New York

EVAN C. LIPSITZ, MD Medical Director of Vascular Diagnostic Laboratory, Division of Vascular Surgery, Montefiore Medical Center; Associate Professor, Division of Vascular Surgery, Albert Einstein College of Medicine, Bronx, New York

FRANK W. LOGERFO, MD Chief, Division of Vascular and Endovascular Surgery, Beth Israel Deaconess Medical Center; William V. McDermott Professor of Surgery, Harvard Medical School, Boston, Massachusetts

SANDY MCAFFEE-BENNETT, RVT Section of Vascular Surgery, Pennsylvania Hospital, Philadelphia, Pennsylvania

JAMES O. MENZOIAN, MD Chief and Professor of Surgery, Section of Vascular Surgery, Boston University Medical Center, Boston, Massachusetts

KENDRA MAGEE MERINE, MD Vascular Surgery Fellow, Department of Vascular Surgery, Washington Hospital Center/Georgetown University Medical Center, Washington, District of Columbia

ALI MESBAHI, MD Resident Physician, Plastic and Reconstructive Surgery, Georgetown University Hospital, Washington, District of Columbia

MICHAEL L. MILLER, MD Staff Vascular Surgeon, Keesler USAF Medical Center, Keesler Air Force Base, Biloxi, Mississippi

JOSEPH L. MILLS, SR., MD Chief, Division of Vascular and Endovascular Surgery, University Medical Center; Professor of Surgery, University of Arizona Health Sciences Center, Tucson, Arizona

MARC E. MITCHELL, MD Chief, Division of Vascular Surgery, University of Mississippi Medical Center; Associate Professor, Department of Surgery and Radiology, University of Mississippi, Jackson, Mississippi

SAMUEL R. MONEY, MD, MBA Head, Department of Vascular Surgery, Ochsner Clinic Foundation; Clinical Associate Professor of Surgery, Tulane University School of Medicine, New Orleans, Louisiana

ALBEIR Y. MOUSA, MD Resident, Department of Surgery, Brookdale University Hospital and Medical Center, Brooklyn, New York

RICHARD F. NEVILLE, MD Chief of Vascular Surgery, Department of Surgery, Georgetown University Hospital, Washington, District of Columbia

GIUSEPPE R. NIGRI, MD, PHD Attending Surgeon, Department of Surgery, Sant'Andrea Hospital; Assistant Professor of Surgery, La Sapienza University, Rome, Italy

ERIC S. NYLÉN, MD Chief of Diabetes, Department of Medicine, Veterans Affairs Medical Center; Professor, Department of Medicine, George Washington University School of Medicine, Washington, District of Columbia

SEAN D. O'DONNELL, MD, COL, MC Director of the Section of Vascular Surgery, Washington Hospital Center, Washington, District of Columbia; Associate Professor of Surgery, Uniformed Services University of the Health Sciences, Bethesda, Maryland

KENNETH OURIEL, MD Chairman, Division of Surgery, Cleveland Clinical Foundation; Professor of Surgery, Cleveland Clinic Lerner College of Medicine, Cleveland, Ohio

FRANK POMPOSELLI, MD Chief, Division of Vascular Surgery, Beth Israel Deaconess Medical Center; Associate Professor of Surgery, Harvard Medical School, Boston, Massachusetts

JOSEPH D. RAFFETTO, MD Assistant Professor of Surgery, Section of Vascular Surgery, Boston University Medical Center, Boston, Massachusetts

TODD E. RASMUSSEN, MD Chief, Vascular and Endovascular Surgery Services, Wilford Hall USAF Medical Center, Lackland Air Force Base, Texas; Assistant Professor of Surgery, Norman M. Rich Department of Surgery, Uniformed Services University of the Health Sciences, Bethesda, Maryland

SEAN P. RODDY, MD Associate Professor, Department of Surgery, Albany Medical College, Albany, New York

SHERRY D. SCOVELL, MD Director, Department of Endovascular Surgery, Beth Israel Deaconess Medical Center; Instructor, Harvard Medical School, Boston, Massachusetts

TEJAS R. SHAH, BS Division of Vascular Surgery, Montefiore Medical Center, Bronx; Department of Vascular Surgery, SUNY Downstate Health Science Center, Brooklyn, New York

GAUTAM SHRIKHANDE, MD Clinical Fellow in Surgery, Harvard Medical School, Beth Israel Deaconess Medical Center, Boston, Massachusetts

CHARLES J. SHUMAN, DPM Assistant Chief, Department of Surgery, Chief of Podiatry, Veterans Affairs Medical Center, Washington, District of Columbia

ANTON N. SIDAWY, MD, MPH Chief, Surgical Services, Veterans Affairs Medical Center; Professor of Surgery, George Washington and Georgetown Universities Medical Centers, Washington, District of Columbia

DAVID L. STEED, MD Director of Wound Healing/Limb Preservation Clinic, Department of Surgery, UPMC Shadyside; Professor of Surgery, Department of Vascular Surgery, University of Pittsburgh, Pittsburgh, Pennsylvania

JANETTE THOMPSON, DPM Assistant Chief, Podiatry, Veterans Affairs Medical Center, Washington, District of Columbia

WILLIAM ANDREW TIERNEY, MD Vascular Fellow, Department of Vascular Surgery, Ochsner Clinic Foundation, New Orleans, Louisiana

FRANK J. VEITH, MD Vice Chairman and William J. von Liebig Chair in Vascular Surgery, Department of Surgery, Montefiore Medical Center; Professsor of Surgery, Montefiore Medical Center–Albert Einstein College of Medicine, Bronx, New York

MATTHEW C. WAKEFIELD, MD Research Fellow, Veterans Affairs Medical Center; Surgical Resident, Walter Reed Army Medical Center, Washington, District of Columbia

JONATHAN M. WEISWASSER, MD Chief, Division of Vascular Surgery, Department of Surgery, Washington Veterans Administration Medical Center; Assistant Professor of Surgery, Department of Surgery, George Washington University Washington, District of Columbia

PAUL W. WHITE, MD Chief Resident, Division of General Surgery, Walter Reed Army Medical Center, Washington, District of Columbia; Instructor, Department of Surgery, Uniformed Services University, Bethesda, Maryland

GABOR A. WINKLER, MD Fellow, Department of Vascular Surgery, Pennsylvania Hospital, Philadelphia, Pennsylvania

THOMAS ZGONIS, DPM Assistant Professor, Department of Orthopedics, University of Texas Health Science Center at San Antonio, San Antonio, Texas

Overview of the Diabetic Foot and Limb Salvage

Cameron M. Akbari   *Anton N. Sidawy*

With the rising incidence and prevalence of diabetes mellitus worldwide, there has been an even greater increase in the prevalence of diabetes-related complications. Foot ulceration is one of the most common and formidable complications of diabetes, affecting almost 20% of all diabetic patients during their lifetime. Despite advances in management, foot problems continue to be the most common cause of hospitalization among patients with diabetes.[1] Diabetes remains the single strongest risk factor for limb loss, contributing to half of all lower extremity amputations in the United States; the relative risk for leg amputation is 40 times greater among diabetic patients. Moreover, up to 50% of diabetic amputees will undergo a second leg amputation within 5 years of the first one.[2]

The spectrum of diabetic foot disease may range from the asymptomatic patient, who may require only preventive foot care, to the unstable and critically ill patient in whom both loss of life and limb are imminent threats. Indeed, the variety of presentations of the diabetic foot often contributes to the clinical confusion and the delays in diagnosis and treatment that unfortunately lead to limb loss. Ultimately, the clinician needs to develop an orderly approach, grounded on firm pathophysiologic principles, in order to prevent limb loss in the patient with diabetes.

PATHOLOGY OF THE DIABETIC FOOT

The principal pathogenic mechanisms involved in diabetic foot disease include ischemia, neuropathy, and infection. Acting synergistically, they contribute to the sequence of tissue ulceration, necrosis, and eventually gangrene. Prevention and treatment of diabetic foot problems should be tailored to these pathogenic factors, either solely or in combination.

Neuropathy

Peripheral neuropathy is a common complication of diabetes mellitus, affecting as many as 60% of all patients in their lifetime, and up to 80% of those presenting with foot lesions.[3] Broadly classified as focal and diffuse, the latter are more common and include both the autonomic neuropathy and chronic sensorimotor polyneuropathies implicated in foot ulceration.

Sensorimotor neuropathy initially involves the distal lower extremities, progresses centrally, and tends to be symmetrical. Sensory nerve fiber involvement leads to loss of the protective sensation of pain, while motor nerve fiber loss results in small muscle atrophy in the foot and flexion of the metatarsals, with subsequent prominence of the metatarsal heads and clawing of the toes. This results in the development of abnormal pressure points on the plantar bony prominence, without protective sensation, and subsequent ulceration at these pressure points. Loss of intrinsic muscle function also results in digital contractures, hammer toe deformity, and ulceration. Because the motor neuropathy may affect the extensor musculature of the leg, deformities can also involve the ankle joint, with resultant so-called equinus deformity and abnormal bending forces.

Autonomic denervation leads to loss of sympathetic tone and increased arteriovenous shunting in the foot with defective nutrient flow. Impaired autonomic regulation of the sweat glands leads to anhidrosis and cracking of dry skin, which creates a predisposition to skin breakdown and possible ulceration. Because of sympathetic innervation to the bone, autonomic neuropathy may also result in an increase in bone blood flow and subsequent osteopenia and "bone washout." This osteoarthropathy of diabetes is more commonly known as Charcot foot, once historically associated with syphilitic tabes dorsalis, and now almost exclusively a complication of diabetes.

The etiology of Charcot foot deformity includes a combination of both sensorimotor and autonomic neuropathies. Continued ambulation on an insensate joint, combined with muscle imbalance and atrophy from motor neuropathy and limited joint mobility, leads to joint instability, loss of joint architecture, and ultimately bone and joint destruction.[4] This destructive process leads to increased bone blood flow and concomitant resorption and softening of normal bone, which in turn leads to further bone destruction and ultimately fracture and Charcot joint.

Infection

The unique anatomy of the foot poses several implications for the presentation and treatment of infection. Recognizing that most infections progress in the plantar aspect, it is useful to understand the three plantar compartments of the foot, which are divided into the medial, central, and lateral compartments.[5] The floor of each compartment is the rigid plantar fascia, while the roof is composed of the metatarsal bones and interosseous fascia. A thick medial intermuscular septum, extending from the medial calcaneal tuberosity to the head of the first metatarsal, defines the medial and central compartments. The intrinsic muscles of the great toe are in the medial compartment, while the central compartment is composed of the intrinsic muscles of the second through fourth toes, as well as the extensor flexor tendons of the toes, the medial and lateral plantar nerves, and the plantar vascular structures. The lateral intermuscular septum, from the calcaneus to the fifth metatarsal, delineates the lateral compartment, which contains the intrinsic muscles of the fifth toe.

Diabetic foot infection may result from a simple puncture wound, a neuropathic ulcer, the nail plate, or from the interdigital web space. Because the intrinsic muscles of each digit are essentially confined within the respective plantar compartment, untreated distal phalangeal infection may progress to a plantar abscess. Infection within these rigid anatomical compartments also creates high intracompartmental pressures, which subsequently impairs capillary blood flow and leads to progressive tissue ischemia and necrosis. Because the roof of each compartment is composed of bone and fascia, deep-space infections show deceptively little abnormality on the dorsal foot. Left untreated, ongoing infection and cellulitis can lead to bacterial spread from one compartment to another through direct perforation of the medial or lateral intermuscular septum, or lead to proximal foot and ankle abscess at the proximal calcaneal convergence of the septum, with an unsalvageable foot.

The microbiology of the diabetic foot infection is dependent on the patient's environment (e.g., outpatient or hospitalized) and the severity of the infection itself.[6] Mild localized and superficial ulcerations, particularly among outpatients, are usually caused by aerobic Gram-positive cocci such as *Staphylococcus aureus* or streptococci. In contrast, deeper ulcers and more generalized, limb-threatening infections are usually polymicrobial. In addition to Gram-positive cocci, the causative organisms in this latter group may include Gram-negative bacilli (*Escherichia coli, Klebsiella, Enterobacter aerogenes, Proteus mirabilis,* and *Pseudomonas aeruginosa*) and anaerobes (*Bacteroides fragilis* and peptostreptococci). Enterococci may also be isolated from the wound, notably among hospitalized patients and, in the absence of other cultured virulent organisms, should probably be considered pathogenic.

Ischemia: Microvascular and Macrovascular Considerations

Two distinct types of vascular disease are seen in patients with diabetes.[7] The first is a nonocclusive microcirculatory impairment, characteristically involving the capillaries and arterioles of the kidneys (nephropathy), eye (retinopathy), and peripheral nerves (neuropathy), and with significant effects in the diabetic foot. The second is a macroangiopathy characterized by atherosclerotic lesions of the coronary and peripheral arterial circulation, which is morphologically and functionally similar in both nondiabetic and diabetic patients.

In the context of the diabetic foot and microvascular dysfunction, the so-called small-vessel disease of diabetes is an inaccurate term, since it suggests an untreatable occlusive lesion in the microcirculation. Prospective anatomic[8] and physiologic studies have demonstrated that there is *no such microvascular occlusive disease.* Dispelling the notion of "small-vessel disease" is fundamental to the principles of limb salvage in patients with diabetes, since arterial reconstruction is almost always possible and successful in these patients.[9]

While there is no occlusive disease in the microcirculation, multiple structural and physiological abnormalities result in a functional microvascular impairment.[10] Endothelial dysfunction and the response to nitric oxide are diminished in patients with diabetes, neuropathy, and vascular disease,[11] and hyperglycemia alone may lead to at least some of these abnormal responses.[12] Thickening of the capillary basement membrane is the dominant structural change in both neuropathy and retinopathy, and alterations of the basement membrane likely contribute to albuminuria and the progression of diabetic nephropathy.[13] In the diabetic foot, capillary basement membrane thickening may theoretically impair the migration of leukocytes and the hyperemic response following injury, thereby increasing the susceptibility of the diabetic foot to infection.[14,15] However, these changes do not lead to narrowing of the capillary lumen, and arteriolar blood flow may be normal or even increased despite these changes.[16]

A variety of other microvascular abnormalities may be demonstrated in the diabetic foot.[17] Both capillary blood flow and the maximal hyperemic response to stimuli are reduced in the diabetic foot, suggesting that a *functional* microvascular impairment is a major contributing factor for diabetic foot problems. Neurogenic vasodilatation is also impaired in the diabetic foot.[18] Normally, injury-mediated nociceptive C fiber stimulation results in adjacent neurogenic release of vasoactive peptides, which subsequently lead to vasodilation and increased blood flow to the area of injury. Absence of this axon reflex further reduces the inflammatory hyperemic response to injury in the diabetic foot.

As noted earlier, macrovascular lower extremity disease in the diabetic patient is morphologically similar to the nondiabetic patient. The major difference between these two populations of patients is the pattern and location of the occlusive lesions.[19] Whereas occlusive lesions of the superficial femoral and popliteal segments are commonly found in the nondiabetic patient with limb ischemia, diabetic patients commonly have occlusive disease involving the infrageniculate, or tibial, arteries. However, the foot arteries are almost invariably patent, which allows for extreme distal arterial reconstruction despite extensive tibial or even proximal multisegmental disease. In addition, the popliteal, superficial femoral, and more proximal arteries are less likely to be affected by atherosclerosis, which allows these vessels to serve as an inflow source for distal arterial bypass grafts.

CLINICAL EVALUATION

As with all other disease processes, the initial evaluation of the patient with any diabetic foot problem begins with a complete history and careful physical examination. Broadly classified, this bedside assessment includes the healing potential of the foot, the details of the foot problem (e.g., ulcer, gangrene, infection, osteomyelitis, etc.), the systemic consequences of diabetes, and any immediate threats to life and/or limb.[20]

History

The history of the foot problem itself can give valuable insight as to the potential for healing, the presence of coexisting infection or arterial occlusive disease, and the need for further treatment. Any patient presenting with a foot ulceration or gangrene should immediately arouse suspicion of underlying arterial insufficiency, even if neuropathy or infection is present. In the patient with diabetes and arterial insufficiency, the inciting event for a nonhealing foot ulcer may be a seemingly benign event such as cutting a toenail, soaking the foot in a warm bath, or using a heating pad.

The duration of the ulcer also provides important clues, insofar as a long-standing, nonhealing ulcer is strongly suggestive of ischemia. Certainly, an ulcer or gangrenous area that has been present for several months is unlikely to heal without some type of further additional treatment, whether it be offloading of weight-bearing areas, treatment of infection, or, most commonly, correction of arterial insufficiency. Did the present ulcer heal previously, and is the present episode a relapsing problem? A history of intermittent healing followed by relapse should raise suspicion of underlying untreated infection, such as recurrent osteomyelitis, or uncorrected architectural abnormality, such as a bony pressure point or varux deformity.

It is helpful to consider past opinions and treatments, while still formulating an objective treatment plan based on presenting data. Many diabetic patients with correctable foot ulceration and limb ischemia have been told that the only option is limb amputation, usually due to "inherited pessimism" and inadequate knowledge of the advances made in limb and foot salvage. In these circumstances, when sought for an additional treatment opinion, it is best to start at the beginning rather than blindly concur with previous actions.

The past history should be first directed to previous foot and limb problems. Recent ipsilateral ulceration or foot surgery that healed in a timely and uncomplicated course, may suggest adequate arterial supply; with a more remote history, however, such information becomes less useful. A history of previous leg revascularization (including percutaneous therapies) also provides an important clue as to underlying arterial insufficiency. Other cardiovascular risk factors, such as cigarette smoking or hyperlipidemia, should also be considered, as their presence increases the likelihood that ischemia is contributing to the present foot problem.

Although claudication or rest pain has traditionally been associated with vascular disease, diabetic neuropathy may obscure those symptoms, and their absence in the diabetic patient certainly does not rule out ischemia. Because even moderate ischemia will preclude healing in the diabetic foot, the absence of rest pain is not a reliable indicator of adequate arterial blood supply; moreover, many patients may not ambulate a sufficient distance to develop true vasculogenic claudication. Conversely, some patients with true ischemic rest pain are dismissed for years as having "painful neuropathy."

Because unrecognized infection in the diabetic patient may rapidly progress to a life-threatening condition, attention should be directed toward detecting the subtle manifestations of an infected foot ulcer. Worsening hyperglycemia, recent erratic blood glucose control, and higher insulin requirements all suggest untreated infection. Due to the microvascular and neuropathic abnormalities in the diabetic foot, classical symptoms of infection such as chills or pain are often absent, and hyperglycemia is often the sole presenting symptom of undrained infection. With ongoing infection and hyperglycemia, impending ketoacidosis or nonketotic hyperglycemic hyperosmolar coma may develop, with symptoms of weakness, confusion, and altered mental status.

The history should also include a comprehensive assessment of the patient's overall health, to help stratify perioperative risk should some type of operative intervention be needed. Knowledge of previous cardiac events, such as myocardial infarction or revascularization, and present cardiac status, anginal severity, and heart failure symptoms are all mandatory components of the history-taking. Similarly, in the patient with suspected infection and ischemia, a history of worsening renal function or impending need for hemodialysis will help determine the dose and choice of antibiotics and may alter plans for standard contrast arteriography. Functional status also becomes an important consideration at this point, and the history should carefully determine the ambulatory and rehabilitative potential of the patient, so that appropriate decisions may be made for limb salvage or amputation.

Physical Examination

Initial evaluation of the diabetic foot ulcer should include a strong suspicion and thorough search for infection. In the patient with cellulitis, the entire foot, including the web spaces and nail beds, should be examined for any potential portals of entry, such as a puncture wound or interdigital ("kissing") ulcer. Encrusted and heavily callused areas over the ulceration should be unroofed, and the wound thoroughly inspected to determine the extent of involvement. A

benign-appearing, dry, gangrenous eschar can often hide an undrained infectious collection. Cultures should be taken from the base of the ulcer, avoiding superficial swabs that may yield only colonizing organisms. Findings consistent with infection might include purulent drainage, crepitus, tenderness, mild erythema, and sinus formation, although these findings may be entirely absent in the neuropathic foot. Close inspection of the ulcer and the use of a sterile probe may also confirm the presence of osteomyelitis, which occurs commonly even in benign-appearing ulcers; if bone is detected with gentle probing, osteomyelitis is presumed to be present. Although not always present, fever and tachycardia are strongly suggestive of deep or undrained infection with impending or already established sepsis.

Because of its prevalence and causative role in diabetic foot ulceration and limb loss, neuropathy should be assessed in every diabetic patient, and appropriate preventive measures taken to ensure against foot ulceration in the high-risk neuropathic foot. Protective sensation may be assessed with a Semmes-Weinstein 5.07 strength monofilament; inability to feel the monofilament when pressed to the skin correlates well with an increased risk of foot ulceration. Advanced sensorimotor neuropathy will lead to the presence of a "claw" foot, due to gradual atrophy of the intrinsic muscles. Charcot deformity, with bone and joint destruction at the midfoot, may also be seen.

Assessment of the arterial perfusion in the diabetic foot is a fundamental consideration, since the diabetic foot needs maximal perfusion to heal. Inadequate or faulty assessment and treatment of underlying ischemia will lead to failure of limb salvage in the patient with diabetic foot ulceration. Mere inspection of the leg and foot, including the ulcer, will often provide suggestive clues. For example, a distal ulceration (on the tip of a digit), an ulceration unassociated with an exostosis or weight-bearing area, and the presence of gangrene are all strongly consistent with underlying ischemia. Multiple ulcerations or gangrenous areas on the foot, absence of granulation tissue, or lack of bleeding with debridement of the ulcer should immediately raise concern for underlying arterial insufficiency. Other signs suggestive of ischemia include pallor with elevation, fissures (particularly at the heel), and absent hair growth. Although poor skin condition and hyperkeratosis may not always be good indicators of arterial disease, they should be noted, as they may help confirm initial clinical impressions.

The pulse examination, most notably the status of the foot pulses, is the single most important component of the physical exam, since, as has been emphasized, ischemia is always presumed to be present in the absence of a palpable foot pulse. As such, great attention should be directed toward the foot pulses, which requires knowledge of the usual location of the native arteries. The dorsalis pedis artery is located between the first and second metatarsal bones, just lateral to the extensor hallucis longus tendon, and its pulse is palpated by the pads of the fingers as the hand is partially wrapped around the foot. If the pulse cannot be palpated, the fingers may be moved a few millimeters in each direction, as the artery may have an occasional slight aberrant course. A common mistake is to place a single finger at one location on the dorsum of the foot. The posterior tibial artery is typically located in the hollow curve just behind the medial malleolus, approximately halfway between the malleolus and the Achilles tendon. The examiner's hand should be contralateral to the examined foot (i.e., the right hand should be used to palpate the left foot and vice versa), so as to allow the hand curvature to follow the ankle.

Noninvasive Arterial Evaluation

Noninvasive arterial testing has a limited role in the diabetic patient with foot ulceration, and should not be used in place of the bedside evaluation. In selected patients, in conjunction with the clinical findings, noninvasive testing may provide useful information. Some examples might include the diabetic patient with absent foot pulses and a superficial ulcer with evidence of healing and a previous history of a healed foot ulcer, or the patient without any foot lesions scheduled to undergo elective foot surgery. However, in the patient with poor healing or gangrene and absent foot pulses, noninvasive testing will add little additional information to the initial clinical evaluation, and will serve only to further delay vascular reconstruction.

All of the noninvasive arterial tests have limitations in the presence of diabetes.[21] Medial arterial calcinosis occurs frequently and unpredictably in patients with diabetes, and its presence can result in noncompressible arteries and artificially elevated segmental systolic pressures and ankle-brachial indices (ABI). Therefore, a "normal" ABI in a patient with diabetes should be interpreted with caution. Measurements may also be affected by inappropriately sized cuffs. For example, too narrow a cuff will result in artifactually high pressures, and so-called narrow cuff artifact is often associated with obese patients. Lower levels of calcification in the toe vessels support the use of toe systolic pressures as a surrogate measure of healing potential; however, despite its advantages in the presence of calcified vessels, toe pressure measurement also have several limitations. The presence of a bandage or toe ulcer often precludes placement of the cuff. In addition, since a plethysmograph is used to detect the pressure at which volume increases, the quality of the tracing may be affected by any vasoconstricted state (e.g., cold weather, cold room, nervous patient, etc.). Last, both the volume and

photo plethysmographs require close calibration, and poor contact of the photocell with the skin will yield poor results.

Segmental Doppler waveforms and pulsed volume recordings are unaffected by medial calcification, but evaluation of these waveforms is primarily qualitative and not quantitative. Although a triphasic Doppler waveform suggests normal arterial perfusion at that level, in the occasional patient, the waveform may be triphasic at the ankle, but there may be occlusive disease more distally. In addition, the quality of the waveforms is affected by peripheral edema and is technically dependent. Similarly, plethysmography (pulsed volume recordings) has several shortcomings, primary among them being that it frequently underestimates the severity of proximal arterial disease (due to the presence of collateral vessels). As with segmental Doppler waveforms, the quality test is affected by several variables, including room temperature (since temperature differences in the air cuff can change the pressure measured by the air-filled plethysmograph), peripheral edema, and obesity. Last, extensive casts or bandages preclude accurate waveform measurement.

Despite the invaluable role of duplex ultrasound in the diagnosis of carotid arterial disease and for postoperative graft surveillance, there are multiple limitations in its use for the diagnosis of lower extremity arterial disease. There is a large variation in the range of "normal" velocities for the leg arteries, and therefore a significant stenosis may be misinterpreted. Although the femoral and popliteal vessels may be visualized relatively easily, the tibial vessels are more cumbersome to scan, and the velocities in the tibial arteries may be even more difficult to interpret. When one considers the usual pattern of vascular disease in diabetes (with a predilection toward atherosclerotic involvement of the tibial vessels), the limitations of duplex in the diagnosis of arterial insufficiency in the diabetic patient are realized. Because the study depends on accurate sonographic localization of the vessel, duplex is quite "operator dependent." Last, multiple other variables can influence the quality of the image, including medial arterial calcification (which can cause artifactual shadowing), obesity, and peripheral edema (which can preclude imaging of the tibial vessels).

Regional transcutaneous oximetry ($TcPO_2$) measurement is also unaffected by medial calcinosis, and some studies have noted its reliability in predicting healing of ulcers and amputation levels.[22] Because hemodynamics are not measured, the test is immune to many of the problems facing other noninvasive tests in the presence of diabetes, such as noncompressible vessels. However, due to the unique considerations of the diabetic foot, $TcPO_2$ measurements are not entirely reliable in the diabetic patient with foot ulceration. Although values <20 and >60 can be predictive, there is a large "gray area" of intermediate values that are of little clinical use. Additionally, patients with diabetes develop foot ulceration at higher $TcPO_2$ values as compared to the nondiabetic population, and a higher $TcPO_2$ value may not correlate with healing potential in the diabetic patient (due to the effects of arteriovenous shunting and microvascular dysfunction). Even in the patient with a normal $TcPO_2$ value, the measurement may not accurately reflect the healing potential at the target area. Because the probe is typically placed at the proximal dorsal foot (near the ankle), more distal ischemia (due to possible distal tibial and paramalleolar occlusive disease) may not be identified. Technical problems, such as poor probe placement, lack of equipment standardization, and user variability and lack of familiarity, may also preclude the reliability of the study.

TREATMENT

Once the initial bedside history and physical evaluation are completed, the astute clinician will have formulated a plan determining the type and urgency of the subsequent treatment and diagnostic tests. Specifically, this timely assessment focuses on the presence and severity of infection, whether the limb is salvageable (which includes an assessment of the underlying medical condition of the patient), and the presence of ischemia.

Infection

Evaluation for and treatment of infection assumes first priority in the management of any diabetic foot problem.[23] Although radiographic tests may confirm initial clinical suspicions, the determination of the severity of infection is almost always made based on the clinical findings, and should be made without undue delay. Infection in the diabetic foot may range from a minimal superficial infection to fulminant sepsis with extensive necrosis and destruction of the foot. Accordingly, the assessment of infection and the subsequent treatment plan should consider the choice of antibiotic (which requires knowledge of the microbiology), the need for drainage, local or even guillotine amputation, and the medical condition of the patient.

In the compliant patient with no evidence of deep-space involvement or systemic infection, treatment may be performed on an outpatient basis, and consists of an oral antibiotic (pending culture results) and non–weight bearing to the involved extremity. Because most pathogens in this group of patients are either *Staphylococcus* or *Streptococcus*, an oral penicillin or first-generation cephalosporin is usually adequate. The patient should be instructed as to appropriate dressing changes to the wound, with frequent follow-up and guidelines to determine improvement or worsening.

Unfortunately, a more common presentation is the patient with ulceration or gangrene and a deep infection involving tendon or bone and possible systemic involvement. These patients require immediate hospitalization, bed rest with elevation of the infected foot, correction of any systemic abnormalities, and broad-spectrum intravenous antibiotics (which may be narrowed once culture results are complete). As noted earlier, the clinical findings of impending sepsis may be subtle, and therefore these patients should have a complete laboratory workup to detect and correct electrolyte and acid-base imbalances.

Duration and choice of antibiotic therapy is dependent on the extent of infection. As noted earlier, deep or chronic, recurrent ulcers are typically polymicrobic, and appropriate empiric antibiotic choices for those infections that are not life-threatening might include clindamycin plus a fluoroquinolone, clindamycin plus a third- or fourth-generation cephalosporin, or an antipseudomonal penicillin. Subsequent culture results will then dictate any further antibiotic coverage. In the absence of osteomyelitis, antibiotics should be continued until the wound appears clean and all surrounding cellulitis has resolved (typically 10 to 14 days). If osteomyelitis is present, treatment should include both surgical debridement and a prolonged (4 to 6 weeks) course of antibiotic, though the course of antibiotic therapy may be abbreviated if the entire infected bone has been removed (as with digital or transmetatarsal amputation). Heel lesions will often present with some degree of calcaneal destruction, and determination of osteomyelitis may be made by either clinical examination alone or in conjunction with other radiographic tests such as plain x-rays or magnetic resonance imaging (MRI).

In the presence of abscess or deep-space infection, immediate incision and drainage to include all infected tissue planes is mandatory. Incisions should be chosen with consideration to the normal anatomy of the foot (including the compartments of the foot) and the need for subsequent secondary (foot-salvage) procedures. Drainage should be complete, with incisions placed to allow for dependent drainage, and all necrotic tissue must be debrided. If an adequate incision and drainage has been performed, placement of drains (such as a Penrose type) is unnecessary, and reliance on such drains should be avoided. Repeat cultures (including both aerobic and anaerobic) should be obtained of the deep tissues. Care is made to avoid drainage incisions on the dorsum of the foot. Abscesses in the medial, central, or lateral compartments should be drained using longitudinal incisions in the direction of the neurovascular bundle and extending the entire length of the abscess. The medial and central compartments are drained through a medial incision, while the lateral compartment is drained through a lateral incision, both just above the plantar surface of the forefoot. Web space infections may be drained similarly through the plantar aspect of the foot. In some instances, open amputation of the foot (such an open-toe or trans-metatarsal amputation) may be necessary to allow for complete drainage and resection of necrotic tissue. Strict adherence to textbook amputations may lead to unnecessary soft tissue removal and possible need for higher amputation during future closure, and therefore all viable tissue should be conserved.

With ongoing, undrained infection, the patient may present with an unsalvageable foot and fulminant sepsis, with hemodynamic instability, bacteremia, and severe acid-base and electrolyte abnormalities. Such a patient should undergo prompt open (guillotine) below-knee amputation. This type of amputation is usually performed at the ankle level, to remove the septic source and to allow for subsequent revision and closure at a later date. Intravenous antibiotics, correction of dehydration and electrolyte abnormalities, and continuous cardiac monitoring are absolutely essential throughout the treatment process.

Once the infection has been drained and tissues debrided, continued wound inspection and management are essential. Ongoing necrosis should raise suspicion of undrained infection or untreated ischemia, and further debridement and treatments may be necessary. Wounds should be kept moist, avoiding caustic solutions, soaks, or whirlpool therapy. Attention should also be focused on avoiding any weight bearing on the affected foot, while also maximizing nutrition and controlling hyperglycemia.

Limb Salvageability

While the infection is being treated and controlled, the surgeon should determine the chances and feasibility of limb salvage. This assessment includes the patient's functional status and the viability of the foot. For example, primary limb amputation may be considered in a nonambulatory, bedridden patient, or in a patient with severe Charcot destruction and degeneration, for whom no further reconstructive foot procedures are possible. "Poor" medical condition is not necessarily an indication for primary limb amputation, considering the higher perioperative morbidity associated with limb amputation. Moreover, in many patients, optimization of the underlying medical comorbidities may be accomplished during treatment of infection and while evaluating for ischemia.

The assessment for limb salvage should be performed as the infection is treated, since appropriate drainage and antibiotics can dramatically change the appearance and perceived viability of the foot. If, however, limb salvage is not deemed possible, the patient should undergo formal below-knee or above-knee amputation.

Ischemia

The determination of ischemia begins with the history and physical exam, and by the conclusion of that initial evaluation, the surgeon should have an accurate assessment of the arterial circulation to the foot. That assessment should remember the treatment goal: To restore maximal, pulsatile arterial perfusion to the foot. The limitations of noninvasive vascular testing in diabetic patients with foot ulceration emphasize the continued importance of a thorough bedside evaluation and clinical judgment. To reiterate, the status of the foot pulse is the most important aspect of the physical exam, and occlusive disease is present if the foot pulses are not palpable. Because restoration of pulsatile flow maximizes the chances of healing in the diabetic foot, non-palpable foot pulses are an indication for contrast arteriography in the clinical setting of tissue loss, poor healing, or gangrene, even if neuropathy may have been the antecedent cause of skin breakdown or ulceration. The arteriogram is obtained to determine and plan the type of arterial reconstruction that will result in restoration of the foot pulse.

Concern about contrast-induced renal dysfunction in the presence of diabetes should not mitigate against the performance of a high-quality arteriogram of the entire distal circulation. Several prospective studies have documented that the incidence of contrast-induced nephropathy is not higher in the diabetic patient without preexisting renal disease, particularly with the judicious use of hydration and renal protective agents.[24] N-acetylcysteine in a 600 mg dose twice daily should be started the day before the arteriogram and continued for 48 hours,[25] and intravenous hydration with 0.45% normal saline (NS) should be run at a rate of 1 mg/kg/hour, beginning 12 hours prior to the scheduled arteriogram. In selected patients, magnetic resonance angiography, carbon dioxide angiography, or both may be used, either in conjunction with or in place of contrast arteriography.

Whatever preoperative imaging modality is chosen prior to arterial reconstruction, it is mandatory that consideration be given to the pattern of lower extremity vascular disease in patients with diabetes, and that the complete infrapopliteal circulation be incorporated, including the foot vessels. Because the foot vessels are often spared by the atherosclerotic occlusive process, even when the tibial arteries are occluded, it is essential that arteriograms not be terminated at the midtibial level.

Principles of Arterial Reconstruction in the Diabetic Foot

The treatment of ischemia in the diabetic foot is to restore maximal perfusion to the foot and, ideally, to restore a palpable foot pulse.[26] Possible approaches include endovascular techniques (angioplasty and stenting), bypass grafting (using autogenous or prosthetic grafts), or a combination of the two.[27] Ultimately, the choice of procedure should be individualized based on the patient's anatomy, comorbidities, and preoperative assessment, with the goal being to provide the most durable procedure with the least risk. For example, angioplasty alone may be of benefit in the patient with an isolated iliac artery stenosis or a focal lesion in the superficial femoral artery, but may also be used in combination with an infrainguinal bypass in the diabetic patient with multilevel disease.

In most patients, restoration of the foot pulse usually mandates infrainguinal arterial bypass grafting. The primary goal of infrainguinal arterial reconstruction in the ischemic diabetic foot is to bypass to an outflow artery that is in direct continuity with the foot, thereby restoring normal arterial pressure to the target area. Although proximal bypass to the popliteal or proximal tibioperoneal arteries may restore foot pulses, more distal revascularization is often needed to achieve this goal, again due to the pattern of occlusive disease in the diabetic patient. Similarly, although excellent results have been reported with peroneal artery bypass, the peroneal artery is not in continuity with the foot vessels and may not achieve the maximal flow required for healing, particularly at the forefoot level. Therefore, the authors believe that peroneal artery bypass should be reserved for those rare circumstances in which there is no dorsalis pedis or posterior tibial artery in continuity with the foot, or when limited venous conduit length mitigates against more distal bypass.

Autogenous vein grafting to the dorsalis pedis, distal posterior tibial, and plantar arteries incorporates knowledge of the anatomic pattern of diabetic vascular disease, satisfies the fundamental goal of restoration of the foot pulse, and provides durable and effective limb salvage.[28] Indeed, extensive experience with arterial reconstruction to the pedal vessels has established the efficacy, durability, and safety of these procedures; improved limb salvage rates in the diabetic patient may be directly attributed to the increasing use of pedal bypass.[29] Ultimately, the choice of outflow artery should be based on availability of conduit, the location of the foot ulcer, and the quality of the outflow vessel. For example, in the patient with an ischemic heel ulcer, first consideration should be given to the posterior tibial or plantar arteries if they are patent by preoperative imaging. However, absence of a posterior tibial artery should not rule against a dorsalis pedis bypass, as comparable rates of healing and limb salvage for heel ulcers have been reported with the dorsalis pedis artery bypass.[30]

Clinical experience has shown a variety of adjunctive techniques to be of advantage in infrainguinal revascularization among diabetic patients. For example, due to the pattern of lower extremity diabetic atherosclerotic disease, the popliteal or distal superficial femoral artery may be used as an inflow site, thereby allowing for a shorter length of vein to be used and avoiding dissection in the groin and upper thigh, a common location for wound complications. In addition, the shorter length of saphenous vein obviates the need for foot extension of the vein harvest incision, which is parallel to the one required to expose the paramalleolar and inframalleolar arteries; this avoids the resultant skin bridge, which may occasionally become ischemic from undue tension.

Although the vein graft may be prepared as in situ, reversed, or nonreversed graft, without any significant difference in outcome, the authors believe that size mismatch may best be minimized with either an in situ or nonreversed technique, particularly for grafts originating from the common femoral artery. Although the valves in the vein graft may be lysed blindly, the authors prefer to cut the valves under direct angioscopic guidance using a flexible valvulotome. This also allows for assessment of the saphenous vein to detect intraluminal abnormalities, and can help direct endoluminal interventions that upgrade the quality of the conduit and improve patency.

Absence of ipsilateral greater saphenous vein is not a contraindication for pedal bypass, as comparable results may be attained using arm vein or lesser saphenous vein grafts. Although prosthetic material may occasionally be used for more proximal reconstructions (as to the above-knee popliteal artery), it should seldom, if ever, be used for extreme distal bypass grafting. When ipsilateral saphenous vein is not available, several alternatives exist for autogenous conduit. Although the contralateral saphenous vein is an obvious alternative, several considerations limit its use in the diabetic patient. Contralateral leg vein may not always be present in this population of patients who often require multiple cardiovascular interventions. More importantly, diabetes is a strong risk factor for subsequent contralateral limb bypass, with almost 60% of patients requiring contralateral bypass at 3 years. Therefore, the authors' approach has been to use arm vein grafts as the first alternative in the absence of ipsilateral saphenous vein.[31] The cephalic, basilic, or upper arm basilic-cephalic loop vein grafts may be harvested. Once the vein has been harvested, angioscopic evaluation is crucial, as many of these patients have undergone multiple venipunctures and cannulations with resultant scarring and weblike synechiae. Angioscopy allows for detection and correction of many of these areas, and allows for precise valve lysis within these thin-walled veins.[32]

Active infection in the foot is not a contraindication to paramalleolar bypass grafting, as long as the infectious process is controlled.[33] Adequate control implies resolution of cellulitis, lymphangitis, and edema, especially in areas of proposed incisions required to expose the distal artery or saphenous vein. Occasionally, severe circumferential calcification of the distal artery may also be encountered. Strategies include the use of special intraluminal bulb-tipped vessel occluders or tourniquet occlusion, with no attempts made at endarterectomy or "cracking" the plaque. Results of bypasses to calcified vessels are comparable to noncalcified vessels.[34]

Several reports have summarized the results of the dorsalis pedis artery bypass, of which the most recent summarizes a decade-long experience of >1,000 cases.[35] In that series, 5-year primary patency rates were 57%, with a limb salvage rate of almost 80%, confirming the efficacy and durability of these procedures. Additionally, concern regarding perioperative morbidity and long-term outcome in diabetic patients has also been dispelled.[36,37]

Secondary Foot Procedures

After successful revascularization, secondary procedures on the foot may be performed for maximal foot salvage. Many of these procedures are discussed in detail in this volume and the reader is referred to those chapters. Fundamentally, these foot procedures should address both the acute problem and the underlying cause, which may be corrected simultaneously or alone. Depending on the location of the ulcer, digital, single metatarsal (ray), or transmetatarsal amputations may be performed. Because of the architecture of the diabetic foot, underlying bony structural abnormalities are often the cause of ulceration and may be corrected with metatarsal head resection or osteotomy. Similarly, ulceration on a previous transmetatarsal amputation may be due to an equinovarus deformity (from disrupted tendons and a decrease in calcaneal inclination). This should be treated by revision of the transmetatarsal amputation (with perhaps ulcer excision) and biomechanical correction (as with an Achilles tendon lengthening). Chronic digit ulcerations may be treated with ulcer excision, arthroplasty, or hemiphalangectomy. In the patient with extensive tissue loss, both local and free flaps may be used in the fully revascularized foot. Heel ulcers may be treated with partial calcanectomy and local or even free flap coverage.

Once healed, attention should be directed toward preventive diabetic foot care. Pressure points may be evaluated and identified with pedobarography, by measuring plantar pressure as the patient walks on a pressure-sensitive platform. Therapeutic footwear and custom orthotics may be prescribed to help offload abnormal pressure points. Regularly scheduled visits to a foot specialist should incorporate counseling, education, shoe inspection, and nail-cutting into the history and physical examination. Ultimately, if we are to realize the nation's stated goal of reducing limb amputations among patients with diabetes by 2010,[38] a comprehensive coordinated and aggressive treatment and preventive plan, as outlined in this book, must be practiced by those caring for patients with diabetes.

REFERENCES

1. Reiber GE, Boyko EJ, Smith DG. Lower extremity foot ulcers and amputations in diabetes. In: *Diabetes in America*. 2nd ed. Bethesda, Md: National Diabetes Data Group, National Institutes of Health, National Institute of Diabetes and Digestive Kidney Diseases; NIH Publication No. 95-1468.1995:409–428.
2. Nathan DM. Long-term complications of diabetes mellitus. *N Engl J Med*. 1993;328:1676–1685.
3. Grunfeld C. Diabetic foot ulcers: etiology, treatment, and prevention. *Adv Intern Med*. 1992;37:103–132.
4. Frykberg RG, Kozak GP. The diabetic Charcot foot. In: Kozak GP, Campbell DR, Frykberg RG, et al., eds. *Management of diabetic foot problems*. 2nd ed. Philadelphia, Pa: WB Saunders; 1995:88–97.
5. Akbari CM, Macsata R, Smith BM, et al. Overview of the diabetic foot. *Semin Vasc Surg*. 2003;16:3–11.
6. Joshi N, Caputo GM, Weitekamp MR, et al. Infections in patients with diabetes mellitus. *N Engl J Med*. 1999;341:1906–1912.
7. Akbari CM, LoGerfo FW. Diabetes and peripheral vascular disease. *J Vasc Surg*. 1999;30:373–384.
8. Strandness DE Jr, Priest RE, Gibbons GE. Combined clinical and pathologic study of diabetic and nondiabetic peripheral arterial disease. *Diabetes*. 1964;13:366–372.
9. LoGerfo FW, Coffman JD. Vascular and microvascular disease of the foot in diabetes. *N Engl J Med*. 1984;311:1615–1619.
10. LoGerfo FW. Vascular disease, matrix abnormalities, and neuropathy: implications for limb salvage in diabetes mellitus. *J Vasc Surg*. 1987;5:793–796.
11. Veves A, Akbari CM, Primavera J, et al. Endothelial dysfunction and the expression of endothelial nitric oxide synthetase in diabetic neuropathy, vascular disease, and foot ulceration. *Diabetes*. 1997;47:457–463.
12. Akbari CM, Saouaf R, Barnhill DF, et al. Endothelium-dependent vasodilation is impaired in both micro- and macrocirculation during acute hyperglycemia. *J Vasc Surg*. 1998;28:687–694.
13. Morgensen CE, Schmitz A, Christensen CR. Comparative renal pathophysiology relevant to IDDM and NIDDM patients. *Diabetes Metab Rev*. 1988;4:453–483.
14. Flynn MD, Tooke JE. Aetiology of diabetic foot ulceration: A role for the microcirculation? *Diabet Med*. 1992;8:320–329.
15. Rayman G, Williams SA, Spencer PD, et al. Impaired microvascular hyperaemic response to minor skin trauma in Type I diabetes. *Br Med J*. 1986;292:1295–1298.
16. Parving HH, Viberti GC, Keen H, et al. Hemodynamic factors in the genesis of diabetic microangiopathy. *Metabolism*. 1983;32:943–949.
17. Akbari CM, LoGerfo FW. Microvascular changes in the diabetic foot. In: Veves A, Giurini JM, LoGerfo FW, eds. *The diabetic foot: Medical and surgical management*. 1st ed. Totowa, NJ: Humana Press; 2002:99–112.
18. Parkhouse N, LeQueen PM. Impaired neurogenic vascular response in patients with diabetes and neuropathic foot lesions. *N Engl J Med*. 1988;318:1306–1309.
19. Menzoian JO, LaMorte WW, Paniszyn CC, et al. Symptomatology and anatomic patterns of peripheral vascular disease: differing impact of smoking and diabetes. *Ann Vasc Surg*. 1989;3:224.
20. Akbari CM, LoGerfo FW. The diabetic foot. In: Wilmore DW, Souba WW, Fink MP, et al., eds. *ACS surgery: Principles and practice*. New York, NY: WebMD Professional Publishing; 2003:1–11.
21. Akbari CM, LoGerfo FW. Peripheral vascular disease in the person with diabetes. In: Porte D, Sherwin RS, Baron AD, eds. *Ellenberg*

and Rifkin's diabetes mellitus. 6th ed. New York, NY: McGraw-Hill; 2003:845–857.

22. Ballard JL, Eke CC, Bunt TJ, et al. A prospective evaluation of transcutaneous oxygen measurements in the management of diabetic foot problems. *J Vasc Surg.* 1995;22:485–492.

23. Akbari CM, Pomposelli FB Jr. Diabetes and diseases of the foot. *IM Internal Medicine.* 2000;21:10–17.

24. Solomon R, Werner C, Mann D, et al. Effects of saline, mannitol, and furosemide to prevent acute decreases in renal function induced by radiocontrast agents. *N Engl J Med.* 1994;331:1416–1420.

25. Tepel M, van der Giet M, Schwarzfeld C, et al. Prevention of radiographic-contrast-agent-induced reductions in renal function by acetylcysteine. *N Engl J Med.* 2000;343:180–184.

26. Akbari CM, LoGerfo FW. Distal bypasses in the diabetic patient. In: Yao JST, Pearce WH, eds. *Current techniques in vascular surgery.* New York, NY: McGraw-Hill; 2001:285–296.

27. Faries PL, Brophy D, LoGerfo FW, et al. Combined iliac angioplasty and infrainguinal revascularization surgery are effective in diabetic patients with multilevel arterial disease. *Ann Vasc Surg.* 2001;15:67–72.

28. Akbari CM, LoGerfo FW. Saphenous vein bypass to pedal arteries in diabetic patients. In: Yao JST, Pearce WH, eds. *Techniques in vascular and endovascular surgery.* Norwalk, Calif: Appleton and Lange; 1998:227–232.

29. LoGerfo FW, Gibbons GW, Pomposelli FB Jr, et al. Trends in the care of the diabetic foot: Expanded role of arterial reconstruction. *Arch Surg.* 1992;127:617–621.

30. Berceli SA, Chan AK, Pomposelli FB Jr, et al. Efficacy of dorsal pedal artery bypass in limb salvage for ischemic heel ulcers. *J Vasc Surg.* 1999;30:499–508.

31. Faries PL, Arora S, Pomposelli FB Jr, et al. The use of arm vein in lower-extremity revascularization: Results of 520 procedures performed in eight years. *J Vasc Surg.* 2000;31:50–59.

32. Akbari CM, LoGerfo FW. Value of arm vein in femoral distal bypass. In: Yao JST, Pearce WH, eds. *Advances in vascular surgery.* New York, NY: McGraw-Hill; 2001:261–269.

33. Tannenbaum GA, Pomposelli FB Jr, Marcaccio EJ, et al. Safety of vein bypass grafting to the dorsal pedal artery in diabetic patients with foot infections. *J Vasc Surg.* 1992;15:982–990.

34. Misare BD, Pomposelli FB Jr, Gibbons GW, et al. Infrapopliteal bypasses to severely calcified outflow arteries: two year results. *J Vasc Surg.* 1996;24:6–16.

35. Pomposelli FB Jr, Kansal N, Hamdan AD, et al. A decade of experience with dorsalis pedis artery bypass: Analysis of outcome in more than 1000 cases. *J Vasc Surg.* 2003;37:307–315.

36. Hamdan AD, Saltzberg SS, Sheahan M, et al. Lack of association of diabetes with increased postoperative mortality and cardiac morbidity. *Arch Surg.* 2002;137:417–421.

37. Akbari CM, Pomposelli FB Jr, Gibbons GW, et al. Lower extremity revascularization in diabetes: Late observations. *Arch Surg.* 2000; 135:452–456.

38. US Department of Health and Human Services. *Healthy people 2010.* Vol. 1. 2nd ed. Washington, DC: US Department of Health and Human Services; 2000.

Diabetic Neuropathy

Jonathan M. Weiswasser   *Anton N. Sidawy*

Since its earliest description, the syndrome of diabetes has always included the development of peripheral neuropathy. Nephropathy, retinopathy, and neuropathy have traditionally encompassed the most significant and predictable sequellae of this ubiquitous disease and, with the aging of our population, most would agree that vasculopathy should be included. Despite its prominence in the sequellae of diabetes, neuropathy has been eagerly classified, but little progress has advanced our understanding of the etiology or mechanism of this syndrome. As a result, we do not currently have any truly powerful treatment strategies.

The syndrome of diabetic neuropathy, or more precisely, polyneuropathy, most often manifests itself secondarily as foot ulceration and injury. The prevalence of distal polyneuropathy affects roughly 30% of people with a diagnosis of diabetes, a figure carried consistently through multiple large studies of these patients.[1-3] Numerous studies have evaluated the development of neuropathy, and in many ways mirroring the factors influencing the progression of vascular disease; progression of neuropathy was associated with exacerbation of cardiovascular risk factors, such as lipemia, hypertension, obesity, and nephropathy.[4] In addition, the progression of neuropathy is directly associated with age, duration of disease, and poor glycemic control.[5]

CLASSIFICATION

Our lack of understanding of the true etiology of diabetic neuropathy has led to a vague classification of this entity. Classification schemes, of which there are many, are based either on clinical presentation or clinical progression. Given the varied clinical presentation of diabetic neuropathy, its classification scheme is similarly complicated. A basic clinical system is presented in Table 2-1. This useful classification schema, based on clinical presentation, was proposed by Low and Suarez,[6] and divides the neuropathies based on symmetry and distribution.

Further classification, especially of the symmetric neuropathies, has been proposed based on the presence or absence of pain. This system developed from the observation that the majority of patients do not present with pain as their predominant symptom.[7] As a way of providing an explanation for the presence of differing symptoms in the most common diabetic neuropathy (distal symmetrical neuropathy), the symptom of pain has been associated with neuropathies that result in a larger degree of small fiber damage; whereas, patients with foot ulceration generally have a greater degree of electrophysiologic dysfunction (representing larger fiber damage) compared to those with pain as their predominant symptom.[8] Additional support for the subcategories of the distal symmetrical neuropathies has been advocated by those who believe that the degree of small fiber relative to large fiber damage determines the type of neuropathy, and that differing etiologies target different fiber types.[9] Others have held the view that painful and painless neuropathies overlap each other and are part of the same overall process.[10] They maintain that, ultimately, vibratory perception threshold determines the type of neuropathy, as both painful and painless types of neuropathies are susceptible to foot ulceration.[11]

FOOT SEQUELLAE OF DIABETIC NEUROPATHY

The direct correlation between diabetic neuropathy and lesions of the foot is well recognized. More than

TABLE 2-1

CLINICAL CLASSIFICATION OF DIABETIC NEUROPATHY

Symmetric neuropathies
Distal sensory and sensorimotor neuropathy
Large fiber type
Small fiber type
Distal small fiber type
Insulin neuropathy
CIDP

Asymmetric neuropathies
Mononeuropathy
Mononeuropathy multiplex
Radiculopathy
Lumbar plexopathy (radiculoplexopathy)
CIDP

CIDP, chronic inflammatory demyelinating polyneuropathy.
Adapted from Veves A, Giurini JM, LoGerfo FW. *The diabetic foot.*
Totowa, NJ: Humana Press; 2002:77.

80% of diabetic patients with foot lesions have demonstrable peripheral neuropathy—lesions which, in conjunction with peripheral vascular disease, lead to the high rates of limb loss among diabetics.[12,13] Other than the lesions formed as a result of trauma unbeknownst to the patient, foot osteoarthropathy as a result of neuropathy is the most common abnormality among the feet of people with diabetes. Otherwise known as Charcot foot from the French physician who denoted this "arthropathy of locomotor ataxia," neuropathic foot arthropathy has several postulated etiologic mechanisms.[14]

The neurotraumatic theory postulates that Charcot foot is a result of repeated trauma, which then leads to joint and bone destruction. Continued use of the extremity exacerbates the process by further injury, generally as a result of the deformation of the foot architecture. The repetitive trauma results in intracapsular effusions, ligamentous laxity, and instability of the joint. While neuropathy is a prerequisite for this process, the neurotraumatic theory does not explain the development of Charcot joint in patients who are nonambulatory. The neurovascular reflex theory of the development of Charcot foot proposes a vascular etiology. As a result of the peripheral arteriovenous shunting that occurs within precapillary arterioles, bone tissue is subjected to increased blood flow. This abnormal increase in flow results in demineralization and weakening. The imbalance of bone resorption and formation among patients with osteoarthropathy was demonstrated recently, especially in patients with acute neuroarthropathy.[15] The actual pathogenesis of Charcot foot most likely is a result of both neurovascular and neurotraumatic etiologies.[16]

Classification of Charcot arthropathy follows the Eichenholtz classification scheme, which divides the destructive process into developmental, coalescent, and reconstructive stages.[17] Fractures, cartilage destruction, and formation of bone spurs and debris characterize the developmental stage. Absorption of much of the debris with reduction in soft-tissue swelling and formation of a callus is characteristic of the coalescent stage. The reconstructive stage is signified by the presence of bony ankylosis and hypertrophic proliferation. Several radiographic findings of Charcot foot are noted but are beyond the scope of this discussion.

Management of Charcot arthropathy is accomplished mainly by immobilization and stress reduction of the affected aspect of the foot. The patient should keep weight off the affected limb for 8 to 12 weeks, using crutches or a wheelchair. Additional benefit may be obtained from use of a light-weight splint or cast to aid in immobilization, or the use of an orthotic device. Surgical intervention is generally indicated when the patient develops instability, gross deformity, or progressive destruction despite immobilization. The reader is directed to text specific to surgical management of Charcot foot for further information regarding operative treatment.

THE NEUROPATHIES

Distal Symmetric Neuropathy

As the most common of the neuropathies associated with diabetes, distal symmetric neuropathy (DSN) is generally what is referred to as "diabetic neuropathy" in the generalized clinical setting. DSN tends to start insidiously, often prior to the diagnosis of frank diabetes, and similar to its vascular counterpart, affects the distal limb first. The pattern of distribution can be of either the "stocking" or "glove" distribution, or both. As the disease progresses, the pattern of distribution extends further proximally, affecting the thigh and, in its most severe form, ultimately affecting the upper extremities and even the face and trunk. Autonomic involvement can also occur but is less common.

Etiology of Distal Symmetric Neuropathy
The etiology of DSN, while extensively studied, remains largely unknown. Theories have emerged from experimental data obtained from many *in vitro* and *in vivo* studies in both animal and human subjects, demonstrating that the etiology of DSN arises from a combination of vascular and metabolic factors.[18] Evidence for a combination theory stems from data describing the interaction between the metabolic results of diabetes with vascular endothelium.[19] Factors that are prominent in the current understanding of the etiology of the disease are related to the formation of oxygen radicals, the polyol pathway, nonenzymatic glycation, protein kinase C activation, and other vascular factors.

Several large-scale, population-based studies have demonstrated a correlation between poor glycemic control (hyperglycemia) and the development of neuropathy.[20,21] This correlation is clear, but whether reversal of neuropathy can be accomplished with improved glycemic control is less clear. Histologically, DSN is characterized by a regression of the nerve root with distal axonal loss[22] and focal reduction in the density of myelinated fibers. Clustered "sprouts" of myelinated and nonmyelinated regenerative axons are observed in some preparations.[23]

Formation of oxygen radicals through hyperglycemia tends to occur through the polyol cascade or through nonenzymatic glycation. In addition, the scavenger nicotinamide adenine dinucleotide phosphate (NADPH) is depleted in states of polyol pathway hyperactivity.[24] With the buildup of oxygen radical species, there exists the potential for nervous damage, either through a directly toxic effect, or by a reduction of epineural blood flow through the depletion of nitric oxide. Further evidence for oxygen radicals affecting diabetic neuropathy comes from the observation that administration of free radical scavengers leads to improvement in nerve conduction velocity in animals.[25]

The activity of the polyol pathway has long been a subject of interest among those studying the etiology of DSN. In addition to promoting damage through the formation of oxygen radicals, the polyol pathway has been implicated in the deposition of sorbitol within peripheral nerves in the setting of hyperglycemia.[26,27] Aldose reductase inhibitors, which have a myriad of significant side effects, have demonstrated improvement in nerve conduction velocity when administered to animal and human subjects with diabetes.[28,29] Though these changes may also be accompanied by morphologic and histologic improvement as well, there is little evidence to demonstrate that aldose reductase inhibitors reverse or prevent clinical neuropathy.[30]

Just as the hemoglobin molecule can be nonenzymatically glycated in the setting of hyperglycemia, so too are other important molecules, at first by reversible means and later by irreversible means. The formation of Amadori products and other molecules that constitute advanced glycation end products represents part of the specter of damage that glucose, in high enough concentrations, can wreak on important substrates in normal metabolism. Based on the observation that nonenzymatically glycated proteins can absorb nitric oxide, some have postulated that nitric oxide–dependent vasodilation is impaired in the epineurium of patients with diabetes, thus leading to ischemia and neuropathy.[31] In addition, demyelination of peripheral nerve has been associated with nonenzymatic glycation,[32] and further disturbances in nerve function are suggested by the finding of increased glycosylated tubulin and advanced glycosylation end products in peripheral nerve.[33]

The effect that hyperinsulinemia has upon the vascular system in the setting of diabetes has led to the hypothesis that these effects may lead to neuropathy through disease in nutritive vessels of the epineurium. This hypothesis is supported by the observation of disease within the neural microvascular network.[34] Clinically, the enhancement in nerve conduction velocity with exercise (which is observed in non-neuropathic diabetic patients) is absent in patients with diabetic neuropathy,[35] an effect that is thought to stem from arteriovenous shunting at the precapillary level leading to nervous hypoxia.[36] Further support is made by the observation that the degree of diabetic neuropathy correlates with tissue capillary oxygen tension.[37] Additionally, histologic changes to the capillary structure, including damage to the endothelium and pericytes, thickening of the basal membrane, and, occasionally, vessel occlusion, are observed. The degree to which these changes occur correlates with the severity of the neuropathy.[38] The severity of neuropathy has been positively correlated to the degree of vascular disease in the same subject.[39] There is debate, however, as to whether revascularization of the macrovessels improves diabetic neuropathy, which is perhaps explained by the hypothesis that neuropathy emanates from disease at the microvessel level.[40,41]

Clinical Presentation of Distal Symmetric Neuropathy

DSN tends to present primarily with sensory loss. The detection of DSN depends on a high clinical suspicion as well as a thorough history and physical examination, including neurologic exam, especially of the lower extremity. The typical patient with DSN tends to be entirely asymptomatic or commonly reports numbness in the affected extremity, although pain is also typical. The numbness is generally reported as most severe with exertion and dependency, and patients will report the sensation of a large callous (in the absence of one) or of "walking on marbles." Paresthesiae are common and this can progress to debilitating pain, particularly at night,[42] leading to insomnia. Burning sensations, aches, allodynia, and cramps can also represent DSN. In addition, symptoms may not encompass the foot in a uniform manner, as they can often involve one or two toes. Alternatively, as the syndrome progresses, involvement of the upper leg may occur, and this is usually associated with involvement of the upper extremity. In perhaps its most debilitating form, DSN can present with both pain and numbness in the limb, a situation that carries the greatest propensity for morbidity.[43]

On further questioning, the patient may report other changes in activities that result from significant DSN. In addition to insomnia (generally from the painful form of the disease), patients may report loss of employment.[44] As the degree of pain progresses, patients will report significant reductions in activities of daily living, especially when autonomic involvement results in the development of postural hypotension.[45] This constellation of effects often leads to depression; fortunately, symptomatic autonomic involvement is rare. The effects of DSN on the pedal and lower extremity muscles involved in maintaining balance, especially in combination with postural hypotension, can lead to several episodes of falling.

On physical examination, thoroughness is key. Shoes and socks should be removed, and careful external examination should ensue with special attention to the possibility of ulceration both on the plantar aspect as well as in the interosseal spaces. Often, in the painless variety of the disease, foot ulceration may be the presenting symptom of DSN with serious consequence.[46] Ulceration and injury is caused by mechanical or thermal insult and can progress to an infection involving bone or fascia without the development of pain or symptoms. The patient may be entirely unaware of the presence of a limb-threatening foot infection, thus physical examination of the feet should be performed at least annually by the primary physician. In addition to the typical examination for sensation to light touch and pinprick, as well as motor strength, particular attention to vibratory sense and proprioception (large fiber function) is required to determine the extent of neuropathy. The use of Semmes-Weinstein filaments, which can very accurately determine the degree and proximal extent of disease, is strongly advised. The loss of proprioception will lead to a positive Romberg sign, and severely diminished or absent deep tendon reflexes at the knee and ankle. The use of nerve conduction studies is useful in questionable cases.[47]

The motor effects are usually apparent later in the course of disease, but early specialized testing with magnetic resonance imaging (MRI) has demonstrated that the motor groups are affected earlier and are clearly part of the functional impairment.[48] As this motor involvement becomes more pronounced, the wasting of lumbricals of the feet and hands (if upper extremity involvement is present) can occur. Unopposed tone of the extensors on the toes may lead to upgoing toes with formation of callous and metatarsal damage on the plantar surface of the foot. This may ultimately lead to the ulceration in this area, commonly referred to as Charcot arthropathy. If the lumbricals of the hands are involved, the patient will report difficulty with fine motor movement and grasp.

In addition to the development of postural hypotension, the involvement of the autonomic nervous system leads to loss of sweat production in the involved foot, and this loss of moisture can lead to flaking, cracking, fissure formation, and ultimately abscess of the foot. Typically, the affected limb is warm and dry, due to the arteriovenous shunting that occurs with disturbance of the autonomic supply to the area.[49] Further evidence for the significance of this phenomenon is reflected in the elevated oxygen tension in these veins.[50] This shunting may actually lead to local tissue ischemia, resulting in a gangrenous toe in the setting of a warm, pulsatile foot. The presence of edema refractory to diuretics in this setting is very often neuropathic in origin and may respond to ephedrine.[51]

Small Fiber Neuropathy

The existence of small fiber diabetic neuropathy (SFN) has been advocated by some as a distinct entity apart from DSN,[52] while others have described it as a phenomenon associated with the early stages of DSN.[53] SFN seems to occur at a younger age, particularly in patients with type I diabetes. As a separate entity, SFN is characterized predominantly by pain greater than numbness. The pain, which at times can be quite severe, entails the same qualities as that seen with DSN, namely, allodynia, paresthesia, localized aches, and cramping pain. Distinguishing SFN from DSN on physical exam is possible by noting the relative sparing of vibratory and proprioceptive senses and the overall greater involvement of the autonomic nervous system. In addition, motor strength and reflexes are largely normal.

Acute Symmetrical Neuropathies

Acute symmetrical neuropathies embody transient neuropathic syndromes that are primarily characterized by severe pain. While relatively uncommon, they tend to present in two distinct forms: Neuropathy of poor glycemic control and the neuropathy associated with insulin neuritis.

The neuropathy of poor glycemic control is a transient, painful neuropathy that has also been termed neuropathic cachexia.[54] As such, it is characterized by the sudden onset of pain, usually in the lower extremity, described as a burning pain, especially along the plantar aspect of the foot. Pain is independent of time, and the character of it can wax and wane, with stabbing and shooting pains emanating from the foot and shooting up the leg on the background of burning pain in the foot. Physical examination is surprisingly normal. The patient generally has little or no motor weakness, and the vibratory senses are largely spared. Reflexes are usually mildly diminished or normal. The hallmark of diagnosis may lie only in the determination of an abnormal temperature sense. Sural nerve biopsy of these patients demonstrates changes consistent with DSN but with active regeneration of both myelinated and demyelinated fibers. Of most interest is the histologic finding of an increased proliferation of the epineurial vessels similar to that seen in diabetic retinopathy. Tesfaye et al.[55] suggest that this network of abnormal vessels creates a "steal" phenomenon, rendering the nerve ischemic and leading to pain, through increased flow through the network precipitated by insulin. Experimental studies have confirmed this observation by demonstrating that insulin reduces nutritive neural blood flow, leading to endoneurial hypoxia by way of the epineurial arteriovenous network.[56] With improved glycemic control, patients can expect that this syndrome will resolve after approximately 10 months.

Neuropathy of rapid insulin control occurs after a poorly controlled diabetic patient undergoes a rapid correction of blood glucose values. This syndrome is typified by the acute onset of allodynia, paresthesias, and burning pain, often worse at night. Unlike the neuropathy of poor glycemic control, the neuropathy of rapid insulin control is worse at night and is not associated with weight loss. Typical nerve conduction studies are largely normal, with some impairment in exercise-induced conduction velocity. There is no motor involvement, and, unlike the typical DSN, the symptoms of neuropathy of rapid insulin control usually resolve after 10 months. Sural nerve biopsy demonstrates active regeneration of fibers, as well as other morphometric qualities consistent with DSN.[57]

Asymmetric Neuropathies

Unlike the symmetric neuropathies, asymmetric neuropathies associated with diabetes tend to be ephemeral, with complete resolution and a more predictable clinical course. In addition to dissimilarity of time course, compared to DSN, asymmetric neuropathies tend to bear no relationship to other factors of diabetic disease severity, such as glucose control.[58,59] These neuropathies tend to affect older men.[60] Given the focal nature and rapid onset of the syndrome, the prudent clinician will eliminate other, potentially more serious, etiologies of the symptoms. The asymmetric neuropathies can be divided into cranial neuropathy, truncal neuropathy, plexopathy, and compression neuropathy.

Plexopathies, or commonly femoral neuropathy, present with severe pain and weakness of proximal motor groups. This condition typically affects patients with either type 1 or type 2 diabetes over 50 years of age.[61] The pain is usually described as a burning pain that is felt deep in the muscle group, such as the thigh. The onset is generally rapid and the symptoms are persistent, resulting in insomnia, depression, and sedentary lifestyle.[62,63] On examination, wasting and loss of bulk of the proximal muscle groups is detected and can involve muscles used in hip flexion and abductors. Sensory loss is not present in the pure form of plexopathy. Once suspected, the patient should undergo evaluation for an underlying malignancy or other

neuropathic lesion, including MRI and electrophysiologic studies. The diagnosis can be confirmed by femoral nerve latency and active denervation of affected muscles. Like other neuropathies, the etiology of diabetic plexopathy is unknown; however, some have postulated that vascular damage to motor nerve roots results in the condition.[64] The course of the disease follows the pattern of similar neuropathies, although little exists to reliably predict its pattern. Generally, symptoms begin to abate at 3 months or so, with gradual resolution over the course of 1 year.[34] Management is supportive, and physiotherapy is encouraged.

Compression neuropathies are common among diabetics. In one large epidemiologic study, the incidence of electrophysiologic signs of carpal tunnel syndrome was as high as 30%, though symptoms were present only in 10%.[65] Compression palsies in people with diabetes have also been noted in the common peroneal nerve (leading to foot drop), and one case of phrenic nerve entrapment in a person with diabetes has been described, although the site of the entrapment could not be absolutely ascertained.[66] Although carpal tunnel release may help in median nerve compression, release of common peroneal nerve entrapment does not guarantee return of function in the lower extremity. The relapse rate of painful symptoms does seem to be higher in people with diabetes than in the unaffected population.[67]

Autonomic Neuropathy

Neuropathy of the autonomic nervous system represents another star in the constellation of nervous disorders among diabetic patients. The prevalence of symptoms related to autonomic dysfunction is less than the symptoms resulting from other forms of diabetic neuropathy, but further physiologic testing of diabetic patients seems to suggest that impairment of the autonomic nervous system may occur more frequently than previously thought, and may affect as many as 24% of all diabetic patients.[68] Cardiovascular and gastrointestinal autonomic neuropathy are the most common manifestations of the disorder, although disorders of other functions of the autonomic nervous system, such as sweating and micturition, can occur.

Autonomic neuropathy may lead to significant capillary arteriovenous shunting, a phenomenon that leads to the observation of a warm neuropathic foot in the presence of Charcot changes consistent with the osteopenic effects that this type of shunting can induce.[69] Treatment includes improved glycemic control, physiotherapy directed at changing the rapidity of postural changes, and support stockings. In severe cases, α-1 agonist pharmacotherapy may be necessary if the symptoms are disabling or are inducing significant cardiac morbidity.

MANAGEMENT OF DIABETIC NEUROPATHY

The options to manage the patient with diabetic neuropathy are meager. Perhaps of foremost importance in the algorithm is the need to rule out other etiologies of pain or numbness involving one or both extremities. Metabolic, neoplastic, and mechanical etiologies abound in the cause of peripheral nervous dysfunction. Of the most import is the determination that the symptoms are not related to a limb-threatening vascular condition, which can usually be diagnosed by a thorough history and physical exam. Once the diagnosis of diabetic neuropathy has been reliably secured, management revolves around treatment of symptoms and the prevention of damage to the foot. The management of the neuropathic foot is covered elsewhere.

Just as hyperglycemia and hyperinsulinemia promote the development of diabetic complications including neuropathy, control of these factors, particularly hyperglycemia, may lead to a reversal or at least to a halting of progression.[14] As with many of the complications of diabetes, the clinician must focus initial therapy on the control of blood glucose through a steady insulin regimen. There is some evidence that an aggressive approach to steady control of blood glucose with insulin, particularly in type 2 diabetics, can in and of itself lead to a reversal in neuropathic symptoms and signs.[70]

The use of tricyclic antidepressant compounds is now considered a first-line therapy in the pharmacologic management of diabetic patients with painful peripheral neuropathy.[42] These compounds act through an unknown mechanism that is independent of their affect on mood.[71] Imipramine or amitriptyline are commonly used, and serious side effects such as dizziness and dry mouth can be avoided by careful and judicious dosing, generally with a gradual increase over a long interval. The side effects are particularly cumbersome among people with autonomic neuropathy in whom the anticholinergic side effects of these drugs may be pronounced.

Other medications that have been used with success in patients with painful diabetic neuropathy include some of the anticonvulsants, such as phenytoin and carbamazepine. Gabapentin has also demonstrated effectiveness.[72] The side effects of these medications is often enough to force patients to discontinue their use. Topical capsaicin may also aid in the long-term management but may result in a short-term exacerbation of symptoms.[73] Last, the use of physioelectric spinal cord stimulation through implantable nerve stimulators has demonstrated long-term effectiveness against painful diabetic neuropathy. This form of therapy is effective against both background as well as neuropathic pain, and one study demonstrated its effectiveness 5 years after implantation.[74]

Surgical revascularization of the lower extremity has demonstrated benefit in the setting of diabetic neuropathy. The correlation between the products of hypoxic metabolism and the development of neuropathy have been described.[75] Histologic studies of endoneurial vessels have demonstrated a proliferative response yet with decreased flow, reflecting favorably on the hypothesis that nonocclusive microcirculatory changes are the culprit in the development of the disease.[76,77] These studies suggest that improvement of arterial circulation in the diabetic extremity with vascular impairment might impact the progression of diabetic neuropathy. Akbari et al.[41] studied peroneal nerve conduction velocity in 55 diabetic patients in need of lower extremity bypass, of whom 21 successfully underwent lower extremity revascularization. They demonstrated that while nerve conduction velocity did not improve with bypass, this parameter did not worsen as did the nonoperative contralateral extremity. The same group demonstrated that, despite an increase in tissue capillary oxygen tensions associated with revascularization, there was no significant increase in sensory nerve function as assessed by Semmes-Weinstein filament test on a similar cohort of patients.[40]

REFERENCES

1. Tesfaye S, Stephens L, Stephenson J, et al. The prevalence of diabetic neuropathy and its relation to glycemic control and potential risk factors: the EURODIAB IDDM Complications Study. *Diabetologia.* 1996;39:1277–1284.
2. Young MJ, Boulton AJ, Macleod AF, et al. A multicentre study of the prevalence of diabetic peripheral polyneuropathy in the United Kingdom hospital clinic population. *Diabetologia.* 1993;36:150–154.
3. Maser RE, Steenkiste AR, Dorman JS, et al. Epidemiological correlates of diabetic neuropathy. Report from Pittsburgh Epidemiology of Diabetes Complications Study. *Diabetes.* 1989;38:1456–1461.
4. Tesfaye S, Chaturvedi N, Eaton SE, et al. Cardiovascular risk factors predict the development of diabetic neuropathy. *Diabetes Med.* 2000;17S:153.
5. Shaw JE, Zimmet PZ. The epidemiology of diabetic neuropathy. *Diabetes Rev.* 1999;7:245–252.
6. Low PA, Suarez GA. Diabetic neuropathies. *Baillieres Clin Neurol.* 1995;4:401–425.
7. Chan AW, MacFarlane IA, Bowsher DR, et al. Chronic pain in patients with diabetes mellitus: comparison with non-diabetic population. *Pain Clin.* 1990;3:147–159.
8. Young RJ, Zhou YQ, Rodriguez E, et al. Variable relationship between peripheral somatic and autonomic neuropathy in patients with different syndromes of diabetic polyneuropathy. *Diabetes.* 1986;35:192–197.
9. Tsigos C, White A, Young RJ. Discrimination between painful and painless diabetic neuropathy based on testing of large somatic nerve and sympathetic nerve function. *Diabetes Med.* 1992;9:359–365.
10. Veves A, Manes C, Murray HJ, et al. Painful neuropathy and foot ulceration in diabetic patients. *Diabetes Care.* 1993;16:1187–1189.
11. Young MJ, Manes C, Boulton AJ. Vibration perception threshold predicts foot ulceration: a prospective study [abstract]. *Diabetes Med.* 1992;9(Suppl 2):542.

12. Caputo GM, Cavanagh PR, Ulbrecht JS, et al. Assessment and management of foot disease in patients with diabetes. *N Engl J Med.* 1994;331:854–860.

13. Pecoraro RE, Reiber GE, Burgess EM. Pathways to diabetic limb amputation. *Diabetes Care.* 1990;13:513–521.

14. Charcot JM. Sur quelques arthropathies qui paraissent dependre d'une lesion du cerveau ou de la moelle epiniere. *Arch Physio Norm Pathol.* 1868;1:161.

15. Gough A, Abraha H, Li F, et al. Measurement of markers of osteoclast and osteoblast activity in patients with acute and chronic diabetic Charcot neuroarthropathy. *Diabetes Med.* 1997;14:527–531.

16. Frykberg RG, Armstrong DG, Giurini J, et al. Diabetic foot disorders: a clinical practice guideline. *J Foot Ankle Surg.* 2000;39 (Suppl 1):2–60.

17. Eichenholtz SN. *Charcot joints.* Springfield, Ill: Charles C Thomas; 1966.

18. Stevens MJ, Feldman EL, Thomas T. Pathogenesis of diabetic neuropathy. In: Veves A, ed. *Contemporary endocrinology: clinical management of diabetic neuropathy.* Totowa, NJ: Humana Press; 1998: 13–48.

19. Ward J, Tesfaye S. Pathogenesis of diabetic neuropathy. In: Pickup J, Williams G, eds. *Textbook of diabetes,* Vol. 2. Oxford, UK: Blackwell Science; 1997:49.1–49.19.

20. United Kingdom Prospective Diabetes Study Group. Intensive blood glucose control with sulphonylureas or insulin compared with conventional treatment and risk of complications in patient with type 2 diabetes. *Lancet.* 1998;352:837–853.

21. Diabetes Control and Complications Trial Research Group. The effect of intensive diabetes therapy on the development and progression of neuropathy. *Ann Intern Med.* 1995;122:561–569.

22. Said G, Slama G, Selva J. Progressive centripetal degeneration of axons in small-fibre type diabetic polyneuropathy. A clinical and pathologic study. *Brain.* 1983;106:791.

23. Malik RA. The pathology of diabetic neuropathy. *Diabetes.* 1997; 46(S2):S50–S53.

24. Cameron NE, Cotter MA. The relationship of vascular changes to metabolic factors in diabetes mellitus and their role in the development and progression of neuropathy. *Ann Intern Med.* 1995; 122:561–568.

25. Cameron NE, Cotter MA, Archbald V, et al. Anti-oxidant and prooxidant effects on nerve conduction velocity, endoneurial blood flow and oxygen tension in non-diabetic and streptozocin-diabetic rats. *Diabetologia.* 1994;37:449–459.

26. Gabbay KH, Merola LO, Field RA. Sorbitol pathway: presence in nerve and cord with substrate accumulation in diabetes. *Science.* 1966;151:209–210.

27. Dyck PJ, Zimmerman BR, Vilan TH, et al. Nerve glucose, fructose, sorbitol, myoinositol, and fiber degeneration in diabetic neuropathy. *N Engl J Med.* 1988;319:542–548.

28. Judzewitsch RG, Jaspan JB, Polonsky KS, et al. Aldose reductase inhibition improves nerve conduction velocity in diabetic patients. *N Engl J Med.* 1983;308:119–125.

29. Tomlinson DR, Moriarty RJ, Mayer H. Prevention and reversal of effective axonal transport and motor nerve conduction velocity in rats with experimental diabetes by treatment with aldose reductase inhibitor sorbinil. *Diabetes.* 1984;33:470–476.

30. Sima AA, Bril V, Nathaniel V, et al. Regeneration and repair of myelinated fibers in sural nerve biopsy specimens from patients with diabetic neuropathy treated with sorbinil. *N Engl J Med.* 1988;319:548–555.

31. Bucala R, Cerami A, Vlassara H. Advanced glycosylation end products in diabetic complications. Biochemical basis and prospects for therapeutic intervention. *Diabetes Rev.* 1995;3:258–268.

32. Bradley JL, Thomas PK, King RH, et al. Myelinated nerve fiber regeneration in diabetic sensory polyneuropathy: correlation with type of diabetes. *Acta Neuropathol Berl.* 1995;90:403–410.

33. Williams SK, Howarth NL, Devenny JJ, et al. Structural and functional consequences of increased tubulin glycosylation in diabetes mellitus. *Proc Natl Acad Sci.* 1982;79:6546–6550.

34. Giannini C, Dyck PJ. Ultrastructural morphometric abnormalities of sural nerve endoneurial microvessels in diabetes mellitus. *Ann Neurol.* 1994;36:408–415.

35. Tesfaye S, Harris N, Wilson RM, et al. Exercise induced conduction velocity increment: a marker of impaired nerve blood flow in diabetic neuropathy. *Diabetologia.* 1992;35:155–159.

36. Newrick PG, Wilson AJ, Jakubowski J, et al. Sural nerve oxygen tension in diabetes. *BMJ.* 1985;193:1053–1054.

37. Young MJ, Veves A, Smith JV, et al. Restoring lower limb blood flow improves conduction velocity in diabetic patients. *Diabetologia.* 1995;38:1051–1054.

38. Malik RA, Newrick PG, Sharma AK, et al. Microangiopathy in human diabetic neuropathy: relationship between capillary abnormalities and the severity of neuropathy. *Diabetologia.* 1998;32: 92–102.

39. Valensi P, Giroux C, Seeboth-Ghalayini B, et al. Diabetic peripheral neuropathy: effects of age, duration of diabetes, glycemic control, and vascular factors. *J Diab Comp.* 1997;11:27–34.

40. Veves A, Donaghue VM, Sarnow MR, et al. The impact of reversal of hypoxia by revascularization on the peripheral nerve function of diabetic patients. *Diabetologia.* 1996;39:344–348.

41. Akbari C, Gibbons G, Habershaw G, et al. The effect of arterial reconstruction on the natural history of diabetic neuropathy. *Arch Surg.* 1997;132:148–152.

42. Tesfaye S, Price D. Therapeutic approaches in diabetes neuropathy and neuropathic pain. In: Boulton AJM, ed. *Diabetic neuropathy.* Carnforth, Lancashire, UK: Marius Press; 1997:159–181.

43. Ward JD. The diabetic leg. *Diabetologia.* 1982;22:141–147.

44. Watkins PJ. Pain and diabetic neuropathy. *BMJ.* 1984;288: 168–169.

45. Watkins PJ, Edmonds MA. Clinical features of diabetic neuropathy. In: Pickup J, Williams G, eds. *Textbook of diabetes,* Vol. 2. Oxford, UK: Blackwell Science; 1997:50.1–50.20.

46. Boulton AJ. Foot problems in patients with diabetes mellitus. In: Pickup J, Williams G, eds. *Textbook of diabetes,* Vol. 2. Oxford, UK: Blackwell Science; 1997:58.1–58.20.

47. Albers JW, Brown MB, Sima AF, et al. Nerve conduction measures in mild diabetic neuropathy in the Early Diabetes Intervention Trial: The effects of age, sex, type of diabetes, disease duration, and anthropomorphic factors. *Neurology.* 1996;46:85–91.

48. Andersen H, Jakobsen J. Motor function in diabetes. *Diabetes Rev.* 1999;7:326–341.

49. Ward JD, Simms JM, Knight G, et al. Venous distension of the diabetic neuropathic foot (physical sign of arterio-venous shunting). *J R Soc Med.* 1983;76:1011–1014.

50. Boulton AJ, Scarpello JH, Ward JD. Venous oxygenation in the diabetic neuropathic foot: evidence of arterio-venous shunting? *Diabetologia.* 1982;22:6–8.

51. Edmonds ME, Archer AG, Watkins PJ. Ephedrine: a new treatment for diabetic neuropathic edema. *Lancet.* 1981;I:548–551.

52. Vinik AI, Parks TS, Stansberry KB, et al. Diabetic neuropathies. *Diabetologia.* 2000;43:957–973.

53. Veves A, Young MJ, Manes C, et al. Differences in peripheral and autonomic nerve function measurements in painful and painless neuropathy: a clinical study. *Diabetes Care.* 1994;17:1200–1202.

54. Archer AG, Watkins PJ, Thomas PJ, et al. The natural history of acute painful neuropathy in diabetes mellitus. *J Neurol Neurosurg Psychiatr.* 1983;46:491–496.

55. Tesfaye S, Malik R, Harris N, et al. Arteriovenous shunting and proliferating new vessels in acute painful neuropathy of rapid glycemic control (insulin neuritis). *Diabetologia.* 1992;35:155–159.

56. Kihara M, Zollman PJ, Smithson IL, et al. Hypoxic effect of endogenous insulin on normal and diabetic peripheral nerve. *Am J Physiol.* 1994;266:E980–E985.

57. Llewelyn JG, Thomas PK, Fonseca V, et al. Acute painful diabetic neuropathy precipitated by strict glycemic control. *Acta Neuropathol (Berl)*. 1986;72:157–163.

58. Boulton AJ, Armstrong WD, Scarpello JH, et al. The natural history of painful diabetic neuropathy—a 4-year study. *Postgrad Med J*. 1983;59:556–559.

59. Eaton SE, Tesfaye S. Clinical manifestations and measurement of somatic neuropathy. *Diabetes Rev*. 1999;7:312–325.

60. Matikainen E, Juntunen J. Diabetic neuropathy: epidemiological, pathogenetic, and clinical aspects with special emphasis on type 2 diabetes mellitus. *Acta Endocrinnol Suppl (Copenh)*. 1984;262:89–94.

61. Garland H, Taverner D. Diabetic myelopathy. *BMJ*. 1953;1:1405.

62. Garland H. Diabetic amyotrophy. *BMJ*. 1955;2:1287–1290.

63. Coppack SW, Watkins PJ. The natural history of femoral neuropathy. *QJ Med*. 1991;79:307–313.

64. Said G, Goulo-Goeau C, Lacroix C, et al. Nerve biopsy findings in different patterns of proximal diabetic neuropathy. *Ann Neurol*. 1994;33:559–569.

65. Dyck PJ, Kratz KM, Karnes JL, et al. The prevalence by staged severity of various types of diabetic neuropathy, retinopathy, and nephropathy in a population-based cohort: the Rochester Diabetic Neuropathy Study. *Neurology*. 1993;43:817–824.

66. White JE, Bullock RF, Hudson P, et al. Phrenic neuropathy in association with diabetes. *Diabetes Med*. 1992;9:954–956.

67. Clayburgh RH, Beckenbaugh RD, Dobyns JH. Carpal tunnel release in patients with diffuse peripheral neuropathy. *J Hand Surg*. 1987;12A:380–383.

68. Tesfaye S, Kempler P, Stevens L, et al. Prevalence of autonomic neuropathy and potential risk factors in type I diabetes in Europe. *Diabetes*. 1998;47(S1):A132.

69. Rayman G. Diabetic neuropathy and microcirculation. *Diabetes Rev*. 1999;7:261–274.

70. Boulton AJ, Drury J, Clarke B, et al. Continuous subcutaneous insulin infusion in the management of painful diabetic neuropathy. *Diabetes Care*. 1982;5:386–390.

71. Max MB, Culnane M, Schafer SC, et al. Amitriptyline relieves diabetic neuropathy pain in patients with normal or depressed mood. *Neurology*. 1987;37:596–598.

72. Backonja M, Beydoun A, Edwards KR, et al. Gabapentin for the symptomatic treatment of painful neuropathy in patients with diabetes mellitus: a randomized controlled trial. *JAMA*. 1998;280:1831–1836.

73. Capsaicin Study Group. The effect of treatment with capsaicin on daily activities of patients with painful diabetic neuropathy. *Diabetes Care*. 1992;15:159–165.

74. Tesfaye S, Watt J, Benbow SJ, et al. Electrical spinal cord stimulation for painful diabetic peripheral neuropathy. *Lancet*. 1996;348:1696–1701.

75. Stevens MJ, Feldman EL, Greene DA. The aetiology of diabetic neuropathy: the combined roles of metabolic and vascular defects. *Diabetes Med*. 1995;12:566–579.

76. Tuck RR, Schmelzer JD, Low PA. Endoneurial blood flow and oxygen tension in the sciatic nerves of rats with experimental diabetic neuropathy. *Brain*. 1984;107:935–950.

77. Yasuda H, Dyck PJ. Abnormalities of endoneurial microvessels and sural nerve pathology in diabetic neuropathy. *Neurology*. 1987;37:20–28.

Biomechanical Impact on the Etiology and Treatment of Neuropathic Ulcerations

3

Charles J. Shuman   *Ian H. Beiser*   *Janette Thompson*

Peripheral neuropathy and peripheral vascular disease (PVD) are the two leading complications of diabetes affecting the feet; both are often causes of limb loss. As a result, complications involving the foot are one of the most common reasons for hospitalization of people with diabetes. Over half of all limb amputations occur in patients with diabetes, and diabetics are 15 times more likely to undergo an amputation.[1]

Vascular insufficiency, infection, or peripheral neuropathy, in conjunction with mechanical factors, often lead to the development of ulcers. Three mechanisms frequently play a part in the development of mechanically induced neuropathic ulcerations. The first mechanism is a result of a traumatic force of elevated pressure over a brief period of time—in other words, a quick traumatic event that results in a piercing of the skin. An example of this is the act of stepping on a sharp object, like a nail or a piece of broken glass.

The second mechanism that leads to mechanically induced ulceration is application of low pressure exerted over a longer period of time. This may occur, for example, when a tight shoe is worn. The shoe pressure causes blanching of the skin over a bony prominence such as a bunion or hammer toe, which leads to a focal area of ischemia. If the pressure is maintained for a significant period of time, the ischemia leads to necrosis and ulceration.

The third mechanism involves a force of repetitive, moderate pressure. This accounts for the majority of diabetic plantar ulcers. Repetitive pressure >10 kg per cm acting on the foot during gait will contribute to the formation of this type of ulcer.[2] In the absence of neuropathy, the repetitive pressure beneath prominent areas produces pain. The pain causes the sensate person to take measures to alleviate the discomfort. Such measures include limping or modification of gait to place weight on a different part of the foot, changing to more comfortable shoes, applying pads, or seeking medical treatment. In the neuropathic patient when there is a loss of protective sensation, these symptoms go undetected. The continued repetitive pressure results in inflammation of that part of the foot. The continued inflammation then leads to an enzymatic autolysis that leads to tissue breakdown and ulceration. The location of this type of ulcer is predictable. Areas of increased pressure are commonly identified by areas of plantar callus formation. The callus usually signifies an area that is bearing more weight than the surrounding areas. The areas of callus are the

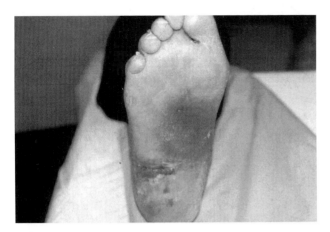

Figure 3-1   Charcot foot ulceration.

locations that are prone to ulceration in the neuropathic patient. In patients with "flatfoot" deformities, there is often excessive pronation and a hypermobile first ray that leads to an excessive amount of pressure beneath the second metatarsal. In neuropathic patients with this foot type, callus formation and subsequent ulcerations often develop beneath the second metatarsal head. In contrast, patients with a rigid cavus foot commonly ulcerate beneath the heel, the first metatarsal, and/or the fifth metatarsal. In patients with a "rocker-bottom" Charcot deformity, the area beneath the cuboid is an area of increased risk (Fig. 3-1).

There have been many advances made with regard to the treatment of ulcers over the past several years. These include many new products and treatments that can be used to encourage wound healing. As good as these products may be, an essential element of treatment is offloading the ulcer. If weight-bearing pressure is not reduced significantly from an ulcer, healing of the ulcer is unlikely. Furthermore, these measures must be continued, even after the ulcer is healed, in order to prevent recurrences. Ideally, the areas prone to the development of ulcerations can be identified and measures can be taken to prevent ulceration in the first place. An understanding of biomechanics and gait is essential to the treatment and prevention of diabetic ulcerations.

BASIC FOOT BIOMECHANICS

There are four major functions that a foot must have for normal gait to occur. It must be (a) flexible and able to adapt to uneven surfaces, yet also have the ability to quickly transform into a (b) rigid lever for propulsion. It must also be able to (c) absorb rotary motion from the hip and leg, and (d) absorb the shock of impact at heel contact. All these functions must occur at the appropriate time in the gait cycle. The ability of the foot to morph from a flexible structure, which is able to adapt to weight bearing on uneven surfaces, to a rigid

lever is accomplished by the realignment of the axis of motion of two major joints, the subtalar joint and the midtarsal joint. The subtalar joint is the joint between the talus and the calcaneus. The midtarsal joint consists of the talus, calcaneus, navicular, and cuboid bones. Abnormal positions of the axis of motion of these major joints or limitations of their normal ranges of motion will significantly affect the foot's ability to efficiently carry out these necessary functions.

There are three anatomic planes. Each plane is associated with a particular motion of the foot, and specific foot pathology is associated with abnormal motion in these planes (Fig. 3-2). Movements of the foot may be uniplane (occurring in one plane) or triplane (occurring in three planes simultaneously). Examples of uniplane motion are inversion and eversion, which occur in the frontal plane; adduction and abduction, which occur in the transverse plane; and plantarflexion and dorsiflexion, which occur in the sagittal plane (Fig. 3-3). Pronation and supination are examples of triplane motion and occur in all three planes at once. Pronation consists of eversion, abduction, and dorsiflexion (Fig. 3-4). Pronation is a normal, important function of the gait cycle. It only becomes abnormal when pronation occurs at a time when the foot should be supinated. Supination consists of inversion, adduction, and plantarflexion. It is this normal movement from pronation to supination at the correct time in the gait cycle that enables the foot to successfully carry out its major functions.

The axes of motion of the subtalar and midtarsal joints reside in all three planes—sagittal, transverse, and frontal—and are therefore triplanar. The interaction of the subtalar joint with the two axes of motion of

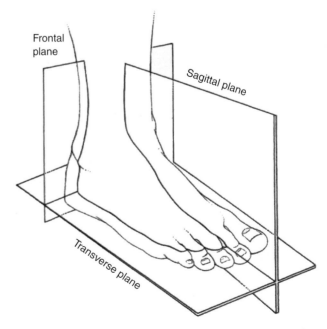

Figure 3-2   Anatomic planes of the foot.

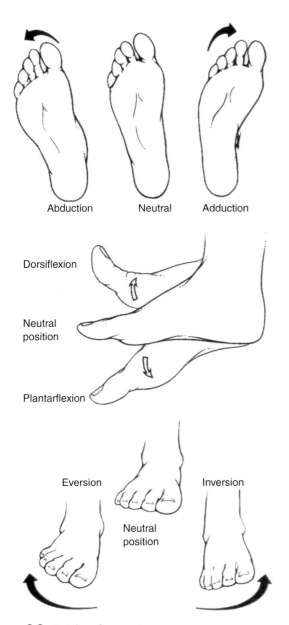

Abduction   Neutral   Adduction

Dorsiflexion

Neutral position

Plantarflexion

Eversion   Inversion

Neutral position

Figure 3-3 Uniplane foot motion.

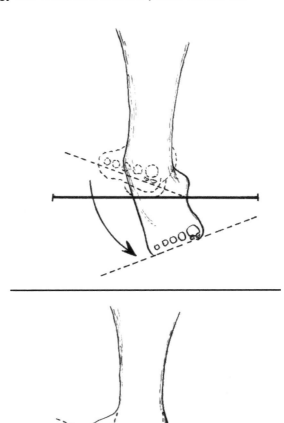

Figure 3-4 Triplanar foot motion.

the midtarsal joint allows the foot to lock and unlock, thus moving in and out of rigidity at the appropriate time in the gait cycle.

NORMAL GAIT CYCLE

The normal gait cycle consists of two components, stance phase (weight-bearing) and swing phase (non–weight-bearing). The stance phase takes up about 60% of the entire gait cycle and is divided into three segments: Contact, midstance, and propulsion or pushoff (Fig. 3-5). The beginning of contact phase is marked by the heel striking the ground. This phase continues until what is known as full forefoot loading. Midstance goes from full forefoot loading until heel lift. The propulsive phase extends from heel lift until pushoff. The gait cycle is initiated when the heel contacts the ground. At the time of impact, the foot is normally supinated several degrees. It then rapidly begins the process of pronation. In the normal foot, the calcaneus goes from a 2-degree inverted position to a 4-degree everted position. The inverted position of the calcaneus at heel strike is why the lateral side of the heel of a shoe wears more than the medial side in a normal foot. Pronatory motion of the subtalar joint allows the foot to absorb shock during heel strike and to adapt to uneven terrain. The anterior crural muscles (tibialis anterior, extensor hallucis longus, extensor digitorum longus, and peroneus tertius) are firing at this time and begin to decelerate the foot as it plantarflexes, preventing the foot from slapping the ground.

Forefoot loading occurs as the body's center of gravity travels forward. Forces move from lateral to medial as the foot pronates, and the center of gravity travels from the lateral side of the heel towards the first metatarsal.

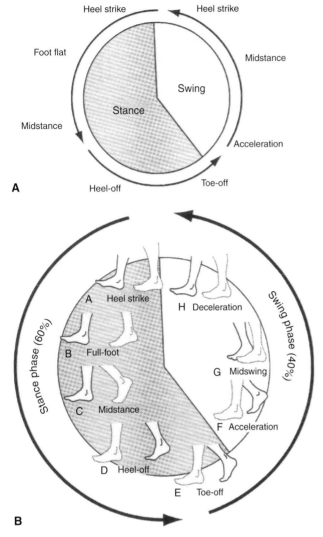

A

B

Figure 3-5   Phases of gait.

Following full forefoot loading, the leg begins to externally rotate relative to the foot and the foot begins to supinate. During this time, the foot must absorb the rotary forces of the leg. Failure to do so can cause a significant stress on other joints, both distal and proximal, which could lead to degenerative joint disease. This is especially noted in the ankle and knee. Patients with fusion of the talar calcaneal joint typically develop significant osteoarthrosis of the ankle joint.

At the time of heel lift, the foot should be supinated. This allows the first ray to act as a rigid lever and allow for propulsion forward. If the foot is not rigid and locked as the propulsive phase begins, the reactive force of the ground elevates the first metatarsal and weight is transferred medially off the foot rather than traveling distally through the hallux. Any abnormal motion or motion at the incorrect time will interfere with normal foot function and result in increased forces on specific areas of the foot. Motion at a time when no motion should occur is referred to as hypermobility.

Swing phase begins after toe-off. At this time, the anterior crurals act to dorsiflex the ankle, preventing the toes from dragging on the ground. They continue to fire throughout the swing phase. This places the foot in a supinated position, setting the foot up to repeat the gait cycle again with the next heel strike.

INTRINSIC FOOT MUSCLE IMBALANCE

Distal symmetrical polyneuropathy is the most common form of neuropathy in people with diabetes. It is primarily the sensory nerves that are affected, but the motor and autonomic fibers are also impacted.[3] The most common result of distal motor neuropathy in the foot is intrinsic muscle wasting. When this occurs, the weakened intrinsic muscles (interossei and lumbricales) are unable to effectively oppose the action of the long extensors, which leads to metatarsal phalangeal joint hyperextension and proximal interphalangeal joint flexion. The result is a retrograde force from the toes to the metatarsal heads, forcing the metatarsal heads to bear more weight. This leads to deformities such as claw toes, hammer toes, and plantarly prominent metatarsal heads (Fig. 3-6).[4,5] Normal digital stability during propulsion is achieved through a delicate balance between the extensors and flexors acting upon the toes. A flexion force is transferred to the

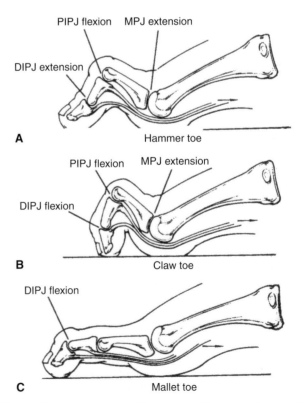

A

B

C

Figure 3-6   Hammer toe (**A**), claw toe (**B**), and mallet toe (**C**) deformities. MPJ, metacarpophalangeal joint; PIPJ, proximal interphalangeal joint; DIPJ, distal interphalangeal joint.

metatarsophalangeal joint when the lumbricales and interossei contract along with an extension force at the proximal interphalangeal joint. The flexion force is opposed by the extensor digitorum brevis and extensor digitorum longus. These muscle forces must remain in balance so neither the extensor forces nor the flexor forces become dominant. As long as there is a balance between these forces, the toes remain parallel to the supporting surface as the metatarsal heads pivot over the plantar plate. In order for the digits to function properly, they must remain aligned in a column, thereby creating stability through compression. Loss of the balance of forces will result in flexion of these joints. When there is a muscle imbalance and consequent loss of stability through compression, the extensor digitorum longus places significant retrograde forces on the affected metatarsal heads in the posterior plantar direction. These forces are quite significant and coupled with the plantar fat pad displacement distally, relative to the metatarsal heads, leave the metatarsal heads with less protection plantarly. This is referred to as anterior displacement of the fat pad. When this occurs, the remaining soft tissue beneath the metatarsal heads is less able to withstand the increased direct pressure and shear pressure associated with weight bearing and gait. The skin's response to excessive pressure is the production of callus. As the callus builds up, plantar pressure increases even further. In the neuropathic patient with loss of protective sensation, areas of callus formation beneath the metatarsal heads or elsewhere are prone to ulceration. Other muscle groups may also be weakened by motor neuropathy. If the anterior crurals are weakened, a drop foot may occur since the long extensors may be unable to extend the foot adequately during the swing phase of gait.

IMPACT OF DIABETES ON JOINT MOTION

Molecular biologic abnormalities associated with diabetes may also contribute to ulcerations in other ways. The skin of diabetic patients is often less resilient than normal, and as a result may be more susceptible to the stresses of shear forces leading to ulcerations. The diminished elasticity of soft tissues, such as skin and tendons, in diabetic patients is thought to be due to abnormal binding of glucose to collagen, which results in an excessive number of cross links.[6,7] Studies using electron microscopy have shown increased packing density of collagen fibrils, diminished fibrillar diameter, and abnormal fibril morphology in the Achilles tendons of long-term diabetic patients with neuropathy.[8] These structural changes could contribute to a tightening of the Achilles tendon and resultant equinus in diabetics that is often associated

with the development of forefoot ulcerations and diabetic neuropathic osteoarthropathy (DNOAP).

Diabetic patients with peripheral neuropathy are susceptible to the development of a condition commonly called Charcot joint or DNOAP. This is often a highly destructive condition resulting in severe deformity of the foot and/or ankle. The classic presentation is of a red, hot, swollen, nonpainful foot with collapse of the arch, and the development of a convex "rocker-bottom." Although the tarso-metatarsal joints are most commonly affected (Fig. 3-7), other joints such as the metatarsal-phalangeal joints, interphalangeal joints, ankle joint, and midtarsal joint may also be affected. Eichenholtz[9] described three stages of Charcot joint. In the first stage, the acute phase, the foot becomes hyperemic and joint destruction begins. In the second stage, there is absorption of osseous debris, fusion, and coalescence of the joints. Last, there is a reconstructive phase in which bone remodeling occurs. This condition is often misdiagnosed as cellulitis or osteomyelitis because of the similar appearance of marked soft-tissue inflammation and associated osseous erosions.

A common presentation of DNOAP is as a rocker-bottom foot in which there is a convexity of the plantar aspect of the foot rather than the normal concave plantar arch. The rocker-bottom Charcot foot is usually associated with a tight Achilles tendon, which raises the posterior portion of the calcaneus. This produces a negative calcaneal inclination angle. The cuboid is often prominent plantarly and is a common location for ulcers.

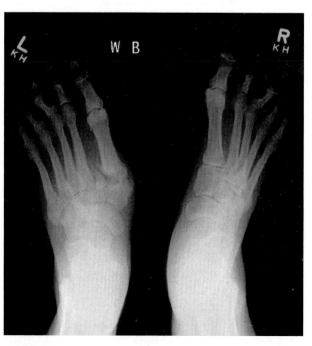

Figure 3-7 Charcot foot x-ray.

THE EFFECT OF COMMON FOOT TYPES AND BIOMECHANICAL DEFORMITIES

No two feet are exactly the same. Although there are often references to the "normal foot," a more proper term to use may be the "ideal" foot since there is such a wide variance in the shape and function of the human foot. We often speak of biomechanical abnormalities when referring to those feet whose structure and function varies significantly from the structure and function of the ideal foot. There are many factors that contribute to these differences, including abnormal osseous development, congenital deformity, abnormal joint fusions, and connective tissue disorders. Some deformities may be directly attributed to complications of diabetes, i.e., a rocker-bottom associated with DNOAP. Other deformities are nonspecific to diabetes but may cause special problems in the diabetic patient when there is concomitant neuropathy or PVD. Some of these deformities may be rigid and thus do not change with weight bearing, while others are flexible. Another way of broadly categorizing some of these deformities is as being cavus (high-arched), cavovarus (high-arched with an inverted heel), planus (flatfooted), or valgoplanus (flatfooted with marked eversion of the heel). Some commonly found foot types in diabetic patients are the hypermobile (flexible) pes planus and the rigid cavovarus foot.

Flexible Pes Planus

The flexible pes planus is a broad category of foot deformities that function similarly during gait. The abnormal biomechanical function that is common to this category of abnormalities is excessive pronation during stance and ambulation. Some examples of deformities and conditions contributing to the existence of this foot type are ligamentous laxity/connective tissue disorders, congenital pes valgus, external tibial or femoral torsion, coxa varum/genu valgum deformities, compensated equinus and tibialis posterior tendon dysfunction or rupture. In many of these conditions, the center of gravity is shifted medial to the subtalar joint axis of motion, thereby causing the heel to pronate excessively when heel contact occurs. If the calcaneus is excessively pronated during heel contact, the foot will not properly absorb the shock of heel contact and will not resupinate at the appropriate time in the gait cycle. A compensated biomechanical equinus is often a contributing factor associated with a flexible pes planus. Biomechanical equinus refers to a limitation of ankle joint dorsiflexion of <10 degrees.[10] Ordinarily, it is necessary to have at least 10 degrees of dorsiflexion available at the ankle joint to compensate for a similar amount of hip extension at the end of midstance. When there is a biomechanical equinus deformity, abnormal compensatory dorsiflexion occurs in the foot rather than at the ankle. When this occurs, the midtarsal joint unlocks and the subtalar joint is forced to pronate to compensate for the limitation of ankle joint dorsiflexion. This causes the foot to continue pronating or to remain pronated at a time when it should be supinating.

Excessive pronation also destabilizes the cuboid, which normally acts as a force multiplier or fulcrum for the peroneus longus. When this occurs, the peroneus longus loses its mechanical advantage and is unable to plantarflex and stabilize the first metatarsal adequately. The first metatarsal subsequently becomes hypermobile (motion at a time when no motion should occur) and elevates relative to the other metatarsals (elevatus). When the first metatarsal is unable to bear its normal load, the weight-bearing forces are transmitted to the second metatarsal. This abnormal weight distribution often results in a callus beneath the second metatarsal. In a sensate foot, this may be painful. In the insensate neurotrophic foot, this area beneath the second metatarsal head is a potential ulcer site.

Hypermobility and first metatarsal elevatus also results in abnormal stress and decreased range of motion at the first metatarsal phalangeal (MTP) joint. This may result in a "jamming" effect at the first MTP joint with resultant degenerative changes at the first metatarsal head. When the hallux cannot dorsiflex adequately, increased pressure is transferred to the hallux interphalangeal joint. This is a common potential ulcer site (Fig. 3-8). When the sagittal plane instability at the first ray is associated with transverse plane instability, the hallux abducts laterally and the first metatarsal adducts medially, resulting in a hallux valgus and bunion deformity. The prominent medial eminence of the first metatarsal and the medial aspect of the hallux interphalangeal joint are potential ulcer sites when these deformities are associated with neuropathy.

Rigid Cavovarus Foot

A foot with a very high longitudinal arch is often referred to as a cavus foot. A cavovarus foot describes a

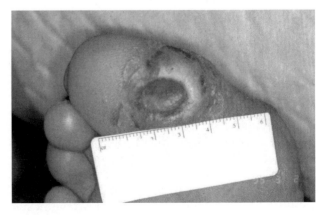

Figure 3-8   Hallux ulceration.

cavus foot in which there is also a marked inversion of the heel. Radiographically, a cavus foot has a high inclination of the calcaneus relative to the ground, as well as a corresponding high declination of the metatarsals. In some cases, the foot appears to have a high arch when it is not bearing weight, but pronates and flattens with stance. However, when reference is made to a classical cavus foot, it is generally applied to a rigid nonreducible or semirigid deformity. These feet typically have limited subtalar joint motion. This results in diminished ability to adapt to ground reactive forces and to absorb shock during gait. This foot type is predisposed to the development of keratoses and ulceration at the heel and laterally at the fifth metatarsal base or cuboid as well as at the ball of the foot beneath the metatarsal heads (Fig. 3-9). Over time, the normal fat pad that provides cushioning at the ball of the foot can become displaced or atrophied, thereby magnifying the potential for metatarsalgia, keratoses, and ulceration beneath the metatarsal heads.

In many cavus feet, the first ray is plantarflexed relative to the lesser metatarsals. When the plantarflexed first ray is rigid, increased pressures will build up under the first metatarsal head (Fig. 3-10) and will lead to the development of keratoses and potential ulceration. After the contact phase of gait, as weight-bearing pressures are being transferred to the forefoot, the rigid plantarflexed first metatarsal forces the foot to rapidly resupinate. This is referred to as a supinatory rock. As the forefoot rapidly supinates, weight is transferred to the plantar aspect of the fifth metatarsal. When this deformity exists, the majority of body weight is borne by the heel, first metatarsal head, and fifth metatarsal head instead of being more equally distributed. The pressure is increased at these three locations since there is more weight distributed over a smaller surface area than in the normal foot. In this foot type, keratoses and potential ulceration are found in this tripod distribution beneath the heel, the first metatarsal head, and the fifth metatarsal head.

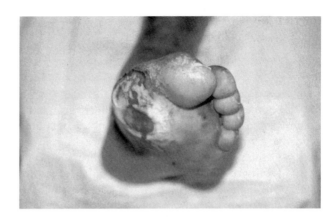

Figure 3-10 First metatarsal ulceration.

EFFECT OF AMPUTATIONS ON FOOT MECHANICS

All amputations have significant biomechanical consequences since they alter the structural integrity of the foot and alter the way the various segments of the lower extremity function together. When dealing with amputations, these biomechanical changes should be addressed so that further complications can be prevented. Different types of amputations will alter the mechanics of motion in predictable ways based on the segment that is amputated.

Hallux Amputations

Ordinarily, the hallux plays a major role during the propulsive phase of gait. When the hallux is lost due to a hallux or first ray amputation, weight is transferred to the second toe and second metatarsal head. Also, since an intact hallux functions as a buttress for the rotation of the first metatarsal head, amputation of the hallux results in a reduction in the first metatarsal head's ability to bear weight. This weight is then transferred to the lesser metatarsals.[11] This increases the risk of lesser metatarsal head ulceration and is associated with a greater risk of lesser metatarsal stress fractures.[12]

Lesser Digital Amputations

The lesser toes do not play as large a role in the gait cycle as the hallux. However, amputation of the second toe results in a loss of the buttress effect it provides for the great toe, and, without it, the hallux usually drifts laterally, creating a hallux valgus deformity. Similarly, a hallux valgus deformity can develop after a loss of the third or fourth toe. A domino effect occurs as each digit drifts laterally to fill the void created by the amputated digit. As the second toe drifts laterally due to loss of the third toe, the hallux also subluxes laterally. A toe filler could be used to try to compensate for the defect following a lesser digital amputation.

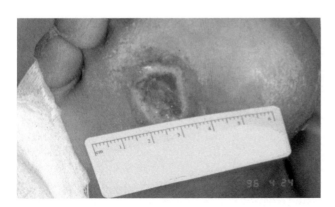

Figure 3-9 Metatarsal ulceration.

Partial Ray Resections

Often, portions of a metatarsal are amputated along with a toe. In addition to the sequelae related to the digital amputation, partial ray resections create increased weight-bearing pressure beneath the remaining bones at the ball of the foot. This often leads to the development of transfer lesions beneath the remaining metatarsal heads. An early sign of this is the appearance of a callus. If this increased pressure is not reduced, an ulcer may eventually develop beneath one or more of the remaining metatarsal heads. Some partial ray amputations are more likely than others to result in transfer lesions because of their normal biomechanical characteristics. The axis of motion of the second, third, and fourth rays are similar and function together as a group, in the same direction. In contrast, the first and fifth rays have independent axes of motion and function separate from the second, third, and fourth metatarsals.[2,10,13] Amputation of the fifth ray will result in increased pressure beneath the fourth metatarsal, which has a different axis of motion. Similarly, first ray amputations will lead to increased pressure beneath the second metatarsal. However, in amputations of the third metatarsal, because of similar axes of motion, weight will be shared more efficiently by the second and fourth metatarsals, thereby having less risk of transfer lesions such as calluses and ulcerations.

Partial ray amputations that extend more proximally can lead to other problems. For example, when the fifth metatarsal base is resected, there is a loss of the insertion of the peroneus brevis. Since this muscle is the strongest everter in the foot, an imbalance is created. This loss of peroneus brevis function will result in a supination deformity of the foot. Lateral keratoses development and ulcer formation can result.

Transmetatarsal Amputations

As with any amputation, the level of the resection will depend on factors such as vascularity, viability of tissue, infection, and the location of ulcers. The level at which a transmetatarsal amputation (TMA) is performed will significantly impact the postoperative biomechanical function of the foot during gait. A longer metatarsal length correlates with a greater lever arm for propulsion.[2] Also, following a TMA, although care can be taken to create new distal attachment points for the ends of the severed extensor tendons, there is usually some degree of functional loss of the extensor tendons. They are no longer able to fully oppose plantar flexion of the foot by the Achilles and tibialis posterior tendons. A plantarflexed attitude often ensues, predisposing the foot to plantar ulceration of the forefoot. Achilles tendon lengthenings or gastrocnemius recessions are often performed to reduce the ulceraton risk and to improve gait.[14] However, care should be taken to avoid overlengthening the Achilles tendon, which could result in a greater risk of calcaneal gait and calcaneal ulceration.

Lisfranc and Chopart Amputations

This level of amputation results in a functional loss of the extensors and flexors as well as a greater loss of lever arm than the TMA. The attachments of the tibialis anterior, peroneus longus, and peroneus brevis are also lost. The functional imbalance created by the loss of these tendons results in an equinovarus deformity. An Achilles tendon lengthening or gastrocnemius recession may help to offset the predictable equinus. Another inherent problem with this level of amputation is difficulty fitting shoes postoperatively. With amputations at the transmetatarsal level, there is usually enough forefoot length remaining to hold a shoe on the foot. At the LisFranc (tarsal-metatarsal joints) and Chopart level (talar-navicular), the stump will tend to slip out of the shoe as the leg is lifted since there is no forefoot to keep the shoe on the foot. In these cases, a brace attached to a shoe is usually required to allow a return to ambulation.

TREATMENT OF BIOMECHANICALLY-INDUCED ABNORMALITIES

Many biomechanical abnormalities can be controlled with orthoses. These are devices that can be placed in shoes to correct or compensate for deformities and functional pathology. Orthotic devices can be broken down into two broad categories: Functional orthoses and accommodative orthoses.

Functional orthoses attempt to hold the foot in a position that allows it to function more normally. Often, the goal of a functional orthotic is to reduce abnormal pronation, such as in the case of a patient who has a pes planus deformity. Functional orthoses often have a rearfoot post that can be wedged to control pronation by limiting subtalar joint motion. The forefoot can also be wedged to compensate for forefoot deformities, such as forefoot varus or valgus deformities. The fabrication of functional orthoses typically begins with taking a cast impression of the foot. Although they may look similar in some ways, functional orthoses are distinguished from over-the-counter arch supports by their ability to address the unique biomechanical needs of the person for whom they are made. In order to maintain their shape and provide control, functional orthoses are generally "hard." However, they may be called semiflexible, semirigid, or rigid depending on how they are made. Examples of common material used to make functional orthoses include fiberglass, carbon fiber composites, and polypropylene.

Functional orthoses are often used by athletes and diabetic patients without neuropathy or significant vascular disease.

Accommodative orthoses are most commonly used to offload areas of increased pressure and reduce shear stress, rather than to alter gait like a functional orthotic device. These devices are most commonly used in sensate patients with painful plantar lesions or in vascular and neuropathic patients with areas of increased pressure, which have a tendency to ulcerate. Several different techniques can be utilized to accomplish the offloading of an at-risk part of a foot. One way is to reduce the thickness of material directly beneath an area that is bearing too much pressure. Another method is to increase the thickness of material around a lesion. Accommodative orthoses are often referred to as "soft." Examples of materials used to make these are leather, Aliplast, Spenco, Sorbothane, PPT, and Plastazote. These materials come in a variety of thicknesses but tend to be bulky. Care should be taken to be sure there is enough room in the shoes to accommodate these orthoses. If the orthosis is too thick relative to the shoe, the dorsum of the toes will rub against the upper part of the shoe and dorsal ulcerations could develop. Deep-depth or "extra-depth" shoes, which have increased room in the toe box, are often used along with orthoses in diabetic patients.

It is not unusual to make an orthosis that is both functional and accommodative. A functional foot orthosis could be covered with accommodative materials to create a combined functional/accommodative device. Or a single intermediate-density material could be used to create an orthosis that provides a modest amount of functional control along with accommodation for plantar lesions.

PREVENTION

Early detection of at-risk diabetic patients with PVD and/or neuropathy is critical to preventing ulcerations, infections, and amputations. There are several tests that can easily be utilized to determine the presence of peripheral neuropathy. A simple, inexpensive, and effective test for neuropathy with a loss of protective sensation is the Semmes-Weinstein monofilament. A comprehensive biomechanical foot exam will help to predict specific parts of the foot that are most susceptible to ulceration. Early correction with either orthoses

or surgical intervention may prevent the development of lesions that often lead to more serious complications. In cases where an ulcer develops and is treated successfully, it is important to follow-up with measures to prevent recurrences. Patients with healed plantar ulcers who return to their usual footwear have a 90% chance of recurrence, compared to a 19% recurrence rate for patients who have modified shoes or orthoses.[15] Identification of biomechanical abnormalities and the use of appropriate orthoses and deep-depth or molded shoes will help to prevent other complications.

REFERENCES

1. Frykberg RG. Diabetic foot ulcerations. In: Frykberg RG, ed. *The high risk foot in diabetes mellitus*. New York, NY: Churchill Livingstone; 1991:151.
2. Schoenhaus HD, Wernick E, Cohen RS. Biomechanics of the diabetic foot. In: Fryberg RG, ed. *The high risk foot in diabetes mellitus*. New York, NY: Churchill Livingstone; 1991:125.
3. Dyck PJ, Thomas PK, Asbury AK et al., eds. *Diabetic neuropathy*. Philadelphia, Pa: WB Saunders; 1987.
4. Cavanagh PR, Ulbrecht JS. Biomechanics of the foot in diabetes mellitus. In: Levin ME, O'Neal LW, Bowker J, eds. *The diabetic foot*. St. Louis, Mo: Mosby–Year Book; 1993:199.
5. Elkeles RS, Wolfe JHN. The diabetic foot. *Br Med J.* 1991;303:1053.
6. Brownlee J, Cerami A, Vlassara H. Advanced glycosylation end products in tissue and the biomechanical basis of diabetic complications. *N Engl J Med.* 1988;318:1315.
7. Brink SJ. Limited joint mobility as a risk factor for diabetic complications. *Clin Diabetes.* 1987;5:122.
8. Grant WP, Sullivan R, Sonenshine DE, et al. Electron microscopic investigation of the effects of diabetes mellitus on the Achilles tendon. *J Foot Ankle Surg.* 1997;36:272–278.
9. Eichenholtz SN. *Charcot joints*. Springfield, Ill: Charles C Thomas Publisher; 1966.
10. Root ML, Orien WP, Weed JH. Forces acting upon the foot during locomotion. In: Root ML, Orien WP, Weed JH, eds. *Normal and abnormal function of the foot, clinical biomechanics*, Vol. 2. Los Angeles, Calif: Clinical Biomehanics Corporation; 1977:165–179.
11. Mann R, Poppen N, O'Konski M. Amputation of the great toe: a clinical and biomechanical study. *Clin Orthop.* 1988;226:197.
12. Ianucci A, Lai King P, Channell R, et al. Spontaneous fractures of the lesser metatarsals secondary to an amputated hallux and peripheral neuropathy. *J Foot Surg.* 1987;26:66.
13. Frykberg RG, Giurini J, Habershaus G. Prophylactic surgery in the diabetic foot. In: Kominsky SJ, ed. *Medical and surgical management of the diabetic foot*. St Louis, Mo: Mosby–Year Book; 1994:399.
14. Nishimoto GS, Attinger CE, Cooper PS. Lengthening of the Achilles tendon for the treatment of diabetic forefoot ulceration. *Surg Clin North Am.* 2003;83:707–726.
15. Levitz SJ, Whiteside LS, Fitzgerald TA. Biomechanical foot therapy. *Clin Podiatr Med Surg.* 1998;5:721.

Management of Diabetic Foot Ulcers

David L. Steed

Lower extremity diabetic foot ulcers are a significant health care problem in the United States. There are as many as 20 million patients with diabetes in the US. Foot ulcers and the complications from these wounds are a major cause of hospitalization in this population of patients. Only 6% to 10% of hospitalizations in diabetic patients are for the care and treatment of foot ulcers, yet these admissions are nearly one quarter of the hospital days in this group.[1] Up to 10% of diabetic patients may develop foot ulcers.[2] This means that as many as 2 million people may require treatment of a diabetic foot wound. Diabetic wounds serve as a portal of entry for bacteria; as long as the wound persists, the patient is at increased risk for amputation.[3] There are 60,000 to 80,000 amputations performed in diabetic patients each year in the US, and the incidence does not appear to be decreasing.[4] It costs $30,000 to care for a diabetic foot ulcer for 2 years. The overall cost of care for these patients is difficult to measure precisely but is probably billions of dollars, considering the cost of office visits, medications, debridements, dressings, hospitalizations, amputations, rehabilitation, and artificial limbs. There is a cost to society in terms of lost wages and long-term care for these patients. The price of pain and suffering cannot be estimated.

PATHOGENESIS

Diabetic foot ulcers are caused by neuropathy and atherosclerotic peripheral vascular disease. Sixty percent to 70% of patients with diabetes and foot ulcers have peripheral neuropathy as the etiology, 15% to 20% have atherosclerotic occlusive vascular disease as the cause, and 15% to 20% have both.[5,6] The peripheral neuropathy is sensory, motor, and autonomic. Prolonged glucose elevation leads to damage of the nerves. Neuropathy is present in 10% of patients when diabetes is diagnosed and is found in up to half of patients who have had diabetes for >10 years. The motor neuropathy occurs when the motor nerves that control motion and position of the foot do not function properly. Nerve signals sent to the small muscles of the foot to hold the bones and joints in the proper position do not occur. As the shape of the foot changes, tendons do not pull in proper alignment and deformities worsen. This abnormality is commonly known as Charcot deformity. There is a "claw" deformity of the toes as they are pulled up and do not touch the ground or bear weight. The metatarsal heads thus become more prominent as they are pushed downward. The metatarsal heads are a very common site of ulceration in diabetic patients, more so for the skin beneath the first and fifth metatarsal heads. As the deformity worsens, the patients develop midfoot collapse with loss of the plantar arch, leading to a "rocker-bottom" contour to the foot.

There is also a sensory neuropathy that leads to loss of protective sensation. The patient thus has a deformed foot in a normal-shaped shoe. This leads to abnormal pressure points. Without the ability to feel the excessive pressure, skin breakdown occurs. Ulcers commonly begin as a minor wound, often from minor trauma. Improperly fitting shoes are responsible for many of these problems. It is also common for the patient to have a foreign body in their foot from walking barefoot. Improper trimming of nails can also occur, as well as burns from putting the foot in water that is too hot or from warming feet on a radiator in cold weather.

Autonomic neuropathy results in inappropriate vasodilatation and vasoconstriction, improper sweating, and drying of the skin. The dry skin is more likely to crack and open. These openings are a potential portal of entry for bacteria.

Diabetes is a risk factor for atherosclerosis, and many of these patients develop peripheral vascular disease. Although there was once a suggestion that diabetic patients had "small-vessel disease" with occlusion of very small vessels, that theory has not been accepted. It is clear that diabetic patients are at increased risk for atherosclerosis. Their pattern of disease commonly involves the tibial arteries. It is common for diabetic patients to have an easily palpable popliteal pulse with no pulse in the foot physical examination. Diabetic patients have other problems leading to foot wounds. They may have thinning of the skin of the plantar surface of the foot in the area where the metatarsal heads are more prominent because of neuropathy. They do not control infection as well. These factors result in a higher amputation rate in diabetic patients.

EVALUATION OF THE PATIENT

The evaluation of the diabetic patient begins with the history and physical examination. Their history may suggest generalized atherosclerosis with coronary artery disease or cerebrovascular disease. Many have had myocardial ischemia with infarction and coronary artery stenting or bypass. They may also have had transient ischemic attack or stroke. They may admit to claudication. Previous amputation is common in this patient population. The level of arterial blockage can usually be determined on physical examination by a careful evaluation of the pulses. Patients must also be examined carefully for peripheral neuropathy. A Charcot deformity of the foot is evidence of significant motor neuropathy. The sensory neuropathy can be quantified with Semmes-Weinstein monofilaments.[7] Lack of sensation to the 5.07 filament suggests the patient is at risk for ulceration.

Factors That Determine the Location of the Ulcer

The cause for the skin breakdown in the diabetic foot can often be determined from the location of the ulcer. Ulcers on the tips of the toes or on the foot laterally are commonly caused by improperly fitting shoes. Ulcers between the toes are known as "kissing ulcers" and may

be from shoes that are too narrow. They are more common in patients with arthritis of their toes and limited joint mobility. Ulcers on the dorsum of the foot and on the tops of the toes are common in patients with a claw deformity of the foot and can be prevented with an extra-depth shoe. Ulcers under the metatarsal heads are very common in patients with a claw toe deformity, which makes the metatarsal heads more prominent. The skin under the first and fifth metatarsal heads is at the greatest risk for ulceration. Ulcers on the plantar surface of the midfoot are found in patients with a rocker-bottom contour to their foot, with maximum weight bearing on the midportion of the plantar surface. Ulcerations of the heel occur in debilitated patients, especially those with vascular disease in the posterior tibial artery.

Noninvasive Evaluation of Arterial Circulation

If the patient does not clearly have a palpable pulse in their foot, they should be evaluated in the noninvasive peripheral vascular laboratory. It is important to assess their pulses before debridement. Local factors such as edema or inflammation may make it difficult to determine the adequacy of blood flow in these patients. Any patient with a foot wound should have noninvasive vascular testing prior to debridement unless a pulse is clearly palpable.

Lower extremity arterial pressures are measured using a blood pressure cuff and a Doppler probe. An ankle-brachial index (ABI) is calculated. A normal ABI is 0.9 to 1.1. In claudication, the ABI is lowered to 0.7. In ischemic rest pain at about 0.4, and in tissue death, the ABI falls to 0.1 to 0.3. Patients with diabetes may have falsely elevated ABIs. Atherosclerosis results in severe calcification of the arteries. When measuring arterial pressure using a Doppler probe and a blood pressure cuff, some of the squeeze of the cuff is used to overcome the hardening of the arterial wall leading to a falsely elevated value. Relying on the ABI alone will miss the severity of the peripheral vascular disease. Other assessments of arterial inflow must be used. Toe pressures reflect the degree of disease more accurately in diabetic patients, but many labs are not equipped with cuffs small enough to measure toe pressures. Arterial waveforms measured by Doppler or pulse volume recording can quantify the amount of atherosclerosis. A normal ABI with a markedly dampened waveform suggests calcified vessels and significant obstruction, and that the ABI is falsely elevated. Transcutaneous oxygen tension measurement ($TcPo_2$) is a measurement of perfusion of the skin. It can be measured noninvasively with an electrode on the skin of the foot. Partial pressure of oxygen measured transcutaneously is about 80% of the arterial Po_2 measured directly by sampling blood by arterial puncture. Normal $TcPo_2$ is defined as 55 mm Hg or greater.

Wound healing usually occurs with $TcPO_2$ of 30 mm Hg or greater, even if the patient has peripheral vascular disease and an absent pulse in their foot on physical examination. Duplex scan is quite accurate in identifying arterial occlusion and calcified atherosclerotic peripheral vascular disease. In some centers, lower extremity arterial reconstruction is being performed based on this test alone.

Diagnosis of Deep Infections, Including Osteomyelitis

Plain x-rays may identify osteomyelitis; however, changes on x-ray are not apparent for 3 weeks or so after osteomyelitis occurs clinically. Thus, a "negative" x-ray means no osteomyelitis or osteomyelitis present for <3 weeks. It may be difficult to separate bony erosions due to previous debridement from the changes of osteomyelitis. Bone scans detect inflammation and increased blood flow, not specifically infection, and may be of limited value in identifying osteomyelitis. Radioactive-labeled white blood cell scans may be used to determine bony involvement, but are expensive and have many false positives and negatives.[8] Magnetic resonance imaging (MRI) is more accurate in determining osteomyelitis, but is expensive. A cost-effective method to screen for osteomyelitis is to probe the wound with a cotton-tipped applicator. If the tip can probe to bone, osteomyelitis may be present in as many as 85% of cases. Debridement is also valuable in determining if osteomyelitis is present.

Infection is frequently present in these patients. If infected, the five signs of inflammation should be present; that is, the foot may be warm, swollen, red, tender, and painful. This is not always the case in certain patients, such as those on steroids or patients who are immunosuppressed. Even though they may not have normal sensation, many diabetic patients still have pain in their foot when infection is present.

Debridement is helpful in finding infection as undrained pockets of pus may be found and unroofed when necrotic tissue is removed. Quantitative bacteriology can be performed to determine if the wound is in "bacterial balance." Wounds with $>10^5$ bacteria per g of tissue have impaired healing. Routine cultures of dry wounds or surface swabs are inaccurate in determining the bacteria responsible for cellulitis. Cultures of dry wounds—that is, those without purulent drainage—grow skin organisms and not the organisms within the tissues causing the infection. Cultures of pus or a piece of tissue taken from the deepest level of debridement are most helpful in determining the infecting organism.

Mild infections may be caused by aerobic Gram-positive cocci. Enteric organisms are more likely to be present in wounds for >1 month. Severe infections are caused by Gram-positive cocci, Gram-negative bacilli, and anaerobes.[9] Diabetic patients commonly have multiple flora in their wounds. One quarter of diabetic patients may have anaerobic bacteria in their wounds. This may go unrecognized as anaerobic bacteria are more difficult to culture. Anaerobic infection may be present even when cultures have not identified these bacteria.

MANAGEMENT

Proper management begins only after a careful history and physical examination (Table 4-1).

Laboratory evaluation, including plain x-rays, noninvasive vascular testing, and cultures, may be necessary. Good wound care minimizes further injury to the tissue, ensures adequate arterial perfusion, eliminates infection, removes necrotic tissue, provides the proper nutrition for healing, and keeps the wound moist. Wounds that close by 50% in the first month are likely to heal completely.[10,11]

The wound should be cleansed to remove necrotic tissue, bacteria, fibrin, foreign substances, and previously applied ointments and dressings. Wounds may be washed with mild bath soap, saline, or a nontoxic wound cleanser. Harsh soaps, surgical scrub soaps, and surgical disinfectants, including iodine, alcohol, and peroxide, may damage cells fundamental to healing, including fibroblasts, keratinocytes, and white blood cells.[12] Washing debrides the wound to some extent and reduces the bacterial colony count. It also removes dead tissue, which can be a culture medium for bacteria. Cleaning the wound also removes bacterial proteases, which can reduce healing by breaking down growth factors.[13]

Reducing weight bearing is critical to the healing of diabetic ulcers,[14] as most wounds occur on the plantar surface of the foot. Complete offloading is best for healing and can be achieved with the use of crutches, a walker, a wheelchair, or other such devices. Ambulatory

---

TABLE 4-1

MANAGEMENT OF DIABETIC FOOT ULCERS

History and physical exam
Vascular laboratory evaluation of arterial supply in question
Revascularization if ischemic
X-ray of foot if osteomyelitis suspected
Debridement
Offloading/protective footwear
Antibiotic therapy, if infected
Assessment therapy, if infected
Control of diabetes
Control of edema
Wound care
    Cleansing
    Topical therapy
    Dressing

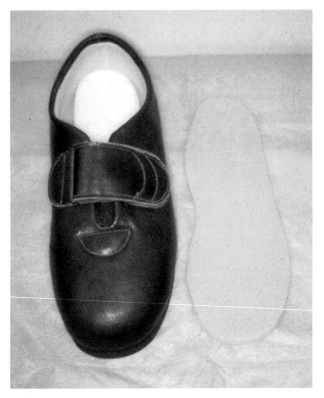

Figure 4-1 Custom diabetic footwear. This shoe is made of soft leather. The shoe and insert are molded to the shape of the foot.

patients prefer to walk with special footwear such as a half-shoe, which will allow them some stability yet not bear weight on the ulcer site. Patients can also use a custom relief orthotic walker, a diabetic boot, or a patella tendon weight-bearing brace. A diabetic shoe with custom insert will reduce pressure significantly, but not completely (Fig. 4-1). This may be adequate for healing. Total contact casting is quite effective in relieving pressure (Fig. 4-2). The cast must be applied by personnel trained in this technique. The correct application of a total contact cast is quite labor intensive. First, the

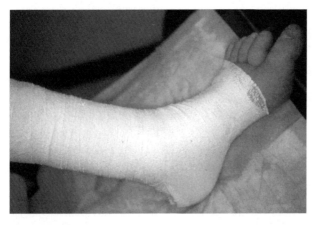

Figure 4-2 Total contact casting. This cast extends from the base of the toes to just below the knee. It is made of moist plaster so as to mold to the foot.

foot is cleansed and dried. Wounds are debrided and bleeding controlled. The ankle and foot are padded over bony prominences. Antifungal powder is placed between the toes. A layer of wet plaster is applied from the toes to the knee. The toes are completely enclosed within the cast. The cast is then reinforced with a harder second layer. The patient may not bear weight on the cast for 24 hours, or until it is completely dry. Walking on the cast before it has hardened may change the shape of the cast, causing rubbing on an insensate foot, resulting in another wound. The cast redistributes weight across the plantar surface as the patient walks, thus preventing high pressure on the ulcerated area. This technique should not be used on infected wounds or patients who are at risk for falling.

Patients are to reduce weight bearing at all times. Walking barefoot at any time or getting out of bed in the middle of the night to use the bathroom without protecting the wound may destroy the healing that has been accomplished that day. Assessment of compliance with non–weight bearing is difficult. As a general rule, however, if patients come to the clinic using appropriate measures to avoid weight bearing, it is likely they are compliant at other times.

If the patient has signs of infection, antibiotics against *Staphylococcus aureus* and β-hemolytic streptococci should be chosen for wounds present for only several weeks or less. Wounds present for >1 month commonly have enteric organisms present.[15–17] Blood glucose monitoring will detect elevated blood glucose levels suggesting uncontrolled infection.

Diabetes and poor nutrition are associated with a delay in wound healing. Poor glycemic control leads to a higher infection rate and more wound complications. Vitamin deficiency can delay wound healing.[18] Few patients, however, are vitamin deficient. Vitamin A is required for normal cell differentiation, epithelialization, and keratinocyte function. Vitamin A deficiency leads to impaired collagen production, collagen cross-linking, and epithelialization. Vitamin A may counteract the negative effects of corticosteroids and wound healing.[19,20] The B vitamins are cofactors for collagen cross-linking. Vitamin B deficiency can delay wound healing. Vitamin C, like vitamins A and B, is also critical for collagen synthesis and cross-linking. It is a cofactor for the hydroxylation of praline and lysine during collagen cross-linking. Patients with vitamin C deficiency have lowered wound tensile strength resulting in wound disruption. Vitamin K is necessary for production of coagulation factors II, VII, IX, and X. Vitamin K–deficient patients have bleeding from their wounds, abnormal provisional matrix formation, and an increased risk of infection. There is no convincing evidence that vitamins are of benefit in wound healing. If there is any question about the nutritional status of the patient, most practitioners will give vitamin

TABLE 4-2
TYPES OF DEBRIDEMENT

Type	Advantages	Disadvantages
Surgical	Efficient; effective	Pain; bleeding; may require anesthesia
Enzymatic	Does not require physician; low risk of bleeding	May be painful; may damage surrounding tissue; slow; necrotic tissue in wound is a potential culture medium for bacteria
Mechanical	Inexpensive; efficient	Slow; may lead to infection
Autolytic	Painless	Slow; inefficient; may lead to infection
Biologic	Efficient	Patient may not accept this therapy

supplementation. These medications are inexpensive and have low risk in standard doses.

Wounds should be debrided early in the course of their management[21] (Table 4-2). Extensive debridement, even completely excising the wound, is of benefit (Figs. 4-3, 4-4, and 4-5).

Keratinocytes do not migrate over necrotic tissue. Debridement is helpful not only in removing dead tissue but also in assessing the depth of the ulcer; determining whether there is bone, joint, or tendon involved; and finding undrained pus.[22,23] If there is bony involvement, the infected, necrotic bone must be removed. Sharp surgical debridement is the most effective method of removing devitalized tissue. In most cases, debridement can often be undertaken using local or regional anesthesia, as these patients have sensory neuropathy. Patients with adequate arterial circulation may have significant bleeding, and the physician performing the debridement must be capable of managing any hemorrhage. To control hemorrhage, platelets enter the wound. Those platelets release growth factors from their α-granules. Those growth factors control wound healing for the first several days. Osteomyelitis

is most efficiently and effectively treated by surgery. Once the infected bone has been excised, antibiotics are necessary only for bacteria control in the soft tissues, and usually for <6 weeks. It may be difficult to determine if there is bony involvement at the time of debridement. A layer of intact viable tissue over bone suggests the bone is not infected. In general, exposed bone is infected bone. Soft, nonbleeding bone is also infected. Debridement should remove this bone back to solid, bleeding bone. Enzymatic debriding agents can be used but are not as efficient as a surgeon's knife. These agents may damage adjacent normal tissue and are often painful. Occlusive dressings such as hydrocolloid dressings, will allow for autolytic debridement. Wet to dry saline-moistened gauze will provide mechanical debridement. Biologic debridement can be accomplished with maggot therapy.

Edema can be controlled with leg elevation in a compliant patient. Patients with severe arterial disease will not tolerate leg elevation because of pain. These patients have less discomfort with the leg in a dependent position. The need to keep their leg in a dependent position may be a clue that they have significant arterial insufficiency. If there is no edema, leg elevation is

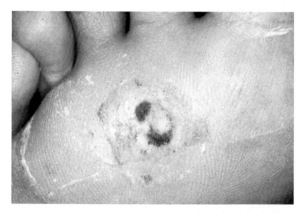

Figure 4-3 Diabetic foot wound. This is a typical wound on the plantar surface of the foot beneath the metatarsal head. There is callus surrounding the ulcer.

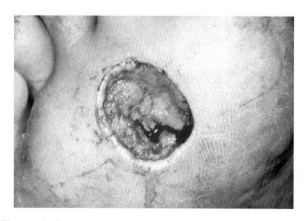

Figure 4-4 Diabetic foot wound. The wound following excisional debridement down to normal tissue.

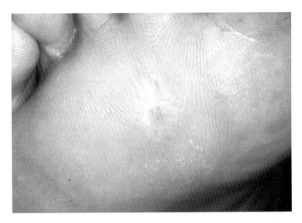

Figure 4-5 Diabetic foot wound. The wound healed in 10 weeks of treatment.

TABLE 4-3
REASONS FOR USING A DRESSING ON A WOUND

Reduce trauma
Reduce contamination
Reduce bacterial load
Prevent desiccation
Absorb moisture
Debride the wound
Deliver medications
Reduce pain

not necessary. The patients probably should keep their leg in whatever position feels most comfortable. Edema can also be controlled with compression wraps, stockings, or pumps.

If the patients do have arterial insufficiency, arteriography may be indicated. Many patients with peripheral vascular disease secondary to diabetes have renal dysfunction as well. Contrast agents used for arteriography may worsen renal function if the patient is not well hydrated or if excessive amounts of contrast are used. Bypass using the saphenous vein to the dorsalis pedis or posterior tibial arteries or even their branches have been successful in salvaging limbs with patency rates approaching or exceeding those of more proximal bypasses. One-year patency rates of 90% have been reported.[24]

Systemic hyperbaric oxygen therapy may offer some benefit in the healing of lower extremity ulcers. There are no randomized, prospective, double-blind trials with sham treatments demonstrating a clear benefit to this form of therapy. There is laboratory evidence in animals that hyperbaric oxygen therapy promotes wound healing in moderately ischemic wounds. Hyperbaric oxygen therapy is probably most effective when the patient is placed in a whole-body chamber. Topical hyperbaric oxygen therapy, provided by placing only the wounded extremity in an oxygen chamber, has also not been proven to be of benefit in randomized, blinded trials. If there is benefit from this therapy, it may be related to compression as well as oxygenation.

Dressings cover the wound and serve several functions (Table 4-3). They function as a barrier and protect the wound from further contamination. They control moisture. They can reduce trauma to the wound or control bleeding. Dressings can be used to supply drugs to the wound bed. In general, wounds heal best in a moist environment. Epithelialization is more likely to occur in a moist wound. A moist dressing will reduce loss of water vapor and heat from the wound. An occlusive dressing will also reduce water loss. If the wound is kept too moist, maceration of the surrounding skin will occur. All dressings reduce bacterial colony counts by washing, debriding, and removing bacteria and dead tissue. Topical antibiotic salves reduce the bacterial colony count while providing a moist wound environment for healing. There have been very few double-blind trials comparing topical antibiotic salves.[25] Saline-moistened gauze provides a moist wound environment with minimal damage to the tissues. If the gauze is allowed to dry, necrotic material will adhere to the gauze and will be removed from the wound with the gauze. New epithelium may also be removed by this technique. In that case, the gauze should be kept moist.

New therapies now offer the ability to manipulate the cellular environment of the wound. Growth factors are present in minute quantities, yet direct and control wound healing. They are found in nearly every tissue of the body. They are in highest concentration in platelets. As platelets enter the wound to initiate the clotting cascade, they also begin the process of healing. Growth factors can be harvested as a "platelet releasate" by extracting the platelet pellet from a peripheral blood sample. The growth factors are found in the α-granules of the platelet and can be released using thrombin. The growth factors found in the platelet then are likely to be the ones involved in wound healing and in the proper ratio. Platelet releasates have been used to treat diabetic foot wounds in randomized trials and have been found to be of benefit in many, but not all, trials.[26–30]

Individual growth factors can be made by recombinant deoxyribonucleic acid (DNA) technology. Platelet-derived growth factor (PDGF) is approved for clinical use. PDGF is a potent chemoattractant and mitogen for fibroblasts, smooth muscle cells, and inflammatory cells. PDGF is produced by platelets, macrophages, vascular endothelium, and fibroblasts.[31] PDGF is stable to extremes of heat, a wide range of pH, and degradation by proteases. Platelets, among the first cells to enter the wound, are the largest source of PDGF in the human body. Circulating monocytes are attracted to the wound and become tissue macrophages. These cells also produce PDGF. PDGF stimulates the production of fibronectin and hyaluronic acid, proteins that are important components of provisional matrix. Collagenase, important in wound remodeling, is also produced in response to PDGF.

When applied topically as a single dose, PDGF has been shown in animals to improve the breaking strength of incisional wounds. Wounds treated with PDGF had a marked increase in inflammatory cells entering the wound, including neutrophils, monocytes, and fibroblasts. Granulation tissue production was also increased. Although PDGF does not directly affect keratinocytes, wounds have an increased rate of epithelialization. PDGF causes an increase in neovascularization, although PDGF does not directly stimulate endothelial cells. Thus, PDGF accelerates the normal sequences of healing.

A randomized, prospective, double-blind trial of recombinant PDGF was performed in patients with diabetic neurotrophic foot ulcers.[32] PDGF doubled the healing rate of diabetic foot ulcers if the arterial blood supply was adequate, the patients were free of infection, and the wounds were extensively debrided. In this study, 48% healed when treated with PDGF, while only 25% healed using vehicle alone ($p < 0.01$). The median reduction in wound area was 98.8% for the PDGF group, but only 82.1% for those treated in the control arm. This was the first clinical trial to suggest that a growth factor, PDGF, applied topically, was effective and safe in accelerating the healing of chronic wounds in humans. In another trial using PDGF in the treatment of similar patients with diabetic foot ulcers, those treated with PDGF had an increase in complete wound closure of 43% as compared with control arm ($p = 0.007$). PDGF also decreased the time to complete wound healing by 32% ($p = 0.013$).[33] PDGF has also been studied in clinical trials in decubitus ulcers.[34] Patients were treated with PDGF topically and followed for 28 days. There was a greater amount of wound closure in patients treated with PDGF. PDGF is approved for use in the US and is sold as Regranex. About one quarter of healed diabetic foot ulcers recur no matter what agent is used to achieve healing.[35]

SUMMARY

In summary, the diabetic ulcer is a significant health care problem affecting more than one million patients in some point in their lives. Inadequate or improper therapy may lead to limb loss. Aggressive treatment including proper footwear, non–weight bearing, appropriate antibiotics, debridement, aggressive revascularization, and careful monitoring may lower the amputation rate in these patients. For the refractory ulcer, new therapies are being developed that might have a significant benefit in lower amputation rate.

REFERENCES

1. Bild DE, Selby SV, Sinnock P, et al. Lower extremity amputation in people with diabetes; epidemiology and prevention. *Diabetes Care.* 1989;12:24–31.
2. Levin ME. Diabetic foot ulcers: pathogenesis and management. *JET Nurs.* 1993;20:191–198.
3. Most RS, Sinnock P. The epidemiology of lower extremity amputation in diabetic individuals. *Diabetes Care.* 1983;6:87–91.
4. Miller OF. Essentials of pressure ulcer treatment, the diabetic experience. *J Dermatol Surg Oncol.* 1993;19:759–763.
5. Pecoraro RE, Reiber GE, Burgess EM. Pathways to diabetic limb amputation: basis for prevention. *Diabetes Care.* 1990;13:513–521.
6. Boulton AJ. The diabetic foot: neuropathic in aetiology. *Diabet Med.* 1990;7:852–858.
7. Sosenko JM, Kato M, Soto R, et al. Comparison of quantitative sensory threshold measures for their association with foot ulceration in diabetic patients. *Diabetes Care.* 1990;13:1057–1061.
8. Keenan AM, Tindel NL, Alavi A. Diagnosis of pedal osteomyelitis in diabetic patients using current scintigraphic techniques. *Arch Intern Med.* 1989;149:2262–2266.
9. Wheat LJ, Allen SD, Henry M. Diabetic foot infections: bacteriologic analysis. *Arch Intern Med.* 1986;146:1935–1940.
10. Robson M, Hill D, Woodske M, et al. Wound healing trajectories as predictors of effectiveness of therapeutic agents. *Arch Surg.* 2000;135:773–777.
11. Robson M, Steed D, Franz M. Wound healing: biologic features and approaches to maximize healing trajectories. *Current Prob Surg.* 2001;38:61–140.
12. Neidner R, Schopf E. Inhibition of wound healing by antiseptics. *Br J Dermatol.* 1986;115:41–44.
13. Yager D, Nwomeh B. The proteolytic environment of chronic wounds. *Wound Rep Regen.* 1999;7:433–441.
14. Boulton AJ, Hardisty CA, Betts RP. Dynamic foot pressure and other studies as diagnostic and management aids in diabetic neuropathy. *Diabetes Care.* 1983;6:26–33.
15. Robson M, Heggers J. Bacterial quantification of open wounds. *Mil Med.* 1969;134:19–24.
16. Robson M. A failure of wound healing caused by an imbalance of bacteria. *Surg Clin North Am.* 1997;77:206–210.
17. Doern GV, Jones RN, Pfaller MA. Bacterial pathogens isolated from patients with skin and soft tissue infections: frequency of occurrence and antimicrobial susceptibility patterns from the SENTRY Antimicrobial Surveillance Program. *Diagn Microbiol Infect Dis.* 1999;34:65–72.
18. Rojas A, Phillips T. Patients with chronic leg ulcers show diminished levels of vitamins A and E, carotenes, and zinc. *Dermatol Surg.* 1999;25:601–604.
19. Ehrlich H, Hunt T. Effects of cortisone and vitamin A on wound healing. *Ann Surg.* 1968;167:324–328.
20. Hunt T. Vitamin A and wound healing. *J Am Acad Dermatol.* 1986;15:817–821.
21. Steed D, Donohoe D, Webster M, et al. The Diabetic Ulcer Study Group. Effect of extensive debridement and rhPDGF-BB (Becaplermin) on the healing of diabetic foot ulcers. *J Am College of Surg.* 1996;183:61–64.
22. Taylor LM, Porter JM. The clinical course of diabetics who require emergency foot surgery because of infection or ischemia. *J Vasc Surg.* 1987;6:454–459.
23. Witkowski JA, Parish LE. Debridement of cutaneous ulcers: medical and surgical aspects. *Clin Dermatol.* 1992;9:585–591.
24. LoGerfo FW, Gibbons GW, Pomposelli FB. Trends in the care of the diabetic foot: expanded role of arterial reconstruction. *Arch Surg.* 1992;127:617–621.
25. Steed D, Moosa H, Webster M. The importance of randomized prospective trials in evaluating therapy for wound healing. *Wounds.* 1991;3:111–115.

26. Steed D, Goslen B, Hambley R. Clinical trials with purified platelet releasate. In: Barbula A, Caldwell M, Eaglstein W, eds. *Clinical and experimental approaches to dermal and epidermal repair: Normal and chronic wounds.* New York, NY: Wiley Liss; 1991:103–113.

27. Knighton D, Ciresi K, Fiegel V. Stimulation of repair in chronic, non-healing cutaneous ulcers using platelet derived wound healing formula. *Surg Gynecol Obstet.* 1990;170:56–60.

28. Krupski WC, Reilly LM, Perez A. A prospective randomized trial of autologous platelet-derived wound healing factors for treatment of chronic nonhealing wounds: a preliminary report. *J Vasc Surg.* 1991;14:526–536.

29. Steed DL, Goslen JB, Holloway GA, et al. Randomized prospective double blind trial in healing chronic diabetic foot ulcers. *Diabetes Care.* 1992;15:1598–1604.

30. Holloway A, Steed D, DeMaraco M. A randomized controlled multicenter dose response trial of activated platelet supernatant topical CT-102 in chronic non-healing diabetic wounds. *Wounds.* 1993;5:198–206.

31. Heldin C, Westermark B. Mechanism of action and *in vivo* role of platelet-derived growth factor. *Physiol Rev.* 1999;79:1283–1316.

32. Steed DL. Diabetic Ulcer Study Group. Clinical evaluation of recombinant human platelet-derived growth factor for the treatment of lower extremity diabetic ulcers. *J Vasc Surg.* 1995;21:71–81.

33. Wieman J, Smiell J, Su Y. Efficacy and safety of recombinant human platelet derived growth factor-bb (Becaplermin) in patients with nonhealing lower extremity diabetic ulcers: A phase III randomized double blind study. *Diabetes Care.* 1998;21:822–877.

34. Rees R, Robson M, Smiell S, et al. Becaplermin gel in the treatment of pressure ulcers: A randomized, double blinded placebo controlled study. *Wound Rep Regen.* 1996;6:A478–A482.

35. Steed D, Edington H, Webster M. Recurrences rate of diabetic neurotrophic foot ulcers healing using topical application of growth factors released from platelets. *Wound Rep Regen.* 1996;4: 230–233.

Management Issues of Diabetes Mellitus and Their Effects on the Progression of Disease

Eric S. Nylén

Diabetes mellitus (DM) is becoming increasingly common, as exemplified by data from the Third National Health and Nutrition Examination Survey (NHANES III)[1]: 29 million Americans (14.4%) over age 20 have diabetes (either diagnosed or undiagnosed) or impaired glucose tolerance. This rate increases to 33.6% in people older than age 60. Diabetes is the leading cause of adult blindness, end-stage renal disease, and amputations; the rate of amputations among people with diabetes is six to ten times that of people without diabetes. Ultimately, most diabetics die from heart disease. The risk of death from cardiovascular causes in a person with diabetes is two to six times the risk of a person without diabetes.[2] Cardiovascular consequences were the most costly complication of diabetes in 2002, accounting for $17.6 billion.

While the rates, suffering, and cost of diabetes are alarming, scientific and clinical expertise has greatly improved to substantially thwart these developments. For example, a significant compounding risk factor is being overweight or obese. While the prevalence of obesity is increasing profoundly, recent studies also show that the onset of diabetes can be forestalled by weight loss and other lifestyle changes.[3,4] Moreover, many of the complications of diabetes can be negated with appropriate glycemic and multifactorial interventions.

DIABETIC COMPLICATIONS

Contrary to expectations, the introduction of insulin in 1922 uncovered serious long-term microvascular complications involving the retina, renal glomerulus, and peripheral nerves. These debilitating disorders afflicted both type 1 (i.e., insulinopenic) and type 2 (i.e., insulin resistant and defective pancreatic β cell secretion) diabetic patients, largely due to their chronic exposure to a hyperglycemic milieu. Diabetics were also shown to be vulnerable to macrovascular complications such as myocardial infarction (MI), congestive heart failure (CHF), peripheral vascular disease (PVD), and strokes; indeed, 75% of people with diabetes die from macrovascular complications. The predominance of cardiovascular consequences has redefined diabetes as "a state of premature cardiovascular death, which is associated with chronic hyperglycemia."[5] While the age-adjusted incidence of cardiovascular disease (CVD) in the United States has declined for both nondiabetic men and women, among people with diabetes, the decline in incidence is much lower (i.e., diabetic men) or has actually increased (i.e., diabetic women).[6]

Microvascular Pathology

The early events associated with microvascular pathology involve abnormal blood flow and vascular leakage. The resulting edema, ischemia, and hypoxia lead to neovascularization of the retina. In the kidney, there is proteinuria, increased mesangial matrix production, and glomerulosclerosis. The peripheral nerves succumb to multifocal axonal degeneration.

Macrovascular Pathology

Although the atherosclerotic process in diabetics appears to be similar to that in nondiabetics (i.e., fatty streaks evolving into fibro-fatty plaques, with subsequent fibrin and calcium deposits leading to plaque fissures and hemorrhage), the lesions occur earlier and are greater in number. There is also an increasing awareness that fatty acids and triglycerides accumulate inappropriately in cardiac and other tissues.

Pancreatic Pathology

The pancreatic β cell is unique in using a metabolic substrate (i.e., glucose) to sense the amount of a hormone (i.e., insulin) to be secreted. Insulin secretion is maximal at an ambient glucose concentration of approximately 115 mg per dL. Higher levels of glucose concentrations that last for longer than 24 hours can lead to decreased insulin secretion, termed glucotoxicity,[7] a process which can be reversed by normalizing the glucose concentration. (Lipids, in the case of free fatty acids, are similarly toxic to the β cell; this is termed lipotoxicity.) In both type 1 and type 2 diabetes, the β-cell mass is reduced. An insulitis reaction is seen in the islets of people with type 1, while 50% of type 2 diabetics have amyloid deposits correlating to severity, duration, and age of the patient.

Pathophysiology

The causative association between hyperglycemia and microvascular complications has now been strongly affirmed by several prospective interventional studies in type 1[8] and type 2[9,10] diabetics. Although the precise mechanism whereby diabetic complications arise is not fully understood, accumulation of several glycolytic intermediate metabolic products appears to be of fundamental importance. Moreover, this may reflect mitochondrial overproduction of reactive oxygen species, which in turn inhibit several glycolytic enzymes.[11]

Advanced Glycation End Products

Excess extra and intracellular glucose combines with free amino acids, leading to early (reversible) and late (irreversible) advanced glycogen end products (AGE) via an Amadori rearrangement. Modified intracellular proteins have altered function and can also alter extracellular matrix components. AGE-modified plasma proteins can interact with AGE receptors on a variety of cells, leading to toxic oxygen species as well as cross linking with collagen, increasing vascular permeability, promotion of mononuclear cell egress, stimulation of cell proliferation, and modification of low density lipoproteins (LDL). Aminoguanidine is a prototype agent that can inhibit AGE formation *in vivo* and *in vitro*; it and many others are undergoing clinical scrutiny.

Sorbitol

Hyperglycemia promotes aldose reductase to convert glucose into sorbitol. Accumulation of sorbitol decreases nicotinamide adenine dinucleotide phosphate (NADPH), increases intracellular osmolarity, and decreases myoinositol, which can interfere with cellular metabolism.

Hexosamine

Excess glucose made into fructose-6-phosphate is diverted away from glycolysis into the so-called hexosamine pathway. This pathway leads to increased gene transcription of several detrimental factors, including plasminogen activator inhibitor-1 (PAI-1).

Protein Kinase C

Hyperglycemia increases diacylglycerol (DAG), which increases certain isoforms of protein kinase C (PKC β and δ), with resultant activation of endothelial nitric oxide synthase (eNOS), endothelin-1 (ET-1), vascular endothelial growth factor (VEGF), PAI-1, and reactive oxygen species. PKC inhibitors have been shown to ameliorate these adverse effects and are currently being tested in clinical trials.

MANAGEMENT ISSUES

Control of Glycemia

It is now clearly recognized that glycemic control by any means results in a salutary microvascular outcome. In the Diabetes Control and Complications Trial (DCCT),[8] retinopathy, nephropathy, and neuropathy risk was reduced by almost 60% by maintaining a near-normal hemoglobin A1c (HgA1c)—7.2% versus 8.3% in the conventionally treated group. A similar effect was seen in type 2 patients in the UK Prospective Diabetes Study (UKPDS),[10] where the overall microvascular complication rate was decreased by 25%. In this study, for every 1% decrease in the HgA1c, there was a 35% reduction in the complication rate.

Glycemic Treatment Strategy

The optimal therapeutic approach to type 2 DM addresses both insulin resistance and β-cell secretion defects. In the case of insulin resistance, diet and exercise have been shown to be effective.[12] Regular aerobic exercise may be particularly beneficial by improving glucose transport and decreasing insulin resistance. Patients initiating an exercise program should, however, first undergo a comprehensive medical evaluation, which may include a cardiovascular stress test.

Diabetic oral agents (Table 5-1) that decrease insulin resistance include biguanides (e.g., metfomin) and thiazolidinediones (e.g., rosiglitazone and pioglitazone). In the case of insulin secretion, restitution of the early phase (first phase) is of considerable importance in modulating excessive hepatic glucose production commonly associated with type 2 DM.[13] Current agents that promote insulin release include sulfonylureas (e.g., chlorpropramide, glyburide, glipizide, glimepiride), meglitinides (e.g., repaglinide), and nateglinides (e.g., starlix); the latter two are considered short-acting agents addressing postprandial hyperglycemia. Acarbose and miglitol are α-glucosidase inhibitors and lower postprandial glucose by delaying intestinal carbohydrate absorption.

Combination therapy using oral agents with different mechanisms not only addresses the underlying dual pathobiology of type 2 diabetes but has also been shown to promote additional reduction in HgA1c (Table 5-2). Several preparations are available with a fixed-dose formulation; for example, Glucovance =

glyburide + metformin; Metaglip = metformin + glipizide; Avandamet = metformin + rosiglitazone.

Insulin continues to be a cornerstone in managing all types of diabetic patients. Molecular modifications of insulin have produced so-called rapid-acting insulin analogs (e.g., humalog and aspart) and long-acting basal insulin analogs (e.g., glargine). The short-acting insulins more closely mimic pancreatic β-cell first-phase secretion, reaching peak levels in 30 to 90 minutes with a duration of no more than 3 hours. Glargine has a gradual and constant release over 24 hours, providing a basal insulin action and avoiding the rise and fall dynamics of the intermediate-acting NPH and Lente insulins.

Treatment Plan

In order to reach the more aggressive glycemic targets outlined in Table 5-3, each patient's vulnerability to develop hypoglycemia and risk of exacerbating comorbid conditions need to be considered, with particular attention to the presence and extent of neuropathy.

TABLE 5-2
EFFECT OF COMBINATION ANTIHYPERGLYCEMIC THERAPY

Combination	Added Reduction in HgA1c
Sulfonylurea + biguanide	1.5% to 2%
Sulfonylurea + thiazolidinedione	0.5% to 1.5%
Sulfonylurea + glucosidase inhibitor	1% to 1.5%
Biguanide + nateglinide	1.5%
Biguanide + glucosidase inhibitor	0.5%

TABLE 5-1
ORAL ANTIHYPERGLYCEMIC AGENTS

Agent	Class	Mechanism	HgA1c Decrease
Sulfonylureas	Sulfonylurea	Increases insulin secretion	1.5% to 2%
Nateglinide	Nonsulfonylurea	Increases prandial insulin secretion	1%
Metiglinide	Nonsulfonylurea	Increases prandial insulin secretion	1% to 2%
Metformin	Biguanide	Decreases hepatic insulin resistance	1.5% to 2%
Pioglitazone	Thiazolidinedione	Decreases peripheral insulin resistance	0.6% to 2%
Rosiglitazone	Thiazolidinedione	Decreases peripheral insulin resistance	0.7% to 2%
Acarbose	Glucosidase inhibitor	Delays glucose absorption	0.5% to 1%
Miglitol	Glucosidase inhibitor	Delays glucose absorption	0.5% to 1%
Orlistat	Lipase inhibitor	Promotes weight loss	1%

TABLE 5-3

SUMMARY OF 2003 AMERICAN DIABETES ASSOCIATION STANDARDS OF MEDICAL CARE OF DIABETIC PATIENTS

Measure	Desirable Value
Glycemic control (HgA1c)	<7.0%
Preprandial glucose	90 to 130 mg/dL
Peak postprandial glucose	<180 mg/dL
Blood pressure	<130/80 mm Hg
LDL	<100 mg/dL
Triglycerides	<150 mg/dL
HDL	>40 mg/dL

LDL, low density lipoprotein; HDL, high density lipoprotein.

Every patient also needs individualized nutrition and exercise counseling. These glycemic targets cannot be met unless the patient is instructed in glucose monitoring, preferably done just before and 2 hours after meals. Early familiarity with the use of insulin is helpful since most people with type 2 diabetes will eventually need insulin, and early education may help overcome the frequent reluctance to use needles. Initial insulin therapy should be considered in diabetics with severe hyperglycemia (e.g., 350 mg per dL, diabetic ketoacidosis, or hyperosmolar hyperglycemia) as well as in any new-onset diabetic with glucose toxicity. Insulin is also preferred for patients with predominant pancreatic insufficiency (e.g., type 1, those with pancreatic damage, and thinner patients with type 2) compared to patients with predominant insulin resistance (e.g., those with obesity).

Macrovascular Improvement

Despite the significant improvement in microvascular outcome, single-factor glycemic intervention has only a modest impact on macrovascular end points. In the follow-up study of patients with type 1 diabetes in DCCT, there was decreased progression of carotid intima media thickness in the intensively treated group.[14] In another glycemic study, intensive insulin management during the postinfarction period was shown to reduce mortality at 1 and 3 years, the effect of which was most pronounced among those without previous use of insulin and a low cardiovascular risk.[15]

Improved macrovascular outcome, however, can be more effectively achieved with a multifactorial intervention strategy using behavioral and pharmacologic therapy to improve hyperglycemia, hypertension, dyslipidemia, and microalbuminuria.[16] In the Steno-2 study, the primary end point was a composite of death from cardiovascular causes, nonfatal MI, coronary

artery bypass grafting, percutaneous coronary intervention, nonfatal stroke, amputation for ischemia, or vascular surgery for peripheral arterial atherosclerosis. After a mean of 7.8 years, the intensive therapy group showed a significant improvement in metabolic parameters (i.e., HgA1c, triglycerides, LDL), blood pressure (BP), nephropathy, retinopathy, neuropathy, and cardiovascular disease (44% experienced events in the control group vs. 24% in the intensively treated group; 95% confidence interval [CI] of 0.24 to 0.73; $p = 0.008$). The number needed to treat to prevent one cardiovascular event was five patients.

In the Steno-2 trial, the HgA1c goal of 6.5% was targeted by diet, exercise, and, if necessary, oral agents or insulin. This successful multifactorial intervention included the following elements:

- Total fat intake <30% of calories and saturated fat intake <10% of calories
- Light-moderate exercise for 30 minutes, 3 to 5 days per week
- Smoking cessation
- Daily supplements, including vitamin C (250 mg), tocopherol (100 mg), folic acid (400 μg), and chromium picolinate (100 μg)
- Angiotensin converting enzyme inhibitor (ACEI), or angiotensin receptor blocker (ARB) if an ACEI was contraindicated
- Thiazides, calcium channel blockers, and/or beta-blockers in addition to the ACEI as needed to maintain BP
- Aspirin, 150 mg per day
- Metformin for patients with a body mass index (BMI) >25
- A statin drug to treat elevated cholesterol
- A fibrate to treat high triglycerides (>350 mg per dL)

Based on Steno-2 and similar trials, comprehensive targets, such as those in Table 5-3, and therapeutic guidelines for the multifactorial intervention of diabetes have been published.[17]

Diabetic Dyslipidemia

The dyslipidemia of diabetes typically involves high triglycerides, lower high density lipoprotein (HDL), and, although LDL is seldom very elevated, it is often abnormally small and dense. In the UKPDS trial,[10] LDL was the major predictor of risk for coronary artery disease (CAD). In the 4S[18] and CARES[19] studies, diabetics had an augmented beneficial response to LDL lowering using a statin. From these and other studies, the target level of LDL should be at least 100 mg per dL, if not lower (<80 mg per dL),[20] which may require combination therapy with drugs such as the cholesterol absorption inhibitor ezetimibe. Alternatively, the routine use of a statin should be considered for all patients with diabetes irrespective of preexisting CAD or cholesterol levels, considering there was an approximately 25% reduction of a major vascular event associated with statin use in one large, recent 5-year trial.[21]

The low HDL level often seen in diabetics is mainly controlled by diet, weight reduction, and exercise. Additional intervention may include a fibric acid or niacin, both of which can increase HDL. Hypertriglyceridemia is often a sign of poor DM control, the effect of alcohol, or excessive carbohydrate intake. This may be an indication for the use of insulin, which is the most effective means to control triglyceride and chylomicron levels. Other additional useful agents include fish oil, fibric acid, and niacin.

Hypertension

Aggressive management of hypertension, with a goal of 130/80 mm Hg or less, not only helps control the progression of diabetic complications such as nephropathy but can also significantly decrease macrovascular events.[10,22] Although diabetics are responsive to diuretics, beta-blockers, and calcium channel blockers, ACEI and ARB both have a unique role in that they can modify the progression of diabetic nephropathy, even in normotensive patients. Moreover, a combination of ACEI and ARB can have additive effects in controlling microalbuminuria.[23]

Antiplatelet Treatment

Multiple trials and one large meta-analysis corroborate the efficacy of aspirin in preventing cardiovascular events, including MI and strokes. A dose of 75 to 325 mg per day have shown an approximately 30% decrease in MI and a 20% decrease in strokes. Those older than 65 years show the most benefit. Clopidogrel has also been shown to reduce cardiovascular events in diabetics.[24]

Smoking Cessation

Diabetics not only smoke more than nondiabetics, but they may also have increased vulnerability to the adverse effects of smoking. It is important to note that cessation improves outcome.[25]

DIABETIC PREVENTION

Although the development of microvascular complications commences with a significant rise in postprandial glucose, the onset of macrovascular complications occurs long before overt type 2 DM is manifest.[26,27] Preventing the onset of diabetes may thus prove to have the most significant impact on diabetic macrovascular complications. Lifestyle changes can reduce the

progression from impaired glucose tolerance (IGT) to type 2 DM by 54%; these changes include improving dietary habits, losing as little as 7% of body weight, and exercising regularly (i.e., brisk walking for 150 minutes per week).[3] This response to lifestyle changes improves insulin sensitivity more so than insulin secretion.[4] Pharmacotherapy, utilizing biguanides, thiazolidinediones, ACEI, and statins, has also been shown to delay the onset of diabetes.[28] For example, volunteers treated with metformin were 31% less likely to develop DM during 3 years.[3] A similar effect was seen using a thiazolidinedione in women with gestational diabetes.[29] In the Study to Prevent Non–insulin-dependent Diabetes Mellitus (STOP-NIDDM) trial, acarbose, a postprandial glucose modulator, was administered to patients with IGT. Over the next 3.3 years, major cardiovascular events (CAD, cardiovascular death, CHF, strokes, PVD) were significantly reduced by 49%. The rate of hypertension also decreased by 34%.[30]

SUMMARY

Although the complications and cost of diabetes are escalating, the management of diabetes has also shown significant evolution. Several pivotal studies reveal that diabetes prevention is achievable and that appropriate management substantially impacts the development of microvascular and macrovascular complications. Perhaps more so than in other chronic diseases, due to its many complexities, diabetes management requires a new, more coordinated treatment paradigm.

REFERENCES

1. Centers for Disease Control and Prevention. National Health and Nutrition Examination Survey 1999–2000 data files. Available at http://www.cdc.gov/nchs/about/major/nhanes/NHANES99_00.htm. Accessed 2005.
2. Kannel WB, McGee DL. Diabetes and cardiovascular disease: the Framingham study. *JAMA*. 1979;241:2035–2038.
3. The Diabetes Prevention Program Research Group. Reduction in the incidence of type 2 diabetes with lifestyle intervention or metformin. *N Engl J Med*. 2002;346:393–403.
4. Uusitupa M, Lindi V, Louheranta A, et al., for the Finnish Study Group. Long-term improvement in insulin sensitivity by changing lifestyles of people with impaired glucose tolerance. *Diabetes*. 2003;52:2532–2538.
5. Fisher BM. Diabetes mellitus and myocardial infarction: a time to act or a time to wait? *Diabet Med*. 1998;15:275.
6. Gu K, Cowie CC, Harris MI. Diabetes and decline in heart disease mortality in US adults. *JAMA*. 1999;281:1291–1297.
7. Leahy JL. Natural history of β-cell dysfunction in NIDDM. *Diabetes Care*. 1990;13:992–1010.
8. The Diabetes Control and Complications Trial Research Group. The effect of intensive treatment of diabetes on the development and progression of long-term complications in insulin-dependent diabetes mellitus. *N Engl J Med*. 1993;329:977–986.
9. Ohkubo Y, Kishikawa H, Araki E, et al. Intensive insulin therapy prevents the progression of diabetic microvascular complications

in Japanese patients with non–insulin-dependent diabetes mellitus. *Diabetes Res Clin Pract.* 1995;28:103–117.

10. UK Prospective Diabetes Study Group. Intensive blood-glucose control with sulfonylureas or insulin compared with conventional treatment and risk of complications in patients with type 2 diabetes. (UKPDS 33). *Lancet.* 1998;352:837–853.

11. Brownlee M. Biochemistry and molecular cell biology of diabetic complications. *Nature.* 2001;414:813–820.

12. Hamdy O, Goodyear LJ, Horton ES. Diet and exercise in type 2 diabetes mellitus. *Endocrinol Metab Clin North Am.* 2001;30:883–907.

13. Bruce DG, Chisholm DJ, Storlien LH, et al. Physiological importance of deficiency in early preprandial insulin secretion in non–insulin-dependent diabetes. *Diabetes.* 1988;37:736–744.

14. Nathan DM, Lachin J, Cleary P, et al. Diabetes Control and Complications Trial; Epidemiology of Diabetes Interventions and Complications Research Group. Intensive diabetes therapy and carotid intima-media thickness in type 1 diabetes mellitus. *N Engl J Med.* 2003;348:2294–2303.

15. Malmberg K, for the DIGAMI Study Group. Prospective randomized study of intensive insulin treatment on long term survival after acute myocardial infarction in patients with diabetes mellitus. *Br Med J.* 1997;314:1512–1515.

16. Gaede P, Vedel P, Larsen N, et al. Multifactorial intervention and cardiovascular disease in patients with type 2 diabetes. *N Engl J Med.* 2003;348:383–393.

17. American Diabetes Association. Clinical practice guidelines. *Diabetes Care.* 2003;26(Suppl 1):S1–S156.

18. Pyorala K, Pedersen TR, Kjekshus J, et al. Cholesterol lowering with simvastatin improves prognosis of diabetic patients with coronary heart disease. A subgroup analysis of the Scandinavian Simvastatin Survival Study (4S). *Diabetes Care.* 1997;20:614–620.

19. Goldberg RB, Mellies MJ, Sacks FM, for the CARES Investigators. Cardiovascular events and their reduction with pravastatin in diabetic and glucose-intolerant myocardial infarction survivors with average cholesterol levels. *Circulation.* 1998;98:2513–2519.

20. Grundy SM, Cleeman JI, Merz CN, et al. Implications of recent clinical trials for the National Cholesterol Education Program Adult Treatment Panel III guidelines. *Circulation.* 2004;110:227–239.

21. Heart Protection Study Collaborative Group. MRC/BHF Heart Protection Study of cholesterol-lowering with simvastatin in 5963 people with diabetes: a randomized placebo-controlled trial. *Lancet.* 2003;361:2005–2016.

22. Hansson L, Zanchetti A, Carruthers SG, et al., for the HOT Study Group. Effects of intensive blood pressure lowering and low dose aspirin in patients with hypertension. Principal results of the Hypertension Optimal Treatment (HOT) randomized trial. *Lancet.* 1998;351:1755–1762.

23. Andersen NH, Knudsen ST, Poulsen PL, et al. Dual blockade with candesartan cilexetil and lisinopril in hypertensive patients with diabetes mellitus: rationale and design. *J Renin Angiotensin Aldosterone Syst.* 2003;4:96–99.

24. Bhatt DL, Marso SP, Hirsch AT, et al. Amplified benefit of clopidogrel versus aspirin in patients with diabetes mellitus. *Am J Cardiol.* 2002;90:625–628.

25. Yudkin JS. How can we best prolong life? Benefits of coronary risk factor reduction in non-diabetics and diabetic subjects. *BMJ.* 1993;306:1313–1318.

26. Haffner SM, Stern MP, Hazuda HP, et al. Cardiovascular risk factors in confirmed prediabetic individuals: does the clock for coronary heart disease start ticking before the onset of clinical diabetes? *JAMA.* 1990;263:2893–2898.

27. Goya K, Kitamura T, Inaba M, et al. Risk factors for asymptomatic atherosclerosis in Japanese type 2 diabetic patients without diabetic microvascular complications. *Metabolism.* 2003;52:1302–1306.

28. Heart Outcomes Prevention Evaluation (HOPE) Study Investigators. Effects of ramipril on cardiovascular and microvascular outcomes in people with diabetes mellitus: results of the HOPE study and MICRO-HOPE substudy. *Lancet.* 2000;355:253–259.

29. Azen SP, Peters RK, Berkowitz K, et al. TRIPOD (TRoglitazone In the Prevention Of Diabetes): a randomized, placebo-controlled trial of troglitazone in women with prior gestational diabetes mellitus. *Control Clin Trials.* 1998;19:217–231.

30. Chiasson JL, Josse RG, Gomis R, et al. Acarbose treatment and the risk of cardiovascular disease and hypertension in patients with impaired glucose tolerance: the STOP-NIDDM trial. *JAMA.* 2003;290:486–494.

Nonoperative Management of Diabetic Foot Infections

Matthew C. Wakefield   Virginia L. Kan   Subodh Arora
Jonathan M. Weiswasser   Anton N. Sidawy

Diabetes mellitus accounts for approximately 50% of all nontraumatic lower extremity amputations performed in the United States.[1,2] The rate of lower extremity amputation for diabetic patients is >40 times higher than for nondiabetics.[3] Foot infections are present in 68% of all diabetics at the time they undergo lower extremity amputation.[4] Osteomyelitis and soft-tissue infections are the most common indications for hospital admission among diabetic patients.[5] These admissions account for at least 25% of all hospital admission for diabetics.[6] The average hospital stay is >1 month, and 44% of these patients are hospitalized for >3 months.[7] The average cost of treating a foot ulcer is $4,595 to $8,988.[8] Factors that are predictive of a diabetic foot infection include sensory neuropathy, immunopathy, and peripheral vascular disease. The primary consideration is to determine whether or not surgical intervention will be required. Management of the diabetic foot infection requires a multidisciplinary approach involving local wound care, directed antimicrobial therapy, medical control of underlying diabetes mellitus, surgical debridement, and, possibly, vascular bypass surgery.

Controlling diabetic foot infection is paramount to the preservation of the lower extremity by obviating the need for amputation or reducing the extent of an amputation that is important for the functional level of the patient. This review focuses on the pathophysiology, diagnosis, microbiology, and medical treatment of diabetic foot infections.

PATHOPHYSIOLOGY

Ischemia, neuropathy, and impaired neutrophil function are the major factors predisposing diabetic patients to foot ulcers and infections. Peripheral arterial disease is present in >50% of diabetics having the disease for >10 years.[9] Atherosclerotic disease appears at an earlier age in people with diabetes and tends to involve the infragenicular vessels.[10] The arteries of the foot, especially the dorsalis pedis artery, are often spared. Diabetics do not have more significant small-vessel occlusions compared to nondiabetics, as previously thought.[11] Peripheral arterial disease also adversely affects antibiotic concentrations in the tissue of interest.[12] Thus, it is very important that evaluation for reconstructable peripheral arterial disease should be undertaken in diabetic patients who have an extremity soft-tissue infection.

Sensory neuropathy is another important factor in predisposing the diabetic patient to infection. Approximately 60% to 70% of diabetic patients have peripheral neuropathy, and this number increases with length of disease.[7,13] This neuropathy often leads to an unrecognized injury that promotes formation of an ulcer and a subsequent foot infection. As diabetic patients may not have pronounced symptoms of foot infection, they often delay seeking medical care.[13] Repetitive trauma and autonomic dysfunction also contribute to the increased risk of infection.[7] Independent predictors of ulcer development include the absence of Achilles deep tendon reflexes, foot insensitivity to a 5.07 Semmes-Weinstein monofilament, and transcutaneous oxygen tension <30 mm Hg.[14]

Diabetes mellitus is also associated with defective humoral and cellular immunity leading to decreased neutrophil chemotaxis, decreased phagocytosis, impaired bacterial killing, and abnormal lymphocyte function.[15–17] These factors lead to increased susceptibility of the diabetic patient to infection.

MICROBIOLOGY

Both aerobic and anaerobic cultures are needed because 40% to 90% of infections contain both types of organisms.[2] The culture technique is crucial to the accurate identification of the pathogen(s) in a diabetic foot infection. Failure to culture for anaerobic organisms can lead to improper treatment. Wheat et al.[5] used a protocol to obtain cultures and transport them immediately to the laboratory in anaerobic transport tubes using established media and methods. They compared the findings of deep-tissue aspiration and tissue or bone biopsy (reliable specimens) with superficial wound cultures (unreliable specimens). The reliable specimens were more likely to contain only a single organism and yielded a higher number of anaerobes. Unreliable specimens were more likely to have greater than four organisms. Based on their data, cultures should be processed appropriately to identify anaerobic bacteria, and specimens from surgical debridement should be submitted for culture. Only 7% of patients actually received inadequate antibiotic treatment based on their unreliable specimen culture results despite poor concordance between the culture data from the reliable and unreliable specimens. These patients received broader antibiotic therapy, which could have subjected them to possible toxic side effects. Aminoglycosides were prescribed unnecessarily due to unreliable culture data in 15% of patients.

Louie et al.[18] also used specific methods to isolate anaerobic bacteria and identified anaerobic bacteria in 18 of 20 diabetic foot ulcer specimens. Furthermore, there was an average of 5.8 bacterial species present per culture. Patients with cellulitis had more bacterial species present than those with stable ulcers (mean of 7.3 vs. 4.9) but there was no difference in the proportion of anaerobes.

These studies illustrate the importance of appropriate culture techniques in order to tailor antimicrobial therapy. The best method for culturing has been shown to be an intraoperative culture from a separate incision and not through the ulcer skin.[6] If osteomyelitis is suspected, a bone biopsy for culture and histologic examination is appropriate. If surgical therapy is not employed, a deep-wound culture should be obtained.

The range of pathogens found in diabetic foot infections is listed in Table 6-1. Staphylococci and streptococci are the most common bacteria isolated. In uncomplicated infections, 89% to 94% of specimens yield aerobic Gram-positive cocci, and they are the sole pathogen in 42% to 43% of these cases.[19,20] Complicated infections also have a predominance of Gram-positive cocci, but isolates of anaerobes[20] and Gram-negative bacteria increase as the severity of infection worsens.[21] The commonly isolated aerobic Gram-negative bacilli are *Klebsiella*, *Proteus*, and *Pseudomonas* species. *Peptococcus* and *Peptostreptococcus* are the most common Gram-positive anaerobes isolated, while *Bacteroides* species are the most prevalent Gram-negative anaerobes.

An exception to these guidelines exists in those who have received prior antibiotic therapy or have risk factors for a nosocomial infection. Such patients often have resistant organisms and may have a higher degree of treatment failure.[2] Among 180 diabetic patients admitted to a specialized diabetic foot unit,[22] 18% foot ulcer cultures grew multidrug-resistant organisms. For this cohort, history of prior hospitalization for the same wound or presence of osteomyelitis were found to be the only significant factors associated with multidrug-resistant organisms in multivariate analysis. However, time to healing was not significantly different for patients with multidrug-resistant organisms

---

TABLE 6-1

COMMON PATHOGENS IN DIABETIC FOOT INFECTIONS

Aerobes
  Gram-negative
    Proteus sp
    Klebsiella sp
    Pseudomonas aeruginosa
  Gram-positive
    Staphylococcus aureus
    Coagulase-negative staphylococci
    Streptococcus
    Enterococci
    Corynebacterium sp

Anaerobes
  Gram-negative
    Bacteroides fragilis
    Bacteroides sp
  Gram-positive
    Peptococcus sp
    Clostridium sp
    Peptostreptococcus sp

during longitudinal follow-up for a subset of 75 patients in this unit. These factors must be taken into account upon making initial management decisions.

DIAGNOSIS

Diabetic patients often present in the advanced stages of a foot infection due to their inability to feel symptoms. Signs associated with an infection include an ulcer, erythema, induration, and pain. Systemic signs include fever, malaise, and poor glycemic control. Most of these patients do not present with fever or leukocytosis.[19] Only 36% of 96 patients with limb-threatening sepsis[2,23] were found to have a temperature >100°F during day one of their admission, and 53% had a white blood cell (WBC) count >10,000 per mm³.[2]

The foot is separated into several compartments by rigid fascial divisions. Dorsal and plantar abnormalities may not be shown in a deep-space infection until late in its course. Any diabetic patient who presents with even mild symptoms and signs in the foot but with systemic indications of ongoing infection should be evaluated carefully with a high index of suspicion for a foot infection.[7]

Once the diagnosis of a diabetic foot infection has been established, there are a variety of classification schemes to grade severity. A treatment protocol has been developed using Wagner's classification system: Grade 0, cellulitis; grade 1, superficial ulcer; grade 2, deep ulcer; grade 3, deep abscess and/or osteomyelitis; grade 4, forefoot gangrene; and grade 5, foot gangrene. Calhoun et al.[24] have shown that treatment based on the Wagner classification scheme can decrease the morbidity and mortality of diabetic foot infections, underscoring the need to accurately determine the severity of the infection.

Another common classification system was developed by Gibbons.[25] This system divides diabetic foot infections into non–limb-threatening or mild infections and limb-threatening or moderate-severe infections. Non–limb-threatening infections are those with <2 cm of cellulitis, superficial, not associated with osteomyelitis, and primarily caused by *Staphylococcus aureus*. Limb-threatening infections have >2 cm of cellulitis accompanied by deep involvement. Life-threatening infections occur in patients who develop systemic toxicity. The microbiology and treatment of these categories are important in the management of these infections.

TREATMENT

Empirical antibiotic choices are listed in Table 6-2. Once culture results are known, antibiotics may be properly tailored for pathogens isolated. The duration of treatment may range from 1 to 2 weeks for mild infections, to >6 weeks for osteomyelitis.

Mild Infections

Mild infections are defined as those with minimal cellulitis and superficial ulcerations without systemic toxicity or osteomyelitis. These infections can generally be treated with outpatient antibiotic therapy and local wound care.[2,19] Cultures should be obtained at the initial visit prior to antibiotic therapy. Antibiotic therapy should be directed against Gram-positive cocci, which are the most common organisms.[19] Follow-up should also be scheduled for 2 to 3 days in order to re-evaluate treatment and tailor antibiotic therapy based on culture results. If improvement is not seen, careful consideration should be given to hospitalization and intravenous therapy. If there are other circumstances, such as prior antibiotic therapy or a nosocomial infection, this initial therapy should be broadened to include methicillin-resistant *S. aureus* and *Pseudomonas aeruginosa*.

TABLE 6-2
ANTIBIOTIC REGIMENS IN DIABETIC FOOT INFECTIONS

Mild infections[a]
Oral therapy
   Amoxicillin-clavulanate
   Cephalexin
   Ciprofloxacin
   Clindamycin
   Dicloxacillin
Parenteral therapy
   Cefazolin
   Clindamycin
   Nafcillin

Moderate/Severe infections
Oral therapy
   Ciprofloxacin + clindamycin
   Levofloxacin
   Linezolid[b]
Parenteral therapy
   Ampicillin-sulbactam
   Cefoxitin
   Ciprofloxacin + clindamycin
   Clindamycin + ceftazidime
   Linezolid[b]
   Piperacillin-tazobactam
   Ticarcillin-clavulanate

Life-threatening infections
Parenteral therapy
   Ampicillin-sulbactam
   Ciprofloxacin + vancomycin + metronidazole
   Imipenem-cilastatin or meropenem or ertapenem
   Piperacillin-tazobactam + vancomycin[c]
   Vancomycin + ceftazidime + metronidazole

[a]No prior antibiotic treatment or risk factors for nosocomial infection.
[b]Linezolid should be added for infections with documented methicillin- or vancomycin-resistant staphylococci or vancomycin-resistant enterococci.
[c]Renal function must be taken into account prior to initiating therapy.

Lipsky et al.[19] have shown that 89% of non–limb-threatening lower extremity infections had aerobic Gram-positive cocci isolated, and they were the sole pathogen in 42%. Aerobic Gram-negative bacilli and anaerobes were found in 36% and 13% of cases, respectively. When patients were randomized to either cephalexin (500 mg four times daily) or clindamycin (300 mg four times daily) for 2 weeks, both agents were equally effective in producing a 75% initial cure rate and an eventual 91% eradication rate following further antibiotic treatment. At a mean follow-up of 15 months, no further therapy was needed in 84% of the cured patients. Adverse reactions were encountered with mild diarrhea in one patient on clindamycin and mild nausea and diarrhea in two patients on cefoxitin. Patients with enterococci isolated improved despite no specific antibiotic therapy directed at these organisms.

Oral ciprofloxacin has also been studied in the treatment of diabetic foot infections. Ciprofloxacin has an extended spectrum for aerobic Gram-negative bacilli of activity with good oral absorption. In Peterson's study,[21] 48 patients with peripheral vascular disease (among whom 46 were also diabetic) received either 750 mg or 1,000 mg of oral ciprofloxacin twice daily. Those with osteomyelitis underwent 3 months of therapy, while those with soft-tissue infection received 3 weeks of ciprofloxacin. Polymicrobial infections represented 77% of cases. Initial success was achieved in 91% of patients. Among 16 cellulitis patients, 50% were defined as having a successful outcome at 1 year; most of the failures were due to Gram-positive bacteria reflecting the limitations of ciprofloxacin as monotherapy. Of the osteomyelitis patients, 65% had a successful outcome at 1 year of follow-up. Only two patients in the high-dose group developed side effects (nausea/vomiting, severe anxiety) requiring cessation of therapy.

Other studies have examined oral ciprofloxacin (750 mg twice daily) in comparison with intravenous cefotaxime (2 g three times daily).[26] The authors concluded that there was no significant difference between the two antibiotic regimens with a 76% to 77% cure rate in both. This study was confounded by the use of clindamycin in some patients from both groups and the fact that less than half of the 59 patients were diabetics.

Amoxicillin-clavulanate has a wide spectrum of bacterial activity, and oral administration allows for outpatient therapy. In Gerards' study[27] of 191 patients with a diabetic foot infection treated with amoxicillin-clavulanate for an average of 15 days, healing or improvement was observed in 76% of cases. Treatment was discontinued in 1.6% of patients due to side effects.

Moderate/Severe Infections

Patients with ulceration, cellulitis, and possible osteomyelitis may have systemic signs of infection present. They are usually candidates for intravenous antibiotics with careful observation, as these infections may have limb-threatening potential. The primary goal in these patients is to ensure that prompt surgical drainage and debridement be performed if necessary.

The common organisms isolated in these infections include *S. aureus*, anaerobes (such as *Bacteroides* sp), and Gram-negative bacilli (such as *Klebsiella* sp, *Pseudomonas* sp). Patients who present with moderate to severe diabetic foot infections have been shown to have a higher incidence of anaerobic pathogens.[28] Initial therapy should be directed at these organisms and should be tailored when culture results are available.

Nosocomial infections are more likely to harbor enterococci, *P. aeruginosa*, or resistant organisms (methicillin-resistant *S. aureus*), and initial therapy should be directed towards these microbes. The antibiotic regimen may be tailored based on culture results. Susceptible enterococci may be treated with ampicillin, an extended-spectrum penicillin, or vancomycin. More resistant enterococci may require quinupristin-dalfopristin or linezolid.[29] If methicillin-resistant *S. aureus* is a possible pathogen, vancomycin therapy should be initiated.

Linezolid,[30] an oxazolidinone, has *in vitro* activity against Gram-positive cocci including those resistant to methicillin, cephalosporins, and vancomycin. In a randomized, open-label trial of 371 diabetic patients,[31] no statistical difference was shown in overall cure rates for foot infections treated with linezolid and ampicillin-sulbactam/amoxicillin-clavulanate (81% vs. 71%, respectively). However, linezolid treatment had significantly higher cure rates for those with infected foot ulcers (81% vs. 68%, respectively; 95% CI, 1.9 to 2.5; $p = 0.018$) and for those without osteomyelitis (87% vs. 72%, respectively; 95% CI, 4.5 to 25.7; $p = 0.003$). In this study, few patients had methicillin-resistant *S. aureus* isolated from their ulcers: 13 of 18 patients in the linezolid arm and four of seven patients in the comparator arm. No reduced vancomycin susceptibility was reported in any bacterial isolates.

Antipseudomonal options include the extended-spectrum penicillins, carbapenems, fluoroquinolones, or the aminoglycosides. However, aminoglycoside use should generally be avoided in these patients given the nephrotoxic effects. Two studies have investigated the use of imipenem-cilastatin as monotherapy for diabetic foot infections.[32,33] Calandra et al.[32] studied 94 patients (32 of whom had osteomyelitis) and found a 47% cure rate at the end of therapy. This retrospective study had a wide variation in dosing regimens (1 to 4 g per day) making conclusions difficult. A prospective, double-blind, randomized trial by Grayson et al.[33] showed that imipenem-cilastatin (2 g per day) produced an 85% cure rate at the end of therapy (mean ±SD, 15 ± 8.9 days). The cure rate at 1 year was 80% in this group. When compared to ampicillin-sulbactam, no significant difference was found between the two antibiotic regimens in cure rates or side effects. Imipenem-cilastatin and ampicillin-sulbactam are good alternatives in patients with moderate to severe diabetic foot infections. Ciprofloxacin should probably not be used as monotherapy in these patients, since 1-year cure rates for cellulitis and osteomyelitis patients were reported to be 52% to 68%.[21] Clinafloxacin, a broader spectrum fluoroquinolone, has been shown to have equivalent efficacy compared with piperacillin-tazobactam, but its utility may be limited by phototoxicity reactions.[34]

Other studies have investigated cefoxitin as single-agent therapy and have found 70% response rates.[35] Furthermore, other extended-spectrum penicillins (ticarcillin-clavulanate and piperacillin-tazobactam) have been studied and found to have similar efficacy in treating these diabetic foot infections.[36,37]

Life-threatening Infections

The primary goals in patients with systemic toxicity from a diabetic foot infection include fluid resuscitation, glycemic control, broad antibiotic therapy, and intensive care support. These patients often require urgent surgical debridement or possibly guillotine amputation. These patients should receive antibiotic directed against *S. aureus*, Gram-negative bacilli—especially *P. aeruginosa*—and anaerobes with special consideration for antibiotic-resistant bacteria. Diabetics may have subcutaneous air present on exam or radiography due to aerobic and anaerobic streptococci, *Proteus* sp, *Escherichia coli*, *Klebsiella*, and enterococci.[38] Although *Clostridium* sp are associated with life-threatening infections characterized by subcutaneous air, clostridia are rare causes of diabetic foot infections.[5,18] Urgent Gram stain of the infected tissue or exudate should differentiate the characteristic Gram-positive bacilli of clostridia from other bacteria to determine proper antibiotic therapy and type of surgical intervention.[7]

Osteomyelitis

Osteomyelitis may be present in up to two thirds of patients with moderate to severe foot infections[13,23] usually from contiguous spread of organisms from an adjacent infected ulcer.[13,39]

Diagnosis of osteomyelitis is often difficult. Grayson et al.[2] suggest the use of a blunt probe to assess for palpable bone at the base of an ulcer. This method has a sensitivity of 69% and a specificity of 78%. Plain radiographs have a sensitivity and specificity of 62% to 100% and <70%, respectively. It may take at least 2 weeks for changes to occur on pedal radiographs,[39] and differentiation from diabetic osteopathy can be difficult. Indium-111–labeled leukocyte scanning has been reported to be highly sensitive for detecting and monitoring therapy in diabetic osteomyelitis.[40] This study also showed that all patients with exposed bone had

osteomyelitis and 68% of ulcers harbored osteomyelitis beneath them. Emphasizing the difficulty in diagnosing osteomyelitis, only 32% of biopsy- or culture-proven osteomyelitis was detected on clinical examination. Magnetic resonance imaging (MRI) has sensitivities and specificities in the 90% to 95% range,[41] and is superior to bone scan.[42]

Osteomyelitis is usually polymicrobial in nature with staphylococci, enterococci, anaerobes, and Gram-negative bacilli present. These patients should undergo surgical debridement of infected bone and have antibiotic therapy for 6 weeks or longer tailored to the organisms isolated.[28]

Bamberger et al.[23] treated 51 cases of osteomyelitis in 42 diabetic patients. Only 13.7% had positive blood cultures. Medical management without need for amputation was accomplished in 53% of these patients with a variety of treatment regimens. Success was associated with culture-directed antimicrobial therapy and 4 weeks of intravenous therapy or 10 weeks of combination oral and intravenous therapy.

Nutrition Therapy

Failure of therapy is associated with a nonhealing wound.[21] Thus, nutrition status and related immunocompetence must be assessed in these patients. In order to ensure proper wound healing to allow the greatest chance of successful therapy and limb salvage, nutrition and glycemic control should be maximized.

Hyperbaric Oxygen Therapy

Hyperbaric oxygen therapy has been proven to be effective in treating radiation-induced hypoxia, and animal studies show it can be helpful in treating osteomyelitis and soft-tissue infections.[43] Diabetic foot ulcers and the associated infections are possible candidates for hyperbaric oxygen therapy given the known association with ischemic disease. To date, there is no conclusive data that suggests hyperbaric oxygen therapy should be standard of care in patients with diabetic soft-tissue infections or osteomyelitis.[43]

SUMMARY

Management of diabetic foot infections requires a multidisciplinary approach.[44] Emphasis should be placed on the prevention of foot ulcers with careful daily examination of the feet and proper footwear. If a foot infection develops, early diagnosis and therapy are paramount. These patients should be classified based on the severity of their infection and the need for surgery at presentation. Medical management can proceed alone or in combination with surgical therapy. Deep cultures are taken prior to initiation of empiric antibiotic therapy in either the outpatient or inpatient setting. These antibiotics may be further tailored based on clinical response and culture results. This approach will minimize the number of patients who have progression and require amputation.

REFERENCES

1. Most RS, Sinnock P. The epidemiology of lower extremity amputations in diabetic individuals. *Diabetes Care.* 1983;6:87–91.
2. Grayson ML. Diabetic foot infections. *Infect Dis Clin North Am.* 1995;9:143–161.
3. Centers for Disease Control. Lower extremity amputations among persons with diabetes mellitus—Washington, 1988. *MMWR Morb Mortal Wkly Rep.* 1991;40:737–739.
4. Reiber GE, Pecoraro RE, Koepsell TD. Risk factors for amputation in patients with diabetes mellitus. *Ann Intern Med.* 1992; 117:97–105.
5. Wheat LJ, Allen SD, Henry M, et al. Diabetic foot infections: bacteriologic analysis. *Arch Intern Med.* 1986;146:1935–1940.
6. Brodsky JW, Schneidler C. Diabetic foot infections. *Orthop Clin North Am.* 1991;22:473–489.
7. Bridges RM, Deitch EA. Diabetic foot infections: pathophysiology and treatment. *Surg Clin North Am.* 1994;74:537–555.
8. Holzer SES, Camerota A, Martens L, et al. Costs and duration of care for lower extremity ulcers in patients with diabetes. *Clin Ther.* 1998;20:169–181.
9. Brandman O, Redisch W. Incidence of peripheral vascular changes in diabetes mellitus. *Diabetes.* 1953;2:194.
10. Menzoian JO, LaMorte WW, Paniszyn CC, et al. Symptomatology and anatomic patterns of peripheral vascular disease: differing impact of smoking and diabetes. *Ann Vasc Surg.* 1989;3:224–228.
11. LoGerfo FW, Gibbons GW. Vascular disease of the lower extremities in diabetes mellitus. *Endocrinol Metab Clin North Am.* 1996;25: 439–445.
12. Seabrook GR, Edmiston CE, Schmitt DD, et al. Comparison of serum and tissue antibiotic levels in diabetes-related foot infections. *Surgery.* 1991;110:671–676.
13. Slovenkai MP. Prevention and treatment of diabetes and its complications. *Med Clin North Am.* 1998;82:949–971.
14. McNeely MJ, Boyko EJ, Ahroni JH, et al. The independent contributions of diabetic neuropathy and vasculopathy in foot ulceration: how great are the risks? *Diabetes Care.* 1995;18: 216–219.
15. Goodson WH, Hunt TK. Wound healing and the diabetic patient. *Surg Gynecol Obstet.* 1979;149:600–608.
16. Morain WD, Colen LB. Wound healing and diabetes mellitus. *Clin Plast Surg.* 1990;17:493–501.
17. Robson MC, Stenburg BD, Heggers JP. Wound healing alterations caused by infection. *Clin Plast Surg.* 1990;17:485–492.
18. Louie TJ, Bartlett JG, Tally FP, et al. Aerobic and anaerobic bacteria in diabetic foot ulcers. *Ann Intern Med.* 1976;85:461–463.
19. Lipsky BA, Pecoraro RE, Larson SA, et al. Outpatient management of uncomplicated lower-extremity infections in diabetic patients. *Arch Intern Med.* 1990;150:790–797.
20. Gerding DN. Foot infections in diabetic patients: the role of anaerobes. *Clin Infect Dis.* 1995;20(Suppl. 2):S283–S288.
21. Peterson LR, Lissack LM, Canter K, et al. Therapy of lower extremity infections with ciprofloxacin in patients with diabetes mellitus, peripheral vascular disease, or both. *Am J Med.* 1989; 86(Pt 2):801–808.
22. Hartemann-Heurtier A, Robert J, Jacqueminet S, et al. Diabetic foot ulcer and multidrug resistant organisms: risk factors and impact. *Diabet Med.* 2004;21:710–715.
23. Bamberger DM, Daus GP, Gerding DN. Osteomyelitis in the feet of diabetic patients. *Am J Med.* 1987;83:653–660.
24. Calhoun JH, Eng M, Cantrell J, et al. Treatment of diabetic foot infections: Wagner classification, therapy, and outcome. *Foot Ankle.* 1988;9:101–106.
25. Gibbons GW, Ellopoulos GM. Infection of the diabetic foot. In: Kozak GP, ed. *Management of diabetic foot problems.* Philadelphia, Pa: WB Saunders; 1984:97–102.
26. Perez-Ruvacaba JA, Quintero-Perez NP, Morales-Reyes JJ, et al. Double-blind comparison of ciprofloxacin with cefotaxime in the treatment of skin and skin structure infections. *Am J Med.* 1987;82(Suppl. 4A):242–246.
27. Gerards V, Schiewe U, Gerards HH, et al. Amoxicillin-clavulanic acid in the therapy of bacterial infections of the diabetic foot. Results of an observational study. *MMW Fortschr Med.* 2000; 142(Suppl. 3):187–194.
28. Lipsky BA, Berendt AR. Principles and practice of antibiotic therapy of diabetic foot infections. *Diabetes Metab Res Rev.* 2000;16(Suppl. 1):S42–S46.
29. Levison ME, Mallela S. Increasing antimicrobial resistance: therapeutic implications for enterococcal infections. *Curr Infect Dis Rep.* 2000;2:417–423.
30. Moellering RC. Linezolid: the first oxazolidinone. *Ann Intern Med.* 2003;138:135–142.
31. Lipsky BA, Itani K, Norden C, et al. Treating foot infections in diabetic patients: a randomized, multicenter, open-label trial of linezolid versus ampicillin-sulbactam/amoxicillin-clavulanate. *Clin Infect Dis.* 2004;38:17–24.
32. Calandra GB, Raupp W, Brown KR. Imipenem/cilastatin treatment of lower extremity skin and soft tissue infections in diabetics. *Scand J Infect Dis Suppl.* 1987;52:15–19.
33. Grayson ML, Gibbons GW, Habershaw GM, et al. Use of ampicillin/sulbactam versus imipenem/cilastatin in the treatment of limb-threatening foot infections in diabetic patients. *Clin Infect Dis.* 1994;18:683–693.
34. Siami G, Christou N, Eiseman I, et al, Severe Skin and Soft Tissue Infections Study Group. Clinafloxacin versus piperacillin-tazobactam in treatment of patients with severe skin and soft tissue infections. *Antimicrob Agents Chemother.* 2001;45:525–531.
35. File TM, Tan JS. Amdcinocillin plus cefoxitin versus cefoxitin alone in therapy of mixed soft tissue infections including diabetic foot infections. *Am J Med.* 1983;75:100–105.
36. Fass RJ, Prior RB. Comparative *in vitro* activities of piperacillin-tazobactam and ticarcillin-clavulanate. *Antimicrob Agents Chemother.* 1989;33:1268–1274.
37. Tan JS, Wishnow RM, Talan DA, et al, The Piperacillin/Tazobactam Skin and Skin Structure Study Group. Treatment of hospitalized patients with complicated skin and skin structure infections: double-blind, randomized, multicenter study of piperacillin-tazobactam versus ticarcillin-clavulanate. *Antimicrob Agents Chemother.* 1993;37:1580–1586.
38. McIntyre KE. Control of infection in the diabetic foot: the role of microbiology, immunopathology, antibiotics, and guillotine amputation. *J Vasc Surg.* 1987;5:787–790.
39. Morrison WB, Lederman HP, Schweitzer ME. MR imaging of inflammatory conditions of the ankle and foot. *Magn Reson Imaging Clin N Am.* 2001;9:615–637.
40. Newman LG, Waller J, Palestro CJ, et al. Unsuspected osteomyelitis in diabetic foot ulcers: diagnosis and monitoring by leukocyte scanning with indium in 111 oxyquinoline. *JAMA.* 1991;266: 1246–1251.
41. Craig JG, Amin MB, Wu K, et al. Osteomyelitis of the diabetic foot: MR imaging-pathologic correlation. *Radiology.* 1997; 203:849–855.
42. Yuh WT, Corson JD, Baraniewski HM, et al. Osteomyelitis of the foot in diabetic patients: evaluation with plain film 99mTc-MDP bone scintigraphy, and MR imaging. *AJR Am J Roentgenol.* 1989; 152:795–800.
43. Bakker DJ. Hyperbaric oxygen therapy and the diabetic foot. *Diabetes Metab Res Rev.* 2000;16(Suppl 1):S55–S58.
44. Frykberg RG. The team approach in diabetic foot management. *Adv Wound Care.* 1998;11:71–77.

7

Operative Management of Diabetic Foot Wounds and Infections: Maximizing Length and Optimizing Biomechanics

Christopher E. Attinger   *Karen Kim Evans*

Advances in vascular, orthopedic, and reconstructive surgery as well as wound care have enabled the salvage of feet in patients with foot ulcers that would have otherwise led to major amputations (below-knee or above-knee amputations). With the use of flaps and biomechanically sound, functional partial foot amputations, the indications for major amputations have been reduced. Patients who present with wet gangrene, dry gangrene, osteomyelitis, Charcot disease, nonhealing ulcers, distal ischemia, and unremitting pain of the foot are candidates for limb salvage using flap coverage or partial foot amputations.

Selecting the proper foot amputation is a complex decision. Reviews of the technical aspects of foot amputations have defined the level of foot amputation as the level of distal necrosis or vascular compromise.[1,2] At times, this cookbook approach can unnecessarily sacrifice foot length and reduce the weight-bearing plantar surface of the foot. Decreasing the total plantar surface area (cm^2) renders the foot more susceptible to recurrent breakdown because the weight of the body must be carried over a smaller surface.

We have previously reviewed our noncookbook approach to foot amputations, which focuses on maximizing blood supply, functional biomechanics, and using reconstructive techniques to save all viable tissue.[3] Although this approach has evolved from treating thousands of diabetic patients with altered foot biomechanics from neuropathy and Charcot disease, it is also applicable to the nondiabetic patient population. Indeed, the nondiabetic patient with foot disease presents less of a reconstructive challenge in terms of having to address the biomechanical aspects of the foot and wound healing issues. We have found that by addressing blood supply, using proper wound management techniques, using all of the reconstructive options, and adhering to biomechanical principles, we can perform functional partial foot amputations and avoid major amputations in >95% of patients who present with foot breakdown.

Prior to closure of any wound, the wound must be prepared surgically through aggressive debridement and by controlling local and systemic infection. In addition, optimizing blood flow to the foot and using the principles of foot angiosomes (Chapter 8) are prerequisites to the success of flap and/or partial foot amputation success. One has to be ready to use all the techniques of wound closure to maximize foot length. Last, the amputation must be designed with sound biomechanical principles to prevent recurrent breakdown.

BIOMECHANICS OF THE FOOT

The biomechanics of foot and gait are discussed in detail in Chapter 3. In brief, changes in the normal biomechanics of the foot include skeletal abnormalities, changes in muscle function, and loss of flexibility in the joint and tendon. Addressing the biomechanics of the foot perioperatively is imperative in the diabetic population.

In the diabetic population, abnormal gait biomechanics lead to high focal plantar pressures. These pressures can be evaluated by foot pressure analysis during gait. These abnormalities can be due to changes in the skeletal framework (long metatarsal, hammer toes, previous bone resection, Charcot collapse, etc.). In addition, high blood glucose levels lead to the glycosylation of connective tissue so that tendons and joints lose their flexibility.[4] If high forefoot plantar pressures are found and/or focal foot ulcerations have developed, the flexibility of the Achilles tendon should be evaluated. The Achilles tendon flexibility is measured by testing the ankle's range of motion in maximal dorsiflexion and plantar flexion with the knee flexed and extended.

Because of the loss of Achilles tendon flexibility in diabetic patients, the foot gradually loses its ability to dorsiflex during gait. The loss of the rolling motion of the ankle creates an abnormally elongated lever arm during the normal gait cycle, placing abnormal forces on the midfoot and forefoot. When one combines these abnormal forces with sensory neuropathy, ulcers occur. In addition, the tight Achilles tendon can also cause a "nutcracker effect" at the ankle joint, which is believed to contribute to the collapse of the midfoot arch seen in Charcot joints.

A simple release of the Achilles tendon corrects this abnormality and can lead to rapid healing of plantar ulcers within 4 to 6 weeks.[5,6] The release also diminishes the risk of recurrent breakdown.[7] Moreover, early release also has the potential to minimize Charcot development in the foot and ankle. In foot amputation, the Achilles tendon must either be lengthened (transmetatarsal amputation) or severed (Lisfranc or Chopart amputation) to prevent the inevitable equinovarus deformity that accompanies these amputations.

While the Achilles tendon is less of a consideration in the nondiabetic patient, routine podiatric evaluation of foot biomechanics to evaluate tendon, skeletal, and muscle function should be preformed in all patients undergoing flap closure or partial foot amputation to prevent recurrent ulceration.

THE IMPORTANCE OF DEBRIDEMENT

Wound debridement is defined as removing necrotic tissue, foreign material, and bacteria from an acute or chronic wound. Because necrotic tissue, foreign material, and bacteria induce the production of proteases, collagenases, and elastases that impede the body's attempt to heal, debridement is a necessary step in controlling an aberrant wound healing process. In addition, bacteria produce their own wound-inhibiting enzymes and consume many of the scarce local resources (oxygen, nutrition, and building blocks) that are necessary for wound healing. During an abnormal wound healing cascade, the building blocks (chemotactants, growth factors, mitogens, etc.) necessary for normal wound healing are destroyed. This hostile environment creates a milieu in which bacteria can proliferate and further inhibit wound healing.

An acute wound is defined as a recent wound that has not yet progressed through the sequential stages of wound healing, while a chronic wound is a wound that is arrested in one of the wound healing stages (usually the inflammatory stage) and cannot progress further. Debriding the acute wound removes damaged tissue or foreign materials that inhibit healing, allowing the normal wound healing phases to evolve (assuming systemic and local factors are normal). Aggressive debridement of a chronic wound converts the chronic wound into an acute wound so that it can progress through the normal phases of wound healing.

Infection of a wound site alters the normal healing process by disrupting and prolonging the inflammatory phase.[8] This inhibits the macrophages' ability to direct the formation of granulation tissue and neovascularization. Clinically, bacterial status of a wound can be assessed by quantitative bacterial counts. A healthy wound with $<10^5$ bacteria per g of tissue should heal successfully either by secondary intention, delayed primary closure, or skin graft.

The lessons of aggressive removal of all necrotic and nonviable tissue learned in burn surgery can be applied with equal effectiveness to chronic wounds. Steed[9] reviewed the data of platelet-derived growth factor's effect on the healing of chronic diabetic wounds and made the seminal observation that wounds heal more successfully when the wound debridement is performed weekly rather than sporadically. The applied growth factor is more effective in promoting wound healing in frequently debrided wounds than in the undisturbed wounds. Most likely, the frequent debridement regularly removes inhibitors of wound healing (such as proteases, collagenases, and elastases) and allows growth factors to exert their positive influence.

The importance of removing the local inhibitory wound healing factors helps explain the success of the vacuum-assisted closure device (VAC) (Kinetic Concepts, Inc., San Antonio, Texas) in converting chronic wounds to healthy healing wounds.[10] The constant suction applied by this device to the surface of the wound prevents an accumulation of proteases and bacteria, resulting in rapid formation of healthy granulation tissue.[11]

There are a multitude of modern wound techniques to stimulate healing and encourage debridement as well as a plethora of various wound dressings. These include growth factors and skin substitutes (such as xenograft, allograft, cultured skin substitutes, Integra [Johnson & Johnson Medical, Arlington, Texas], and Alloderm [LifeCell Corporation, Branchburg, New Jersey]) as well as living skin equivalents (Apligraf [Organogenesis, Inc., Canton, Massachusetts, and Novartis Pharmaceutical Corporation, East Hanover, New Jersey]). In addition, wound healing adjuncts, such as the use of hyperbaric oxygen, can be beneficial in certain cases. The subject of this chapter initially focuses on the importance of surgical debridement in the management of wounds.

WOUND ASSESSMENT

After a careful medical history is obtained, the wound is assessed by measuring its size and depth, and then photographed. If cellulitis is present, the border of the erythema should be marked with indelible ink. This permits immediate bedside assessment of whether subsequent antibiotics and/or debridement are immediately successful in controlling the cellulitis. If, after 4 to 6 hours, the cellulitis has extended beyond the inked boundary, the antibiotics are inadequate and/or the wound has been inadequately debrided.

It is important not to confuse cellulitis with dependent rubor. If the erythema disappears when the lower leg is elevated above the level of the heart, then the erythema is due to dependent rubor. With dependent rubor, inflammation is usually absent and the skin should have visible wrinkling. If the erythema persists despite elevation, the wound likely has surrounding cellulitis and needs antibiotic treatment and/or debridement. In the immediate perioperative state, dependent rubor is often seen and should not be confused with postoperative cellulitis. Again, rapid resolution of the erythema with elevation and presence of wrinkled skin at the incision edge indicate dependent rubor rather than cellulitis.

The depth of the wound should be assessed for bone, tendon, and/or joint involvement. A metallic probe is used to assist in the evaluation of the depth of the wound. If the probe touches bone, there is an 85% chance that osteomyelitis[12] is present. An x-ray should be obtained to assist with the evaluation of the underlying bone; however, it is important to remember that it can take up to 3 weeks for osteomyelitis to appear on x-ray. A magnetic resonance imaging (MRI) scan or nuclear scan is usually superfluous if the surgeon plans to evaluate the bone during debridement. These studies are useful when the extent of osteomyelitis in the suspected bone is unclear or when there is suspicion that other bones may be involved.

If a tendon is involved, the infection is very likely to have tracked proximally or distally. One should evaluate the character of the tendon sheaths proximally and distally, and check for bogginess. If the suspicion is strong that a distal infection has spread proximally, the proximal areas where the tendon sheaths are readily accessible should be checked (i.e., dorsal or volar wrist, extensor retinaculum, tarsal tunnel, etc.).

The blood flow to the area is then evaluated by palpation and/or handheld Doppler.[13] If the quality of flow is questionable, a formal, noninvasive vascular evaluation must be performed. If the flow is inadequate, the patient should then be referred to a vascular surgeon. In the face of undetermined or inadequate blood flow, debridement should be delayed until blood flow status has been assessed and corrected, if possible. Immediate debridement is indicated (regardless of the vascular status) if wet gangrene, ascending cellulitis from a necrotic wound, or necrotizing fasciitis is present. Revascularization should follow as soon as possible thereafter.

Sensation and motor function must also be assessed. A careful nerve exam is critical when ruling out possible compartment syndrome. In diabetic patients or those with neurologic disorders, the neurologic exam is also helpful in explaining the wound's etiology and critical in preventing potential recurrences. Lack of protective sensation can be established if the patient is unable to feel 10 g of pressure (Semms-Weinstein filament 5.08). This prevents patients from noticing potential damage from excessive local pressure; prolonged decubitus position; tight shoes, clothes, or dressings; biomechanical abnormalities; or the presence of foreign bodies. The repetitive trauma of ambulation in neuropathic patients makes matters worse when biomechanical abnormalities exist in these patients. Abnormally high focal plantar pressures result and the tissue breaks down under the stress of ambulation.

DEBRIDEMENT

General Technical Considerations

The wound should be debrided in the operating room if the patient cannot be adequately anesthetized with a regional block and/or the debridement will lead to bleeding that may be difficult to control. The wound should be debrided without a tourniquet so that the quality of bleeding at the freshened wound edges can be accurately assessed.

The most important step in treating any wound is performing an adequate debridement to remove all foreign material and unhealthy or nonviable tissue until the wound edges and base consist only of normal and healthy tissue. Only excellent atraumatic surgical techniques[14] should be used to avoid damaging the healthy tissue left behind. The remaining healthy tissue establishes the necessary surface for successful wound healing and ensures that the wound is free from gross infection, and necrotic tissue to inhibit healing.

A useful approach to surgical debridement is to view a wound much like an oncology surgeon would approach a tumor, without focus on the subsequent reconstruction. The goal is to excise the wound completely until only normal, soft, well-vascularized tissue remains. An acute wound must be devoid of all questionably viable tissue and foreign material so that it can either progress through the normal healing phases or be ready to close safely. A chronic wound has to be converted by debridement to an acute wound so that it can proceed through the normal healing phases or be closed surgically.

After debridement, it is important to cleanse the wound with a pulsed lavage system.[15] The pressure from the pulsating liquid is very effective in getting rid of any loose tissue and superficial bacteria. There has been no convincing scientific evidence that there is benefit to adding antibiotics to the saline or water used in lavage. It is important to first tag any important structures (nerve and tendon ends) with monofilament suture because these structures tend to swell during the pulse lavage and are difficult to identify.

If the wound is going to be closed immediately after debridement, then it is important to use a double instrument setup in the operating room to avoid recontaminating the newly debrided wound. There should be two separate sets of instruments, gloves, gowns, drapes, suction, and electrocautery: One for debridement and one for wound closure. New instruments are then used to close the wound. The reasoning behind this extra setup is that cultures of the instruments used in debriding wounds have a residual concentration of bacteria $>10^4$ per g of tissue.[16] Reintroducing bacteria into the wound that has just been debrided prior to closure is an unnecessary infectious risk and can be avoided with the double instrument setup.

Debriding Skin

Debriding skin consists of removing nonviable, nonbleeding skin. If the injured skin does not blanch, is insensate, and has blistered, it is not likely to be alive. There is no advantage to waiting for this dead skin to redevelop circulation. At the edges and under the dead skin, there is a high concentration of harmful proteases and/or bacteria that inhibit subsequent healing. The protracted course necessary for the dead skin to separate itself from the underlying tissue may lead to functional loss, bad scarring, deeper tissue damage, and disseminated infection.

Therefore, the approach to nonviable skin should be to remove it as soon as possible. If the border between live and dead tissue is clearly demarcated, then the skin should be excised along that border. If the border is not clearly demarcated, then one should start at the center and remove concentric circles of skin until viable tissue is reached. When excising skin, one should look for bleeding at the normal skin edge. Clotted venules at the skin edge reflect a complete interruption in the local microcirculation and are an excellent indicator that further excision is necessary. Only when there is normal arterial bleeding at the edge of the wound and absence of clotted veins can one be satisfied that the cutaneous debridement has been adequate.

When removing the skin, it is important to examine the subcutaneous tissue. A culture should be obtained and a temporary biologic dressing or VAC should be placed on the debrided site after it has been pulse lavaged. If the remaining viable tissue appears infected, then a topical antibiotic, such as silver-sulfadiazine, or moist pure silver sheeting[17,18] should be placed on the wound. For *Pseudomonas* infections, 0.25% acetic acid or gentamycin ointment may be more appropriate. For methicillin-resistant *Staphylococcus aureus* (MRSA), mupirocin (bactroban) is an appropriate initial topical antibiotic, keeping in mind that resistance can develop quickly.[19] If the tissue is not viable, deeper debridement is necessary.

Debriding Subcutaneous Tissue

Subcutaneous tissue consists of fat, vessels, and nerves, but because of the decreased concentration of blood vessels in the subcutaneous fat, bleeding is not always a reliable indicator of healthy tissue. Viable fat is soft and resilient with a shiny yellow color, while necrotic fat is hard and nonpliable with a grey pallor. Fat should be debrided until soft, yellow, normal-looking fat is attained. Undermining should be avoided because it threatens the viability of the overlying skin. It is very important to use a moist dressing after debridement to prevent dessication of the fat.

Small blood vessels should be coagulated using bipolar cautery to minimize damage to the surrounding tissue. If the vessels are >3 mm in diameter, they should be ligated. Surgical clips are the least reactive foreign body material to accomplish this. If a suture is to be used, then a small-diameter, monofilament suture should be used to minimize the risk of facilitating further infection. Silk suture is a foreign body that stimulates a vigorous inflammatory reaction. In addition, bacteriostatic polyglycolic woven suture has multiple recesses within which bacteria can survive in a semiprotected state.

Viable nerves are shiny with a white, glistening appearance. In the subcutaneous tissue, the nerves are typically sensory and can be very painful when exposed. If a healthy exposed nerve is to be preserved, it should be kept moist until it can be covered with adequate tissue. Consideration should be given to burying the nerve underneath other tissue or a flap. In addition, sewing the epineurium over the nerve fascicles using 8-0 or 9-0 nylon can minimize neuroma formation. If the nerve is to be sacrificed, then longitudinal traction should be used to allow the nerve to retract within normal tissue when it is cut at the edge of the wound.

Debriding Fascia, Tendon, and Muscle

Healthy fascia has a white, glistening, hard appearance and should be preserved if it looks viable. When necrotic and liquefying, the appearance is dull, soft, and stringy. All necrotic fascia should be debrided until solid normal-looking bleeding fascia is reached. Since neurovascular bundles can be close to overlying fascia, debridement should proceed with caution. Again, the viable fascia must be kept moist in the postdebridement period to avoid dessication.

The underlying muscle must also be examined for a bright red, shiny, and resilient appearance. Healthy muscle contracts when grasped with forceps or touched with cautery. In neuropathic patients, the muscle may have a pale, even yellowish, color that may initially appear nonviable. However, it will display some degree of tone and will bleed when cut.

Necrotic muscle will be swollen, dull, and grainy when palpated and falls apart when pinched. If viability of the muscle is questionable, it is best to be cautious and remove only what is not bleeding and appears dead. Subsequently, the wound should be serially debrided until only viable muscle remains. If only a portion of the muscle is necrotic, it is best to remove only the dead portion, because removing the entire muscle involves further dissection that might compromise blood flow to the surrounding tissues (i.e., overlying skin).

Tendon debridement is always a difficult question because sacrifice of the tendon leads to loss of function. Attempts should be made to preserve viable paratenon, which supplies nutrients to the tendon. The tendon must be kept moist postdebridement, especially when the paratenon is removed, and should be covered with viable tissue as soon as the wound is stable (infection-free with adequate blood supply). Without adequate coverage, the tendon may desiccate or become infected. If infected, the tendon looks dull, soft, and grainy with parts separating and/or liquefying. It is important to make a proximal and distal incision above and below the exposed tendon to ensure that any hidden necrotic tendon is also removed.

If the tendon is small and part or all of it is infected, all of the exposed tendon should be removed. When the extensor tendons on the dorsum of the foot become exposed, it is difficult to preserve them unless they are quickly covered with healthy tissue. If the tendons remain in place while the wound progresses to the point of closure, they usually become infected and will impede further wound healing until they are removed.

When the tendon is larger (e.g., Achilles tendon, anterior tibial tendon), only the necrotic portion should be debrided. Again, great care and attention should be directed at keeping the remaining viable tendon moist, and it should be covered as soon as the wound is stable with a local, pedicled, or free flap.

A commonly encountered wound at the posterior ankle may lead to exposure of the Achilles tendon. The Achilles tendon receives excellent blood supply from both the posterior tibial and peroneal arteries allowing it to remain viable. If part of the tendon is necrotic, it should be debrided to a hard, shiny tendon. Serial debridement may be necessary. It should be kept moist using silver-sulfadiazine and an occlusive dressing while granulation tissue forms. Granulation formulation can be accelerated with either the VAC (first covering the tendon with a Vaseline mesh gauze) or with the combined usage of hyperbaric oxygen treatments and topical growth factor. Once a healthy bed of granulation tissue has formed, the tendon can then be skin grafted.

Debriding Bone

Debridement of necrotic or dead bone is relatively straightforward. All soft, nonbleeding bone should be removed. Useful handheld tools include the rongeur, curettes, and rasps. Power tools, such as the sagittal saw and the cutting burr, are also necessary. One should remove only what is dead and infected and leave bleeding bone behind, without shattering proximal viable bone. In this regard, power tools are safer to use than rongeurs or chisels. The best way to debride the osteomyelitic smaller long bones (phalanx, metacarpals, or metatarsals) is to serially cut slices of bone until healthy bone is reached. In the larger bones (tibia, fibula, radius, ulna), a cutting burr is more useful to remove layer by layer of the osteomyelitic bone until healthy, bleeding bone is reached. Copious irrigation should be used to ensure that the heat generated by the burr does not damage the healthy bone. When burring the cortical bone, the process is continued until punctate bleeding is visualized emanating from the cortical bone (the Papineau sign). This signifies that healthy bone has been reached.

When debriding cancellous bone, look for bleeding and normal-appearing marrow. Biomechanical considerations should not deter the surgeon from debriding enough bone to ensure that all osteomyelitis has been eradicated. Correction of the resultant biomechanical abnormality can be made once the wound has healed. Current orthopedic techniques, including bone grafting and Ilizarov frames, allow repair of most bone defects.

Obtaining cultures of what appears to be normal bone proximal to the area of debridement and of the debrided osteomyelitic bone are crucial. Once the infected bone has been removed and only bleeding, healthy bone is left behind, the wound is ready to close, assuming surrounding soft tissue is likewise healthy. Subsequent prolonged antibiotic therapy (i.e., 6 weeks) for the infected osteomyelitis is not only unnecessary but also excessive once the involved infected bone is removed. It places the patient in further jeopardy to the complications of prolonged antibiotic therapy (*Clostridia difficilis*, resistant organisms, allergic reactions, etc.). When only healthy bone remains, only 1 week of appropriate antibiotics is necessary after wound closure. The exception to a 1-week course of antibiotics postclosure is when the surgeon suspects that the bone left behind may still harbor osteomyelitis (e.g., calcaneus or tibia). In that instance, a longer course of antibiotics is indicated.

SPREAD OF INFECTION ALONG TISSUE PLANES

When the deeper structures are involved, it is always important to rule out proximal or distal spread. With necrotizing fasciitis, the infection spreads along the fascia and deeper structures. The key is to remove all questionable tissue, consider using hyperbaric oxygen as adjunct, and redebride every 24 to 48 hours until the wound has stabilized. With necrotic and purulent ulcers overlying tendon or muscle, infection can spread along tendon sheaths and/or fascial planes.

It is very important to evaluate any suspected route along which the infection could spread. For example, the flexor tendon sheaths, peroneal tendon sheaths, and extensor tendon sheaths are possible avenues of spread in any necrotic plantar foot ulcer. Evaluation of infection within those possible routes includes feeling for bogginess of the overlying tissue as well as needle aspiration or direct exploration of the actual tendon sheath. A small incision in the skin directly over the suspect tendon sheath followed by gentle spreading with straight clamp will reveal whether purulence is present. It is also very useful to milk the suspected area of spread along the underlying tendon sheath and look for purulence at the ulcer site.

Once the spread of infection has been located, make an incision directly over the most proximal or distal site of spread and remove all necrotic paratenon and tendon tissue. Great care should be taken to ensure that the incision and dissection have extended far enough proximally. The proximal exploration should stop only when the surrounding tissue is normal. This may require filleting the foot, ankle, and leg all the way up to the popliteal fossa or the hand, wrist, and arm all the way to the antecubital fossa. With extensive infection, repeat debridements should be performed every 12 to 48 hours until the wound is infection-free. This aggressive approach is often the only chance to save the diffusely infected limb.

THE ACUTE WOUND

The acute wound is fresh and has not yet begun the normal healing phases. The wound should be stabilized and cleansed of as much contaminants and dead tissue as soon as possible. This may be done in the emergency room or the operating room. Giving the patient a peripheral nerve block can facilitate the emergency room debridement. The actual cleansing of the wound is best done with pulsed lavage using at least 2 L of saline.

In the emergency room, cultures[20] of the debrided tissue and loose bone fragments should be sent to the lab. These have been shown to best correlate with future osteomyelitis, should it develop. The wound is then dressed with a sterile moist normal saline and cotton gauze dressing while the patient awaits surgery.

Once the cultures have been sent, the patient should be started on broad-spectrum antibiotics.[21] In the case of gross contamination such as garbage truck or farm injuries, penicillin and an aminoglycoside or a more potent combination should be added for better coverage of anaerobic and Gram-negative bacteria. Antibiotics can then be adjusted for more specific coverage as soon as the initial wound culture results are back. An infectious disease consult can be very useful to optimally manage the antibiotic regimen in any contaminated wound.

In the operating room, the goal of the initial debridement is to remove all obvious dead skin, subcutaneous tissue, fascia, muscle, and bone, while leaving behind all potentially viable tissue to reevaluate in 12 to 24 hours. If the skin and subcutaneous tissue is avulsed, there is an overwhelming chance that the majority of it will die. Therefore, avulsed tissue should be trimmed until actual bleeding at the skin edge is seen. Cultures of the wound are again obtained. The anatomic damage should be fully evaluated, including avulsed nerves and/or tendons. Cut nerves should be tagged with a fine monofilament suture so that they do not become lost in the subsequent soft-tissue swelling. The wound should then be cleansed with pulse lavage to remove all foreign debris and dressed in a continuously moist, nonirritating bandage that keeps exposed tendons, fascia, and bone moist.

Serial debridements every 24 to 48 hours are recommended until the wound is ready for closure. The wound is ready for closure when it contains only viable tissue, and is soft, without erythema, and minimally painful. It is important to facilitate reconstruction within 7 days of the date of injury to minimize complications.[22] Good results, however, can still be achieved after that time if the wound is clean and fully debrided to normal tissue at the time of reconstruction.

THE INFECTED WOUND

In the infected wound, it is important to know the source and extent of the infection. Obtaining an x-ray of the area underlying the wound lets the physician know whether the bone is involved and whether gas is present in the soft tissue. If gas is seen within the tissue planes on the x-ray, then gas gangrene is present and the wound becomes a surgical emergency. This gas is usually a byproduct of anaerobic bacteria (usually *Clostridium perfringens)* that has traveled along the fascial planes. The wound needs to be debrided very aggressively and immediately to prevent limb loss or death. The involved compartments of the foot and/or leg must be evaluated for high pressure and released if there is any question that the pressure is abnormal. Hyperbaric oxygen should be considered postoperatively to help control the anaerobic infection.[23] The wound should be re-explored in 24 to 48 hours if there is any question of residual infection.

It is critical to quickly assess whether there is sufficient blood supply to eradicate the infection. Insufficient blood flow inhibits the body from delivering the necessary white blood cells, nutrients, oxygen, and antibiotics to the wound site. Palpable pulses usually signify sufficient inflow. Otherwise, noninvasive vascular studies should be performed. If the flow is deemed insufficient, the affected extremity should be urgently revascularized. Unless there is gas gangrene or a rapidly ascending infection, debridement should be limited until the limb has been adequately revascularized.

Again, it is important to obtain aerobic and anaerobic cultures of the wound as soon as possible by obtaining a piece of deep, initially unexposed tissue. A swab or superficial tissue culture is of limited use because it only reflects surface flora rather than the actual underlying bacteria responsible for the infection. For quantitative bacterial culture lab, a minimum of 0.3 cm^3 of tissue specimen is necessary for the culture to be processed. A concentration of $>10^5$ bacteria per g of tissue reflects a significant infection that will inhibit healing.[8] The wound should then be debrided as specified above. Broad-spectrum antibiotics can then be started after the deep-tissue cultures have been obtained.

The edge of the erythema around the wound is then marked with an indelible ink marker and followed closely. If, subsequently, the redness extends beyond the drawn margins, either the broad spectrum antibiotic is insufficient or the wound has not been adequately debrided. The surgeon should not hesitate to return to the operating room every 12 to 24 hours to redebride the wound if there is suspicion that there is undrained purulence or necrotic tissue inhibiting the resolution of the infection. The antibiotics are then changed and/or the wound is re-explored to ensure that only healthy viable tissue remains.

Hydrogen peroxide, 1% Dakin's solution, Povidone iodine, or chlorhexidine are bacteriocidal and help sterilize the wound. However, these agents also destroy normal tissue and should therefore only be used when there is residual gangrene or necrotic tissue in the wound.[24] If only viable tissue lies at the base of the wound, topical therapy should be gentle enough to promote, rather than hinder, healing. Appropriate topical antibiotics may be useful because they can help control the local infection while minimizing damage to normal tissue.

THE CHRONIC WOUND

Chronic wounds are at times more difficult to treat because the etiology is often not known. Moreover, these wounds are typically infected topically and may harbor a deeper infection. In contrast to the acute wound, debridement is not always the first step in treatment.

The etiology of the wound determines the initial step. If the wound is due to vasculitis, the initial treatment is aimed at controlling the vasculitis by pharmaceutical intervention. One half of these patients also suffer from a coagulopathy, which should be treated prior to addressing the wound successfully.[25] If the wound is due to cancer, it should be biopsied to determine the extent of resection that will be needed to have the best chance for a cure. If the wound is due to venous stasis disease, the venous system should be assessed for venous incompetence or thrombosis and treated surgically, if appropriate, before addressing the wound. If the wound is due to radiation, pretreating it with hyperbaric oxygen should be considered.[26] If the wound is due to a hematologic abnormality (e.g., clotting abnormalities, sickle cell, thrombocytosis, cryoglobulinemia, etc.), it should be medically managed until the patient's condition is optimized. Of course, if the wound is due to vascular insufficiency, the affected limb should first be revascularized.

Debridement of a chronic wound will recreate the acute wound milieu. The chronic wound surface is debrided until normal-appearing, vascularized tissue is reached. This can be difficult in extensive chronic venous stasis disease or in radiation wounds with a large amount of cicatrix. The amount of resection necessary to remove all the involved tissue may make reconstruction difficult or impossible. In those instances, rather than debriding until normal tissue is reached, it is preferable to debride to the edge of bleeding scar tissue. This scar tissue, although indurated and stiff, can granulate in and eventually be covered with a skin graft or a flap. However, if a flap is eventually going to close the defect, then as much abnormal tissue should be removed as can be replaced by the size of the chosen flap.

Because thorough and careful wound debridement is the crucial first step in allowing a successful foot reconstruction, mastering the above techniques and principles will make closure and reconstruction easier. There are a multitude of reviews to add to the above emphasis on debridement techniques and various wound dressings.[8,27–44] Once the wound is clean, the gamut of reconstructive options to optimize amputations and rebuilding a functional foot are available.

CLOSURE AND RECONSTRUCTION

General Technical Considerations

Only when the wound shows no further sign of infection or inflammation (i.e., no erythema, induration, or swelling) can the definitive closure be performed. To close the wound prematurely leads to a minimum 20% complication rate including dehiscence of the incision and infection.[45] Applying a strict atraumatic technique during debridement and closure is vital to ensure that the often very fragile tissues will not become damaged, necrotic, or infected. Even the simple crushing action of a tissue forceps on the skin can be enough to cause skin edge necrosis. The skin should be retracted with skin hooks and bleeding controlled with bipolar cautery or clips. Sharp, decisive incisions without beveling should be made with the Bard Parker blade.

Freshened soft wound edges must be apposed without tension. Blanching along the suture line is a worrisome sign, suggesting that there is too much tension and eventual tissue necrosis will occur. Any nonvascular structures (such as residual volar plates, not usable tendons, or joint capsule) that inhibit the pliability of the soft-tissue envelope should be removed prior to closure. Frequently the simple removal of these structures releases a significant amount of tension on the final closure. If the skin closure is still tight, additional bone may have to be resected to develop a larger soft-tissue envelope. In other words, converting a long transmetatarsal amputation to a short transmetatarsal amputation, or a short transmetatarsal amputation to a Lisfranc amputation, or Lisfranc amputation to a Chopart amputation is preferable to risking poor wound healing and infection due to a tight closure.

In general, few if any deep sutures are used because they potentiate the risk of infection. For skin closure, nonabsorbable monofilament suture such as Prolene or nylon is preferred over braided suture material to minimize the tissue inflammatory response to foreign body. The skin incisions are closed with vertical mattress sutures rather than a running suture. We have found that this closure ensures excellent skin eversion, which is especially important in plantar incisions to avoid tissue depression at the healed sutured line. Interrupted sutures also allow the surgeon to address localized infection or hematoma at the bedside by removing one or two sutures rather than having to disrupt an entire running suture line. Great care is taken to ensure that the closure is well contoured and will, upon healing, easily fit into a normal shoe or custommade shoe.

Skin Grafts Coverage

Primary closure is the simplest of all reconstructive closure techniques. This is followed, in complexity, by delayed primary closure or secondary closure, skin grafts, local flaps, pedicled flaps, and last, microsurgical transfer of tissue. In general, the simplest mode of reconstruction that will achieve a stable soft-tissue envelope for the amputation is selected. We have found that 90% to 95% of wounds or amputations can be closed with the simpler options of delayed primary closure, skin graft, and/or local flap(s). For any of the reconstructive options, the success is also dependent upon

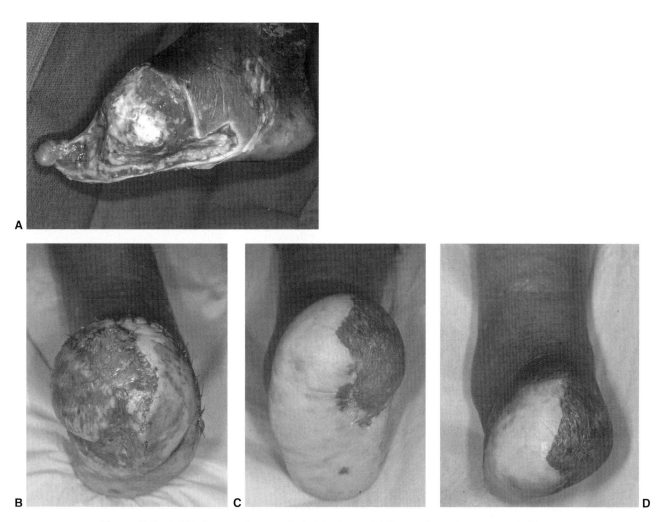

Figure 7-1 **A:** This is a poorly controlled diabetic, renal failure patient who presented with gangrene and osteomyelitis of his medial forefoot. He was debrided multiple times and a proximal transmetatarsal amputation was performed. **B:** To preserve length, a lateral flap and a split-thickness skin graft were performed for closure. **C, D:** Three-year postoperative photos. (From Attinger C, Venturi M, Kim K, et al. Maximizing length and optimizing biomechanics in foot amputations by avoiding cookbook recipes for amputation. *Semin Vasc Surg.* 2003;16:44–66, with permission.)

ensuring that the direction of the blood flow to the wound edge is adequate.[46]

Skin grafts are an excellent way to preserve length in an amputation if there is sufficient healthy granulation tissue covering bone or tendon (Fig. 7-1). The superficial layer of granulation tissue, however, should be curetted or shaved off prior to skin grafting because it may harbor bacteria within its interstices. For non–weight-bearing sites, a split-thickness skin graft should be used, whereas for plantar surfaces, a glabrous skin graft should be used to ensure better long-term durability.[47] To achieve a 95% take rate, a negative pressure device such as the VAC should be applied for the first 3 to 5 days post grafting.[48]

For split-thickness skin grafts, a medium thickness should be harvested (15/1,000 in.). Donor sites include the dorsal instep, calf, and thigh. If the skin graft donor site is flaccid, it can be preinjected with normal saline so that the surface is firm enough for the dermatome to harvest skin without skipping. In elderly patients, donor site healing can become a problem. If the skin graft is from the thigh and the skin around the site is loose, the donor site after harvesting can be excised and closed primarily. The skin graft can be stabilized on the recipient site with staples or a running suture. The skin graft is covered with Vaseline gauze or a perforated silicone sheet such as Mepitel (Mölnlycke Health Care Limited, Bedfordshire, United Kingdom), a layer containing silver such as Acticoat (Smith & Nephew, Cambridge, United Kingdom) followed by the VAC for 3 to 5 days. If the granulation bed is inadequate, it can be made thicker by adding a layer of dermis such as Integra (Johnson & Johnson, Hamburg, Germany) prior to skin grafting.[49] The use of Integra can preserve structures such as joints, bone, or tendon that would otherwise have to be sacrificed because of inadequate soft-tissue coverage.

Local Flap Closure Techniques

When there is no granulation tissue covering tendon or bone, and dermal substitutes are not indicated, skin grafts cannot be used and local flaps should be considered. The design of local fasciocutaneous or cutaneous rotation or advancement flaps is centered on the blood supply at the base of the flap. To avoid distal necrosis, the length-to-width ratio of the designed flap should not exceed a ratio of 1:1. In addition, the design of the flap should be large enough to ensure that there is no tension on the closure.

Random local flaps such as V-Y advancement flaps, rotation flaps, or transposition flaps are all useful in the foot and ankle (Fig. 7-2).[50] They can be as large as to include the entire lateral or medial half of the forefoot if needed to cover a wound on the other side. If using large advancement or rotation flaps, the donor site can either be closed primarily or skin grafted.

In addition to random local flaps, pedicled flaps have a defined and hence more reliable blood flow. The 1:1 length-to-width ratio does not apply. These flaps can either be muscle flaps, musculocutaneous flaps, or fasciocutaneous flaps. The use of these pedicled flaps requires a detailed knowledge of their vascular anatomy, because one small error can not only sacrifice the blood flow to the flap, but also jeopardizes the flow to the rest of the foot and ankle.

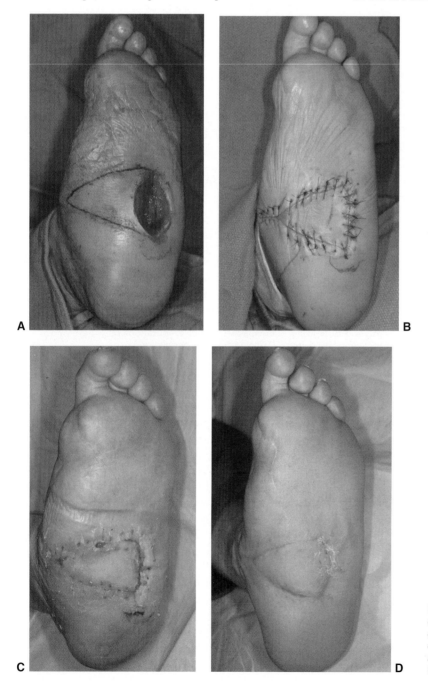

A

B

C

D

Figure 7-2 **A:** This diabetic patient with Charcot disease presented with a large chronic ulcer and osteomyelitis of his lateral midfoot. **B:** After three operative debridements and long-term antibiotics, a V-Y fasciocutaneous flap was designed. **C, D:** Postoperative photos at 3 and 6 months.

Pedicled muscle flaps are very useful for closing smaller defects of the foot and ankle.[51] All muscles of the foot and ankle are classified in the standard Mathes and Nahai classification as type II muscles (one dominant pedicle and multiple smaller minor pedicles).[52] This means that they can be divided distally and rotated on their proximally based dominant pedicle.

For coverage of mid and posterior lateral defects of the sole of the foot and the lateral calcaneus and distal ankle, the abductor digiti minimi muscle (ADM) is useful. This muscle's dominant vascular pedicle arises from the lateral plantar artery and enters the muscle just distal to its origin at the medial process of the calcaneus. We caution that this is a small muscle and its distal muscle bulk can be disappointing. Slightly larger and bulkier, the abductor hallucis brevis (AHB) muscle receives its dominant pedicle at the takeoff of the medial plantar artery. It can be rotated to cover medial defects of the midfoot and hindfoot and the medial calcaneus and distal ankle. If there is a larger defect of the midfoot and the heel, the AHB and the ADM can be used together.

The flexor digitorum brevis (FDB) muscle can be used to cover small, deep plantar heel ulcers with exposed calcaneus. This muscle receives its dominant vascular pedicle from the proximal lateral plantar artery near its origin at the medial tubercle of the calcaneus. The muscle can be flipped 180 degrees to fill the ulcer, and a skin graft can be applied on top for skin closure.

The extensor digitorum brevis (EDB) muscle has little bulk but can be used for local defects around the anterior and lateral ankle and proximal dorsum of the foot. The muscle can be rotated either in a limited fashion on its dominant pedicle, the lateral tarsal artery, or in a wider arc by also taking the proximal dorsalis pedis artery.

Although muscle flaps are useful to fill deep ulcers or to supply vascularized tissue to areas of osteomyelitis, these foot muscles are quite small. Pedicled fasciocutaneous flaps of the foot and ankle are more useful for larger defects. The most versatile and reliable fasciocutaneous flap of the foot is the medial plantar flap, which is used to cover heel defects and medial ankle wounds. This flap can survive on the superficial or deep branch of the medial plantar artery and can be as large as 6 cm by 10 cm. It has sensibility, and has a wide arc of rotation if it is taken with the proximal part of the medial plantar artery.

Other useful fasciocutaneous flaps are the lateral calcaneal flap, the supramalleolar flap, and the fillet of toe flap. The lateral calcaneal flap is based on the calcaneal branch of the peroneal artery and is harvested with the lesser saphenous vein and sural nerve to cover defects of the Achilles tendon and posterior heel. The supramalleolar flap is based on the anterior perforating branch of the lateral plantar artery and can be used for anterolateral ankle defects. The fillet of toe flap essentially involves deboning the toe while preserving the digital arteries. It is useful to cover gaps left after removal of its own or adjacent metatarsophalangeal joint.

Free Flaps Reconstructive Techniques

If the patient is not a candidate for local flap coverage or the foot or ankle defect is too large for local flap coverage, microsurgical transfer of tissue is indicated. Free flaps involve the transportation of a distal flap (muscle, fasciocutaneous, bone, and any variation thereof) to the foot and ankle, and the use of microsurgical techniques to anastamose the vascular pedicle into the arteries and veins of the foot.[53]

Free flaps are more technically challenging and require a longer operative time and longer hospital stay than do simpler techniques. Preoperative cardiac clearance is essential. Because the ulcerated or gangrenous foot usually has diseased vessels, magnified angiographic views of the distal arterial tree are helpful in surgical planning. An end-to-side anastomosis to the recipient artery is performed and preferably two end-to-end venous anastomoses are performed. The flap is then carefully trimmed so that when it heals, there is minimal, if any, residual unwanted bulk.

Proper free flap selection depends on the location of the defect and the length of the flap's vascular pedicle. For the non–weight-bearing portion of the foot, fasciocutaneous free flaps work well (radial forearm flap, lateral arm flap, parascapular flap, or anterolateral thigh flap). For weight-bearing portions, free muscle flaps covered with skin graft work best (rectus abdominus muscle, gracilis muscle, or serratus muscle).

PARTIAL FOOT AMPUTATIONS

General Principles

Partial amputations of the foot and ankle are used to address soft-tissue wounds, osteomyelitis, or infections that encompass an entire anatomical subunit such as the toe, forefoot, or midfoot. The technical aspects of a successful partial foot amputation parallel the principles of local flaps that focus on optimizing blood flow to the wound edge. Incisions should preferably be made along the angiosome boundaries so that each side of the incision or the created soft-tissue flaps has optimal blood flow.[46] Undermining tissue should be minimized as this may damage perforating vessel and affect cutaneous blood supply. The level of amputation should be higher if the bleeding at the skin edge is deemed inadequate. Creativity is the key in designing flaps for these amputations. Skeletal length should be preserved so that when there is inadequate plantar tissue, alternative dorsal-, medial-, or lateral-based skin flaps may be required for closure.

Proper technique for bone cuts ensures optimal healing and biomechanical function. Newly exposed cartilage during the amputation need not be addressed if it appears normal. However, all previously exposed cartilage at the base of the wound should be removed because it may be infected. Periosteal blood supply should be spared by making the osteotomy with minimal tissue dissection. Bone cuts should be made with an oscillating saw to avoid splintering the proximal bone. Any sharp or prominent edges on the osteotomy will interfere with ambulation and may result in recurrent ulceration, so the shape and contour of the osteotomy is important. Bone cuts should be angled in dorsal-distal to plantar-proximal direction, laterally in a medial-distal to lateral-proximal direction, and medially in a lateral-distal to medial-proximal.

Toe Amputations

Toe amputations are among the most commonly performed amputations. These may be performed at any level, at the phalangeal bone, phalangeal joints, or metatarsophalangeal joint; however, resultant foot biomechanical changes occur.[54] For example, proximal amputation of any of the central toes (second, third, or fourth) will result in medial drifting of the lateral toes and lateral drifting of the medial toes. Second, amputation of the hallux leaves the foot without adequate pushoff during the propulsive phase of gait, and prolongs the amount of time spent on the metatarsophalangeal (MTP) heads during gait cycle. Overcompensation by the flexors and intrinsic muscles can lead to claw toe deformity of the other toes and further increases the pressure on the metatarsal heads and distal phalangeal tips during gait. Third, the loss of the second toe leads to a hallux valgus deformity (bunion) because the hallux loses its lateral support.

Distal toe amputations require attention to the nail bed and tendon attachments. Great care should be taken to ensure complete removal of the nail bed matrix to avoid the later emergence of the residual nail plate. Attempts should be made to keep the proximal portion of the distal phalanx and thus preserve the attachments of the long flexors and extensors. The bone cuts should be performed with a power saw rather than a bone cutter to avoid cracking or splitting the proximal bone. As in all amputations, the bone should be cut at a level where the remaining bone is hard and bleeding and the marrow appears normal. Because the digital blood vessels run along either side of the flexor tendon, the toe can be closed with either side-to-side flaps or dorsal-plantar flaps. The latter flaps give the toe a smoother pushoff surface. The key is to ensure that the flap ends are bleeding and that there is no tension when the edges are

approximated. Again, bone length should always be sacrificed to achieve a tension-free closure. The flaps should be closed with interrupted monofilament suture and the dog-ears should be removed. Good skin eversion is the key to avoid poor healing and depressed scar with subsequent localized callus formation.

For more proximal toe amputations, one can either cut the phalanx or disarticulate the toe at the distal, proximal, or MTP joint. For the lesser toes, the preferred method of amputation is a partial amputation leaving enough of the proximal phalanx so that drifting of the toes on either side does not occur. A vertical or horizontal fish-mouth or tennis racket pattern incision may be used to excise the amputated part and close the amputation. However, sometimes these patterns are not usable because the goal is to preserve bone length with an adequate soft-tissue envelope for closure. The incision may have to be modified if the pattern of viable tissue does not fit within a standard incision pattern. In that circumstance, one adjusts the planned closure by removing just enough bone so that the unusual designed flap can be mobilized to cover the distal end of bone without tension. This flap is usually a medially- or laterally-based flap.

For hallux amputations, it is best to try to preserve the proximal centimeter of the proximal phalanx for biomechanical stability. By preserving this small portion of proximal phalanx, the functions of the plantar fascia, intrinsic muscles, and flexor hallucis brevis, as well as the plantar flexion of the first metatarsal are partially preserved.[55,56] This minimizes the increased transferred pressure that the second and third metatarsal head subsequently experiences during gait. Because of continued motion at the joint, the suture line can be difficult to heal, and it may be worthwhile to pin the joint temporarily to avoid this complication.

The hallux amputation skin closure must be durable enough for repetitive weight bearing. A plantar flap rotated superiorly provides the best surface for long-term durability especially if there is a toe filler built onto the orthotic. For the plantar flap to be more malleable and easier to inset, the flexor tendon and volar plate at the interphalangeal joint should be removed. This should be done carefully so that the digital arteries are not damaged in the process. Incidentally, if the entire hallux has to be amputated, there is no reason to remove the sesamoids as they tend to retract behind the head of the metatarsal. It is important to remove any dog-ears so that the final contour is as close to normal as possible (Fig. 7-3).

Ray Amputations

A ray amputation involves partial or complete removal of the metatarsal bones. Any questionable portion of the metatarsal bone should be resected to ensure complete removal of any diseased area. In addition, only

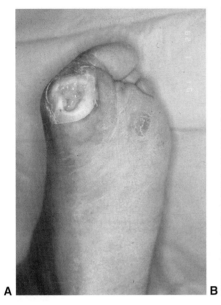

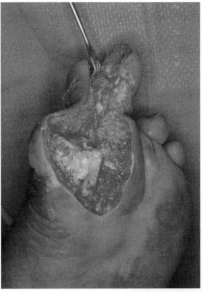

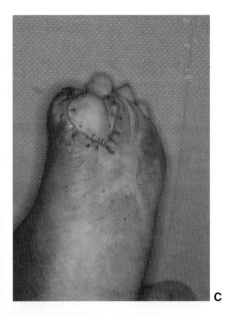

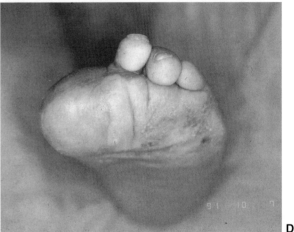

Figure 7-3 **A:** This patient presented with osteomyelitis of the first metatarsal head. **B:** The patient underwent operative debridements including resection of the first metatarsal head. The hallux was filleted. **C:** The filleted toe flap was rotated to close the defect. **D:** Postoperative, healed photograph. (From Attinger C, Venturi M, Kim K, et al. Maximizing length and optimizing biomechanics in foot amputations by avoiding cookbook recipes for amputation. *Semin Vasc Surg.* 2003;16: 44–66, with permission.)

enough should be resected to achieve an adequate soft-tissue envelope for closure of the wound. Filleting the distal toe can help in creating additional soft tissue for better distal coverage.

Preserving metatarsal length is crucial for skeletal stability. Preservation of the muscular attachments to the proximal metatarsal is important to minimize resulting pronation or supination abnormalities. The first and fifth rays are relatively independent of the other metatarsals and can be amputated and usually closed easily. The metatarsals of the central column (two, three, and four), however, act as a unit and removal of one or more disrupts that unit. When more than two metatarsal bones are involved, it is preferable to perform a panmetatarsal head resection if the toes are uninvolved or a transmetatarsal amputation if the toes are involved (Fig. 7-4).

First metatarsal ray resections should be approached via a medial incision along the glabrous junction between dorsal and plantar skin (Fig. 7-5). The cut should be triplanar and beveled so that the medial and

plantar sides are shorter than the lateral and dorsal sides. Great care should be taken to preserve the attachment of the tibialis anterior tendon. If the entire metatarsal has to be sacrificed and the anterior tibial tendon is normal, then it should be reattached to the medial cuneiform. Loss of the tibialis anterior will cause pronation of the foot and transfer of excessive pressure to the second metatarsal head that will eventually break down.

Fifth metatarsal ray resections should be approached via a lateral incision along the glabrous junction between dorsal and plantar skin (Fig. 7-6). The cut should be triplanar and beveled so that the lateral and plantar sides are shorter than the medial and dorsal sides. Great care should be taken to preserve that attachment of the peroneus brevis tendon. If the entire metatarsal has to be sacrificed and the peroneus brevis tendon is normal, then it should be reattached to the cuboid. Loss of the peroneus brevis will cause supination of the foot and the fourth metatarsal head will be overloaded and eventually break down.

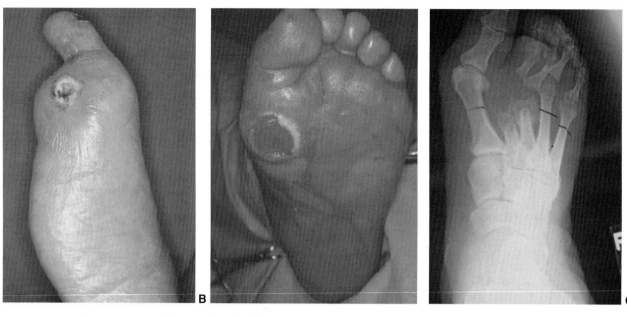

Figure 7-4 A: This patient presented with an ulcer over the second metatarsal head after ray amputations of the lateral three metatarsals. This placed abnormally high pressure on the remaining medial two metatarsal heads. **B:** This patient developed an ulcer over the first metatarsal head after resection of the second and third metatarsal heads. There was too much pressure over the first metatarsophalangeal head during ambulation. **C:** The solution is to perform a panmetatarsal head resection or a transmural-tarsal amputation. (From Attinger C, Venturi M, Kim K, et al. Maximizing length and optimizing biomechanics in foot amputations by avoiding cookbook recipes for amputation. *Semin Vasc Surg.* 2003;16:44–66, with permission.)

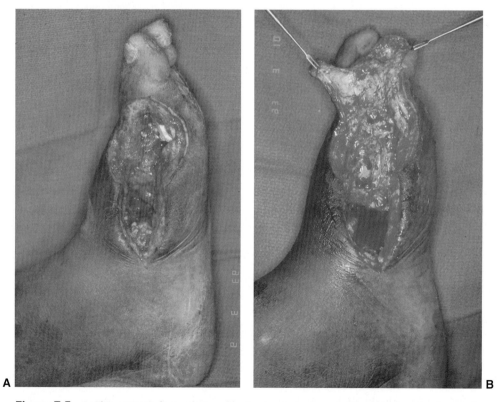

Figure 7-5 A: This patient's first metatarsal had extensive osteomyelitis, which was inadequately treated over a 9-month period. **B:** The foot was debrided and the hallux was filleted to create a flap to fill the medial forefoot.

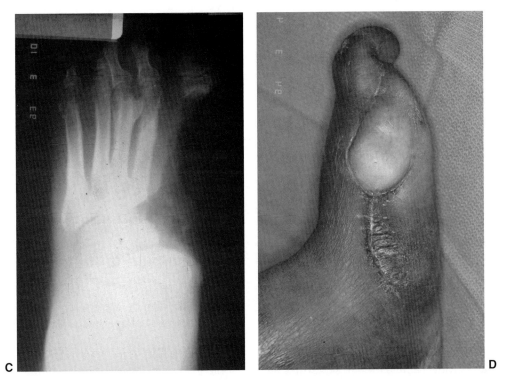

Figure 7-5 (*continued*) **C:** Postdebridement radiograph. **D:** The healed foot is shown. (From Attinger C, Venturi M, Kim K, et al. Maximizing length and optimizing biomechanics in foot amputations by avoiding cookbook recipes for amputation. *Semin Vasc Surg.* 2003;16:44–66, with permission.)

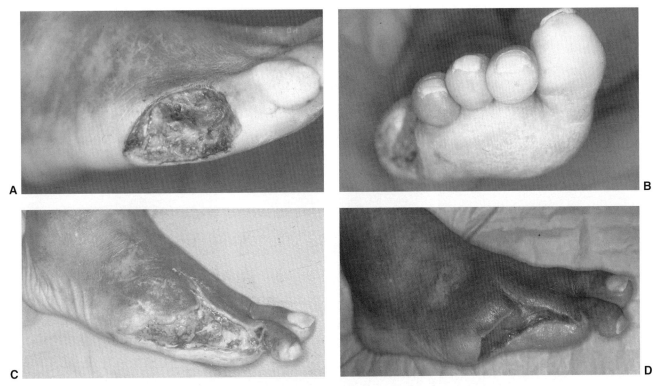

Figure 7-6   A: This is a renal failure, diabetic patient with gangrene and osteomyelitis of the fifth metatarasal head. **B:** The infection then progressed to the fourth and third toes. **C:** The entire area had to be debrided and the patient was placed on long-term intravenous antibiotics. **D:** Once the wound stabilized, the area was skin grafted. This foot is unstable with only two metatarsal heads and would have been more biomechanically stable if a formal transmetatarsal amputation was preformed instead. (From Attinger C, Venturi M, Kim K, et al. Maximizing length and optimizing biomechanics in foot amputations by avoiding cookbook recipes for amputation. *Semin Vasc Surg.* 2003;16:44–66, with permission.)

Central metatarsal ray amputations are best approached dorsally if the plantar tissue is unaffected. Distal ray amputations can be covered with filleted toes. Leaving the unattached toe intact will not prevent medial and lateral migration of the neighboring toes. In addition, a floppy toe will eventually ride dorsally and become an impediment to shoeing.

Panmetatarsal Amputations

If ulcers are under several metatarsal heads or if transfer lesions have occurred from one resected metatarsal head to a neighboring metatarsal, consideration should be given to performing a panmetatarsal head resection (Fig. 7-7). The benefit of the panmetatarsal amputation is preservation of the long flexors and extensors of the foot that prevent the foot from an equinovarus deformity. This deformity will result in the eventual breakdown over the lateral forefoot.

Following the panmetatarsal head amputation, the toes may migrate into a dorsiflexed position, but there is enough protective soft-tissue redundancy that this is not a problem (as long as the patient wears shoes with an adequate toe box). This operation has proved to be extremely successful in diabetics even though it is never listed as an option in texts on diabetic foot amputations.

The panmetatarsal amputation is performed via three dorsal incisions over the first, third, and fifth metatarsals. Great care is taken to preserve the proportional lengths of each metatarsal; i.e., the normal distal metatarsal head parabola is preserved, with the second metatarsal being the longest. The cut of the fifth metatarsal head should be triplanar and beveled so that the lateral and plantar side are shorter than the medial and dorsal side. The central metatarsal heads are beveled so that the plantar side is shorter than the dorsal side. The cut of the first metatarsal head should be triplanar and beveled so that the medial and plantar sides are shorter than the lateral and dorsal sides.

Transmetatarsal Amputation

If both the toes and the metatarsal heads are involved, the transmetatarsal amputation (TMA) is performed at the level of the metatarsal shafts (Fig. 7-8). There is no formula for closure because the goal is to preserve as much metatarsal length as possible (Fig. 7-9). This maximizes the amount of plantar tissue preserved and decreases the load per cm^2 that the foot experiences during weight bearing. It is ideal to create as large a plantar flap as possible so that the anterior portion of the foot is covered with plantar tissue. If there is missing tissue along the plantar foot, then the remaining normal plantar tissue can be rotated toward the defect to provide adequate coverage. In addition, when the lateral plantar tissue is missing, filleting the hallux can provide necessary plantar tissue to rotate laterally to close the wound. Filleting the hallux

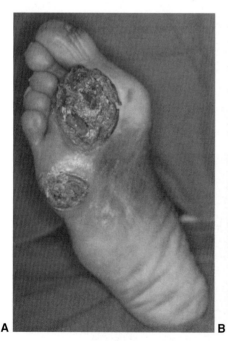
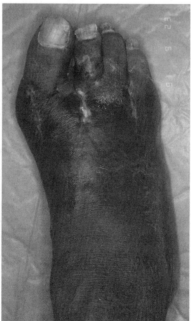
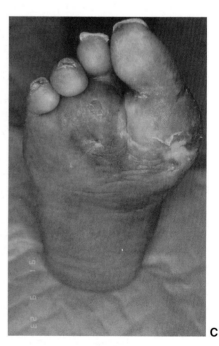

A   B   C

Figure 7-7   A: This renal failure, diabetic patient presented with chronic ulcers and osteomyelitis over most of his metatarsal heads. **B:** Dorsal incisions were used to perform a panmetatarsal head resection. **C:** The foot healed in 6 weeks. (From Attinger C, Venturi M, Kim K, et al. Maximizing length and optimizing biomechanics in foot amputations by avoiding cookbook recipes for amputation. *Semin Vasc Surg.* 2003;16:44–66, with permission.)

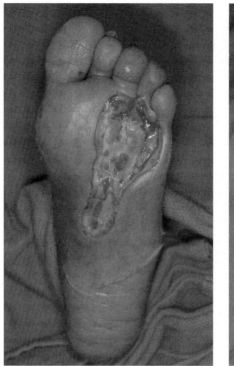
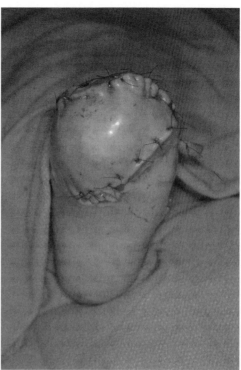

Figure 7-8   A: This patient presented with gangrene and osteomyelitis of his plantar midfoot and forefoot. The third, fourth, and fifth metatarsal heads had extensive osteomyelitis. **B:** A transmetatarsal amputation was preformed using medial tissue to cover the lateral metatarsals in order to preserve as much length as possible. (From Attinger C, Venturi M, Kim K, et al. Maximizing length and optimizing biomechanics in foot amputations by avoiding cookbook recipes for amputation. *Semin Vasc Surg.* 2003;16:44–66, with permission.)

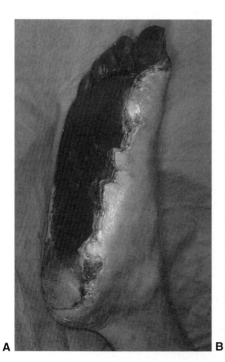
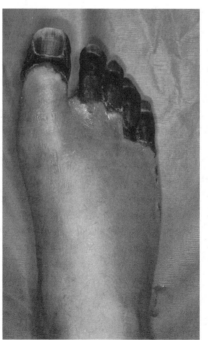
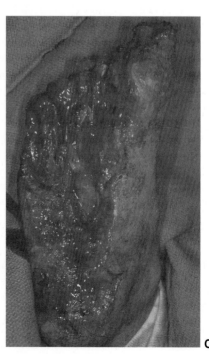

Figure 7-9   A, B: This renal failure, diabetic patient presented with gangrene of his entire plantar foot and osteomyelitis of all metatarsal heads. **C:** The area was debrided and the patient was treated with hyperbaric oxygen.

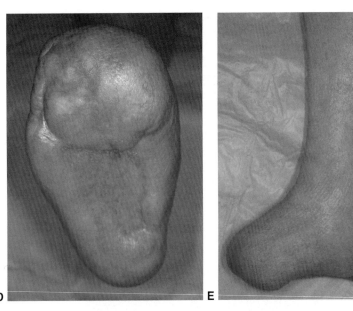

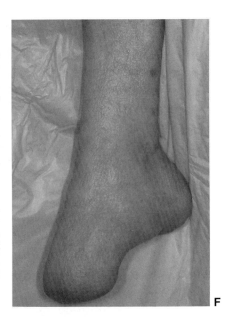

Figure 7-9 (*continued*) **D:** A transmetatarsal amputation was preformed at the midmetatarsal level with remaining dorsal tissue. **E, F:** The patient also underwent a percutaneous Achilles tendon–lengthening procedure. These photographs were taken 2 years after closure showing plantar and dorsiflexion. (From Attinger C, Venturi M, Kim K, et al. Maximizing length and optimizing biomechanics in foot amputations by avoiding cookbook recipes for amputation. *Semin Vasc Surg.* 2003;16:44–66, with permission.)

can also be useful in covering distal medial dorsal defects so that a minimum amount of length has to be sacrificed. In the interest of preserving length when there is insufficient plantar tissue to cover the anterior foot, a split-thickness skin graft over the distal end of the amputation is an excellent solution (Fig. 7-1).

The incision for the TMA is variable depending on the available local tissue. The dorsal incision is made at the base of the proximal phalanges. The plantar incision is made along the proximal digital crease, preserving as much plantar tissue as possible. The incisions are extended proximally along the glabrous junction over the first and fifth metatarsal heads. The dorsal flap is then elevated off the metatarsal heads. The metatarsal heads are then cut in such a way as to recreate the normal metatarsal head arcade. The cut of the fifth metatarsal head should be triplanar and beveled so that the lateral and plantar sides are shorter than the medial and dorsal sides. The central metatarsal heads are beveled so that the plantar side is shorter that the dorsal side. The cut of the first metatarsal head should be triplanar and beveled so that the medial and plantar sides are shorter than the lateral and dorsal sides. If there is so little soft tissue remaining that the metatarsals have to be cut close to their base, great care should be taken to preserve the proximal perforators at the Lisfranc joint to optimize distal blood flow and prevent flap necrosis.

Once the bony cuts are made and the surface irrigated to remove any bone debris, the plantar flap is brought up to cover as much of the stump as possible. To increase the flexibility of the plantar flap, the digital flexors and

the metatarsalphalangeal volar plates are removed. The incision is closed without any deep sutures to minimize the risk of subsequent infection. Simple interrupted vertical mattress sutures with monofilament suture are all that is required. All dog-ears should be trimmed so that the distal amputation is ideally shaped. The foot is then dressed and splinted in neutral position. The patient should be non–weight-bearing until the wound is completely healed (usually 4 to 6 weeks). Orthotics and molded shoes should then be ordered.

The major complication of the transmetatarsal amputation is the resultant equinovarus deformity that develops from the loss of the digital extensors.[57] This leaves the tendo-Achilles complex and anterior tibial tendon unopposed, which will lead to eventual breakdown under the lateral fifth metatarsal (Fig. 7-10). To avoid this, the flexors and extensors of the lateral fourth and fifth toes should each be tenodesed together while the foot is in the neutral position. In those feet in which tenodesis is not possible (infected tendon) or in which there is already an equinovarus deformity, a percutaneous Achilles tendon–lengthening procedure should be performed.[58] The routine performance of Achilles tendon lengthening and/or tenodesis has reduced our transmetatarsal reulceration rate from 50% to 4%.

Lisfranc Amputation

The Lisfranc amputation is the most proximal forefoot amputation, performed at the tarsalmetatarsal joint,

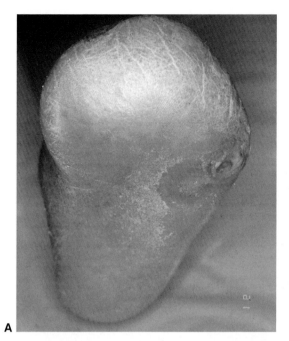
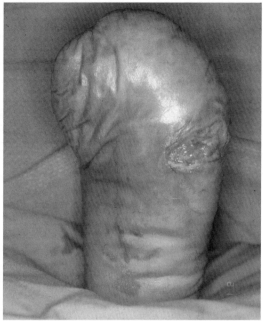

A

B

Figure 7-10 A, B: Both of these patients underwent transmetatarsal amputations and suffered recurrent breakdown over the remaining portion of the fifth metatarsal due to the biomechanical result of losing the extensors. This complication should be avoided by tenodesing the flexor and extensor tendons of the fourth and fifth toes or lengthening the Achilles tendon. (From Attinger C, Venturi M, Kim K, et al. Maximizing length and optimizing biomechanics in foot amputations by avoiding cookbook recipes for amputation. *Semin Vasc Surg.* 2003;16:44–66, with permission.)

removing all of the metatarsal bones. Amputation at this level is indicated if there is skeletal instability and/or inadequate soft tissue to cover a short TMA. Preservation of the most proximal portion of the second metatarsal (that acts as a keystone stabilizer of the midfoot) should be attempted. In addition, it is also important to retain the most proximal first and fifth metatarsals so that the respective tibialis anterior, peroneus brevis, and tertius attachments are preserved. This will help prevent the nearly inevitable equinovalgus or equinovarus deformities that develop from this amputation. Unfortunately, if a short amputation is performed, those tendons are usually involved and have to be resected. However, if they are uninvolved, they should be reattached to the medial cuneiform (anterior tibial tendon) and cuboid (peroneus brevis). If only the anterior tibialis tendon is intact, it can be divided so that one part can be attached to the cuboid to restore balance.

Again, it is important to create as large a plantar flap as possible to cover the anterior portion of the amputation because plantar tissue adds to the amputation's long-term viability (Fig. 7-11). Because the connections between the dorsal and plantar circulation are divided, one must ensure that there is sufficient dorsal and plantar flow for both the dorsal and plantar flaps to survive. In order to obtain better adherence of the soft tissue to the underlying bone, it is important to shave off all of the exposed cartilage with a sagital saw. The

flap is closed with simple interrupted vertical mattress sutures using monofilament suture. All dog-ears are trimmed so that the amputation is ideally shaped for shoe wear (Fig. 7-12).

While the equinovarus deformity is a consideration in the TMA, more proximal amputations such as the Lisfranc lead to an even further loss of stability, inevitable equinovarus deformity, and the development of ulcers. Adequate tendon transfers, whenever possible, are imperative to prevent this deformity.[59] If this is not possible, a 1- to 2-cm piece of the Achilles tendon should be resected to help rebalance the foot. The foot must be splinted in neutral postoperatively. When healed, a high-top molded shoe that provides added ankle stability has to be made. A final option to preventing equinovarus deformity and stabilizing the ankle is to place a calcaneal-tibial nail when the amputation has healed (Fig. 7-13).

Chopart Amputation

More proximal than the Lisfranc joint, the Chopart joint defines the articulation of the talus and calcaneus with the tarsal bones. The Chopart amputation is only indicated when disease involves the tarsal bones or joints, or there is inadequate soft tissue and skeletal stability for a more distal amputation. The skin incision is made on the dorsal aspect of the foot extending from the navicular tubercle to the midline of the cuboid, and all tissue is dissected to the talonavicular

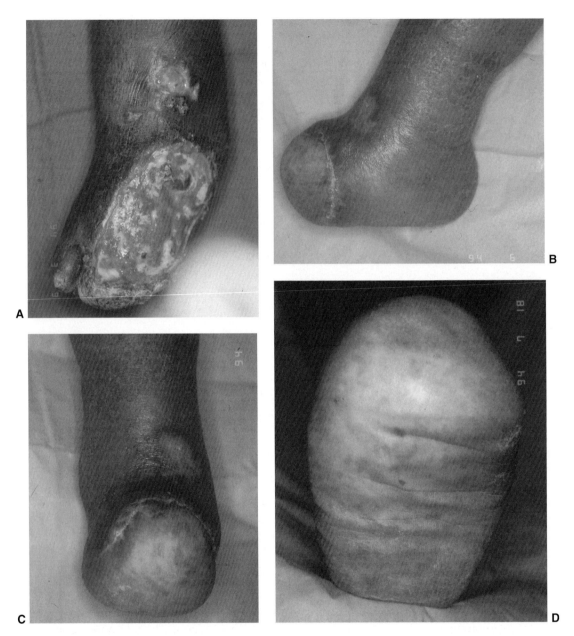

Figure 7-11 **A:** This poorly controlled diabetic patient presented with gas gangrene and osteomyelitis of his medial forefoot. He underwent operative debridements, removing the first and second necrotic metatarsals. **B, C:** The lateral forefoot was then filleted and deboned and the soft tissue was used to cover the cuneiforms and cuboid bones. **D:** There was excellent distal and plantar surface created by this flap. (From Attinger C, Venturi M, Kim K, et al. Maximizing length and optimizing biomechanics in foot amputations by avoiding cookbook recipes for amputation. *Semin Vasc Surg.* 2003;16:44–66, with permission.)

and calcaneocuboid joints. The talonavicular and calcaneocuboid joints are then separated. At this point, any bony prominences and the cartilaginous surfaces of the talus and calcaneus are removed to create a smooth adherent surface. The plantar skin flap is developed by removing the tarsal and metatarsal bones without damaging the underlying blood flow. The plantar flap is then rotated superiorly and sewn into the dorsal tissue.

Because the tissue loss that necessitates the use of a Chopart amputation is typically extensive, the standard dorsal and plantar flaps cannot always be designed. One should be ready to modify both the dorsal and plantar flaps to cover the exposed anterior rear foot. The keys to having enough available tissue to close the wound are rotating the available plantar flap medially or laterally, and preserving as much length to the dorsal flap as possible (Fig. 7-14). The flaps are

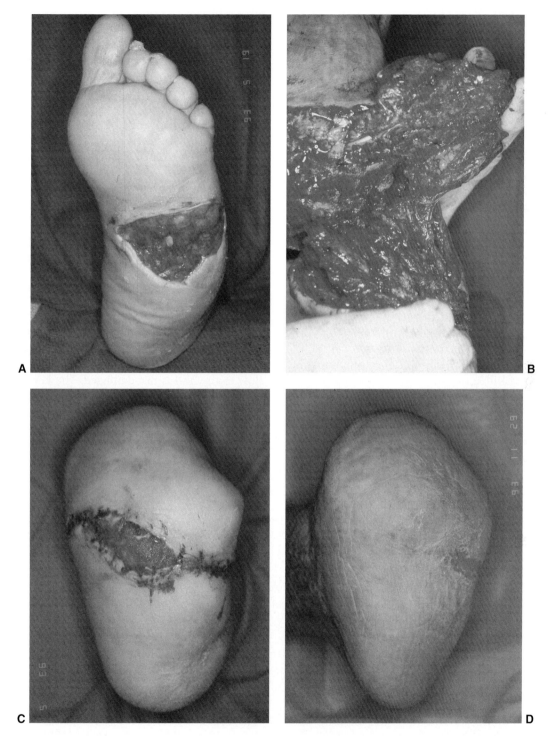

Figure 7-12   A: This morbidly obese diabetic man presented with an infected Charcot Lisfranc joint. The infected bone was removed, and the patient was treated conservatively until the infection resolved. **B:** At the time of reconstruction, the forefoot was filleted and deboned and then closed as a Lisfranc amputation. **C:** On the fourth postoperative day, the wound dehisced when the patient walked on his foot. **D, E:** The wound was washed out and resutured in the operating room and the patient went on to heal. (From Attinger C, Venturi M, Kim K, et al. Maximizing length and optimizing biomechanics in foot amputations by avoiding cookbook recipes for amputation. *Semin Vasc Surg.* 2003;16:44–66, with permission.)

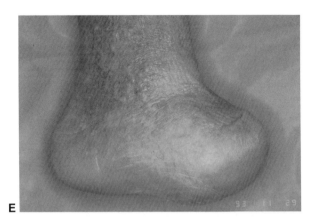

Figure 7-12 (continued)

then shaped so that there is no redundancy or dog-ears that could complicate the design of appropriate shoe wear.

If possible, the tibialis anterior tendon, at the antero-lateral portion of the talus, should be identified and preserved, again, to prevent the equinus deformity.[59,60] Similar to the Lisfranc, an Achilles tenectomy must be preformed to stabilize the amputated foot in a neutral position. Alternatively, a calcaneal-tibial nail can be placed to fuse the ankle in neutral after the amputation has healed. Again, the patient will need a high-top shoe that stabilizes the ankle and gives adequate anterior and lateral support.

Syme Amputation

The Syme amputation is essentially an ankle disarticulation and is contraindicated if the heel is ulcerated.[61,62] A dorsal incision is usually marked at the level of each malleoli and then extends in a plantar direction beneath the heel pad. The ligaments of the ankle are divided, and the periosteum of the talus and calcaneus are stripped as the foot is disarticulated from the tibia. The medial and lateral malleoli are removed with a saw, taking care not to thin the tibia. All tendons are removed, and plantar and anterior tibial neurovascular bundles should be cut under tension and allowed to retract to prevent later neuroma formation. The plantar fascia of the empty heel pad is sutured to the extensor retinaculum prior to skin closure. Alternatively, holes can be drilled to the anterior tibia and the fat pad can be sutured to it (Fig. 7-15).

At closure, there are usually large dog-ears on either side of the amputation that make the amputation bulky and difficult for the fit of shoes. The dog-ears can be revised at the time of surgery provided that the blood flow to the heel is not damaged. The key is to preserve both the calcaneal branches of the posterior tibial artery and peroneal artery for adequate heel perfusion. If there is any question about jeopardizing the heel, the correction of the dog-ears can be performed when the amputation has healed.

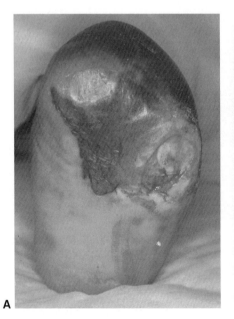
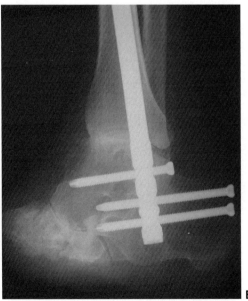

Figure 7-13   **A:** This patient underwent a Lisfranc amputation with subsequent equinovarus deformity because the Achilles tendon was not addressed. In addition, the peroneal attachments to the lateral fifth metatarsal were removed and the anterior tibial tendon was not divided and reattached to the cuboid. **B:** The ankle had to be fused in neutral using a calcaneal-tibial nail. (From Attinger C, Venturi M, Kim K, et al. Maximizing length and optimizing biomechanics in foot amputations by avoiding cookbook recipes for amputation. *Semin Vasc Surg.* 2003;16:44–66, with permission.)

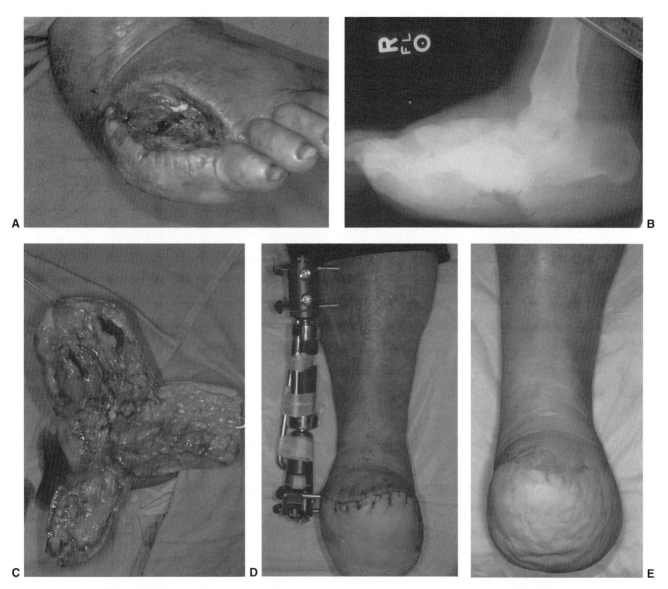

Figure 7-14 A, B: This obese diabetic patient developed Charcot osteomyelitis in his midfoot. **C:** The forefoot and midfoot bones were removed, and three flaps were created. **D:** The foot reconstruction was performed by assembling these three flaps. The foot was stabilized with an external fixation device to prevent equinovarus deformity. **E, F:** Photographs taken 2 years after closure.

Although this amputation is advocated as an alternative to below-knee amputation, its effectiveness is solely determined by the prosthetist's ability to design an adequate prosthesis. Because the amputation is often poorly designed and too bulky, many prosthetists in the United States are uncomfortable with the fitting of this amputation. However, the Syme amputation, when well performed, is an excellent amputation because it minimizes the energy of ambulation and it allows the patient to ambulate for short distances without having to put on a prosthesis.

CONCLUSION

In summary, debridement, local flaps, pedicled muscle flaps, free flaps, and partial amputations of the foot all share similar reconstructive principles. Careful handling of tissue, attention to blood supply, and a constant focus on function determines the success of these operations. Prior to considering reconstruction, the wound must be prepared surgically with thorough debridement to ensure the success of these techniques. Mastering these techniques empowers the surgeon to avoid major leg amputations for foot pathology.

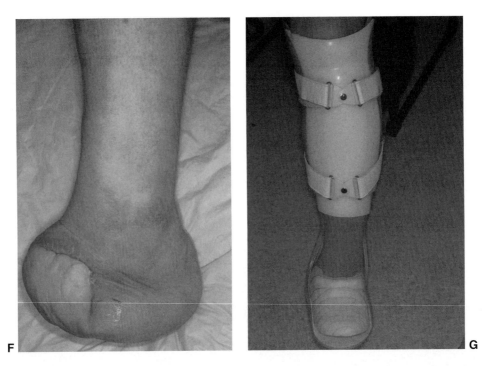

Figure 7-14 *(continued)* **G:** The patient wears a patellar weight-bearing brace to protect the Chopart amputation. (From Attinger C, Venturi M, Kim K, et al. Maximizing length and optimizing biomechanics in foot amputations by avoiding cookbook recipes for amputation. *Semin Vasc Surg.* 2003;16:44–66, with permission.)

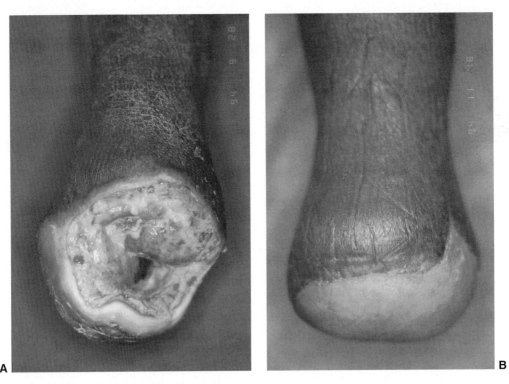

Figure 7-15 **A:** This patient presented with an open incomplete Syme amputation in which a portion of the talus was remaining. **B:** The amputation was completed and closed without dog-ears so that the patient could wear a patellar weight-bearing brace. (From Attinger C, Venturi M, Kim K, et al. Maximizing length and optimizing biomechanics in foot amputations by avoiding cookbook recipes for amputation. *Semin Vasc Surg.* 2003;16:44–66, with permission.)

REFERENCES

1. Edmonson AS, Crenshaw AH, eds. *Campbell's orthopedics.* 6th ed. St. Louis, Mo: CV Mosby; 1980.

2. Evarts CM. *Surgery of the muskuloskeletal system.* 2nd ed. New York, NY: Churchill Livingstone; 1990.

3. Attinger C, Venturi M, Kim K, et al. Maximizing length and optimizing biomechanics in foot amputations by avoiding cookbook recipes for amputation. *Semin Vasc Surg.* 2003;16:44–66.

4. Grant WP, Sullivan R, Sonenshine DE, et al. Electron microscopic investigation of the effects of diabetes mellitus on the Achilles tendon. *J Foot Ankle Surg.* 1997;36:272–278.

5. Armstrong DG, Stacpoole-Shea S, Nguyen H, et al. Lengthening of the Achilles tendon in diabetic patients who are at high risk for ulceration of the foot. *J Bone Joint Surg.* 1999;81-A:535–538.

6. Lin SS, Lee TH, Wapner KL. Plantar forefoot ulceration with equinus deformity of the ankle in diabetic patients: the effect of tendo-Achilles lengthening and total contact casting. *Orthop.* 1996;19: 465–475.

7. Mueller MJ, Sinacore DR, Hastings MK, et al. Effect of Achilles tendon lengthening on neuropathic plantar ulcers. A randomized clinical trial. *J Bone Joint Surg.* 2003;85a:1436.

8. Robson MC, Stenberg BD, Heffers JP. Wound healing alterations caused by infection. *Clin Plast Surg.* 1990;17:485–492.

9. Steed DL, Donohoe D, Webster MW, et al Effect of extensive debridement and treatment on the healing of diabetic foot ulcers. *J Am Coll Surg.* 1996;183:61–64.

10. Argenta LC, Morykwas MJ. Vacuum-assisted closure: a new method for wound control and treatment: clinical experience. *Ann Plast Surg.* 1997;38:563–576.

11. Morykwas MJ, Argenta LC, Shelton-Brown EI, et al. Vacuum assisted closure: a new method for wound control and treatment: animal studies and basic foundation. *Ann Plast Surg.* 1997;38: 553–562.

12. Grayson ML, Gibbons GW, Balogh K, et al. Probing to bone in infected pedal ulcers: a clinical sign of osteomyelitis in diabetic patients. *JAMA.* 1995;273:721–723.

13. Attinger CE, Cooper P, Blume P. Vascular anatomy of the foot and ankle. *Op Tech Plast Reconstr Surg.* 1997;4:183–198.

14. Edgerton MT. *The art of surgical technique.* Baltimore, Md: Williams & Wilkins; 1988.

15. Rodeheaver GT, Pettry D, Thacker JG, et al. Wound cleansing by high pressure irrigation. *Surg Gynecol Obstet.* l975;141:357–362.

16. Bulan EJ. personal communication, 1999.

17. Tredget EE, Shankowsky HA, Goeneveld A, et al A matched-pair, randomized study evaluating the efficacy and safety of Acticoat silver coated dressing for treatment of burn wounds. *J Burn Care Rehabil.* 1998;19:531–537.

18. Yin HQ, Langford R, Burrell RE. Comparative evaluation of the antimicrobial activity of Acticoat antimicrobial dressing. *J Burn Care Rehabil.* 1999;20:195–200.

19. Vasquez JE, Walker ES, Franzus BW, et al. The epidemiology of mupirocin resistance among methicillin-resistant Staphylococcus aureus at a Veterans' Affairs hospital. *Infect Control Hosp Epidemiol.* 2000;21:459–464.

20. Gustilo RB, Anderson JT. Prevention of infection in the treatment of 1025 open fractures of long bones. *J Bone Joint Surg.* l976;58A: 453–458.

21. Patzakis MJ, Wilkins J, Moore TM. The use of antibiotics in open tibial fractures. *Clin Orthop Rel Res.* 1983;178:31–35.

22. Byrd HS, Spicer TE, Cierny G III. Management of open tibial fractures. *Plast Reconstr Surg.* l985;76:719.

23. Brummelkamp WD, Hogendijk J, Boerema I. Treatment of anaerobic infections (clostridial myositis) by drenching the tissues with oxygen under high pressure. *Surgery.* 1961;49:299.

24. Rhodeheaver GT. Wound cleansing, wound irrigation, and wound disinfection. In: Krasner K, Kkane D, eds. *Chronic wound care: a clinical source book for health professionals.* 2nd ed. Wayne, Pa: Health Management Publications; 1997:97–108.

25. Cupps T, et al. The importance of identifying and treating coexisting pro-coagulant states in patients with recalcitrant inflammatory skin ulcers and underlying autoimmune disease [Abstract]., San Fransisco, Calif: American College of Rheumatology; 2001.

26. Hart GB, Strauss MB. Hyperbaric oxygen in management of radiation injury. In: Schmutz J, ed. *Proceedings 1st Swiss symposium on hyperbaric medicine.* Basel, Switzerland: Stiftung fur Hyperbare Medizin; 1986:31–35.

27. Attinger CE, Bulan EJ. Debridement the key initial first step in wound healing. *Foot Ankle Clin N Am.* 2001;6:627–660.

28. Heimbachs DM, Engrave L. *Surgical management of the burn wound.* New York, NY: Raven Press; 1985.

29. Krizek TJ, Robson MC. The evolution of quantitative bacteriology in wound management. *Am J Surg.* 1975;130:579–584.

30. Robson MC, Heggers JP. Delayed wound closure based on bacterial counts. *J Surg Oncol.* 1970;2:379–383.

31. Haimowitz JE, Margolis DJ. Moist wound healing In: Krasner D, Kane D, eds. *Chronic wound care: a clinical source book for health care professionals.* 2nd ed. Wayne, Pa: Health Management Publications, Inc; 1997:49–56.

32. Daltrey DC, Rhodes B, Chattwood JG. Investigations into microbial flora of healing and non-healing decubitus ulcers. *J Clin Pathol.* 1981;34:701–705.

33. Vilijanto J. Disinfection of surgical wounds without inhibition of normal wound healing. *Arch Surg.* 1980;115:253–256.

34. Kannon GA, Garret AB. Moist wound healing with occlusive dressing: a clinical review. *Dermatol Surg.* 1995;21:583–590.

35. Mertz PM, Ovington LG. Wound healing microbiology. *Dermatol Clin.* 1993;11:739–747.

36. Hinman CD, Mailbach H. Effect of air exposure and occlusion on experimental human skin wounds. *Nature.* 1962;200:377–378.

37. Alvarez OM, Hefton JM, Eaglstein WH. Healing wounds: occlusion or exposure. *Infect Surg.* 1984;3:173–181.

38. Alvarez OM, Mertz PM, Eaglstein WH. The effect of occlusive dressings on collagen sythesis and re-epithelialization in superficial wounds. *J Surg Res.* 1983;35:142–148.

39. Mertz PM, Davis SC, Oliveira-Gandia M, et al. The wound environment: implications from research studies for healing and infection In: Krasner D, Kane D, eds. *Chronic wound care: a clinical source book for health care professionals.* 2nd ed. Wayne, Pa: Health Management Publications, Inc; 1997:57–63.

40. Linsky CB, Rovee DT, Dow T. Effects of dressings on wound inflammation and scar tissue. In: Hildick-Smith G, ed. *The surgical wound.* Philadelphia, Pa: Lea & Feibiger; 1981:191–205.

41. Falanga V. Occlusive wound dressings. Why, when, which? *Arch Derm.* 1988;124:872–877.

42. Bromberg BE, Song IC, Mohn MP. The use of pigskin as a temporary biological dressing. *Plast Reconstr Surg.* 1965;36:80.

43. Falanga V, Margolis D, Alvarez O, et al. Rapid healing of venous ulcers and lack of clinical rejection with an allogeneic cultured human skin equivalent. *Arch Dermato.* 1998;134:293–300.

44. Veves A, Falanga V, Armstrong DG. Graftskin, a human skin equivalent, is effective in the management of non-infected neuropathic diabetic foot ulcers. *Diabetes Care.* 2001;24:290–295.

45. Fisher DF Jr, Clagett GP, Fry RE, et al. One-stage versus two-stage amputation for wet gangrene of the lower extremity: a randomized study. *J Vasc Surg.* 1988;8:428–433.

46. Attinger CE, Cooper P, Blume P, et al. The safest surgical incisions and amputations using the angiosome concept and Doppler on arterial-arterial connections of the foot and ankle. *Foot Ankle Clin North Am.* 2001;6:745–799.

47. Banis JC. Glabrous Skin Grafts for plantar defects. *Foot Ankle Clin.* 2001;6:827.

48. Scherer LA, Shiver S, Chang M, et al. The vacuum assisted closure device: a method of securing skin grafts and improving graft survival. *Arch Surg.* 2002;137:930–934.

49. Jeschke MG, Rose C, Angele P, et al. Development of new reconstructive techniques: use of integra in combination with fibrin Glue and negative–pressure therapy for reconstruction of acute and chronic wounds. *Plast Reconstr Surg.* 2004;113:525–530.

50. Paragas LK, Attinger CE, Blume PA. Local flaps. *Clin Podiatr Med Surg.* 2000;17:267.

51. Attinger CE, Ducik I, Zelen C. The use of local muscle flaps in foot and ankle reconstruction. *Clin Podiatr Med Surg.* 2000;17:681–711.

52. Mathes SJ, Nahai F. Reconstructive surgery: principles, anatomy and technique. Churchill Livingstone; 1997.

53. Attinger CE, Colen L. The role of microsurgical free flaps in foot and ankle surgery. *Clin Podiatr Med Surg.* 2000;17:649.

54. Funk C, Young G. Subtotal pedal amputations: biomechanical and intra-operative considerations. *JAPMA.* 2001;91:6.

55. Bowker JH. Partial foot amputations and disarticulations. *Foot Ankle.* 1997;2:153.

56. Mann RA, Poppen NK, O'Konski M. Amputation of the great toe: a clinical and biomechanical study. *Clin Ortho Relat Res.* 1998; 226:192.

57. Chrzan JS, Giurini JM, Hurchik JM. A biomechanical model for the transmetatarsal amputation. *JAPMA.* 1993;83:82.

58. Barry DC, Sabacinski KA, Habershaw GM, et al. Tendo Achillis procedures for chronic ulcerations in diabetic patients with transmetatarsal amputations. *JAPMA.* 1993;83:97.

59. Reyzelman AM, Hadi S, Armstrong DG. Limb salvage with Chopart's amputation and tendon balancing. *JAPMA.* 1999; 89:100.

60. Letts M, Pyper A. The modified Chopart's amputation. *Clin Ortho Relat Res.* 1990;256:44.

61. Harris RI. Syme's amputation: the technical details essential for success. *J Bone Joint Surg.* 1956;38B:614–632.

62. Gaine WJ, McCreath SW. Syme's amputation revisited: a review of 46 cases. *J Bone Joint Surg.* 1956;78B:461–467.

Angiosomes of the Foot and Angiosome-Dependent Healing

8

Christopher E. Attinger   *Karen Kim Evans*   *Ali Mesbahi*

Knowledge of vascular anatomy and an understanding of the dynamic nature of the vasculature is essential to the success of any planned surgical procedure. The angiosome principle was defined by Ian Taylor's anatomic study that divides the body into individual angiosomes: Three-dimensional blocks of tissue fed by "source" arteries. The foot and ankle is composed of five such distinct angiosomes. As in other parts of the body, the main arteries of the foot and ankle have direct arterial–arterial connections that allow alternative routes of blood flow to develop if the direct route is disrupted or compromised.

An understanding of the angiosome principles and detailed vascular anatomy provides a road map for planning safe incisions that preserve blood flow for the surgical wound to heal. This enables the surgeon to better predict whether a given amputation will heal or which pedicled flap can successfully be harvested. Last, this knowledge should help guide the vascular surgeon in choosing bypass procedures that have the best chance of healing existent ischemic ulcers.

ANGIOSOMES OF THE FOOT AND ANKLE

Ian Taylor expanded on the work of previous anatomists to further our understanding of muscle and skin vascular anatomy in his landmark paper on angiosomes.[1–9] He defined an angiosome as an anatomic unit of tissue (which has skin, subcutaneous tissue, fascia, muscle, and bone) fed by a source artery (Fig. 8-1). He defined at least 40 angiosomes in the body, including five in the foot and ankle.[10] Adjacent angiosomes are bordered by choke vessels, which link neighboring angiosomes to one another and demark the border of each angiosome.[11,12] In addition, these choke vessels are important safety irrigation conduits that allow a given angiosome to provide blood flow to an adjacent angiosome if a source artery is damaged.

The choke vessel system links each angiosome to one another. A unified network is created so that one source artery can provide blood flow to multiple angiosomes beyond its immediate border. Occluding or interrupting one source artery surgically manipulates the system so that blood will eventually be forced to flow through the neighboring choke vessels. This is one explanation of the "delay phenomenon," and is best demonstrated by Figure 8-2.[13,14] While the choke vessels are small interconnections, there are also larger arterial–arterial connections and collaterals that can allow blood flow to more immediately bypass local obstructions.

The five angiosomes of the foot and ankle originate from the three main arteries in the lower extremity. The

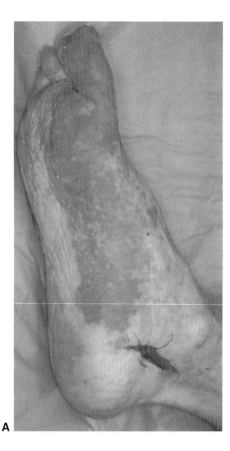

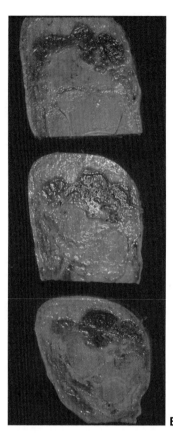

Figure 8-1 A: The angiosome supplied by the medial plantar artery is shown here in an injected cadaver specimen. In this case, the angiosome also includes the hallux. Due to normal vascular anatomic variations, the hallux can also be part of the angiosome supplied by the first dorsal metatarsal artery (FDMA) and/or the lateral plantar artery. **B:** Note that the angiosome is three-dimensional and includes the skin, underlying fascia, muscle, and bone. (From Attinger CE, Cooper P, Blume P, et al. The safest surgical incision and amputations applying the angiosomes principle and using the Doppler to assess the arterial–arterial connections of the foot and ankle. *Foot Ankle Clin North Am.* 2001;6:745–801, with permission.)

A

B

posterior tibial artery supplies the sole of the foot, the anterior tibial artery feeds the dorsum of the foot, and the peroneal artery supplies the lateral supramalleolar area and the heel. More specifically, the calcaneal branch, the medial plantar branch, and the lateral plantar branch, all branches of the posterior tibial artery, supply the sole of the foot. The peroneal artery has the anterior perforating branch (which supplies the lateral anterior upper ankle) and a calcaneal branch (which supplies the plantar heel). The anterior tibial artery supplies the anterior ankle and then becomes the dorsalis pedis artery that supplies the dorsum of the foot. Detailed descriptions of the vascular anatomy and angiosomes of the lower leg, foot, and ankle have been thoroughly illustrated elsewhere.[15–18]

Angiosomes from the Posterior Tibial Artery: The Calcaneal Artery, the Medial Plantar Artery, and the Lateral Plantar Artery

In the leg, the posterior tibial artery supplies the medial lower leg starting from the anterior border of the tibia and moving posteriorly to the medial half of the calf along the central raphe of the Achilles tendon (Fig. 8-3). There are smaller perforator arteries along the course of

the posterior tibial artery that perforate through the flexor digitorum longus (FDL) and/or soleus to supply the overlying skin. In addition, there are smaller serial branches to the deep flexor muscles, the medial half of the soleus muscle, and the Achilles tendon.[16,18]

In the foot, the posterior tibial artery gives off the posterior medial malleolar branch at the medial malleolus. The posterior medial malleolar branch joins the anterior medial malleolar branch from the dorsalis pedis artery, giving rise to an important interconnection between the posterior tibial artery and the anterior tibial artery. This system supplies the medial malleolar area. At the same level, the medial calcaneal artery branches off of the posterior tibial artery and arborizes into multiple branches that travel in a coronal direction to supply the heel. The medial calcaneal artery's angiosome boundary includes the entire plantar heel and extends from the posteromedial heel to the glabrous junction of the lateral posterior and plantar heel (Fig. 8-4).[19]

The posterior tibial artery then enters the calcaneal canal underneath the flexor retinaculum and bifurcates into the medial and lateral plantar arteries at the level of the transverse septum between the abductor hallucis longus and the flexor digitorum brevis (FDB) muscles. The medial plantar artery's angiosome encompasses

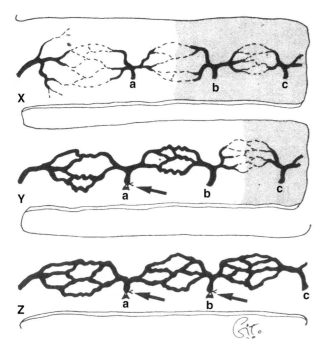

Figure 8-2 Choke vessels mark the boundary of any angiosome depicted in dotted lines. The dynamic role of choke vessels as the boundary between adjacent angiosomes is best demonstrated by considering the delay phenomenon. In the **top** drawing, artery X has the potential to immediately supply blood to the adjacent territory (fed by artery a) via the open choke vessels between them, if artery a loses its blood supply. In the **middle** panel, the vessel a has been tied off. In the ensuing 72 hours, the choke vessels linking the angiosome a to angiosome b on opposite sides have opened up. The flap has been delayed so that artery X's blood flow (which is artery Y in the **middle** panel) can now support the territory once fed by artery a and has the potential also to supply the angiosome fed by artery b. In the **bottom** panel, the reach of artery X (now named artery Z) has been further extended because now artery b has been tied off and an additional 72 hours have passed. This sequential delay (tying off artery a and then artery b) allows artery X to carry the territories fed by artery a, artery b, and artery c because the choke vessels have had time to open up. (From Taylor GI, Corlett RJ, Caddy CM, et al. An anatomic review of the delay phenomenon: II. Clinical applications. *Plast Reconstr Surg.* 1992;89:408, with permission.)

the instep (Fig. 8-1). Its boundaries are as follows: Posteriorly, the anteromedial edge of the plantar heel; laterally, the midline of the plantar midfoot; distally, the posterior edge of the plantar forefoot; and medially, an arc 2 to 3 cm above the glabrous junction, with its highest point being the anterior border of the navicular-cuneiform joint. The distal border can vary depending on anatomic variation and can extend to include the hallux as seen in Figure 8-1.

It is important to understand the route of the medial plantar artery because the course defines how the angiosome boundaries are formed. The medial plantar artery gives off two main branches, the superficial and the deep branch (Fig. 8-5). The superficial branch of the medial plantar artery travels obliquely up to the navicular-cuneiform joint, then along the superior

border of the cuneiform and the first metatarsal bone before descending to the medial plantar aspect of the distal metatarsal. Interconnections with the anterior tibial tree exist, as cutaneous branches connect proximally with medial cutaneous branches from the dorsalis pedis artery and distally with branches of the first dorsal metatarsal artery (FDMA). The artery then extends plantarly and laterally where it joins with the deep branch of the medial plantar artery and the first plantar metatarsal (a branch of the lateral plantar artery).

The second major branch of the medial plantar artery, the deep branch, travels deep and along the medial intramuscular septum between the abductor hallucis muscle (AHB) and the FDB. Perforating branches supply the medial sole of the foot. At the neck of the first metatarsal, it passes underneath the flexor tendons and anastomoses with the first plantar metatarsal artery and/or the distal lateral plantar artery.

The lateral plantar artery's angiosome includes the lateral plantar surface as well as the plantar forefoot (Fig. 8-6). The borders are as follows: Posteriorly, the anterior-lateral edge of the plantar heel; medially, the central raphe in the plantar midfoot; laterally, the glabrous junction between the lateral dorsum of the foot and plantar surface of the foot; and medially, the glabrous juncture between the medial plantar forefoot and medial distal dorsal forefoot (Fig. 8-4). The distal border includes the entire plantar forefoot. Note that while the hallux is usually part of the lateral plantar angiosome, it can also be part of the medial plantar artery angiosome or the dorsalis pedis angiosome.

Again, the course of the lateral plantar artery is descriptive of the angiosome's boundaries. This artery enters the middle compartment of the foot where it travels obliquely between the FDB muscle and the quadratus plantae muscle towards the base of the fifth metatarsal. Then, it travels distal to the proximal fifth metatarsal underneath the flexor digiti minimi muscle and turns medially where it crosses the proximal (two, three, and four) metatarsals. It finally anastomoses with the perforating branch of the dorsalis pedis in the proximal first interspace. Here, the important deep plantar arch is formed. Specifically, the deep plantar arch is formed by the transverse portion of the lateral plantar artery and a connection with the dorsalis pedis (Fig. 8-7).

The four plantar metatarsal arteries emanate from the deep plantar arch to nourish the plantar forefoot. They travel along each metatarsal shaft deep to the interossei and the transverse adductor muscles but superficial to the deep transverse carpal ligament. According to Murikami,[20] they bifurcate and are joined by the deep plantar arteries and the plantar intermetatarsal arteries to form an arcade of arterial triangles.

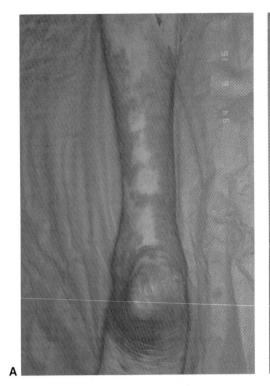

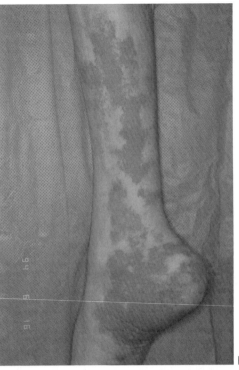

A

B

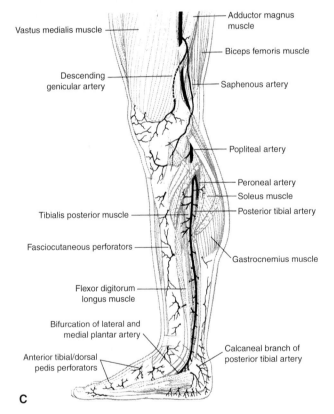

C

Labels on figure C:

- Vastus medialis muscle
- Adductor magnus muscle
- Biceps femoris muscle
- Descending genicular artery
- Saphenous artery
- Popliteal artery
- Peroneal artery
- Soleus muscle
- Posterior tibial artery
- Tibialis posterior muscle
- Fasciocutaneous perforators
- Gastrocnemius muscle
- Flexor digitorum longus muscle
- Bifurcation of lateral and medial plantar artery
- Calcaneal branch of posterior tibial artery
- Anterior tibial/dorsal pedis perforators

Figure 8-3 A, B, C: The posterior tibial artery gives off perforators that arise between the flexor digitorum longus (FDL) and soleus muscle. They split into anterior and posterior branches to supply the overlying skin. This injection study shows the angiosome fed by the posterior tibial artery (*shaded*). Note that the island of shaded skin just above the anterior medial malleolus comes from the peroneal via one of the arterial–arterial interconnections that will be discussed later. (From Attinger C. Vascular anatomy of the foot and ankle. *Op Tech Plast Reconstr Surg.* 1997;4:183–198, with permission.)

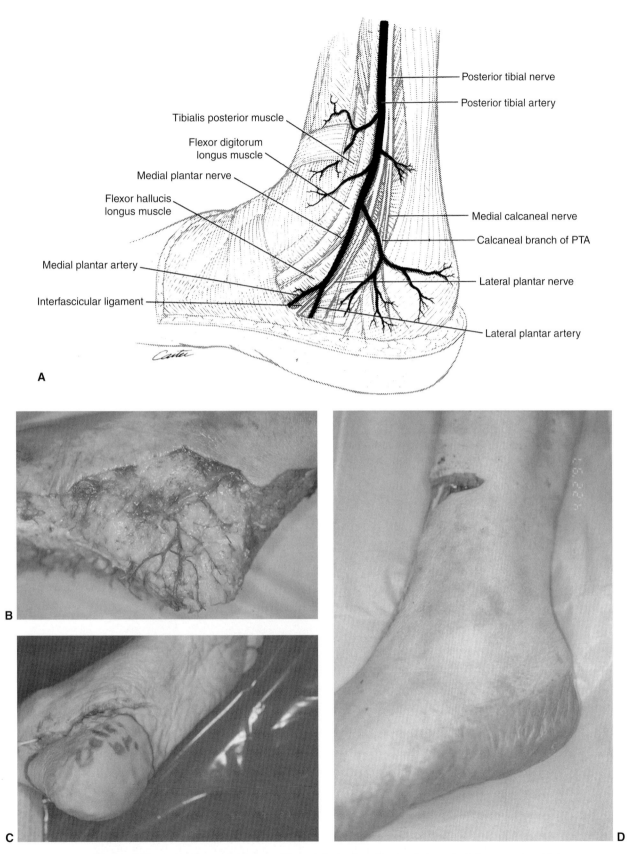

Figure 8-4   A, B: The medial calcaneal branch is the first distal main branch of the posterior tibial artery (PTA). Its angiosome includes the medial heel **(C)** and the plantar heel all the way to the contralateral glabrous junction **(D)**. (From Attinger C. Vascular anatomy of the foot and ankle. *Op Tech Plast Reconstr Surg.* 1997;4:183–198, with permission.)

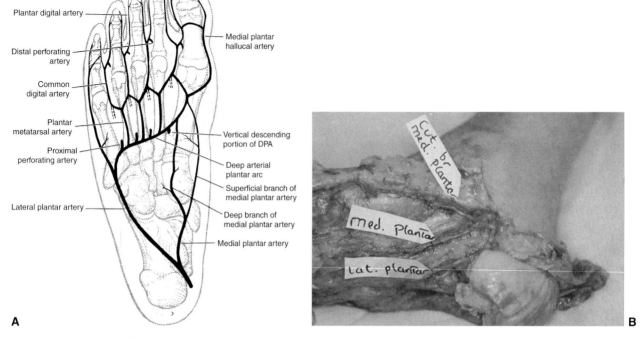

A

B

Figure 8-5   A: The plantar arteries of the foot. **B:** The medial plantar artery gives off two main branches: The superficial branch (labeled *cut. br. med. plantar*) and deep branch (labeled *med. plantar*). The superficial branch travels obliquely up toward the navicular-cuneiform joint and then travels along the superior border of the cuneiform and first metatarsal bone before descending to the medial plantar aspect of the distal metatarsal. The deep branch travels along the medial intramuscular septum deep and along the fibular side of the abductor hallucis muscle (AHB). DPA, distal perforating artery. (From Attinger C. Vascular anatomy of the foot and ankle. *Op Tech Plast Reconstr Surg.* 1997;4:183–198, with permission.)

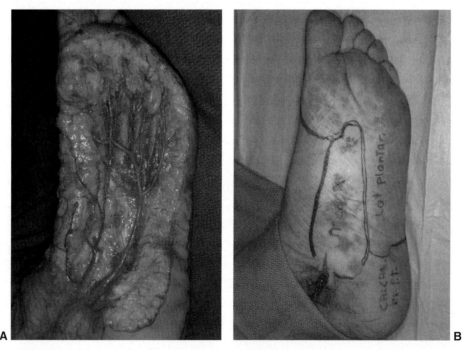

A

B

Figure 8-6   A: Cadaver dissection of lateral plantar artery. (From Attinger CE, Cooper P, Blume P, et al. The safest surgical incision and amputations applying the angiosomes principle and using the Doppler to assess the arterial–arterial connections of the foot and ankle. *Foot Ankle Clin North Am.* 2001;6:745–801, with permission.) **B:** The lateral plantar artery supplies the lateral plantar surface as well as the plantar forefoot. Its posterior border is the anterior border of the plantar heel, its medial border is the central raphe of the plantar midfoot and the glabrous juncture between the medial plantar forefoot and medial distal dorsal foot, and its lateral border is the glabrous junction between the lateral dorsum of the foot and plantar surface of the foot.

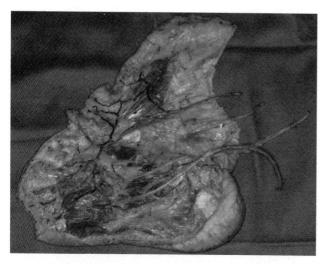

Figure 8-7 In this cadaver specimen, all bones except for the calcaneus have been removed. Note the direct connection between the dorsalis pedis artery and lateral calcaneal artery just distal to where the Lisfranc joint was. (From Attinger CE, Cooper P, Blume P, et al. The safest surgical incision and amputations applying the angiosomes principle and using the Doppler to assess the arterial–arterial connections of the foot and ankle. *Foot Ankle Clin North Am.* 2001;6:745–801, with permission.)

The common digital arteries arise at the apices of these triangles in the proximal web spaces.

The common digital arteries bifurcate into two digital arteries for each toe and are joined by distal perforating branches that originate from the dorsal metatarsal arteries. The proper plantar digital arteries are the predominant blood supply to the lesser toes except for the medial side of the second toe that is supplied by the first metatarsal artery.[19]

Angiosomes from the Anterior Tibial Artery: The Lateral and Medial Malleolar Arteries

In the leg, the anterior tibial artery's angiosome includes the area overlying the anterior compartment with the fibula as the lateral boundary and the anterior tibia as the medial boundary (Fig. 8-8). This artery originates from the popliteal artery and pierces the interosseus membrane to travel deep in the anterior compartment between the tibialis anterior (TA) muscle and extensor hallucis longus (EHL) muscle. During its course, it contributes multiple small pedicles[10–14] to the TA muscle, EHL muscle, and extensor digitorum longus (EDL) muscle.

At the ankle, the anterior tibial artery gives off the lateral malleolar artery at the level of the lateral malleolus that joins with the anterior perforating branch of the peroneal artery (Fig. 8-9). At the same level, it also branches into the medial malleolar artery, which anastomoses with the posteromedial artery of the posterior tibial artery. The anterior tibial artery then emerges under the extensor retinaculum of the ankle to become the dorsalis pedis artery.

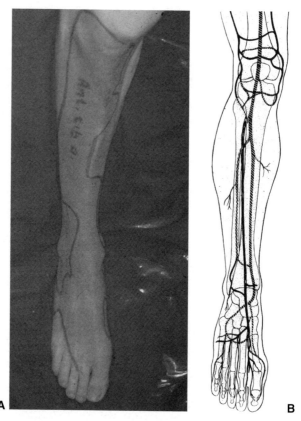

A **B**

Figure 8-8 **A:** The three main arteries of the leg, including the anterior tibial artery. **B:** The anterior tibial artery angiosome encompasses the anterior part of the leg overlying the anterior compartment with the fibula as the lateral boundary and the anterior tibia as the medial boundary. (From Attinger C. Vascular anatomy of the foot and ankle. *Op Tech Plast Reconstr Surg.* 1997;4:183–198, with permission.)

Angiosomes from the Dorsalis Pedis Artery: The Tarsal Arteries, the Arcuate Artery, and the First Dorsal Metatarsal Artery

The dorsalis pedis artery's angiosome encompasses the entire dorsum of the foot (Fig. 8-10) and the toes. This artery receives contributions from the superficial medial plantar artery medially, from the perforators of the lateral plantar artery distally, and from the calcaneal branch of the peroneal artery laterally. The dorsalis pedis artery arises at the level of the ankle joint, travels underneath the EHL, and then curves between the EHL and EDL along the dorsum of the first interspace. As Huber[21] has pointed out, the dorsalis pedis artery is absent or extremely attenuated in 12% of cases, and there are many anatomic variations to its course.

Typically, the dorsalis pedis artery branches into three lateral arteries: The proximal and distal tarsal arteries and the arcuate artery. These are often linked together to form an interconnecting "rete" (net) pattern

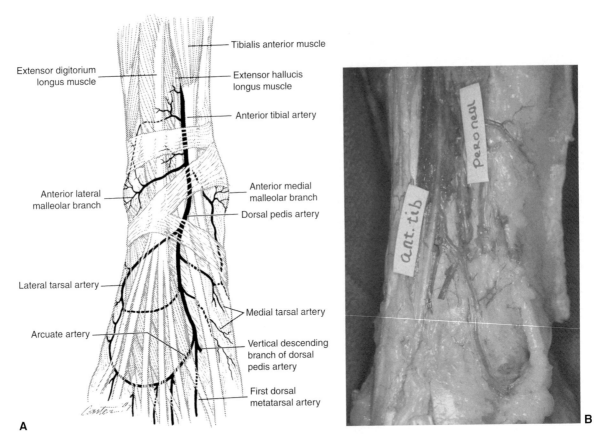

Figure 8-9 labels:
- Extensor digitorium longus muscle
- Tibialis anterior muscle
- Extensor hallucis longus muscle
- Anterior tibial artery
- Anterior lateral malleolar branch
- Anterior medial malleolar branch
- Dorsal pedis artery
- Lateral tarsal artery
- Medial tarsal artery
- Arcuate artery
- Vertical descending branch of dorsal pedis artery
- First dorsal metatarsal artery

A

B (ant. tib / peroneal)

Figure 8-9 A, B: At the ankle, the anterior tibial artery gives off the lateral malleolar artery at the level of the lateral malleolus. It anastomoses with the anterior perforating branch of the peroneal artery. (From Attinger C. Vascular anatomy of the foot and ankle. *Op Tech Plast Reconstr Surg.* 1997;4:183–198, with permission.)

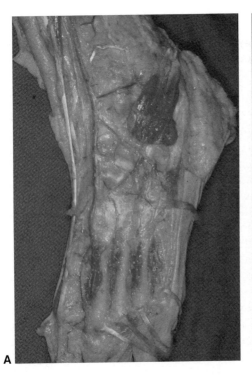

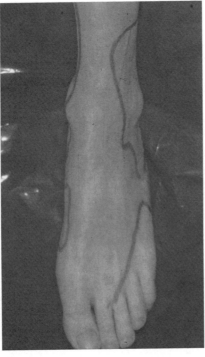

A

B

Figure 8-10 A: The dorsalis pedis artery and its branches are dissected out in this cadaver specimen. **B:** The dorsalis pedis artery angiosome supplies the entire dorsum of the foot, although it gets contributions from the superficial medial plantar artery medially, the perforators of the lateral plantar artery anteriorly, and both the calcaneal and anterior perforating branches of the peroneal artery laterally. (From Attinger CE, Cooper P, Blume P, et al. The safest surgical incision and amputations applying the angiosomes principle and using the Doppler to assess the arterial–arterial connections of the foot and ankle. *Foot Ankle Clin North Am.* 2001;6:745–801, with permission.)

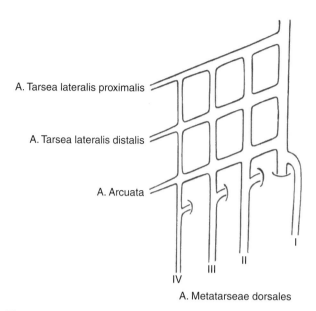

A. Tarsea lateralis proximalis

A. Tarsea lateralis distalis

A. Arcuata

I

II

III

IV

A. Metatarseae dorsales

Figure 8-11 The "rete" or net of the dorsalis pedis' lateral branches ensures redundant lateral dorsal blood flow patterns from the sinus tarsi to the Lisfranc joint. The "rete" is also connected laterally to the calcaneal branch of the peroneal artery and superiorly to the lateral malleolar artery and, by extension, to the anterior perforating branch of the peroneal artery. (From Sarrafian SK. *Anatomy of the foot and ankle*. Philadelphia, Pa: JP Lippincott Co; 1993:300, with permission.)

(Fig. 8-11).[22] The tarsal arteries and the arcuate arteries are worth describing.

The proximal lateral tarsal artery originates at the lateral talar neck. It travels underneath the extensor digitorum brevis muscle giving off one or more branches to this muscle as well as branches to the distal arcuate artery. Laterally, it communicates with the calcaneal branch of the peroneal artery. It may also connect superiorly to the lateral malleolar artery and

inferiorly to the arcuate artery. Medially, the dorsalis pedis artery (usually) gives off two tarsal arteries. One tarsal artery is located at the middle of the navicular bone and the other at the cuneonavicular joint. Usually, one of these joins with the superficial branch of the medial plantar artery.

The third branch of the dorsalis pedis, the arcuate artery, takes off at the level of the first tarsal-metatarsal joint and travels laterally over the bases of the second, third, and fourth metatarsals. It gives off the second, third, and fourth dorsal metatarsal arteries before it joins the lateral tarsal artery.

After giving off the arcuate artery, the dorsalis pedis artery enters into the proximal first intermetatarsal space giving rise to the FDMA, which courses over the first dorsal interossei muscles. The dorsalis pedis artery then takes a 90-degree turn deep followed by another 90-degree turn laterally to join the lateral plantar artery (Fig. 8-12). In 22% of cases, the FDMA originates after the dorsalis pedis has made the downward 90-degree turn.[23] In these instances, the FDMA rises toward the dorsum by traveling through the first interosseus muscle until it lies on top of the interosseus muscle at or near the metatarsophalangeal (MTP) level. Regardless of its course, this artery is important because it supplies the first interosseus muscle, the skin overlying it, and the first web space. In addition, the FDMA gives off medial and lateral branches that supply blood to the hallux and second digit (Fig. 8-13).

The dorsal metatarsal arteries, which supply the toes, originate from both the dorsal system (the arcuate artery) and the deep plantar system (the proximal perforating arteries). At the metatarsal heads, the dorsal metatarsal arteries divide into two dorsal digital arteries and then travel to the plantar area via the distal perforating arteries (also called anterior perforating

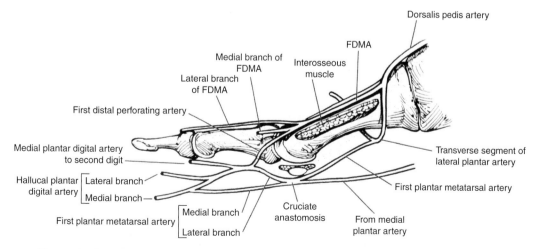

Dorsalis pedis artery

FDMA

Medial branch of FDMA

Interosseous muscle

Lateral branch of FDMA

First distal perforating artery

Medial plantar digital artery to second digit

Hallucal plantar digital artery — Lateral branch

Medial branch

First plantar metatarsal artery

Medial branch

Lateral branch

Cruciate anastomosis

Transverse segment of lateral plantar artery

First plantar metatarsal artery

From medial plantar artery

Figure 8-12 After giving off the arcuate artery, the dorsalis pedis artery dives into the proximal first intermetatarsal space at a 90-degree angle and then turns another 90 degrees laterally to join the lateral plantar artery. FDMA, first dorsal metatarsal artery. (From Attinger C. Vascular anatomy of the foot and ankle. *Op Tech Plast Reconstr Surg*. 1997;4:183–198, with permission.)

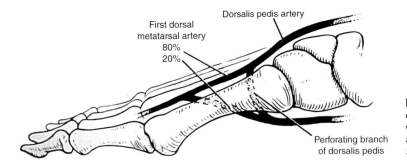

Figure 8-13 The most common pattern of the first dorsal metatarsal artery (FDMA) and its connections with the plantar circulation. (From Attinger C. Vascular anatomy of the foot and ankle. *Op Tech Plast Reconstr Surg.* 1997;4:183–198, with permission.)

arteries). These perforating arteries join the plantar metatarsal artery to supply the plantar digits. In this way, the web space and the toes on either side of the web space receive dorsal and plantar blood supply from a dual system: The dorsalis pedis artery and the plantar system (from the medial and lateral plantar arteries).

Angiosomes from the Peroneal Artery: The Calcaneal Branch and the Anterior Perforating Branch

The peroneal artery is derived from the tibial peroneal trunk and courses along the medial side of the fibula supplying the posterolateral lower leg, ankle, and heel (Fig. 8-14). The peroneal artery's angiosome is bounded laterally by the central raphe overlying the Achilles tendon and medially by the anterior edge of the lateral compartment (Fig. 8-15). It supplies the deep posterior compartment muscles (flexor hallucis longus [FHL], FDL), the osseous blood supply to the fibula, the lower portion of the soleus muscle, the lateral half of the Achilles tendon, and the lower distal two thirds of the peroneus longus and brevis muscles. The posterior lateral skin of the leg is supplied by peroneal perforators (at 3- to 5-cm intervals), which travel close to, alongside, or through the posterolateral intramuscular septum.[24,25]

Before the peroneal artery emerges at the level of the lateral malleolus, it bifurcates into the anterior perforating branch and the lateral calcaneal branch (Fig. 8-16). The lateral calcaneal branch's angiosome includes the plantar and lateral heel (Fig. 8-17). More specifically, the boundaries extend medially to the medial glabrous junction of the heel, distally to the proximal fifth metatarsal, and superiorly to the lateral malleolus. The course of the lateral calcaneal artery begins at the level of the lateral malleolus as it emerges laterally between the Achilles tendon and the peroneal tendons. It curves with peroneal tendons 2 cm distal to the lateral malleolus, and gives rise to four or five small calcaneal branches. The lateral calcaneal artery terminates at the level of the fifth metatarsal tuberosity where it connects with the lateral tarsal artery.

The anterior perforating branch's angiosome is made of the skin overlying the distal interosseus membrane (this area encompasses the area from which the well-known supramalleolar flap can be harvested).[26]

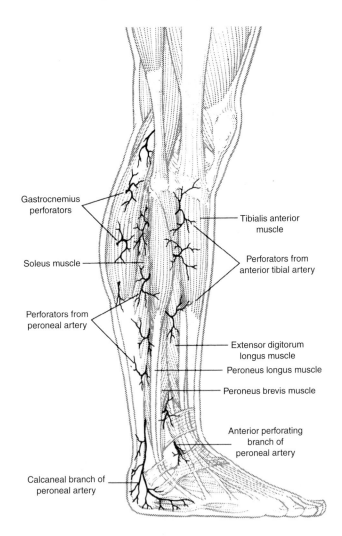

Figure 8-14 The peroneal artery arises from the tibial peroneal trunk and travels along the medial side of the fibula in the deep compartment and supplies the posterolateral lower leg, ankle, and heel. Perforators (at 3- to 5-cm intervals) travel close to, alongside, or through the posterolateral intramuscular septum before supplying the posterolateral skin. (From Attinger C. Vascular anatomy of the foot and ankle. *Op Tech Plast Reconstr Surg.* 1997;4:183–198, with permission.)

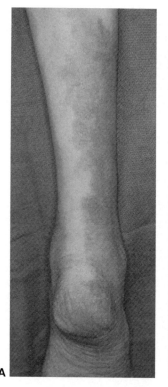
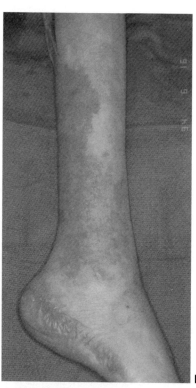

Figure 8-15   A, B: The peroneal artery angiosome extends from the midline of the posterior calf to just the anterior edge of the lateral compartment. It extends inferiorly to the anterolateral ankle and lateral heel. (From Attinger CE, Cooper P, Blume P, et al. The safest surgical incision and amputations applying the angiosomes principle and using the Doppler to assess the arterial–arterial connections of the foot and ankle. *Foot Ankle Clin North Am.* 2001;6:745–801, with permission.)   **A**   **B**

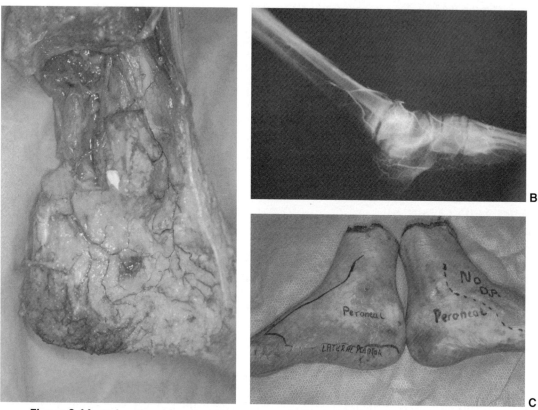

Figure 8-16   Before the peroneal artery emerges at the level of the lateral malleolus, it bifurcates into the anterior perforating branch and the lateral calcaneal branch. **A:** The cadaver dissection shows the bifurcation after the fibula was removed. **B:** The angiogram view of the same bifurcation is shown. **C:** These two injections show the boundaries of the angiosome fed by the two terminal branches of the peroneal artery. (From Attinger CE, Cooper P, Blume P, et al. The safest surgical incision and amputations applying the angiosomes principle and using the Doppler to assess the arterial–arterial connections of the foot and ankle. *Foot Ankle Clin North Am.* 2001;6:745–801, with permission.)

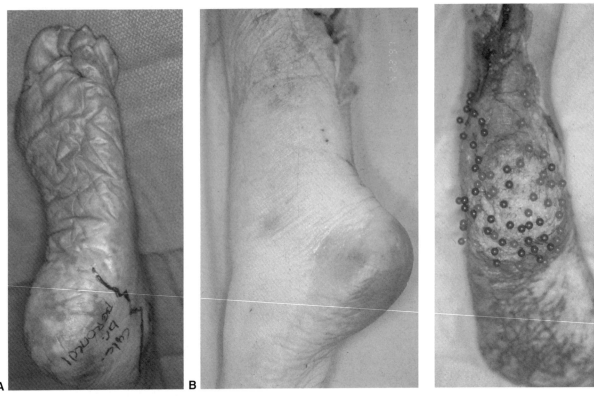

A   **B**   **C**

Figure 8-17   A: The calcaneal branch of the peroneal artery supplies the entire plantar heel as well as the lateral ankle. Note that the heel is privileged in that it has two source arteries—the medial and lateral calcaneal arteries. **B:** The overlap is best shown in this cadaver specimen where each was injected with a different color and they completely overlap. **C:** The skin was then removed, and the different colored perforators were marked with different colored pins, further emphasizing the overlap. (From Attinger CE, Cooper P, Blume P, et al. The safest surgical incision and amputations applying the angiosomes principle and using the Doppler to assess the arterial–arterial connections of the foot and ankle. *Foot Ankle Clin North Am.* 2001;6:745–801, with permission.)

Last, the anterior branch pierces through the anterior intermuscular septum to connect directly with the anterior lateral malleolar artery.

ANATOMIC AND CLINICAL EVALUATION OF ARTERIAL–ARTERIAL CONNECTIONS

Arterial–arterial connections allow for uninterrupted blood flow to the entire foot despite the occlusion of one or more arteries. By understanding the location of these arterial connections in the foot and ankle, the surgeon can determine both the presence of flow from the source artery and which artery is predominately supplying the angiosome. The use of the handheld Doppler instrument at specific anatomic locations as described above (or in any anatomic text) is invaluable.[15]

To evaluate the direction of flow, apply selective occlusion with finger-applied pressure either above or below the area being Dopplered.[27] The resulting character of the Doppler sound helps to evaluate the quality of flow present in the artery. Triphasic flow indicates normal arterial flow. Biphasic flow indicates mildly compromised flow. Monophasic flow indicates arterial compromise unless the patient suffers from sympathetic neuropathy (a complication of diabetes) and the distal vessels have lost their tone. A blunt, short, monophasic, spittinglike sound indicates complete distal occlusion with no runoff.

For example, it should be straightforward to determine whether the flow to the dorsum of the foot is derived from the anterior tibial artery, the peroneal artery (via the anterior perforating branch), or from the posterior tibial artery (via the lateral plantar artery) by listening and selectively occluding these areas. In addition, one should be able to determine whether the blood flow to the heel is coming directly from the calcaneal branch of the posterior tibial artery or the calcaneal branch of the peroneal artery, or indirectly from the anterior tibial artery via the lateral malleolar branch or from the dorsalis pedis via the lateral plantar artery. Incidentally, this directional flow assessment and arterial predominance provides additional information to that obtained by routine angiography.

In the patient with diabetes mellitus and/or peripheral vascular disease who presents with a foot ulcer or rest pain, this clinical assessment can aid enormously in choosing which incisions to make if the patient requires a debridement or closure. In these patients, it is crucial that the critically redirected blood flow is not compromised by a poorly planned surgical incision. Moreover, this information aids the vascular surgeon in ensuring that his bypass will actually reach the angiosome that is ischemic. It has been reported that 15% of bypasses fail to heal the foot despite remaining patent because the bypass failed to revascularize the affected angiosome.[28]

Connections around the Ankle

Arterial connections around the ankle are complex and difficult to evaluate. All three main arteries of the leg communicate with each other around the ankle. The peroneal artery communicates with the anterior tibial artery via the anterior perforating branch and lateral malleolar branch, and the peroneal and the posterior tibial artery share three transverse communicating branches. The anterior tibial artery and posterior tibial artery communicate directly via the anastomoses of the dorsalis pedis with the lateral plantar arteries.

Peroneal and Posterior Tibial Connections

The peroneal artery communicates distally with the posterior tibial artery via one to three transverse communicating branches that are located along the fat pad deep to the Achilles tendon (Fig. 8-18). These branches are located 5 to 7 cm above the ankle joint, at the ankle joint, and just above the insertion of the Achilles tendon. As we have previously reported, because one cannot selectively occlude the deep peroneal or posterior tibial artery underneath the Achilles tendon, it is impossible by Doppler to know whether the flow along the distal posterior tibial artery originates directly from the proximal posterior tibial artery or indirectly from the distal peroneal artery via the above perforators. Likewise, one cannot tell whether the flow along the peroneal artery originates from the peroneal artery or from the posterior tibial artery via perforators.[18]

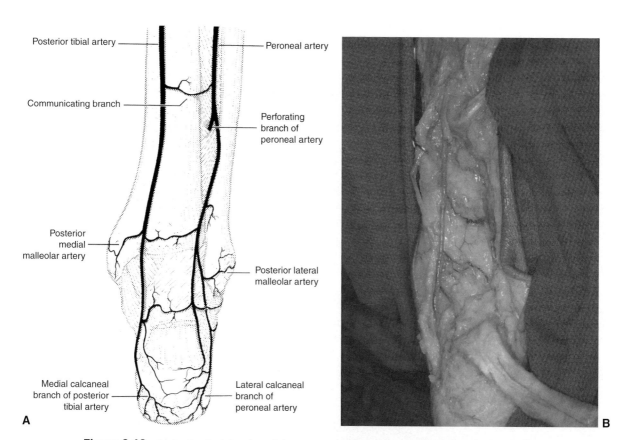

Posterior tibial artery

Communicating branch

Posterior medial malleolar artery

Medial calcaneal branch of posterior tibial artery

A

Peroneal artery

Perforating branch of peroneal artery

Posterior lateral malleolar artery

Lateral calcaneal branch of peroneal artery

B

Figure 8-18   **A:** Anatomical drawing of the communications between the peroneal artery and posterior tibial artery. **B:** Cadaver specimen showing that the peroneal artery communicates distally with the posterior tibial artery via one to three transverse communicating branches and with the anterior tibial artery via anterior perforating branch. (From Attinger C. Vascular anatomy of the foot and ankle. *Op Tech Plast Reconstr Surg.* 1997;4:183–198, with permission.)

Anterior Tibial and Posterior Tibial Connections

The anterior tibial artery and posterior tibial artery are also directly connected. This communication occurs distal to the Lisfranc joint where the dorsalis pedis artery enters into the proximal first interspace to join directly with the lateral plantar artery (Figs. 8-7 and 8-12).

To evaluate whether the flow along the anterior tibial artery is antegrade or retrograde, place the Doppler probe over the anterior tibial artery and occlude the more distal dorsalis pedis artery. If the signal persists despite occlusion, there is antegrade flow. However, if the sound disappears, the flow along the anterior tibial artery is retrograde from the posterior tibial artery via the lateral plantar and dorsalis pedis arteries. In this instance, interruption of this connection could lead to ischemia or even tissue loss.

Moreover, if there is a Doppler signal over the anterior tibial artery, the flow could be from the lateral malleolar artery (Fig. 8-9). It is therefore important when evaluating the flow at the anterior tibial artery to occlude the lateral malleolar artery at the same time as the dorsalis pedis artery. This eliminates the possible contributions from the peroneal artery via its anterior perforating branch and lateral malleolar branch, as will be described later (Fig. 8-19).

Using the Doppler to assess the direction and character of flow of the posterior tibial artery is preformed at the tarsal tunnel. The posterior tibial artery can be occluded distally (Fig. 8-20), and if the signal remains, there is antegrade flow along the posterior tibial artery. If there is no signal with the distal occlusion, the flow is retrograde from the anterior tibial artery via the dorsalis pedis and lateral plantar arteries. The blood flow travels from the anterior tibial artery into the dorsalis pedis where it joins the lateral plantar artery, and then it travels retrograde into the posterior tibial artery. If there is no antegrade flow along the posterior tibial artery, it also suggests that the peroneal artery is either occluded or the arterial connections between the posterior tibial and peroneal arteries are occluded (Fig. 8-18).

Anterior Tibial and Peroneal Connections

The importance of evaluating the patency of the distal connection between the anterior and posterior tibial artery cannot be emphasized enough. If that connection is critical to supplying either the dorsal or plantar surface of the foot, interruption of that connection while performing an amputation can lead to gangrene on the portion of the foot that was dependent on retrograde flow (Fig. 8-21).[18]

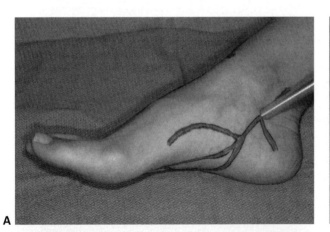

A

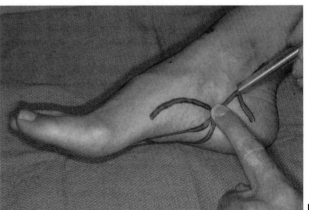

B

C

Figure 8-19 A: The Doppler probe is placed over the tarsal tunnel to listen to the posterior tibial artery. **B:** Finger pressure applying distal occlusion can be used to test for antegrade or retrograde flow. If the signal remains despite distal occlusion, then there is antegrade flow. If the signal disappears, then there is only retrograde flow from the anterior tibial artery via the dorsalis pedis and lateral plantar artery. **C:** Listen to the posterior tibial artery while occluding the dorsalis pedis artery. If the signal disappears, then there is only retrograde flow over the posterior tibial artery from the dorsalis pedis artery. (From Attinger CE, Cooper P, Blume P, et al. The safest surgical incision and amputations applying the angiosomes principle and using the Doppler to assess the arterial–arterial connections of the foot and ankle. *Foot Ankle Clin North Am.* 2001;6:745–801, with permission.)

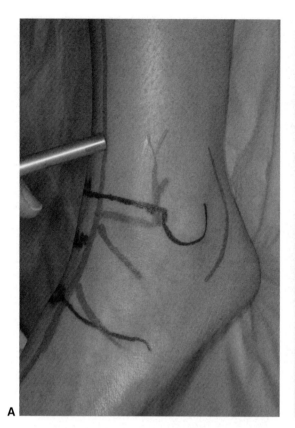
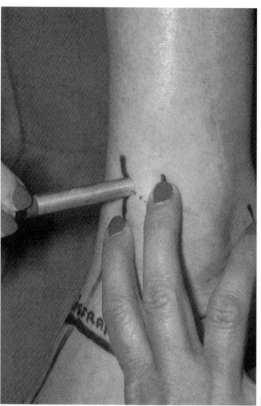

Figure 8-20   A: The Doppler probe is placed above the ankle joint over the anterior tibial artery. **B:** The anterior tibial artery is occluded at the level of the lateral malleolar artery to prevent the retrograde flow from both the peroneal artery and the posterior tibial artery. (From Attinger CE, Cooper P, Blume P, et al. The safest surgical incision and amputations applying the angiosomes principle and using the Doppler to assess the arterial–arterial connections of the foot and ankle. *Foot Ankle Clin North Am.* 2001;6:745–801, with permission.)

Again, the anterior tibial artery and the peroneal artery are connected through the anterior perforating branch of the peroneal artery and the lateral malleolar branch of the anterior tibial artery (Fig. 8-9); thus, the flow of the peroneal artery can be retrograde from the anterior tibial artery via the lateral malleolar artery.

To evaluate the direction of flow at the peroneal artery, Doppler the anterior perforating branch of the peroneal artery, which is usually found in the lateral soft area just above the ankle joint between the tibia and fibula (Fig. 8-22). Next, occlude the anterior tibial artery at the takeoff of the lateral malleolar branch. If the Doppler sounds continue, there is antegrade flow along the anterior perforating branch of the peroneal artery. As we previously stated, whether that flow actually originates from the peroneal artery or the posterior tibial artery is impossible to determine because one cannot selectively occlude the flow of the interconnecting branches anterior to the Achilles tendon. However, if the Doppler sound stops, then there is no antegrade flow and the distal peroneal artery depends on the anterior tibial artery via the lateral malleolar artery for retrograde flow. Disruption of that connection can put the lateral ankle soft tissue in jeopardy.

To assess whether the peroneal artery is contributing significantly to the anterior tibial artery flow, the anterior perforating branch is occluded while the Doppler is placed on the anterior tibial artery. Because of possible retrograde flow from posterior tibial artery via the dorsalis pedis artery, it is important to also occlude the anterior tibial artery distal to the takeoff of the lateral malleolar artery. If there is no Doppler sound, then the pressure over the anterior perforating branch is lifted. If flow returns, then the anterior tibial artery and dorsalis pedis arteries receive their blood flow in part (or all) from the peroneal artery.

Connections around the Heel

The heel is unique in that it is the only angiosome that receives inflow from two source arteries: The calcaneal branch of the posterior tibial artery and the calcaneal branch of the peroneal artery. The posterior tibial calcaneal branch supplies the medial aspect of the heel, while the peroneal calcaneal branch supplies the lateral aspect of the heel. The former runs directly toward the heel pad along the center of the medial heel, while the latter curves around the lateral malleolus 2 cm distal

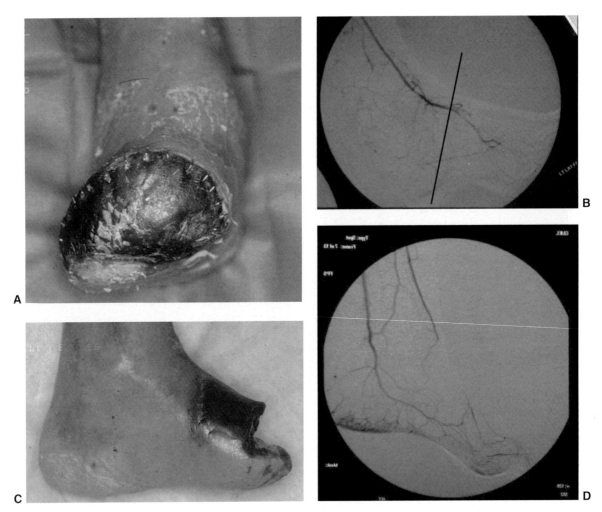

Figure 8-21   A, B: This patient's plantar blood supply came from the dorsalis pedis artery in a retrograde fashion. When an amputation was performed and that connection was sacrificed, the distal plantar surface became necrotic. **C, D:** This patient's dorsal blood supply came from the lateral plantar artery in a retrograde fashion. When the amputation was performed and that connection was severed, the distal dorsal surface became necrotic. (From Attinger CE, Cooper P, Blume P, et al. The safest surgical incision and amputations applying the angiosomes principle and using the Doppler to assess the arterial–arterial connections of the foot and ankle. *Foot Ankle Clin North Am.* 2001;6: 745–801, with permission.)

to the malleolar tip and travels toward the proximal fifth metatarsal head. There are no anatomic arterial–arterial connections to these arteries, and, therefore, a Doppler signal obtained in this location represents only antegrade flow. However, it is important to assess the flow in both the calcaneal branch of the posterior tibial artery and the peroneal artery (Fig. 8-23) to determine if one artery predominates over the other.

Connections on the Plantar Surface

There are multiple levels of arterial–arterial interconnections in the plantar foot. Proximally, the dorsal and plantar circulation is linked together at the Lisfranc joint via proximal perforators. Proximally and medially there are the connections between the branches of the medial tarsal artery and the superficial medial plantar artery, although the medial tarsal artery is often too small to

accurately Doppler. At the Lisfranc joint, the dorsal and plantar circulation is linked together via proximal perforators. Medially the dorsalis pedis links directly with the lateral plantar artery (Figs. 8-7 and 8-12). More laterally, the dorsal and plantar metatarsal arteries are linked at their takeoff by the proximal perforating branches (Fig. 8-5). At the web spaces, distal perforating arteries again link the dorsal and plantar metatarsal arteries.

Dorsalis Pedis and Lateral Plantar Connections

In the plantar foot, the principle connection to evaluate is that between the dorsalis pedis and lateral plantar artery. First, Doppler the lateral plantar artery proximal to the base of the proximal first interspace (Fig. 8-24). Then, occlude the dorsalis pedis proximal to tarsal-metatarsal joint and the takeoff of the arcuate artery (the arcuate artery is located at the level of the first tarsal-metatarsal joint and travels laterally over the

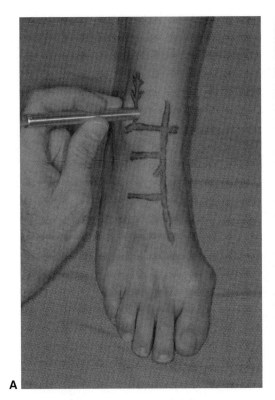
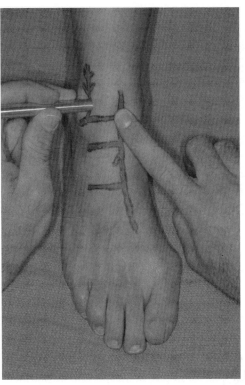

A   B

Figure 8-22 **A:** The anterior perforating branch of the peroneal artery is located in the lateral soft area just above the ankle joint between the tibia and fibula. **B:** Then, the anterior tibial artery is occluded at the takeoff of the lateral malleolar branch. If the Doppler sounds remain, then there is antegrade flow along the anterior perforating branch of the peroneal artery. (From Attinger CE, Cooper P, Blume P, et al. The safest surgical incision and amputations applying the angiosomes principle and using the Doppler to assess the arterial–arterial connections of the foot and ankle. *Foot Ankle Clin North Am.* 2001;6:745–801, with permission.)

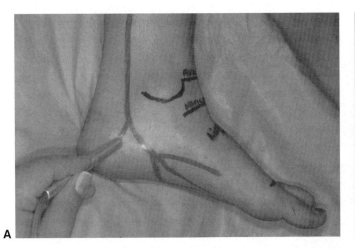
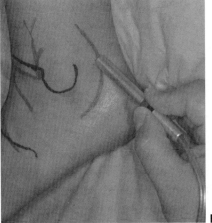

A   B

Figure 8-23 **A:** The calcaneal branch of the posterior tibial artery can be Dopplered at the heel pad along the center of the medial heel. **B:** The calcaneal branch of the peroneal artery curves around the lateral malleolus 2 cm distal to the malleolar tip and then travels towards the proximal fifth metatarsal head. (From Attinger CE, Cooper P, Blume P, et al. The safest surgical incision and amputations applying the angiosomes principle and using the Doppler to assess the arterial–arterial connections of the foot and ankle. *Foot Ankle Clin North Am.* 2001;6:745–801, with permission.)

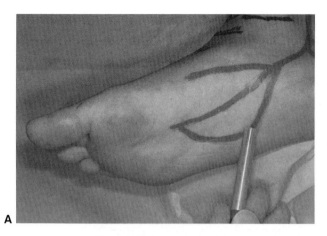

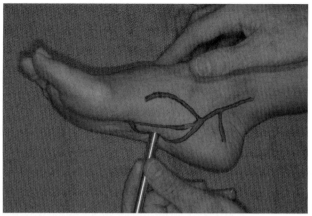

A   B

Figure 8-24   A: The lateral plantar artery is Dopplered out on the plantar surface. **B:** The dorsalis pedis is then occluded proximal to the tarsal-metatarsal joint, taking care to also occlude the takeoff of the arcuate artery. If the signal disappears, then the flow to the lateral plantar artery depends on the dorsalis pedis arterial flow. However, if the sound remains, it means that there is antegrade flow from the distal posterior tibial artery to the lateral plantar artery. (From Attinger CE, Cooper P, Blume P, et al. The safest surgical incision and amputations applying the angiosomes principle and using the Doppler to assess the arterial–arterial connections of the foot and ankle. *Foot Ankle Clin North Am.* 2001;6:745–801, with permission.)

bases of the second, third, and fourth metatarsals). If the signal disappears, then flow in the lateral plantar artery depends on the dorsalis pedis arterial flow. However, if the sound remains, it means that there is antegrade flow from the posterior tibial artery to the lateral plantar artery.

In the very rare circumstance, this scenario represents occlusion of the proximal lateral plantar artery with a still-patent medial plantar artery that is supplying plantar retrograde flow via the cruciate anastomosis (Fig. 8-12). This very rare circumstance could be established by Dopplering out the lateral plantar artery (Fig. 8-25)

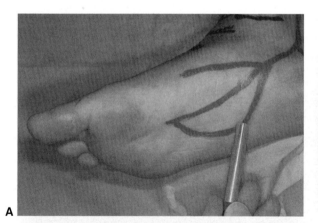

A

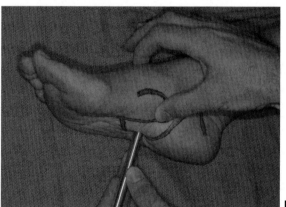

B

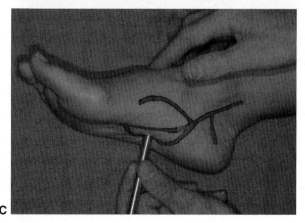

C

Figure 8-25   A: To determine whether the medial plantar artery is providing retrograde flow to the lateral plantar artery, Doppler the lateral plantar artery. **B:** Then occlude the medial column (to prevent retrograde flow along the medial plantar artery) and the dorsalis pedis artery. If the signal disappears, then there is no antegrade flow. **C:** If the signal returns when the pressure is lifted off the medial column but maintained on the dorsalis pedis artery, then the flow to the lateral plantar artery is retrograde from the medial plantar artery. (From Attinger CE, Cooper P, Blume P, et al. The safest surgical incision and amputations applying the angiosomes principle and using the Doppler to assess the arterial–arterial connections of the foot and ankle. *Foot Ankle Clin North Am.* 2001;6:745–801, with permission.)

and then occluding the medial column (to prevent retrograde flow along the medial plantar artery) and the dorsalis pedis artery. If the signal disappears, then there is no antegrade flow from the medial plantar artery. If the signal returns when the pressure is lifted off the medial column but maintained on the dorsalis pedis artery, then the flow to the lateral plantar artery is retrograde from the medial plantar artery.

Connections at the Cruciate Anastamosis

As we just mentioned, a second source of arterial–arterial anastomosis occurs proximal to the first metatarsal head, at the cruciate anastomosis, when the superficial and deep medial plantar arteries join (Fig. 8-5, 8-12). The first plantar metatarsal artery also joins the cruciate anastomosis. The cruciate anastomosis links the medial plantar artery with the lateral plantar artery. The blood supply to the first toe depends on which arteries anastomose at the cruciate anastomosis—the medial plantar artery, lateral plantar artery (Fig. 8-26), or FDMA (Figs. 8-6 and 8-8).

To determine the flow at the cruciate anastomosis, Doppler the deep medial plantar artery proximally

(Fig. 8-27). Then, apply pressure at the cruciate anastomosis just proximal to the first metatarsal head and at the proximal lateral plantar artery simultaneously. If the signal persists, then there is antegrade flow. If it

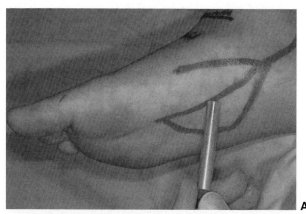
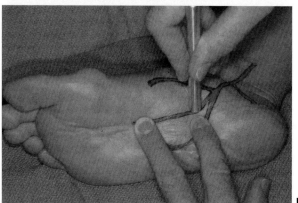
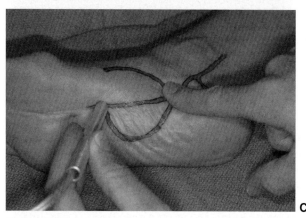

Figure 8-27 **A:** The deep medial plantar artery is Dopplered proximally. **B:** Pressure is applied at the cruciate anastomosis just proximal to the first metatarsal head and to the proximal lateral plantar artery simultaneously. If the signal persists, then there is antegrade flow. If it disappears, then the flow is retrograde. Occluding the medial plantar arteries at their takeoff, and then selectively occluding and releasing the dorsalis pedis artery and the lateral plantar artery can establish which of the two arteries can provide retrograde flow. **C:** Here the proximal medial plantar arteries and the distal lateral plantar arteries are being occluded while the Doppler is placed on the distal deep medial plantar artery. If there is a signal, then the dorsalis pedis is the source of the retrograde flow. (From Attinger CE, Cooper P, Blume P, et al. The safest surgical incision and amputations applying the angiosomes principle and using the Doppler to assess the arterial–arterial connections of the foot and ankle. *Foot Ankle Clin North Am.* 2001;6:745–801, with permission.)

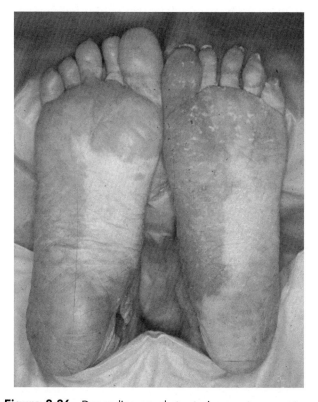

Figure 8-26 Depending on what arteries anastomose at or around the cruciate anastomosis, the hallux can be primarily nourished by the medial plantar artery, lateral plantar artery, or first dorsal metatarsal artery (FDMA). This injected cadaver shows the dual blood supply to the forefoot. (From Attinger CE, Cooper P, Blume P, et al. The safest surgical incision and amputations applying the angiosomes principle and using the Doppler to assess the arterial–arterial connections of the foot and ankle. *Foot Ankle Clin North Am.* 2001;6:745–801, with permission.)

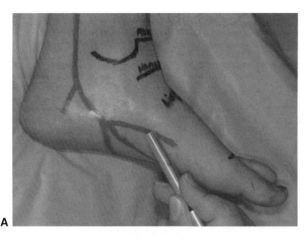
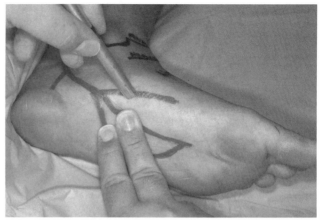

A   B

Figure 8-28   A: The superficial plantar artery is Dopplered out to establish its course, which can be variable. **B:** The lateral plantar artery and deep medial plantar artery are occluded at their takeoff to make sure that the flow along the superficial plantar artery is antegrade. In addition, the superficial medial plantar artery can be occluded at its takeoff to see if there is retrograde flow from the cruciate anastomosis (not pictured here). The retrograde flow can be from one or more of these arteries: The first dorsal metatarsal artery (FDMA), the deep medial plantar artery, or the lateral plantar artery. (From Attinger CE, Cooper P, Blume P, et al. The safest surgical incision and amputations applying the angiosomes principle and using the Doppler to assess the arterial–arterial connections of the foot and ankle. *Foot Ankle Clin North Am.* 2001;6:745–801, with permission.)

disappears, then the flow is retrograde. To determine if the dorsalis pedis or the lateral plantar artery provides the retrograde flow, occlude the medial plantar arteries at their takeoff and then selectively occlude and release the dorsalis pedis artery and the lateral plantar artery, respectively. The superficial medial plantar artery can be tested in a similar manner (Fig. 8-28).

Dorsalis Pedis and Lateral Plantar Arteries Linked by the Subdermal Plexus

The final arterial–arterial interconnection was first described by Hidalgo and Shaw,[29] who showed a fine subdermal arteriolar plexus linking the dorsalis pedis with the lateral plantar artery in a circumferential wraparound pattern about the plantar foot (Fig. 8-29). These arteries are of extremely fine caliber (0.1 to 0.2 mm) and are too small to assess by the Doppler probe. They span the angiosome boundaries of the dorsalis pedis artery, medial plantar artery, and lateral plantar artery. Because their presence has not masked the defined boundaries of the plantar angiosomes, it is thought this subdermal circulation provides an additional but very limited source of blood flow. However, this circulation undoubtedly proves to be crucial for the sole to recover from the daily trauma of walking or if there is damage to the principal blood supply.

Connections on the Dorsum of the Foot

As just discussed, the dorsal and plantar arterial systems are closely linked at multiple levels. The most proximal is located in the medial foot where the medial tarsal artery communicates with the superficial

(medial branch) of the medial plantar artery. It is usually too difficult to Doppler this small connection. Laterally, there is the "rete" (net) that connects the proximal lateral tarsal artery to the distal tarsal and arcuate arteries and to the lateral malleolar artery and the anterior perforating branch of the peroneal superiorly. In addition, the calcaneal branch of the peroneal artery connects with the lateral tarsal artery.

Because of this complex network of connections, it is very difficult to determine the source of retrograde flow over the major tarsal artery when it is occluded proximally. Of course, antegrade and retrograde flow along the proximal tarsal artery can be established by occluding it proximally and distally and assessing the sound. But determining where the blood flow comes from is a more complex question. If retrograde flow along the proximal lateral tarsal artery is discovered, it signifies an intact network of connections that can include the following: The anterior perforating branch of the lateral plantar artery, the lateral malleolar artery, the calcaneal branch of the peroneal artery, the distal tarsal artery, and the arcuate artery.

Another important arterial connection occurs just distal to the Lisfranc joint where the dorsalis pedis artery joins the lateral plantar artery in the proximal first interspace (Figs. 8-7 and 8-12). The dorsalis pedis can be Dopplered proximal to the Lisfranc joint (Fig. 8-30). If the Doppler sound continues when pressure is applied to the posterior tibial artery at the tarsal tunnel, then there is antegrade flow. If the Doppler sound disappears, then the flow to the dorsalis pedis artery is retrograde from the posterior tibial artery via the lateral plantar artery.

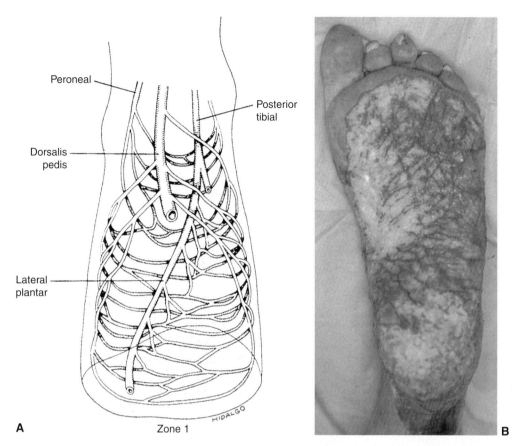

Figure 8-29 A, B: Hidalgo and Shaw showed that there was a subdermal arteriolar plexus linking the dorsalis pedis with the lateral plantar artery in a circumferential wrap-around pattern. This system consists of a very fine network of minute arterioles. It further protects the sole of the foot by providing another source, albeit small, of vascular inflow to the plantar skin. This flow is not of sufficient caliber to disturb the angiosome boundaries described above or to feed the entire sole of the foot, but it reinforces the choke vessels to provide an additional as well as alternative vascular pathway. (From Hidalgo DA, Shaw WW. Anatomic basis of plantar flap design. *Plast Reconstr Surg.* 1986;78:267, with permission.)

At the distal web spaces, the distal perforating arteries link the distal dorsal and plantar metatarsal arteries (Fig. 8-5). The direction(s) of flow along the dorsal metatarsals can be easily determined. By Dopplering the artery proximally and occluding distally, one can establish whether there is antegrade flow. By Dopplering the artery distally and occluding proximally, one can establish whether retrograde flow is present. This method also establishes the patency of the distal perforators in the web space (Fig. 8-31). This close linkage ensures that collateral flow will nourish the entire foot despite occlusion to either the dorsalis pedis or posterior tibial artery.

USING THE PRINCIPLES OF ANGIOSOMES TO MAKE SAFE INCISIONS IN THE NORMAL AND VASCULARLY COMPROMISED PATIENT

As we have previously reported, there are four important factors to be considered and balanced when choosing where to place an incision.[18] Of course, the incision must

provide adequate exposure for the planned procedure. In addition, there must be adequate blood supply on either side of the incision to maximize healing. Third, the incision should spare the sensory and motor nerves. Last, the incision should not be placed perpendicular to a joint due to the risk of causing scar contracture and resultant joint immobility. While adequate exposure, nerve location, and scar contracture are important factors, we will focus primarily on the vascular ramifications of typical incisions in the foot and ankle.

We have described above in detail the importance of assessing the blood flow to each angiosome. As we stated, the presence of a palpable pulse or a Dopplerable triphasic sound over the source artery to a given angiosome indicates adequate blood flow to that angiosome. If there is good blood flow from the source artery feeding each angiosome, the safest incisions to make are along the borders between two adjacent angiosomes because each side of the incision has maximal blood flow. Therefore, incisions along the central raphe over the Achilles tendon, along the glabrous junction separating the sole of the foot from the dorsum of the foot,

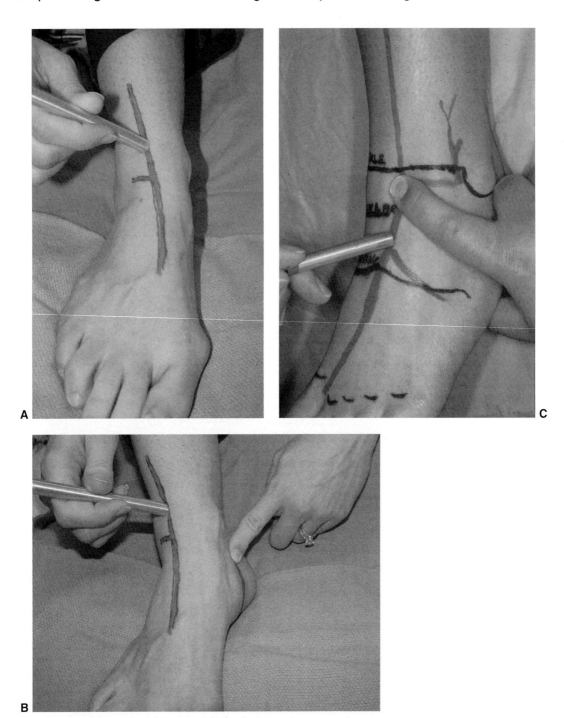

Figure 8-30   A: The anterior tibial artery is Dopplered out just proximal to the Lisfranc joint. **B:** If pressure is applied to the posterior tibial artery at the tarsal tunnel, and the Doppler sound continues, then there is antegrade flow. **C:** If pressure is applied to the proximal dorsalis pedis artery, and the Doppler sound continues, then there is good retrograde flow from the posterior tibial artery via the lateral plantar artery. (From Attinger CE, Cooper P, Blume P, et al. The safest surgical incision and amputations applying the angiosomes principle and using the Doppler to assess the arterial–arterial connections of the foot and ankle. *Foot Ankle Clin North Am.* 2001;6:745–801, with permission.)

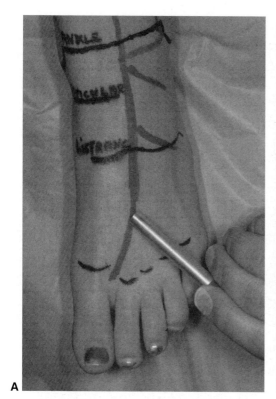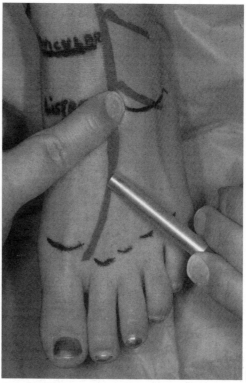

A   **B**

Figure 8-31   A: The antegrade and retrograde flow of the first dorsal metatarsal artery (FDMA) is being evaluated. The Doppler is placed over the FDMA. **B:** The dorsalis pedis is then occluded at the proximal first interspace. If there still is a signal, then there is retrograde flow from the first web space. (From Attinger CE, Cooper P, Blume P, et al. The safest surgical incision and amputations applying the angiosomes principle and using the Doppler to assess the arterial–arterial connections of the foot and ankle. *Foot Ankle Clin North Am.* 2001;6:745–801, with permission.)

or along the midline of the sole of the foot are very safe incisions.[18]

Unfortunately, one cannot reach all areas of the foot through these incisions, and blood flow to each angiosome is not always satisfactory; thus, well-deliberated compromises need to be made. When the signal of a source artery to one of two adjacent angiosomes is absent, the affected ischemic angiosome depends on the surrounding angiosomes for blood flow via the choke vessels. Because the choke vessels require 4 to 10 days after a given angiosome becomes ischemic to become patent, incisions placed too soon after an arterial occlusion for collateral circulation to develop run the risk of poor healing, necrosis, or gangrene.[13,30] However, in patients with arteriosclerosis, the occlusion is gradual and the choke vessels are usually patent by the time the source vessel closes.

When faced with abnormal blood flow, mapping out the direction of blood flow along the main arteries of the foot and ankle is critical. Again, important information regarding arterial vessel predominance and directional flow can be obtained with the handheld Doppler. This is not to minimize the extreme importance of angiography in assessing vascular

pathology. In the vascular patient, there may be collateral flow keeping the affected angiosome vascularized and incisions must be planned so that this collateral flow is not disturbed. In the more extreme ischemic cases where there are no palpable pulses and the Doppler sounds are monophasic, then possible surgical revascularization should be entertained before proceeding.

Incisions at the Achilles Tendon

Incisions over the Achilles tendon are the safest if made along the midline that divides the peroneal angiosome from the posterior tibial angiosome (Fig. 8-32). As we have previously reported, this ensures that perforators from the peroneal artery keep the tissue lateral to the central incision alive while perforators from the posterior tibial artery keep the medial tissue alive.[18] Incisions on either side of the Achilles tendon to expose the distal tibia or fibula, respectively, are also safe provided that both the posterior tibial artery and peroneal artery are patent. The rich interconnecting vascular plexus around the Achilles tendon keeps the skin above the Achilles tendon viable.

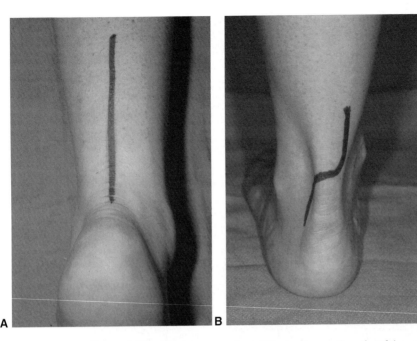
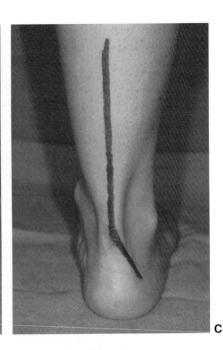

Figure 8-32 **A:** Incisions over the Achilles tendon are the safest if they are made along the midline that divides the peroneal angiosome from the posterior tibial angiosome. **B:** If there is a good Doppler signal over the posterior tibial artery and the calcaneal branch of the peroneal artery, an S-shaped incision can be made starting medially and finishing laterally to avoid the sural nerve and lesser saphenous vein. **C:** If the incision must continue distally to the level of the posterior heel, it should veer laterally along the posterior heel pad glabrous junction. (From Attinger CE, Cooper P, Blume P, et al. The safest surgical incision and amputations applying the angiosomes principle and using the Doppler to assess the arterial–arterial connections of the foot and ankle. *Foot Ankle Clin North Am.* 2001;6:745–801, with permission.)

When either of the two arteries is damaged, we described above the difficulty of assessing existing arterial–arterial connections. However, if there is a triphasic Doppler signal over the posterior tibial artery and over the calcaneal branch of the peroneal artery, one can then assume that both sides of the central incision are adequately vascularized.

While a medially to lateral S-shaped incision minimizes injury to the sural nerve and lesser saphenous vein (Fig. 8-32), direct transverse incisions over the Achilles tendon are also safe. If an incision is made at the glabrous junction of the posterior heel, the medial portion of the incision should not extend much distal to the medial edge of the Achilles tendon to avoid damaging the medial calcaneal neurovascular structures. It is safe to continue the incision laterally along the glabrous junction, which represents the distal boundary of the calcaneal branch of the posterior tibial artery.

If the incision must continue distally through the posterior heel, the incision can be placed straight down to the midline of the heel. However, this may be problematic distally where a sensitive scar can be irritated by the heel counter of a shoe. A useful alternative is to curve laterally along the posterior heel pad glabrous junction (Fig. 8-32). The lateral curve ensures that the usual predominate blood supply (from the calcaneal artery of the posterior tibial artery to the plantar heel rather than the peroneal artery) is preserved. It also avoids the risk of damaging either the posterior tibial calcaneal artery or the medial calcaneal nerve. Of course, if the peroneal artery proves to be superior in a patient, one could curve the incision medially. This design, however, increases the risk of damaging the branches of the medial calcaneal nerve and artery.

When one of the pulses is not present, it is best to place the incision away from the patent source artery, as we have previously reported.[18] This is the safest location because there is minimal risk to damaging the patent source artery or the crucial choke vessels. For example, if the peroneal artery has no signal, the incision should be placed quite lateral to the Achilles (within the peroneal artery angiosome) to allow the posterior tibial artery to feed the posterior side of the incision via the choke vessels over the central raphe of the Achilles tendon. The anterior tibial artery (via choke vessels between the peroneal and anterior tibial angiosome) feeds the anterior side of the incision. The patency of the anterior tibial artery should be checked before making the incision. Despite all these precautions, there are still no assurances that the tissue lateral to the incision will heal uneventfully.

Incisions at the Lateral Calcaneus

The need for exposure of the lateral calcaneus for calcaneal fractures is common. The L-shaped incision, as

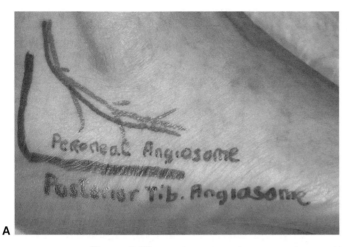

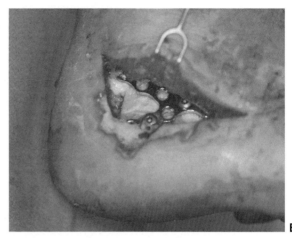

A   B

Figure 8-33   A: The L-shaped incision, advocated by Benirschke, to expose the lateral calcaneus in calcaneus fractures should be designed with the lower portion of the incision along the glabrous junction between the plantar heel and lateral heel. The lateral heel glabrous juncture is the boundary that represents the lateral extent of angiosome fed by the calcaneal branch of the posterior tibial artery. An incision above the glabrous juncture into the lateral heel proper leaves the tissue between the glabrous junction and the incision in jeopardy because that tissue lies in the just-divided angiosome of the calcaneal branch of the peroneal artery. **B:** This patient's incision was located above the glabrous border for internal fixation of a calcaneal fracture. The skin necrosed and hardware became exposed. (From Attinger CE, Cooper P, Blume P, et al. The safest surgical incision and amputations applying the angiosomes principle and using the Doppler to assess the arterial–arterial connections of the foot and ankle. *Foot Ankle Clin North Am.* 2001;6:745–801, with permission.)

advocated by Benirschke,[19,31] is safest if the lower portion of the incision is made along the glabrous junction between the plantar heel and lateral heel (Fig. 8-33). Because the lateral heel glabrous juncture is the lateral border of the angiosome fed by the calcaneal branch of the posterior tibial artery, an incision above that glabrous juncture into the lateral heel proper leaves the intervening tissue between the glabrous junction and the incision in jeopardy. This is because that intervening tissue lies within the angiosome of the calcaneal branch of the peroneal artery (Fig. 8-33B). In the usual trauma patient with a calcaneal fracture, the choke vessels between the posterior tibial and peroneal angiosome have not opened up to allow the calcaneal branch of the posterior tibial artery to feed the tissue. As we stated above, it usually takes 3 to 10 days for the choke vessels to become patent and potentially even longer in the setting of overlying soft-tissue damage and inflammation.[30]

The vertical portion of the L incision can be safely placed anterior to the lateral Achilles tendon because there is blood flow via arterioles from the posterior tibial artery that wrap around the Achilles to keep the tissue vascularized. Moreover, we advocate using a sharply curved incision over the 90-degree angle at the corner of the L incision to aid in closure.[19] Note that if the calcaneal branch of the peroneal artery is acutely thrombosed or damaged, then any incision over the lateral heel will likely lead to tissue loss. However, if that branch has been occluded for any considerable time and the calcaneal branch of the posterior tibial

artery and the anterior tibial artery are open, then the incision may be safe if it is made in the center of the peroneal artery angiosome, which lies closer to the lateral malleolus.

Incisions at the Hindfoot

The standard horizontal incisions over the sinus tarsi used commonly for hindfoot arthrodesis procedures are safe.[32] They overlie a "rete" (net) of arteries that arise from the continuation of the anterior tibial artery, the dorsalis pedis artery, the perforating branch of the peroneal artery, and lateral calcaneal artery.[22] The incision should be placed parallel to the direction of the lateral dorsal vessels traveling in a medial to lateral direction. This minimizes the disruption of the blood flow without inhibiting exposure.

Both the perforating branch of the peroneal artery and the lateral malleolar artery typically supply the tissue proximal to the incision. The proximal tarsal artery, the calcaneal branch of the peroneal artery, the distal tarsal artery, and the arcuate artery all provide blood flow to the tissue distal to the incision. Depending on the exact placement of the incision, the artery of the sinus tarsi and the lateral talar artery may be above or below the incision. The proximal tarsal artery is usually below the incision. The incision can be extended anteriorly to expose the calcaneocuboid joint. Care must to be taken not to damage the arcuate artery.

In patients with vascular disease, the incision must be modified. If the peroneal artery is absent, attention must be focused on preserving branches of the anterior tibial artery and dorsalis pedis artery when making the incision. In addition, great care should be taken to preserve any of the medial to lateral directed branches of dorsalis pedis artery. The incision is horizontal and placed between the lateral malleolar and lateral tarsal artery. Using the Doppler to optimally place the incision is recommended.

Incisions at the Medial Calcaneus

The medial calcaneus lies within the posterior tibial angiosome. The flow inferior to the tarsal tunnel is provided by the calcaneal branch of the posterior tibial artery, while the flow superior to the tarsal tunnel is provided by the posterior medial malleolar artery, medial talar artery, and medial tarsal artery. In addition, the anterior medial malleolar artery (a branch of the anterior tibial artery) connects anteriorly in this area with the posterior medial malleolar artery.

For access of the medial calcaneus, incisions around the tarsal tunnel are useful. If the posterior tibial artery and its branches are patent, an incision directly over the tarsal tunnel is safe (Fig. 8-34). Incisions anterior to the tarsal tunnel are only safe if the anterior tibial artery and its medial branches are patent. Although it is preferable if the incision is placed parallel to the course of the medial malleolar arteries, it can also be parallel to the curve of the tarsal tunnel. Incisions inferior to

and parallel to the tarsal tunnel should be avoided because they will damage the medial calcaneal neurovascular bundle; in addition, the tissue between the glabrous junction of the heel and the incision will be vascularly compromised.

When there is no posterior tibial pulse, one has to make sure that both the anterior tibial artery and peroneal artery are open, that the occlusion is chronic, and that there is no acute trauma or chronic scarring in the area. In addition, the transcutaneous oxygen tension over the planned incision should be >40 mm Hg. Under these circumstances, an incision over the tarsal tunnel may be safe. Straying to either side of the tarsal tunnel may lead to some tissue slough. If the posterior tibial artery and one of the other two main arteries are occluded, incisions are then fraught with healing complications. Collateral flow must be mapped out by Doppler to ensure that the planned incision will not interfere with that flow.

Incisions at the Plantar Heel

In general, these incisions are reserved for hindfoot limb salvage in the presence of osteomyelitis. Safe incisions over the plantar heel from a vascular perspective can be coronal or sagittal in orientation if both the posterior tibial and peroneal arteries are patent (Fig. 8-35). Whether the resultant scar is acceptable is another question altogether.[33] Recall that the blood flow to the heel lies primarily in a coronal direction from both the calcaneal branch of the posterior tibial artery and the peroneal artery supplying blood flow from the medial and lateral side, respectively. The coronal incision will not disturb the coronal flow or the sensory nerves that travel in the same direction.

If the incision is in the sagittal direction, then the flow comes to each side of the incision from the respective calcaneal arteries. However, the sensory nerves will be damaged, which of course is no concern if the patient is neuropathic. If this is the case, a Gaenslen incision down the central heel pad is the ideal choice to expose the calcaneus for calcanectomy (Fig. 8-35).[34] Great care to adequately evert the edges when closing the incision will avoid an inverted and chronically callused scar.

If one of the two calcaneal source arteries is occluded, the incisions have to be planned more carefully. In this circumstance, a coronal incision is safer because it does not damage the coronally directed flow from whichever open calcaneal artery is supplying the heel. However, a sagittal incision interrupts the coronal direction of flow, putting the side away from the patent source artery at risk. Again, in order for a sagittal incision to be safe, one has to be sure that the side away from the patent artery is being supplied by collateral arteries, and there must be adequate time for the collateral circulation to develop. Listening for Doppler flow over the heel with the still

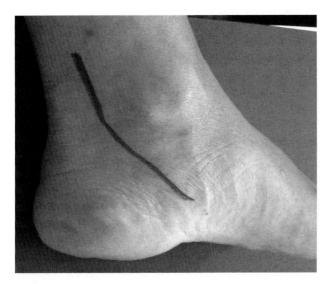

Figure 8-34 An incision directly over the tarsal tunnel is safe if the posterior tibial artery and its branches are patent. Incisions anterior to the tarsal tunnel are safe if the anterior tibial artery and its medial branches are also patent. Although it is preferable if the incision is placed parallel to the course of the medial malleolar arteries, it can also be parallel to the curve of the tarsal tunnel. Incisions inferior to and parallel to the tarsal tunnel should be avoided because they will damage the medial calcaneus neurovascular bundle. In addition, the tissue between the glabrous junction of the medial heel and the incision will be vascularly compromised.

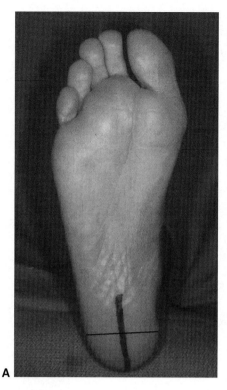
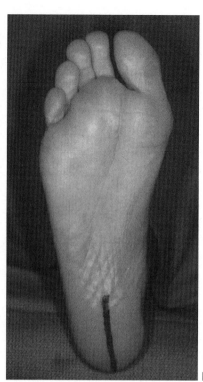

Figure 8-35 **A:** A safe incision over the plantar heel from a vascular perspective can be along either a coronal or sagittal direction if both arteries are patent. Coronally placed incisions avoid damage to the sensory nerve. **B:** The midline sagittal incision (Gaenslen) offers excellent calcaneal exposure for calcanectomy. (From Attinger CE, Cooper P, Blume P, et al. The safest surgical incision and amputations applying the angiosomes principle and using the Doppler to assess the arterial–arterial connections of the foot and ankle. *Foot Ankle Clin North Am.* 2001;6:745–801, with permission.) **A** **B**

patent source artery occluded can give an indication of the quality of the collateral flow.

Incisions at the Plantar and Medial Midfoot

To review, the blood flow to the midfoot plantar sole comes from perforators from the medial and lateral plantar arteries that travel on either side of the plantar fascia (Fig. 8-36). In addition, there is a subdermal arteriolar plexus over the plantar midfoot and proximal forefoot that connects the dorsal to the plantar circulation via minute arterioles coursing in a coronal direction (Fig. 8-29).[29] This subdermal circulation is also connected to the perforators that arise from the medial and lateral plantar arteries.

If both plantar arteries are open, the safest incision is along the plantar midline separating the medial plantar angiosome from the lateral plantar angiosome. Care has to be taken to preserve the perforators along either side of the plantar fascia. Coronal incisions are also equally secure if the proximal and distal perforators or the underlying neurovascular bundles are not damaged. If many of the perforators are damaged, a full excision of the threatened skin (which can be assessed with intravenous fluorescene and a Wood lamp) is recommended to avoid significant skin slough.

For removal of plantar fibromatosis, a straight incision down the midline of the sole of the foot is the safest from a vascular perspective (Fig. 8-37). One can also use a curved or Z-shaped incision with the top two limbs following more or less along the boundary of the medial plantar artery angiosome (Fig. 8-37). If a curved incision is chosen, it

should have its apex laterally based in order to better follow the angiosome boundary between the medial and lateral plantar artery (Fig. 8-37).

If flow in one of the plantar arteries has been acutely interrupted, the flow over the other plantar artery and the dorsal circulation must be assessed. While a central sagittal plantar incision may still be safe because of the coronally directed subdermal flow, the choke vessels at the glabrous junction between the dorsal and plantar angiosomes have not had time to develop. In this case, the side of the incision away from the patent plantar artery is at risk. If there is any question, a coronal incision may be safer because it does not interrupt the subdermal flow.

If one plantar artery's flow has been chronically absent, then a careful Doppler exam has to be performed. Only if flow into both sides of the planned incision is Dopplerable can a relatively reliable incision be designed. Plantar midline incisions are probably safer because the plantar angiosome whose source artery has no flow can be fed by the dorsal circulation via the choke vessels along the glabrous juncture as well as by arterial–arterial connections.

For approaches to the medial midfoot, the safest incision (Fig. 8-38) is along the border between the medial plantar artery angiosome and the dorsalis pedis angiosome (Fig. 8-1A), 2 to 3 cm above the medial glabrous junction. To accurately map out the border, one should Doppler out the course of the superficial medial plantar artery (Fig. 8-28) and design the incision dorsal to its course. The plantar side of the incision is

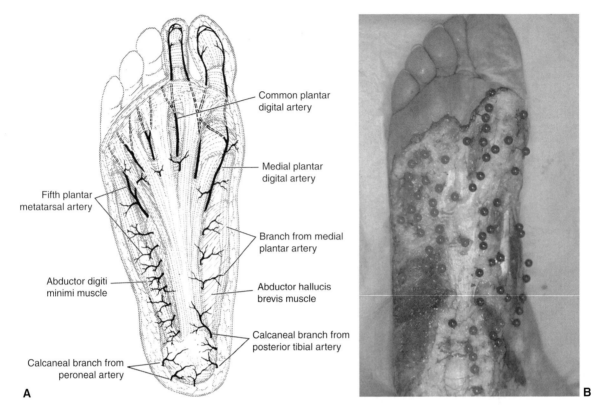

Figure 8-36 **A:** Most of the perforators that feed the plantar midfoot arise along each side of the plantar fascia from the lateral plantar artery and deep medial plantar artery. **B:** The pins show the location of the perforators on either side of the plantar fascia. (From Attinger CE, Cooper P, Blume P, et al. The safest surgical incision and amputations applying the angiosomes principle and using the Doppler to assess the arterial–arterial connections of the foot and ankle. *Foot Ankle Clin North Am.* 2001;6:745–801, with permission.)

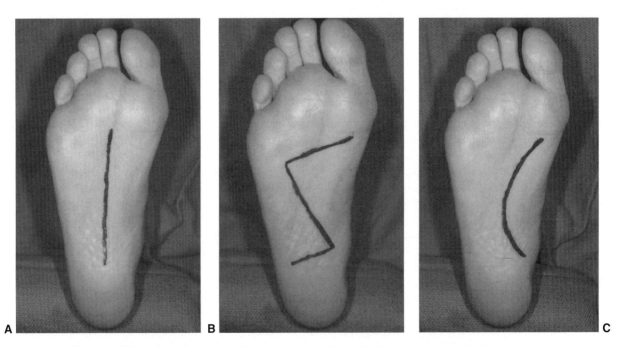

Figure 8-37 **A:** A straight incision down the midline of the sole of the foot is the safest from a vascular perspective. **B:** One can also use a curved or Z-shaped incision with the top two limbs following more or less along the boundary of the medial plantar artery. **C:** If a curved incision is chosen, it should have its apex laterally based so as to better follow the angiosome boundary between the medial and lateral plantar arteries. (From Attinger CE, Cooper P, Blume P, et al. The safest surgical incision and amputations applying the angiosomes principle and using the Doppler to assess the arterial–arterial connections of the foot and ankle. *Foot Ankle Clin North Am.* 2001;6:745–801, with permission.)

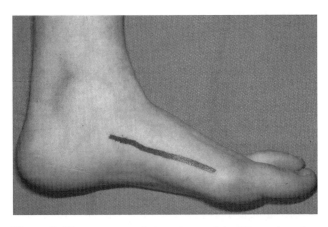

Figure 8-38 For approaches to the medial midfoot, the safest incision is along the border between the medial plantar artery angiosome and the dorsalis pedis angiosome. This incision is 2 to 3 cm above the medial glabrous border. The plantar side of the incision is carefully lifted off the underlying bone, taking care not to damage the superficial medial plantar artery. (From Attinger CE, Cooper P, Blume P, et al. The safest surgical incision and amputations applying the angiosomes principle and using the Doppler to assess the arterial–arterial connections of the foot and ankle. *Foot Ankle Clin North Am.* 2001;6:745–801, with permission.)

then carefully lifted off the underlying bone, taking care not to damage the superficial medial plantar artery. Because two medial plantar arteries provide blood supply to the medial plantar angiosome, it is safe to make an incision between them, providing they are both patent.

Incisions at the Plantar Forefoot

The angiosome of the plantar forefoot is supplied by the metatarsal arteries that come off the lateral plantar artery, and reinforced by the proximal and distal perforators between the dorsal and plantar metatarsal arteries (Fig. 8-5A). Incisions in any direction are safe if both the dorsalis pedis and the lateral plantar arteries are open and care is taken to interrupt as few of the perforators as possible.

Coronal incisions just distal to the metatarsal heads (as advocated for rheumatoid lesser toe procedures) avoid the primary weight-bearing areas (Fig. 8-39), but may interrupt the distal perforators linking the plantar to the dorsal circulation. If the metatarsal antegrade

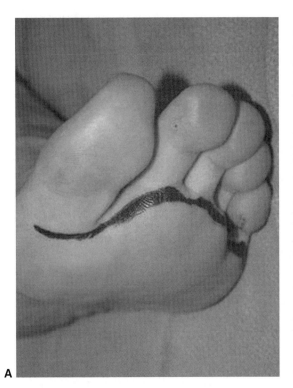

A

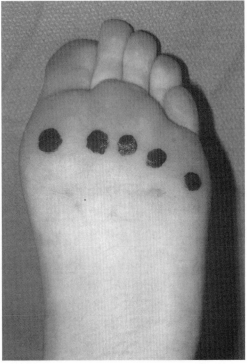

Figure 8-39 **A:** Because of the dual blood flow the plantar forefoot enjoys, incisions in any direction are safe from a vascular perspective, but subsequent scarring may pose a problem with some incisions. Coronal directed incisions distal to the metatarsal heads (depicted here) avoid the primary weight-bearing areas but may interrupt the distal perforators linking the plantar to the dorsal circulation. This should not be a problem if the metatarsal antegrade arterial flow is intact and the digital arteries are spared. Moreover, coronal incisions proximal to the metatarsal heads lie along the border between the medial and lateral plantar angiosome and are safe if the underlying lateral plantar and metatarsal arteries are not damaged. Note that sagittal directed incisions will risk less harm to the underlying metatarsal/digital arteries, but run across the weight-bearing portion of the forefoot. **B:** Location of the metatarsal heads, an important landmark in plantar forefoot incisions.

arterial flow is intact and the digital arteries are spared, this should not be a problem. Sagittal incisions will risk less harm to the underlying metatarsal/digital arteries, but cross the weight-bearing portion of the forefoot (Fig. 8-39). These incisions should be placed between the metatarsal heads for better healing.

If either the lateral plantar artery or dorsalis pedis arteries is/are absent, then the proximal or distal perforators must not be damaged when designing the incision. Interruption of those perforators may lead to insufficient dorsal blood flow if the dorsalis pedis artery is compromised or insufficient plantar flow if the lateral plantar artery is diseased. Careful Doppler examination to accurately locate the perforators is necessary in planning any incision under these circumstances and the surgical approach should focus on avoiding damage to the perforators.

Incisions on the Dorsum of the Foot

When considering dorsal foot incisions, recall that the dorsal circulation proximal to the Lisfranc joint travels in a coronal direction, while circulation distal to the Lisfranc joint travels in a sagittal direction (Fig. 8-9). The lateral proximal dorsum of the foot is composed of a "rete" (net) of coronally interconnected arteries of the lateral malleolar, tarsal (proximal and distal), and arcuate arteries (Fig. 8-11). This rete is laterally linked to the anterior perforating branch and calcaneal branch of the peroneal arteries. Medial to the proximal dorsalis pedis is the medial tarsal artery that may join the medial plantar circulation.

Again, we advocate the principle of placing the incision parallel to the direction of the arterial supply. Coronal incisions in the lateral dorsal midfoot are parallel to the coronally directed arteries (proximal tarsal, distal tarsal, arcuate arteries, and their perforators). In addition, the dorsalis pedis artery should be identified and spared unless it is clear that the antegrade and retrograde flow is strong.

On the other hand, sagittal incisions over the rete are also safe if both the peroneal artery and dorsalis pedis are intact, and the medial and lateral sides of the rete are left undisturbed. In addition, lateral incisions can be made along the glabrous junction between the dorsal and plantar circulation assuming the flow along the dorsalis pedis and lateral plantar arteries is intact.

For approaches to the medial midfoot, the safest incision is along the border between the medial plantar artery angiosome and the dorsalis pedis angiosome (Fig. 8-38). This border is usually 2 to 3 cm above the medial glabrous junction. One should Doppler the course of the superficial medial plantar artery (Fig. 8-28) and make the incision dorsal to its course.

Dorsal incisions in the proximal dorsum of the foot can become problematic if the anterior tibial artery or posterior tibial arteries are occluded and the peroneal is not providing adequate alternative flow. If the posterior tibial is occluded, then the dorsalis pedis flow is antegrade, and if the anterior tibial is occluded, then the flow is retrograde. Interrupting the major flow can lead to significant tissue necrosis. For example, if the anterior tibial artery flow is retrograde (from the lateral plantar artery) and the peroneal artery is out, then any incision that interrupts the distal to proximal blood flow will lead to tissue death proximal to the incision (Fig. 8-21).

If the peroneal artery is occluded, it is important to protect the tarsal and arcuate arteries because they are the sole blood supply to the lateral dorsal midfoot. If choke vessels have opened, the lateral plantar artery can help contribute to the lateral dorsal blood flow. In addition, if the dorsalis pedis artery is occluded, then the dorsum of the foot is being supplied by the arcuate artery blood flow, which is coming from the proximal perforators and from the tarsal artery (being supplied by the peroneal artery). Moreover, if the posterior tibial artery is out, the incision must not disrupt the arcuate artery because this may damage the proximal perforators that are supplying the plantar foot.

For incisions of the distal forefoot, it is important not to place an incision through the metatarsal arteries unless they both have antegrade flow (from the arcuate artery and proximal perforators) and retrograde flow (from the distal perforators). Recall that the metatarsal arteries arise from the arcuate artery, travel along the interosseus space, and are connected to plantar circulation both proximally and distally by perforators. If the metatarsal artery flow is bidirectional, then coronally directed incisions are safe but are seldom needed. However, if the flow is unidirectional, the incisions should be in the sagittal direction, over the metatarsal bones themselves, in order to not disturb the dorsal metatarsal arteries. Multiple parallel sagittal incisions over the distal dorsal forefoot can be performed as long as the dorsal metatarsal arteries are preserved (Fig. 8-40). Incidentally, only three incisions are necessary to gain access to all metatarsals, and the incisions should be short, with little undermining of the skin overlying the interosseus muscles.

Incisions at the First Metatarsophalangeal Joint

The first MTP joint is a common area for plantar ulcerations and dorsal traumatic wounds, as well as bony disease requiring access to this area. This region is supplied by contributions from the dorsalis pedis artery via the

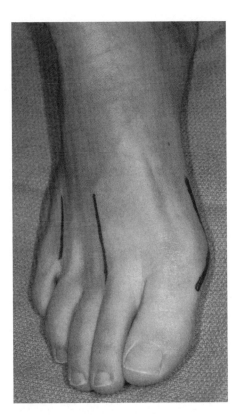

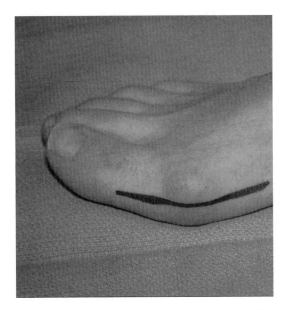

Figure 8-41 The safest incision over the first metatarsal joint is at the medial glabrous junction because it does not disturb either the dorsal or plantar circulation.

Figure 8-40 Multiple parallel sagittal incisions over the distal dorsal forefoot can be performed as long as the dorsal metatarsal arteries are patent and preserved. (From Attinger CE, Cooper P, Blume P, et al. The safest surgical incision and amputations applying the angiosomes principle and using the Doppler to assess the arterial–arterial connections of the foot and ankle. *Foot Ankle Clin North Am.* 2001;6:745–801, with permission.)

Incisions for Amputations

In general, performing forefoot and midfoot amputations in patients who have intact circulation with both the dorsal and plantar antegrade blood flow has minimal risk. All incisions should be designed at the angiosome boundaries to maximize blood flow at the edges of the amputation. Medial and lateral incisions should be at the glabrous juncture between the dorsal and plantar circulation, while dorsal and plantar incisions should be straight down to bone, preserving metatarsal arteries in the flaps.

When there is compromised flow and a forefoot or midfoot amputation is planned, it is very important that the remaining blood flow and arterial–arterial connections are completely elucidated. If the dorsal circulation depends on the plantar circulation or vice versa, then connections between the two regions cannot be disturbed (Fig. 8-21). That is, the connection between the dorsalis pedis and lateral plantar artery at the proximal first interspace must be maintained. Therefore, when performing a short transmetatarsal or Lisfranc amputation, the lateral four metatarsals are removed laterally while the first metatarsal is removed medially.

FDMA, from the medial plantar artery (via the medial first plantar metatarsal artery), and from the lateral plantar artery (via the lateral first plantar metatarsal artery) (Figs. 8-12 and 8-13). As stated above, the dorsal and plantar circulations are closely linked proximally by the juncture of the dorsalis pedis artery and lateral plantar artery (Fig. 8-7), and distally by the distal perforator in the first interspace. Of course, there are many anatomic variations, and the dominant flow can come from one of the three main arteries: The FDMA or the medial or lateral plantar arteries.

When designing incisions over the first MTP, the medial glabrous junction is the safest incision because it does not disturb either the dorsal or plantar circulation (Fig. 8-41). This incision can safely be extended more distally if both the dorsal and plantar circulation are open. Likewise, an incision over the extensor hallucis tendon is safe if the dorsal and plantar circulations are intact (Fig. 8-41). However, an incision in the first interspace can be fraught with danger because it can damage the principal flow to the hallux. This is especially true if either the dorsal or plantar circulation is compromised and depends on the other for blood flow.

USING THE ANGIOSOME PRINCIPLE IN PLANNING THE OPTIMAL REVASCULARIZATION

Despite the current advances in revascularization techniques, vascular bypass surgery fails to heal approximately 15% of ischemic lower extremity wounds with a patent bypass.[35–46] Gooden et al.[47] found that up to 25% of patients with heel ulcers ultimately succumbed to a proximal leg amputation despite a palpable pedal pulse. A portion of these failures may be due to inadequate treatment of the wound postoperatively.[48] Part of the problem, however, may also be due to the inadequate revascularization of the local ischemic area because of inadequate vascular connections between the revascularized vessel and the source vessel nourishing the ischemic area. Thus, successful limb salvage for ischemic wounds involves more than simply restoring circulation to any vessel in the distal lower extremity.

The literature states that bypassing to one distal artery should be sufficient to heal any foot wound. Unfortunately, there is a 15% failure rate when bypassing to the dorsalis pedis artery for heel ulcers. It stands to reason that the new blood flow to the dorsalis pedis artery has to reach the heel for healing to occur. If the arterial connections between the dorsal and plantar circulation are not present, the wound is unlikely to heal. Direct revascularization of either the posterior tibial artery or the peroneal artery (both of which have calcaneal branches that supply the plantar heel) is more likely to succeed than bypassing to the more remote dorsalis pedis artery. Therefore, the most effective revascularization is directed to the source artery of the angiosome containing the ulceration.

We investigated whether limb salvage was more successful when revascularization was to the major artery directly supplying the ischemic and ulcerated angiosome rather than to one of the other two major arteries.[49] Sixty consecutive distal lower extremity wounds were retrospectively reviewed from 56 consecutive patients who required vascular bypass for an ischemic foot wound prior to wound closure from 1994 through 1998. The wounds were divided into two groups: Direct revascularization (direct bypass to the major blood vessel supplying the source vessel to the angiosome where the ulcer was located) or indirect revascularization (bypass to a major vessel unrelated to the affected angiosome). Eight wounds were excluded due to incomplete follow-up. Outcome of the remaining 52 wounds was rated as healed, failure to heal leading to amputation, or death unrelated to wound. We found that 51.1% of the limbs were directly bypassed, while 48.9% underwent indirect revascularization. Among the 52 wounds, 33 (63.5%) progressed to complete healing after closure; ten (19.2%) failed to heal and went on to proximal amputation (below-knee amputation [BKA]/above-knee amputation [AKA]); nine legs (17.3%) could not be adequately assessed due to premature death of the patient unrelated to the wound. Time to heal between the two groups (162.4 days [direct] vs. 159.8 days [indirect]) was not statistically significant ($p = 0.95$). There was also no difference in time to heal when bypass was above the tibioperoneal

trifurcation (179.4 days) versus distally (156.5 days) ($p = 0.81$).

When looking at outcome of all cases relative to the bypass received, there was a 9.1% failure rate when wounds were directly revascularized versus a 38.1% failure rate in the wounds indirectly bypassed ($p = 0.03$). Those who failed to heal went on to a major leg amputation. The amputation rate, therefore, in the indirectly bypassed group was four times that of the directly bypassed group. This study supports the suggestion that direct revascularization of the affected angiosome leads to higher limb salvage rates.

If the vascular surgeon has more than one vessel to bypass to or has the choice of opening more than one vessel, he/she should preferentially open the vessel that directly feeds the affected angiosome. For heel wounds, the peroneal or posterior tibial artery should be revascularized. For plantar foot wounds, the posterior tibial artery should be preferentially revascularized. For lateral ankle wounds, the peroneal artery should be preferentially revascularized. For dorsal foot wounds, the anterior tibial artery should be preferentially revascularized.

If the vascular surgeon cannot revascularize the source artery to the affected angiosome, he/she can then predict a certain failure rate from an alternative bypass unless he/she can demonstrate that the arterial–arterial connections between the artery to be revascularized and the source artery of the affected angiosome are open.

CONCLUSION

In the normal patient, blood flow to the foot and ankle is plentiful, from three major arteries of the leg, complete with their multiple arterial–arterial connections. With a thorough understanding of this anatomy, the consequences of arterial insufficiency, and the angiosome principle, safe incisions can be designed that minimize healing complications. Because this anatomy varies from patient to patient, the Doppler allows the surgeon to map out the vascular tree that exists preoperatively. Using the angiosome principles, appropriate adjustments can be made to the planned incisions. Last, bypassing to the source artery of an ulcerated angiosome ensures the highest possible salvage rate.

REFERENCES

1. Morain WD, Ristic J. *Manchot: the cutaneous arteries of the human body.* New York, NY: Springer Verlag; 1983.
2. Taylor GI, Tempest MN, Salmon M, eds. *Arteries of the skin.* Edinburgh: Churchill Livingston; 1988.
3. McGregor IA, Morgan G. Axial and random pattern flaps. *Br J Plast Surg.* 1973;26:202.

4. Daniel RK, Cunningham DM, Taylor GI. The deltopectoral flap: an anatomical and hemodynamic approach. *Plast Reconstr Surg.* 1975;55:275.

5. Mathes SJ, Nahai F. *Clinical atlas of muscle and musculocutaneous flaps.* St. Louis, Mo: CV Mosby; 1979.

6. Ger R. Operative treatment of the advanced stasis ulcer using muscle transposition. *Am J Surg.* 1970;120:376.

7. Orticochea M. The musculocutaneous flap method—an immediate and heroic substitute for the method of delay. *Br J Plast Surg.* 1972;25:106–110.

8. McCraw JB, Dibell DG. Experimental definition of independent myocutaneous vascular territories. *Plast Reconstr Surg.* 1977;60: 341–352.

9. Taylor GI, Palmer JH. The vascular territories (angiosomes) of the body: experimental studies and clinical applications. *Br J Plast Surg.* 1990;43:1.

10. Taylor GI, Minabe T. The angiosomes of the mammals and other vertebrates. *Plast Reconstr Surg.* 1992;89:181–215.

11. Calligari PR, Taylor GI, Caddy CM, et al. An anatomic review of the delay phenomenon: I. Experimental studies. *Plast Reconstr Surg.* 1992;89:397–407.

12. Taylor GI, Corlett RJ, Caddy CM, et al. An anatomic review of the delay phenomenon: II. Clinical applications. *Plast Reconstr Surg.* 1992;89:408–416.

13. Morris SF, Taylor GI. The time sequence of the delay phenomenon: when is a surgical delay effective? An experimental study. *Plast Reconstr Surg.* 1995;95:526–533.

14. Dhar SC, Taylor GI. V The delay phenomenon: the story unfolds. *Plast Reconstr Surg.* 1999;104:2079–2091.

15. Sarrafian SK. *Anatomy of the foot and ankle.* Philadelphia, Pa: JP Lippincott Co; 1993:294–355.

16. Taylor GI, Pan WR. Angiosomes of the leg: anatomic study and clinical implications. *Plast Reconstr Surg.* 1998;102:599.

17. Attinger CE, Cooper P, Blume P. Vascular anatomy of the foot and ankle. *Op Tech Plast Reconstr Surg.* 1997;4:183–198.

18. Attinger CE, Cooper P, Blume P, et al. The safest surgical incision and amputations applying the angiosomes principle and using the Doppler to assess the arterial-arterial connections of the foot and ankle. *Foot Ankle Clin North Am.* 2001;6:745–801.

19. Attinger C, Cooper P. Soft tissue reconstruction for calcaneal fractures or osteomyelitis. *Orthop Clin North Am.* 2001;32:135.

20. Murakami T. On the position and course of the deep plantar arteries, with special reference to the so-called plantar metatarsal arteries. *Okajimas Folia Anat Jpn.* 1971;48:295.

21. Huber JF. The arterial network supplying the dorsum of the foot. *Anat Rec.* 1941;80:373.

22. Adachi B. *Das arteriensystem der japaner.* Kyoto: Maruzren; 1928: 246–248.

23. May JW, Chait LA, Cohen BE. Free neurovascular flap from the first web of the foot in hand reconstruction. *J Hand Surg.* 1977; 5:387.

24. Shusterman MA, Reece GP, Milller MJ. The osteocutaneous free fibula flap: is the skin paddle reliable? *Plast Reconstr Surg.* 1992; 90:787.

25. Jones NF, Monstrey MD, Gambier BA. Reliability of the fibular osteocutaneous flap for mandibular reconstruction: anatomical and surgical confirmation. *Plast Reconstr Surg.* 1996;97:707.

26. Masqualet AC, Beveridge J, Romana C. The lateral supramalleolar flap. *Plast Reconstr Surg.* 1988;81:74.

27. Taylor GI, Doyle M, McCarten G. The Doppler probe for planning flaps: anatomical study and clinical applications. *Br J Plast Surg.* 1990;43:1–16.

28. Berceli SA, Chan AK, Pomposelli FB, et al. Efficacy of dorsal pedal artery bypass in limb salvage for ischemic heel ulcers. *J Vasc Surg Sept.* 1999;30:499–508.

29. Hidalgo DA, Shaw WW. Anatomic basis of plantar flap design. *Plast Reconstr Surg.* 1986;78:267.

30. Dhar SC, Taylor GI. The delay phenomenon: the story unfolds. *Plast Reconstr Surg.* 1999;104:2079–2091.

31. Benirschke SK, Sangeorzan BJ. Extensive intra-articular fractures of the foot: surgical management of calcaneal fractures. *Clin Orthop.* 1993;291:128.

32. Gelberman RH, Mortensen WW. The arterial anatomy of the talus. *Foot Ankle.* 1983;4:64.

33. Jahss MH. Surgical principles and the plantigrade foot. In: Jahss MH, ed. *Disorder of the foot and ankle: medical and surgical management.* 2nd ed. Philadelphia, Pa: WB Sauders Co; 1991:236–279.

34. Gaenslen FJ. Split heel approach in osteomyelitis of the os calcis. *J Bone Joint Surg.* 1931;13:759–772.

35. Berceli SA, Chan AK, Pomposelli FB, et al. Efficacy of dorsal pedal artery bypass in limb salvage for ischemic heel ulcers. *J Vasc Surg.* 1999;30:499.

36. Treiman GS, Oderich GS, Ashrafi A, et al. Management of ischemic heel ulceration and gangrene: an evaluation of factors associated with successful healing. *J Vasc Surg.* 2000;31:1110.

37. Carsten CG III, Taylor SM, Langan EM III, et al. Factors associated with limb loss despite a patent infrainguinal bypass graft. *Am Surg.* 1998;64:33.

38. Edwards JM, Taylor LM, Porter JM. Limb salvage in end-stage renal disease (ESRD), comparison of modern results in patients with and without ESRD. *Arch Surg.* 1998;123:1164.

39. Chang BB, Paty PK, Shah DM, et al. Results of infrainguinal bypass for limb salvage in patients with end-stage renal disease. *Surgery.* 1990;108:742.

40. Andros G, Harris RW, Dulawa LB, et al. The need for arteriography in diabetic patients with gangrene and palpable foot pulses. *Arch Surg.* 1984;119:1260.

41. Johnson BL, Glickman MH, Bandyk DF, et al. Failure of foot salvage in patients with end-stage renal disease after surgical revascularization. *J Vasc Surg.* 1995;22:280.

42. Elliot BM, Robison JG, Brothers TE, et al. Limitations of peroneal artery bypass grafting for limb salvage. *J Vasc Surg.* 1993;18:881.

43. Bergamini TM, George SM, Massey HT, et al. Pedal or peroneal bypass: which is better when both are patent? *J Vasc Surg.* 1994; 20:347.

44. Seeger JM, Pretus HA, Carlton LC, et al. Potential predictors of outcome in patients with tissue loss who undergo infrainguinal vein bypass grafting. *J Vasc Surg.* 1999;30:427.

45. Darling RC III, Chang BB, Paty PS, et al. Choice of peroneal or dorsalis pedis artery bypass for limb salvage. *Am J Surg.* 1995;170:109.

46. Abou-Zamzam AM, Moneta GL, Lee RW, et al. Peroneal bypass is equivalent to inframalleolar bypass for ischemic pedal gangrene. *Arch Surg.* 1996;131:894.

47. Gooden MA, Gentile AT, Mills JL, et al. Free tissue transfer to extend the limits of limb salvage for lower extremity tissue loss. *Am J Surg.* 1997;174:644.

48. Attinger CE, Ducic I, Neville RF, et al. The relative roles of aggressive wound care versus revascularization in salvage of the threatened lower extremity in the renal failure diabetic patient. *Plast Reconstr Surg.* 2002;109:1281–1290.

49. Bulan EJ, Attinger CE, Ducic I, et al. Implications of direct versus indirect revascularization of the ulcerated ischemic angiosome in limb salvage. Presented 16th American Soc. for Reconstructive Microsurgery, Coronado, California Jan 2001.

Angiogenesis in Wound Healing

Albeir Y. Mousa   Peter Henderson   K. Craig Kent

Angiogenesis is a dynamic process that involves the sprouting of new capillaries from preexisting vessels. Multiple steps are involved, including retraction of pericytes from the abluminal surface of existing capillaries, release of proteases from activated endothelial cells, degradation of the extracellular matrix that surrounds preexisting vessels, endothelial migration towards an angiogenic stimulus, and subsequent proliferation of these cells to form tubelike structures (Fig. 9-1). This process is completed by fusion of these structures with existing vessels and ultimately the initiation of blood flow through newly formed capillaries. Angiogenesis is held delicately in balance by the interplay of both positive and negative regulators. There are >20 known angiogenic growth factors and >30 known angiogenic inhibitors. Under normal physiologic conditions, angiogenesis is "turned off" because the influence of inhibitors outweighs that of activators (Fig. 9-2). Consequently, the replication rate for adult endothelial cells is one of the lowest of all cells in the body, with 0.01% engaged in cell division at any given time. However, angiogenesis is an important part of normal and abnormal human physiology. In normal adults, angiogenesis is required for healing wounds, the menstrual cycle, and pregnancy. Pathologic angiogenesis results in the spread and growth of tumors as well as conditions such as rheumatoid arthritis and diabetic retinopathy.

Angiogenesis is also an important component of wound healing. In fact, angiogenesis is the source of granulation tissue. John Hunter[1] used the term "granulation tissue" in 1787 to describe the appearance of prominent blood vessels within the initial connective tissue formed in the wound space. The process of wound healing can be divided into four well-defined, overlapping phases: Hemostasis, inflammation, proliferation, and maturation. During inflammation, the capillaries become permeable to leukocytes and plasma proteins, which, within hours, fill the wound with an inflammatory exudate of neutrophils, monocytes, and proteins. Meanwhile, the wound begins the process of epithelialization with basal epithelial cells migrating in from the wound margins. On approximately the third day, fibroblasts appear in the wound in significant numbers, marking the beginning of the proliferative phase. Fibroblasts begin to multiply in number and release collagen and interstitial matrix. Meanwhile, endothelial cells begin the angiogenic process of proliferation and new vessel formation. This is a critical point in wound healing, as it marks the initiation of the development of granulation tissue. This is followed by wound contraction, which is carried out by myofibroblasts. After approximately 3 weeks, the fibroblasts and macrophages gradually disappear from the wound, and relatively acellular collagen begins the continuous process of remodeling and maturation.

"Therapeutic angiogenesis" is the exogenous application of angiogenic agents to a target tissue for the purpose of achieving a therapeutic benefit. Since angiogenesis is central to the process of wound healing, therapeutic angiogenesis has been proposed as a method of enhancing healing of chronic wounds. In this chapter, we will explore this concept in detail and relay the findings of a number of studies where therapeutic angiogenesis has been employed.

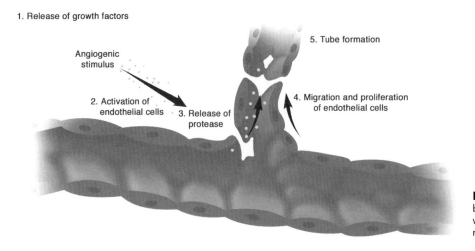

1. Release of growth factors

Angiogenic stimulus

5. Tube formation

2. Activation of endothelial cells

3. Release of protease

4. Migration and proliferation of endothelial cells

Figure 9-1 The angiogenesis process begins with release of growth factors which provide the angiogenic stimulus required by endothelial cells.

ANGIOGENIC STIMULI

There are a variety of growth factors that have been evaluated in animal and human trials of angiogenesis. Although all of these proteins are similar in that they can initiate or propagate the angiogenic process, there are marked differences in their behavior and function. Ultimately, therapeutic angiogenesis may be best produced by using a combination of these various angiogenic proteins.

Vascular Endothelial Growth Factor

Vascular endothelial growth factor (VEGF) is a family of six 34- to 46-kDa dimeric glycoproteins. These proteins were initially determined to be vascular permeability factors, although in 1989, VEGF was characterized and cloned as an angiogenic factor.[2] Splicing of the VEGF-A gene results in five isoforms ($VEGF_{121}$, $VEGF_{145}$, $VEGF_{165}$, $VEGF_{189}$, and $VEGF_{206}$), differing in total amino acid number; the most commonly expressed proteins are $VEGF_{121}$ and $VEGF_{165}$. VEGF has a signaling sequence that permits its secretion by intact cells. Thus, VEGF produced in transfected cells has the ability to be secreted and become biologically active. It is probable that these various isoforms have different functions. VEGF appears to be the most potent regulator of angiogenesis. This protein is synthesized by a variety of cell types in and around the vessel wall; however, VEGF specifically stimulates endothelial cell proliferation and migration and enhances endothelial cell survival by binding to two transmembrane tyrosine-kinase receptors: fms-related tyrosine kinase 1 (flt-1)/vascular endothelial growth factor receptor-1 (VEGFR-1), and kinase insert domain–containing receptor/fetal liver kinase (KDR/flk-1) (VEGFR-2).[3] Although VEGF does not have a direct effect on smooth muscle cells (SMC) or pericytes, VEGF can stimulate SMC migration and proliferation indirectly through factors released by the endothelial cell. Hypoxia is a potent stimulus for VEGF expression.[4] Transcription of VEGF messenger ribonucleic acid (mRNA) is mediated in part by the binding of hypoxia-inducible factor 1 to a binding site located on the VEGF promoter.[5] Furthermore, VEGF mRNA is intrinsically labile; however, in response to hypoxia there is stabilization of its mRNA.[6,7] VEGF also increases expression of plasminogen activator and collagenase in endothelial cells, which in turn degrade extracellular matrix, allowing endothelial cell migration and sprouting. Thus, VEGF plays a number of distinct roles in the angiogenic process.

Fibroblast Growth Factor

Fibroblast growth factor (FGF) is a family of structurally homologous 16- to 24-kDa proteins that enhance proliferation of endothelial cells, fibroblasts, and SMC. At present, there are at least 20 known proteins in the FGF family.[8] Unlike VEGF, FGF lacks the signaling

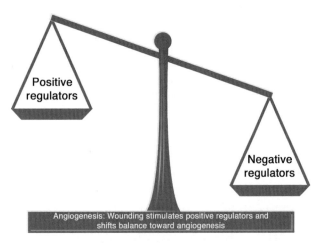

Positive regulators

Negative regulators

Angiogenesis: Wounding stimulates positive regulators and shifts balance toward angiogenesis

Figure 9-2 The shifting balance between positive and negative angiogenesis regulators.

sequence that allows direct cellular secretion of this protein.[9] Thus, techniques to overexpress FGF must be accompanied by a mechanism that promotes protein secretion from the cell. The biologic effects of FGF are mediated by four structurally related tyrosine kinase receptors that are broadly expressed.[10,11] FGF regulates the expression of several molecules that are critical during angiogenesis including interstitial collagenase, urokinase-type plasminogen activator, plasminogen activator inhibitor, the plasminogen activator receptor, and the beta-1 integrin. It should be noted that systemic treatment with FGF has been associated with renal and hematologic toxicity, both of which may affect the potential therapeutic use of this protein.[12]

Tissue Hypoxia and Tissue Hypoxia Factor

Tissue hypoxia is the most important physiologic stimulus of angiogenesis. Moreover, hypoxia is critical to the development of granulation tissue in a wound. It has been demonstrated that a hypoxic tissue gradient is mandatory for the angiogenesis that contributes to wound healing. Hypoxia-inducible factor-1 (HIF-1) is a heterodimeric transcription factor that regulates the expression of a number of oxygen-dependent genes such as VEGF. The VEGF gene contains a hypoxia response element (HRE) within its promoter that is responsive to this factor.[13] Thus, a novel approach to promote angiogenesis in chronic wounds might be through gene transfer of HIF-1. Although an interesting hypothesis, to date, no animal or clinical trials of HIF-1 have been initiated.

Transforming Growth Factor β

Transforming growth factor β (TGFβ) is a polypeptide growth factor with a multiplicity of diverse biologic effects. Many cell types, including monocytes, macrophages, and platelets, produce it. TGFβ affects the growth, survival, and phenotype of many cells and is a very important mediator of vascular development and hematopoiesis. In soft-tissue wounds, TGFβ has been shown to stimulate wound contraction and induce the formation of granulation tissue and extracellular matrix.

Hepatocyte Growth Factor/Scatter Factor

Recent studies have identified the protein hepatocyte growth factor (HGF) as a member of the family of angiogenic agents. HGF is a mesenchyme-derived pleiotropic factor, which regulates growth, motility, and morphogenesis of various cell types.[14] Moreover, HGF is similar to VEGF in that it contains a sequence that allows secretion of the protein from cells, and is also an endothelium-specific growth factor.

METHODS OF DELIVERING ANGIOGENIC PROTEINS

Angiogenic proteins can be delivered to chronic wounds using several different approaches. The simplest is to directly administer the protein, which then has the potential to both rapidly and directly stimulate angiogenesis. However, proteins generally have short half-lives and therefore frequent or continuous protein administration is necessary to achieve sustained biologic activity. Alternatively, gene therapy or gene transfer results in a "turned-on" gene that leads to the continuous release of high concentrations of therapeutic protein over a sustained period of time. For gene transfer to be successful, however, the foreign gene must cross the outer membrane of the host cell. To accomplish this, the gene is first inserted into a plasmid, a naturally occurring circular deoxyribonucleic acid (DNA) molecule. The plasmid (or naked DNA) can be directly applied to tissues. Since the uptake of naked DNA by cells is limited, high concentrations of naked DNA are required and expression of the transfected gene is often weak. Alternatively, a carrier, referred to as a vector, can be used to deliver recombinant DNA into a host cell. Viruses are commonly used vectors. Transfection efficiencies can be achieved with adenoviruses that are many-fold greater than what can be achieved by exposing cells to naked DNA.[15] Unfortunately, when an adenovirus is used to infect a target cell, a host immune response is incited against the adenovirus. Neutralizing antibodies to the adenovirus are formed, and these antibodies limit the duration of DNA expression[16] and also eliminate the possibility of using an adenoviral vector on subsequent occasions.[17] Thus, the advantage of naked DNA is that it can be injected on multiple occasions (but transfection efficiencies and protein production may be low). Alternatively, the advantage of adenoviral vectors is the high levels of gene and protein production that can be achieved (but immune responses limit the durability of the effect). The optimal approach to therapeutic angiogenesis is yet to be determined and may vary with the growth factor or the tissue being treated.

ANIMAL STUDIES

Angiogenic growth factors have been used in a variety of animal models of wound healing with varying results.

Vascular Endothelial Growth Factor

An association between VEGF and wound healing has been established, particularly in the diabetic condition. VEGF expression is decreased in the wounds of genetically diabetic mice. These findings suggest that impaired wound healing in diabetes may, at least in part, be due to altered regulation of VEGF gene expression. These data also lead to the hypothesis that VEGF supplementation of diabetic wounds may restore healing to its usual pace.

In a diabetic mouse model, wound healing was stimulated by the 165-amino acid isoform of VEGF-A delivered via an adeno-associated virus. An incisional skin wound was made in female diabetic mice, and their normal littermates and animals were randomized to receive intradermal injection of either a control or the VEGF$_{165}$ gene. In the VEGF-treated animals, there was a remarkable induction of new vessel formation, the synthesis and maturation of extracellular matrix, as well as an increase in the rate of healing. In a second study, genetically diabetic mice and their nondiabetic littermates received full-thickness wounds. Mice were then treated with recombinant VEGF$_{165}$ protein or placebo. The length of time to achieve 50% wound closure in the nondiabetic animals was 8.5 days for controls versus 7.8 days for the VEGF-treated animals. Alternatively, the length of time to achieve 50% wound healing in the diabetic animals was 15.8 days in control and 11.8 days with VEGF treatment. Thus, VEGF was a potent stimulant of healing in the presence of diabetes. The mechanism for this effect appears to be the enhancement of neovascularization in diabetic wounds.[18] Adding further support for a role for VEGF in wound healing, the breast cancer chemotherapeutic agent SU5416, an antiangiogenic agent that inhibits VEGF, has a potent inhibitory effect on wound healing.[19] Thus, VEGF gene transfer might represent a novel approach for the treatment of the wound-healing disorders associated with diabetes.[20]

Platelet-derived Growth Factor and Fibroblast Growth Factor

There have been several recent evaluations of the effect of platelet-derived growth factor (PDGF) on wound healing. In one study, cultured mouse dermal fibroblasts, retrovirally transduced with the *PDGF-B* gene, were seeded onto polyglycolic acid scaffolds. These matrices were then used to treat full-thickness excisional dorsal skin wounds in diabetic mice. *In vitro* production of PDGF-β protein by these transduced cells reached steady-state levels of 1,000 ng per 10^6 cells per 24 hours. At 21 days, there was a significant acceleration of the healing of wounds treated with PDGF-transduced cells. Immunohistochemical staining revealed intense staining for PDGF.[21] In a second study, large, full-thickness skin wounds were made on the backs of genetically diabetic C57 Black mice. In diabetic mice, there is a delay in the entry of inflammatory cells into wounds, a diminution in the amount of granulation tissue, and impaired wound healing. Recombinant PDGF-B or FGF proteins, alone or in combination, were applied topically for 5 to 14 days after wounding. Wounds treated with PDGF or FGF had more fibroblasts and capillaries in the wound bed at 10 and 21 days. Animals treated with growth factors also had significantly improved wound healing at 21 days. Combining the growth factors did not increase the rate of wound healing above what could be achieved with either growth factor alone. These and other studies demonstrate the potential use of topically applied growth factors in the treatment of patients with deficient wound repair.[22]

Werner et al.[23] assessed the role of endogenous FGF in tissue repair. One day following skin injury, there was 160-fold induction of the mRNA encoding keratinocyte growth factor (KGF), a member of the FGF family. Interestingly, mRNA levels for acidic and basic FGF and FGF-5 were only slightly increased during wound healing. There were no increases in the expression of FGF-3, -4, or -6 at baseline or following wounding. The highest levels of KGF mRNA were identified in the dermis and hypodermis at the wound edge. mRNA encoding the receptor of this growth factor (a splice variant of FGF receptor 2) was also predominantly expressed in the epidermis. These results suggest a unique role for the KGF member of the FGF family in wound repair.

Hepatocyte Growth Factor/Scatter Factor

Hepatocyte growth factor/scatter factor (HGF/SF) is a potent stimulant of angiogenesis. In a transgenic mouse model exhibiting overexpression of HGF, excisional wounds were associated with increased quantities of granulation tissue and marked angiogenesis compared to controls. VEGF expression in the skin of these animals was also significantly increased at baseline and robustly upregulated during wound healing. Elevated levels of VEGF protein were detected predominantly in endothelial cells and fibroblasts within the granulation tissue. Serum levels of VEGF were also elevated in HGF/SF transgenic mice. Thus, HGF/SF appears to have a significant role in angiogenesis and granulation tissue formation during wound healing, a process that appears to be mediated by the induction of VEGF.[24]

Nitric Oxide

Healing of excisional wounds was significantly delayed in endothelial nitric oxide synthase (eNOS) knockout mice compared to wild-type controls. Because diabetes is associated with a deficiency in nitric oxide (NO) at the wound site, it was proposed that exogenous NO supplementation with the NO donor, molsidomine, might reverse impaired wound healing found in diabetics. Studies revealed that treatment with molsidomine does, at least in part, reverse the effect of diabetes on chronic wounds.[25]

Stem Cells

The role of stem cells is being explored in a variety of different arenas, including wound healing. In a recent study, the ability of mesenchymal stem cells to enhance wound healing was explored in a diabetic mouse model. Eight-mm flank wounds were created in diabetic and nondiabetic mice. Wounds were then treated with mesenchymal stem cells, unprocessed bone marrow cells, and saline control. At 7 and 30 days, there was a greater density of fibroblasts and enhanced re-epithelization in the wound bed of animals treated with mesenchymal stem cells. Trichrome stain of these wounds demonstrated increased collagen deposition as well as increased levels of VEGF in the mesenchymal cell cohort. This is a provocative study that suggests the use of cells derived from autogenous bone marrow may enhance the healing of chronic wounds.[26]

HUMAN CLINICAL TRIALS

Vascular Endothelial Growth Factor

A recent study from Germany demonstrated proteolysis of $VEGF_{165}$ by plasmin in fluid collected from chronic nonhealing wounds, suggesting that VEGF degradation and the loss of its biologic activity may contribute to the impairment in wound healing.[27] Therefore, to prevent degradation of VEGF, an alteration of the amino acid sequence at the plasmin-sensitive cleavage site of $VEGF_{165}$ was performed. This altered protein maintained its growth-promoting properties but was plasmin resistant. In an exploratory study, three patients with chronic nonhealing wounds were treated with topical application of plasmin-resistant VEGF, and wound healing appeared accelerated in all three. Recombinant VEGF RhVEGF (Telbermin; Genentech) is currently in a phase I trial to evaluate its safety in the healing of chronic diabetic foot ulcers.

Platelet-derived Growth Factor

Becaplermin (Regranex, 0.01% gel, Johnson & Johnson Wound Management, Somerville, NJ), a once-a-day topical gel that contains human recombinant PDGF-BB, was the first drug approved by FDA to actively stimulate wound healing. Although there are many mechanisms of action of PDGF, this growth factor does appear to increase the quantity of granulation tissue or angiogenesis. Four clinical trials[28,29] of multicenter, randomized, blinded, and parallel-group design were conducted to compare the efficacy and safety of becaplermin gel with placebo or good wound care alone in the healing of chronic, neuropathic, or ischemic ulcers. The main differences among these trials were the treatment arms and the types of ulcers

studied. These clinical trials included, in total, 922 patients with foot (93%), or ankle or leg ulcers (7%). Complete wound healing occurred after 20 weeks in 47% of patients with becaplermin 0.01% gel, 42% with becaplermin 0.003% gel, 35% with vehicle gel, and 30% with good wound care alone ($p = 0.001$). Time to complete ulcer healing was also significantly shorter in the becaplermin 0.01% group compared to vehicle gel (92 vs. 131 days; $p = 0.008$). No outcome data is available in these patients on the rate of amputation, mortality, or the long-term durability of healing. However, ongoing studies of cost-effectiveness, quality of life, and treatment duration will help to clarify these issues. It is clear that in combination with debridement and careful wound care, regranex does promote wound healing. However, it perhaps was best stated by the European Agency for evaluation of the Medicinal Products when they concluded that becaplermin gel possesses "modest efficacy" in the treatment of chronic wounds.[30]

One of the limitations of becaplermin is the durability of its action. As mentioned above, adenoviral or gene therapy techniques can be used to produce more sustained protein release. Phase I clinical trials have begun to evaluate the safety of topical applications of a gene for PDGF-BB contained within an adenoviral vector and delivered through a bovine type I collagen gel. Whether or not genetic delivery of PDGF will improve upon the results of becaplermin remains to be seen.

Transforming Growth Factor β

The efficacy of TGFβ in the treatment of chronic diabetic foot ulcers was recently evaluated in a randomized, double-blinded, placebo-controlled, multicenter trial.[31] Patients with chronic diabetic foot ulcers were randomized to receive standard care with or without repeated therapeutic doses of TGFβ. Time to complete wound closure and durability of wound closure were the outcomes measured.

The TGFβ groups fared significantly better than placebo; the frequency of complete wound closure was nearly twice as great. The results of this study support the notion that repeated topical delivery of TGFβ may have a beneficial effect on the healing of chronic wounds in the diabetic patient.

Keratinocyte Growth Factor/Fibroblast Growth Factor

KGF-2 is a naturally occurring protein that is a member of the fibroblast growth factor family.[23] As mentioned before, KGF-2 selectively stimulates proliferation of normal epithelial keratinocytes. A truncated KGF-2 protein (repifermin) has been designed that retains full biologic activity compared with the parent molecule. Moreover, animal studies with repifermin demonstrated the ability of this growth factor, administered either topically or systemically, to stimulate keratinocyte cell proliferation in both full- and partial-thickness cutaneous wounds.

Thus, a randomized, double-blinded, parallel-group, placebo-controlled, multicenter study was initiated recently to evaluate the efficacy and safety of repifermin (KGF-2) in subjects with venous ulcers. Two different doses of repifermin were compared with placebo following twice weekly topical application for up to 26 weeks. The endpoint of this study was the percentage of subjects achieving complete wound closure within 20 weeks of therapy. Three hundred subjects with venous ulcers, 3 to 25 cm in size, were evaluated. Unfortunately, data from the phase II portion of this study did not demonstrate a statistically significant benefit of KGF-2 over placebo.

Bilayered Cellular Matrix

In a recent trial, the effectiveness of bilayered cellular matrix (BCM) in the healing of neuropathic diabetic foot ulcers was evaluated. These matrices are composed of normal human allogeneic skin cells (epidermal keratinocytes and dermal fibroblasts), which are cultured in two separate layers within type I bovine collagen sponge. Cells in this matrix are thought to secrete a variety of growth factors that have the potential to stimulate angiogenesis. Patients were randomized between BCM treatment and control. Patients in the control group received standard therapy for up to 12 weeks, or until the ulcer was completely healed. Patients in the BCM treatment group received standard therapy plus an application of fresh BCM weekly for up to six applications or until the ulcer was completely healed. If healing had not occurred after six applications of BCM, standard care was provided to the ulcer for an additional 6 weeks or until the wound healed completely. During the 12-week study period, 35% of all ulcers in the BCM treatment group healed versus 20% in the control group. The mean rate of wound closure in the BCM group was significantly greater than that of the standard treatment group.[32] The accelerated wound healing was thought to have resulted from an angiogenic response to growth factors released from the biologic dressing.

SIDE EFFECTS AND DANGERS OF ANGIOGENIC THERAPY

There are potential drawbacks to the use of growth factors and angiogenic agents in the treatment of wound healing. VEGF is a vascular permeability factor and can potentially produce edema adjacent to the treatment area. Angiogenic agents also carry the risk of stimulating neovascularization in nontarget tissues such as the eyes or joints. Because tumor growth is dependent upon angiogenesis, there is potential risk with administration of angiogenic factors of accelerating the progression of latent tumors. Moreover, angiogenic factors may also cause unnatural cellular proliferation leading to the initial development of malignant lesions. There is also concern that VEGF and other growth factors could lead to progression of atherosclerosis as well as plaque instability and rupture. The actual risk of any of these untoward events is unknown. Fortunately, most normal tissues do not express measurable levels of the receptors for many of these proteins. Moreover, to date, none of these effects have been observed in animals or in human clinical trials.

SUMMARY

The importance of angiogenesis in wound healing has been well established. It is therefore logical to assume that treatments that accelerate this process will be beneficial in the treatment of chronic wounds. Human clinical studies of therapeutic angiogenesis are in their infancy. A number of trials employing a variety of agents are either under development or being initiated. We anticipate that these trials will eventually lead to an effective, minimally invasive biologic strategy for the treatment of patients suffering from chronic wounds.

REFERENCES

1. Hunter J. Lectures on the principles of surgery. In: Palmer J, ed. *The works of John Hunter.* 1st ed. London: Longman Press; 1835–1837.
2. Ferrara N, Henzel WJ. Pituitary follicular cells secrete a novel heparin-binding growth factor specific for vascular endothelial cells. *Biochem Biophys Res Commun.* 1989;161:851–858.
3. Shibuya M, Ito N, Claesson-Welsh L. Structure and function of vascular endothelial growth factor receptor-1 and -2. *Curr Top Microbiol Immunol.* 1999;237:59–83.
4. Levy AP, Levy NS, Wegner S, et al. Transcriptional regulation of the rat vascular endothelial growth factor gene by hypoxia. *J Biol Chem.* 1995;270:13333–13340.
5. Semenza GL. HIF-1, O (2), and the 3 PHDs: How animal cells signal hypoxia to the nucleus. *Cell.* 2001;107:1–3.
6. Ross J. mRNA stability in mammalian cells. *Microbiol Rev.* 1995; 59:423–450.
7. Paulding WR, Czyzyk-Krzeska MF. Hypoxia-induced regulation of mRNA stability. *Adv Exp Med Biol.* 2000;475:111–121.
8. Cross MJ, Claesson-Welsh L. FGF and VEGF function in angiogenesis: signalling pathways, biological responses and therapeutic inhibition. *Trends Pharmacol Sci.* 2001;22:201–207.
9. Barbul A. Immune aspects of wound healing. *Clin Plast Surg.* 1990;17:433–442.
10. Jaye M, Schlessinger J, Dionne CA. Fibroblast growth factor receptor tyrosine kinases: molecular analysis and signal transduction. *Biochimica et Biophysica Acta.* 1992;1135:185–199.
11. Szebenyi G, Fallon JF. Fibroblast growth factors as multifunctional signaling factors. *Int Rev Cytol.* 1999;185:45–106.
12. Unger EF, Epstein SE, Chew EY, et al. Effects of a single intracoronary injection of basic fibroblast growth factor in stable angina pectoris. *Am J Cardiol.* 2000;85:1414–1419.

13. Semenza GL. Hypoxia inducible factor 1: master regulator of oxygen homeostasis. *Curr Opin Genet Dev.* 1999;8:588–594.

14. Matsumoto K, Nakamura T. Emerging multipotent aspects of hepatocyte growth factor. *J Biochem (Tokyo).* 1996;119:591–600.

15. Nabel EG, Nabel GJ. Complex models for the study of gene function in cardiovascular biology. *Annu Rev Physiol.* 1994;56:741–761.

16. Wilson JM. Adenoviruses as gene-delivery vehicles. *N Engl J Med.* 1996;334:1185–1187.

17. Zabner J, Petersen DM, Puga AP, et al. Safety and efficacy of repetitive adenovirus-mediated transfer of CFTR cDNA to airway epithelia of primates and cotton rats. *Nat Genet.* 1994;6:75–83.

18. Kirchner LM, Meerbaum SO, Gruber BS, et al. Effects of vascular endothelial growth factor on wound closure rates in the genetically diabetic mouse model. *Wound Repair and Regen.* 2003;11:127–131.

19. Roman CD, Choy H, Nanney L, et al. Vascular endothelial growth factor-mediated angiogenesis inhibition and postoperative wound healing in rats. *J Surg Res.* 2002;105:43–47.

20. Galeano M, Deodato B, Altavilla D, et al. Adeno-associated viral vector-mediated human vascular endothelial growth factor gene transfer stimulates angiogenesis and wound healing in the genetically diabetic mouse. *Diabetologia.* 2003;46:546–555.

21. Breitbart AS, Laser J, Parrett B, et al. Accelerated diabetic wound healing using cultured dermal fibroblasts retrovirally transduced with the platelet-derived growth factor B gene. *Ann Plast Surg.* 2003;51:409–414.

22. Greenhalgh DG, Sprugel KH, Murray MJ, et al. PDGF and FGF stimulate wound healing in the genetically diabetic mouse. *Am J Pathol.* 1990;136:1235–1246.

23. Werner S, Peters KG, Longaker MT, et al. Large induction of keratinocyte growth factor expression in the dermis during wound healing. *Proc Natl Acad Sci U S A.* 1992;89:6896–6900.

24. Toyoda M, Takayama H, Horiguchi N, et al. Overexpression of hepatocyte growth factor/scatter factor promotes vascularization and granulation tissue formation *in vivo. FEBS Lett.* 2001;509:95–100.

25. Lee PC, Salyapongse AN, Bragdon GA, et al. Impaired wound healing and angiogenesis in eNOS-deficient mice. *Am J Physiol.* 1999;277:H1600–H1608.

26. Keswani SG, Javazon EH, Kozin ED, et al. Novel effects of adult murine mesenchymal stem cells in diabetic wound healing. St. Louis, Mo: Society of University Surgeons; Paper presented on Feb. 12, 2004.

27. Lauer G, Sollberg S, Cole M. Generation of a novel proteolysis resistant vascular endothelial growth factor165 variant by a site-directed mutation at the plasmin sensitive cleavage site. *FEBS Lett.* 2002;531:309–313.

28. Steed DL. Clinical evaluation of recombinant human platelet-derived growth factor for the treatment of lower extremity diabetic ulcers. Diabetic Ulcer Study Group. *J Vasc Surg.* 1995;21:71–88; discussion 79–81.

29. Wieman TJ, Smiell JM, Su Y. Efficacy and safety of a topical gel formulation of recombinant human platelet-derived growth factor-BB (becaplermin) in patients with chronic neuropathic diabetic ulcers. A phase III randomized placebo-controlled double-blind study. *Diabetes Care.* 1998;21:822–827.

30. Committee for Proprietary Medicinal Products. European Public Assessment Report (EPAR) Regranex, 29th March 1999 Available at: http://www.eudra.org/emea.html. Accessed: May 2004.

31. Robson MC, Steed DL, McPherson JM, et al. Effects of transforming growth factor ß2 on wound healing in diabetic foot ulcers. Paper presented at: *3rd Joint Meeting of the European Tissue Repair Society and the Wound Healing Society; 1999,* Bordeaux, France.

32. Lipkin S, Chaikof E, Isseroff Z, et al. Effectiveness of bilayered cellular matrix in healing of neuropathic diabetic foot ulcers: Results of a multicenter pilot trial. *Wounds.* 2003;15:230–236.

The Diabetic Charcot Foot

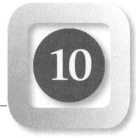

Robert G. Frykberg   *Thomas Zgonis*

The diabetic Charcot foot (neuropathic osteoarthropathy) can be defined as a progressive joint destructive condition affecting single or multiple joints and characterized by dislocation, pathologic fractures, and severe destruction of the pedal architecture.[1] Osteoarthropathy may therefore result in severe deformity with attendant high plantar pressures, ulceration, and subsequent amputation. The condition is closely associated with severe peripheral neuropathy and the most common etiology today is diabetes mellitus.

It has been estimated that <1% of diabetic patients will develop Charcot arthropathy.[2] The true incidence of osteoarthropathy in diabetes is limited by the small number of prospective or population-based studies currently available. Much of the data we rely on is based on retrospective studies of small, single-center cohorts. Whereas many cases go undetected (especially in their early stages), the frequency of Charcot cases reported is therefore very likely an underestimation.[1,3,4] The prevalence of this condition is variable, ranging from 0.15% of all diabetic patients to as high as 29% in a population of only neuropathic diabetic subjects.[1] In a recent prospective study of a large cohort of diabetic patients in Texas followed for 2 years, the incidence of pedal Charcot arthropathy was 8.5 per 1,000 patients per year. Charcot foot was also more common in non-Hispanic whites than in Mexican Americans.[5] With an increased awareness of this entity's signs and symptoms, there appears to be an increased frequency of diagnosis in recent years.[4,6]

THE ETIOLOGY OF NEUROPATHIC OSTEOARTHROPATHY

The primary risk factors for this potentially limb-threatening deformity are the presence of dense peripheral sensory and autonomic neuropathy, relatively normal or abundant circulation, and a history of preceding trauma that often may be minor in nature.[7,8] Trauma is not necessarily limited to injuries such as sprains or fractures, but can even include joint infections or surgical trauma.[9] Foot deformities, including prior partial foot amputations, may result in sufficient biomechanical stress that can lead to Charcot joint disease (Fig. 10-1). However, not all patients with neuropathy who sustain trauma will go on to develop neuropathic arthropathy; there appears to be other undefined risk factors that may predispose patients to this disorder.

The actual etiology of Charcot arthropathy most likely is a combined effect of both the neurovascular and neurotraumatic theories.[10-12] It is generally accepted that trauma superimposed on an insensate extremity can precipitate the development of an acute Charcot foot in susceptible people. With the development of autonomic neuropathy, there is an increased blood flow to the foot, resulting in osteopenia, and a relative weakness of the bone (neurovascular theory).[11,13,14] The presence of sensory neuropathy renders the patient unaware of the precipitating trauma and often profound osseous destruction taking place during ambulation. Despite the severe bone changes, fractures, and dislocations, the patient will continue to walk on the

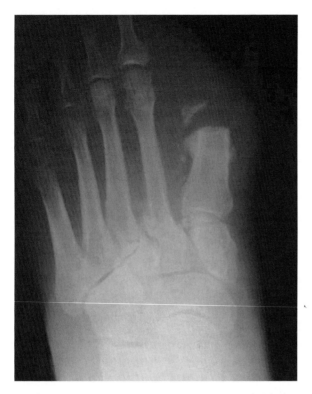

Figure 10-1 Osteoarthropathy at the Lisfranc joint developed after first ray resection.

injured foot, usually only noting the appearance of edema, deformity, and minor pain or aching as further damage occurs (neurotraumatic theory).[6,7,15,16]

CLINICAL DIAGNOSIS OF ACUTE CHARCOT ARTHROPATHY

Diagnosis of acute Charcot arthropathy can usually be based on characteristic clinical findings in corroboration with plain radiographs. It is especially important, therefore, that the clinician have a high index of suspicion for this disorder.

Marked unilateral swelling, increased skin temperature, erythema, and a subtle change in the shape of the foot with or without precipitating trauma in an insensate foot will most often suggest the appropriate diagnosis.[1,7,8,17] Radiographic findings (Table 10-1) may include fractures, subtle or gross dislocations, joint effusions, loss of normal joint and pedal architecture, periosteal new bone formation, and soft-tissue edema.[3,14] These clinical and radiologic signs are often pathognomonic of acute Charcot arthropathy. In >75% of cases, the patient will present with some degree of pain in an otherwise insensate extremity.[7]

Patient demographics also play an important role in establishing this diagnosis, since studies have shown rather consistent findings in this regard (Table 10-2). Typically, the majority of patients will be in their sixth decade (50 to 59 years) and have had diabetes mellitus for a duration of 10 to 20 years.[1,3,7,18] All patients will have peripheral neuropathy of some degree, and most should have an identifiable history of antecedent trauma. A recent report from London distinguishes the characteristics of type 1 diabetic patients with osteoarthropathy from those of type 2 diabetes patients.[18] In their cohort of 85 acute Charcot patients, 44 (51.7%) had type 1 diabetes. Of note, these patients were significantly younger (mean age 42 years) and had diabetes for a longer duration (24 years) than those with type 2 diabetes (mean age 59 years; diabetes duration 13 years). Although the entire group was characteristic of the usual demographic profile as previously mentioned, this report suggests that we need to further characterize Charcot patients according to their type of diabetes.

When diabetic patients present with a warm, edematous, insensate foot, plain radiographs are invaluable

TABLE 10-1
RADIOGRAPHIC FINDINGS IN THE DIABETIC CHARCOT FOOT TYPICAL OF EACH REGION

Forefoot	Midfoot	Rearfoot
Osteolysis	Osteopenia	Osteopenia
"Sucked candy" metatarsals	Osteolysis	Severe osteolysis
Phalangeal hourglassing	Joint subluxations	Joint subluxations
Toe/MTP subluxations	Periosteal new bone	Ankle deformity or collapse
Neuropathic fractures	Neuropathic fractures	Neuropathic fractures
Periosteal new bone	Osseous hypertrophy	Ankle, talus, calcaneus
Medial arterial calcification	Midfoot collapse	Edema
Soft-tissue edema	"Rocker-bottom deformity"	Medial arterial calcification
Joint effusions	Edema	Equinus contracture
	Plantar ulceration	
	Medial arterial calcification	

MTP, metatarsophalangeal.

TABLE 10-2

CHARACTERISTICS OF PATIENTS PRESENTING WITH CHARCOT ARTHROPATHY

Patient Characteristics	Acute	Chronic
Diabetes duration >10 y	Edema	Deformity usually present
Mean age: Mid 50s (type 1 diabetes, younger)	Erythema	May have edema
	Warmer than other foot	May be slightly warm
	Deformity may be present	
History of trauma	Bounding pulses	Pulses usually palpable
Painful or painless foot	Neuropathic	Neuropathic
		Loss of protective sensation
Trouble fitting shoe on foot	Loss of protective sensation	Sensory, motor, autonomic
Instability when walking	Diminished vibratory, thermal, and pain perception	manifestations
	Anhidrotic (dry) skin	Anhidrotic (dry) skin
	Callus or ulcer may be present	Callus or ulcer often present

in ascertaining the presence of osteoarthropathy (Fig. 10-2). In most cases, plain films will be the only imaging studies required to make the correct diagnosis. With a concomitant wound, it is often difficult to differentiate between acute Charcot arthropathy and osteomyelitis (or to confirm both) solely based on plain radiographs.[16,17] If the wound probes directly to bone or if bone is visible at the base of the wound, concomitant osteomyelitis is highly likely.[19–21]

A bone biopsy and culture in this case should be considered as the most specific method of determining the presence of osteomyelitis. Additional laboratory studies may also prove useful in arriving at a correct diagnosis. The white blood cell count (WBC) may not even be elevated in acute osteomyelitis, since this parameter is often blunted in persons with diabetes.[20,22] Similarly, while the erythrocyte sedimentation rate and C-reactive protein (CRP) are variably reactive in the presence of diabetic foot infection, they are nonspecific and can be elevated solely due to the osteoarthropathy and attendant inflammatory response.

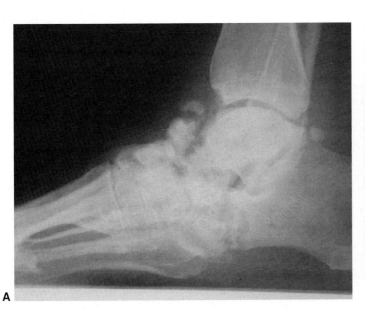

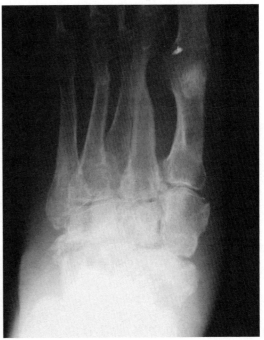

A   B

Figure 10-2   A: Radiograph of acute Charcot foot. **B:** Anterior-posterior view of midfoot/midtarsal joint Charcot.

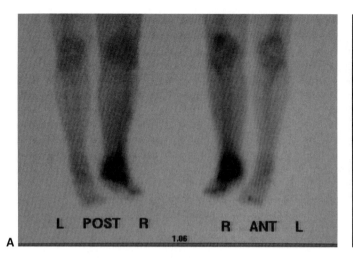
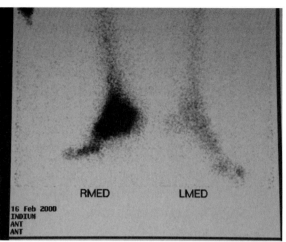

Figure 10-3   **A:** Bone scan of patient with acute Charcot arthropathy. **B:** False-positive Indium scan of same patient. There was no history of infection.

Technetium bone scans are highly sensitive but generally nonspecific in assisting in the differentiation between osteomyelitis and acute Charcot arthropathy.[20,23–25] Bone scans (Fig. 10-3A), however, are sometimes very useful in arriving at an early diagnosis of neuroarthropathy when radiographs are still without changes, but when clinical suspicion is high.[1] Indium or technetium-99m-d,l-hexamethyl-propylene amine oxime (Tc-HMPAO)-labeled leukocyte scans have shown somewhat more specificity for bone infection, although they still can result in false-positive readings, as shown in Figure 10-3B.[26,27] Magnetic resonance imaging (MRI) may be the diagnostic modality of choice in this regard (Fig. 10-4), although it is still difficult to distinguish marrow changes due to infection from those related to osteoarthropathy.[27–30]

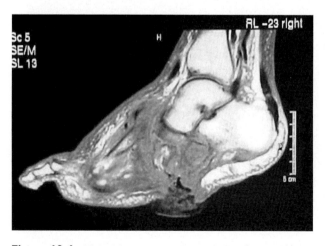

Figure 10-4   Magnetic resonance image (MRI) of acute Charcot foot with plantar ulcer.

CLASSIFICATION OF CHARCOT ARTHROPATHY

The simplest and perhaps the most common classification scheme for Charcot arthropathy is the one proposed in 1966 by Eichenholtz.[31] This system is based on radiographic appearance as well as physiologic stages of the process wherein it is divided into the developmental, coalescent, and reconstructive stages. The developmental stage is characterized by significant soft-tissue edema, joint effusions, osteochondral fragmentation, fractures, and dislocation of varying degrees.[8,31] The stage of coalescence is noted by a reduction in soft-tissue swelling, bone callus proliferation, and consolidation of fractures. Last, the reconstructive stage is indicated by bone healing, joint ankylosis, and osseous hypertrophy without further clinical signs of inflammation.[3] While this system is very descriptive, from a radiologic standpoint, its clinical usefulness is less so. Therefore, most clinicians will simply consider the initial stage as being active, while the coalescent and reconstructive stages combined are regarded the quiescent or reparative stages. There are several other schemes in the literature as well, although none has been uniformly adopted as being superior or predictive of outcome.[32–34] The authors' preferred classification system, shown in Figure 10-5, is based upon five anatomic sites of involvement, but does not describe the activity of the disease.[1,3]

MANAGEMENT OF ACUTE CHARCOT ARTHROPATHY

First and foremost, the acute Charcot foot must be rested and immobilized.[1,3,4,7,16] We advocate complete non–weight bearing through the use of wheelchair,

The high-risk foot in diabetes mellitus

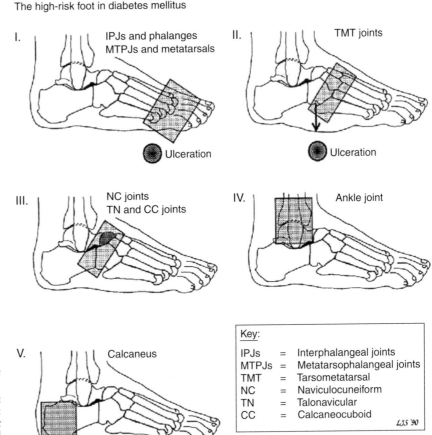

Figure 10-5 Classification of patterns of involvement in the diabetic Charcot foot. (From Sanders LJ, Frykberg RG: Diabetic neuropathic osteoarthropathy: The Charcot foot. In: Frykberg RG, ed. *The high risk foot in diabetes mellitus.* New York, NY: Churchill Livingstone; 1991:297, with permission.)

crutches, or other assistive modalities during the initial acute period. When offloading one foot entirely, care must be taken to protect the other foot because of added stress to the weight-bearing extremity and the potential for contralateral osteoarthropathy.[35] Following a period of offloading with mild compression or casting, a reduction in skin temperature and edema heralds the stage of quiescence.[7] Although there are no firm data specifying the length of time that a patient needs to be offweighted, we recommend a general time frame of approximately 3 months for conversion to the reparative stage. Progression to protected weight bearing is then permitted, usually with the aid of a cane or crutches. Some centers prescribe an initial ambulatory total contact cast (TCC) without necessitating a period of non–weight bearing.[36,37] Currently, there are no comparative studies between these two approaches from which we can determine what approach, if any, is best. Nonetheless, when weight bearing is permitted, TCCs or other offloading modalities (i.e., fixed ankle walker, total contact prostheses, Charcot restraint orthotic walkers, patellar tendon-bearing braces, etc.), will allow patients to safely ambulate while healing

progresses.[7,10,16,38] The mean time of rest and immobilization (casting followed by removable cast walker) prior to return to permanent footwear is approximately 4 to 6 months.[3,4,7,15]

Several reports in the recent literature suggest that the adjunctive use of bisphosphonates (osteoclastic inhibitors) may help expedite the conversion of the acute process to the quiescent, reparative stage.[39,40] Although these studies have found a significant reduction of osteoclastic markers and more rapid reduction of skin temperature in treated patients, they have not demonstrated a more rapid consolidation of fractures nor quicker return to footwear. Adjunctive bone-growth stimulation has also been proposed as a means to promote rapid consolidation of fractures in acute osteoarthropathy.[41] Both of these ancillary treatments (in addition to standard care) are very attractive in theory, but need to be conclusively proven effective through large, multicenter, prospective, randomized, and controlled clinical trials before we can incorporate them into standard treatment protocols. Table 10-3 highlights the basic tenets for managing both acute and chronic Charcot foot disorders.

TABLE 10-3

PRIMARY CONSIDERATIONS FOR MANAGING THE CHARCOT FOOT

Acute	Chronic
Offload	Therapeutic footwear with customized
Complete non–weight bearing	pressure-relieving insoles
Crutches, wheelchair	Commercially available
Immobilization	Custom fabricated (for severe deformity)
Soft compression bandage	Bracing for unstable deformities
Posterior splint	PTTB
Cast or total contact cast	CROW
Or	Surgery for severe instability, nonplantigrade
Partial weight bearing with assistive devices	feet, recurrent ulcers, or deformities not
Crutches, walker, wheelchair	amenable to footwear therapy
And	Plantar exostecomy
Total contact cast or removable cast walker	Osteotomies
Manage associated wounds	Arthrodeses
Manage medical comorbidities	Amputation (selected cases only)
Continue weight-bearing restrictions until	Lifetime surveillance
edema recedes, temperature normalizes,	
and osseous healing progresses (3 to 6 mo)	
May consider bisphosphonates or bone	
stimulators to expedite consolidation	
Surgery *might be* considered in cases with	
severe dislocations and deformity	
(Caution—this has not been widely reported)	

PTTB, patellar tendon bearing brace; CROW, Charcot restraint orthotic walker.

SURGICAL RECONSTRUCTION OF THE DIABETIC CHARCOT FOOT

In recent years, reconstructive foot surgery has assumed an important role in the management of Charcot feet that cannot be effectively treated by casting, bracing, or footwear therapy.[6,10,34,36,37,42–44] While in optimal circumstances surgical treatment for Charcot deformities will be unnecessary, such patients often initially present in the active stage with rather severe or unstable deformities. It has long been held that surgery in the acute stage is unadvisable due to the extreme edema, hyperemia, and osteopenia present during this phase.[1,3,7,9,36,43–45] However, in the presence of acute subluxation without significant fractures (typified by talonavicular dislocation) one report suggests that primary fusion might in fact be the recommended treatment.[35] Another small, retrospective study challenged the prevailing opinions by performing successful primary midfoot arthrodeses in patients with acute osteoarthropathy.[46] While the appropriateness of reconstructive surgery during the acute phase is still a matter of debate, surgery on the chronically deformed

or unstable quiescent Charcot foot has become rather common in current practice.[36,37,44,47,48] While the majority of operations consist of plantar exostectomies to remove bony prominences associated with recurrent ulcers, joint fusions are more frequently reserved for realignment and stabilization of severely deformed feet.[3,48]

It is well accepted that patients with diabetic Charcot neuroarthropathy have reduced bone mineral densities in the bones of their feet.[13,14,49] As a result of this osteopenia, rigid internal fixation becomes a rather poor option in any reconstructive procedure of the foot and ankle and particularly in patients with Charcot neuroarthropathy (Fig. 10-6). However, by using thin wires in a multiplanar array, rigid fixation to the foot and leg can be accomplished without significant risk of loosening of the implants.

Multiplanar frames have been introduced for the treatment of Charcot neuroarthropathy in the last decade.[50–53] As previously noted, treatment of acute Charcot events has traditionally been conservative, as physicians used casting and offloading with no attempt to reduce the deformity. In addition, the treatment of

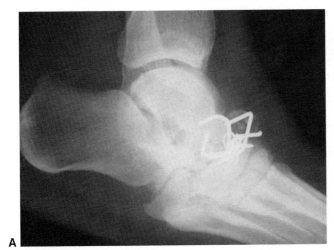

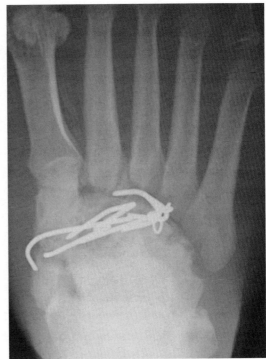

Figure 10-6 Evidence of radiographic nonunion and inadequate fixation in an attempted surgical Charcot foot reconstruction. **A:** Lateral view. **B:** Anterior-posterior view.

chronic deformities has involved the use of below-knee casting, non–weight bearing for a long period of time, and reconstruction via internal fixation.[37,54–56] Only recently have surgeons considered reconstruction via tarsal osteotomies, as evidenced by the few papers that

have appeared in peer-reviewed journals describing the use of external fixation for such treatment.[50–53,57–59]

External fixation reduces the need for extensive surgical exposure in reconstruction, and may provide a means of reducing acute Charcot deformities while

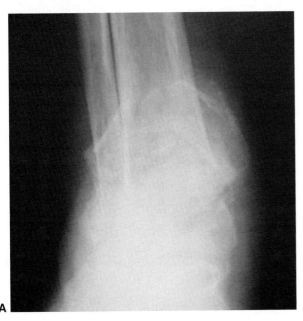

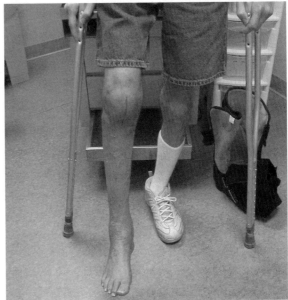

Figure 10-7   **A–F:** Conservative treatment of an acute Charcot ankle with immobilization and non–weight bearing.

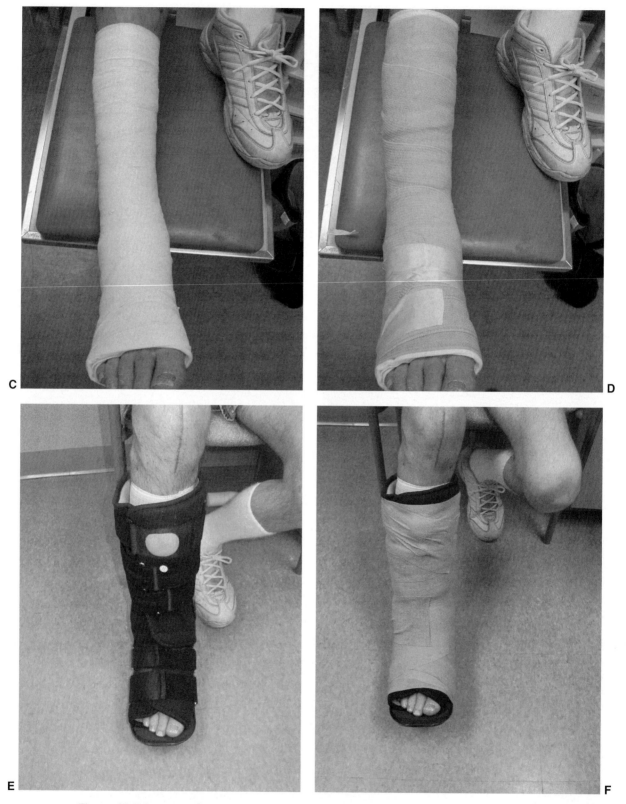

Figure 10-7 (continued)

maintaining the reduction during consolidation. Single medial incisions and compression via a multiplanar frame are performed to address the forefoot abduction deformities for the chronic Charcot deformities. It has been shown that the Lisfranc joint is the most common one developing a foot collapse during the Charcot process.[2,7,33,60] External fixation is also ideal in infected acute and chronic Charcot deformities for stabilization and arthrodesis of the joints after the infection has been appropriately managed.

Regardless of the degree or duration of the Charcot deformity, the foot is usually casted until such time as the clinician feels that sufficient consolidation has been achieved to permit guarded weight bearing. Skin thermography is often used as a criterion for the discontinuation of treatment.[3,7] Deformities that

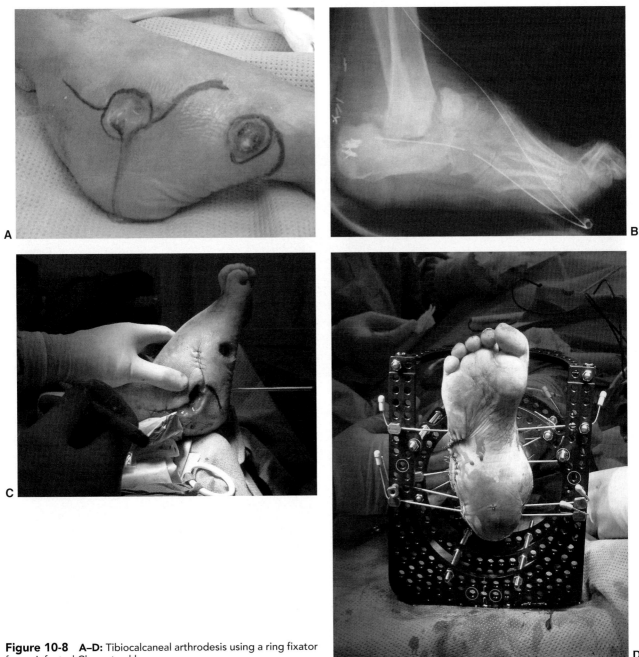

Figure 10-8   A–D: Tibiocalcaneal arthrodesis using a ring fixator for an infected Charcot ankle.

develop as a result of collapse should be treated conservatively first before any surgical intervention (Fig. 10-7).

In acute and chronic deformities with avascular necrosis, osteomyelitis, or severe dislocation of the talus, a tibiocalcaneal fusion with an external skeletal frame is indicated. While the incidence of nonunion of a tibiocalcaneal fusion is variable, a stable, fibrous nonunion is an acceptable alternative to the below-knee amputation[10] (Fig. 10-8).

Generally, midfoot disruption that results in a complete dissociation of the tarsometatarsal joints or plantar subluxation of the cuboid or navicular should be considered for operative intervention. Similarly, destruction of the ankle or subtalar joint that results in

a significant varus or valgus deformity that would be difficult to brace and shoe should also be considered for operative treatment (Fig. 10-9).

Lower extremity reconstruction for the acute and chronic Charcot deformity should be a viable option to the experienced surgeon after all the conservative treatments have been utilized. The goal of treating a patient with a Charcot foot deformity is to avoid skin breakdown and restore a stable foot. External fixation use and appropriate postsurgical treatment, including immobilization after frame removal and use of bone stimulation, will have a successful impact to the reconstructed Charcot foot. The surgeon should be aware of all treatment options, and surgical intervention should be considered when it is indicated.

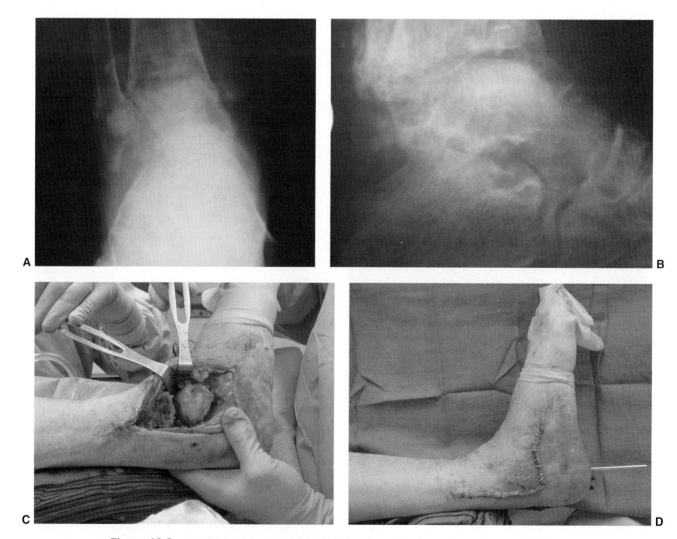

Figure 10-9   A–G: Tibio-talo-calcaneal arthrodesis using a ring fixator for an acute ankle Charcot with a fracture dislocation.

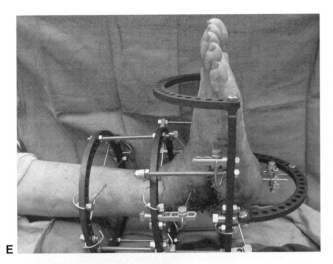

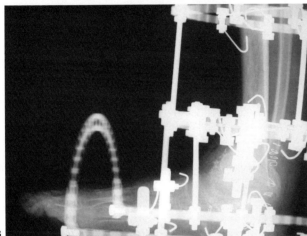

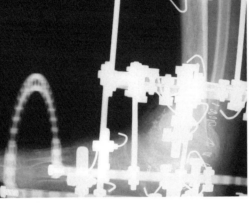

Figure 10-9 (*continued*)

REFERENCES

1. Sanders LJ, Frykberg RG. Diabetic neuropathic osteoarthropathy: the Charcot foot. In: Frykberg RG, ed. *The high risk foot in diabetes mellitus.* New York, NY: Churchill Livingstone; 1991:297.

2. Sinha S, Munichoodappa C, Kozak GP. Neuro-arthropathy (Charcot joints) in diabetes mellitus: clinical study of 101 cases. *Medicine (Baltimore).* 1972;52:191.

3. Sanders L, Frykberg RG. Charcot foot. In: Levin ME, O'Neal LW, Bowker JH, et al., eds. *The diabetic foot,* 6th ed. St. Louis, Mo: Mosby–Year Book; 2000.

4. Frykberg RG, Kozak GP. The diabetic Charcot foot. In: Kozak GP, Campbell DR, Frykberg RG, et al., eds. *Management of diabetic foot problems,* 2nd ed. Philadelphia, Pa: WB Saunders; 1995:88–97.

5. Lavery LA, Armstrong DG, Wunderlich RP, et al. Diabetic foot syndrome: evaluating the prevalence and incidence of foot pathology in Mexican Americans and non-Hispanic whites from a diabetes disease management cohort. *Diabetes Care.* 2003;26: 1435–1438.

6. Frykberg RG. Charcot foot: an update on pathogenesis and management. In: Boulton AJM, Connor H, Cavanagh PR, eds. *The foot in diabetes,* 3rd ed. Chichester: John Wiley and Sons; 2000:235–260.

7. Armstrong DG, Todd WF, Lavery LA, et al. The natural history of acute Charcot's arthropathy in a diabetic foot specialty clinic. *Diabet Med.* 1997;14:357–363.

8. Frykberg RG, Kozak GP. Neuropathic arthropathy in the diabetic foot. *Am Fam Physician.* 1978;17:105.

9. Frykberg RG, Armstrong DG, Giurini J, et al. Diabetic foot disorders; a clinical practice guideline. *J Foot Ankle Surg.* 2000; 39(Suppl 1):2–60.

10. Johnson JTH. Neuropathic fractures and joint injuries: pathogenesis and rationale of prevention and treatment. *J Bone Joint Surg.* 1967;49A:1.

11. Brower AC, Allman RM. Pathogenesis of the neurotrophic joint: neurotraumatic vs. neurovascular. *Radiology.* 1981;139:349.

12. Edelman SV, Kosofsky EM, Paul RA, et al. Neuro-osteoarthropathy (Charcot's joint) in diabetes mellitus following revascularization surgery. *Arch Int Med.* 1987;147:1504.

13. Young MJ, Marshall A, Adams JE, et al. Osteopenia, neurological dysfunction, and the development of Charcot neuroarthropathy. *Diabetes Care.* 1995;18:34–38.

14. Herbst SA, Jones KB, Saltzman CL. Pattern of diabetic neuropathic arthropathy associated with the peripheral bone mineral density. *J Bone Joint Surg Br.* 2003;86-B:378–383.

15. Caputo GM, Ulbrecht J, Cavanagh PR, et al. The Charcot foot in diabetes: six key points. *Am Fam Physician.* 1998;57:2705–2710.
16. Banks AS. A clinical guide to the Charcot foot. In: Kominsky SJ, ed. *Medical and surgical management of the diabetic foot.* St. Louis, Mo: Mosby–Year Book; 1994:115–143.
17. Frykberg RG, Mendeszoon ER. Management of the diabetic Charcot foot. *Diabetes Metab Res Rev.* 2000;16(Suppl 1):S59–S65.
18. Petrova NL, Foster A, Edmonds ME. Difference in presentation of Charcot arthropathy in type 1 compared to type 2 diabetes. *Diabetes Care.* 2004;27:1235–1236.
19. Grayson ML, Gibbons GW, Balogh K, et al. Probing to bone in infected pedal ulcers: a clinical sign of underlying osteomyelitis in diabetic patients. *JAMA.* 1995;273:721–723.
20. Lipsky BA, Berendt AR, Embil J, et al. Diagnosing and treating diabetic foot infections. *Diabetes Metab Res Rev.* 2004;20(Suppl 1): S56–S64.
21. Frykberg RG. An evidence-based approach to diabetic foot infections. *Am J Surg.* 2003;186(5A):44S–54S.
22. Eneroth M, Apelqvist J, Stenstrom A. Clinical characteristics and outcome in 223 diabetic patients with deep foot infections. *Foot Ankle Int.* 1997;18:716–722.
23. Keenan AM, Tindel NL, Alavi A. Diagnosis of pedal osteomyelitis in diabetic patients using current scintigraphic techniques. *Arch Intern Med.* 1989;149:2262–2266.
24. Johnson JE, Kennedy EJ, Shereff MJ, et al. Prospective study of bone, Indium-111-labeled white blood cell, and Gallium-67 scanning for the evaluation of osteomyelitis in the diabetic foot. *Foot Ankle Int.* 1996;17:10–16.
25. Lipsky BA. Osteomyelitis of the foot in diabetic patients. *Clin Infect Dis.* 1997;25:1318–1326.
26. Schauwecker DS, Park HM, Burt RW, et al. Combined bone scintigraphy and Indium-111 leukocyte scans in neuropathic foot disease. *J Nucl Med.* 1988;29:1651–1655.
27. Lipsky BA. Medical treatment of diabetic foot infections. *Clin Infect Dis.* 2004;39:S104–S114.
28. Croll SD, Nicholas GG, Osborne MA, et al. Role of magnetic resonance imaging in the diagnosis of osteomyelitis in diabetic foot infection. *J Vasc Surg.* 1996;24:266–270.
29. Morrison WB, Ledermann HP, Schweitzer ME. MR imaging of the diabetic foot. *Magn Reson Imaging Clin N Am.* 2001;9:603–613.
30. Schweitzer ME, Morrison WB. MR imaging of the diabetic foot. *Radiol Clin North Am.* 2004;42:61–71.
31. Eichenholtz SN. *Charcot joints.* Springfield, Ill: Charles C Thomas Publisher; 1966.
32. Harris JR, Brand PW. Patterns of disintegration of the tarsus in the anaesthetic foot. *J Bone Joint Surg.* 1966;48B:4.
33. Brodsky JW. The diabetic foot. In: Coughlin MJ, Mann RA, eds. *Surgery of the foot and ankle,* 6th ed. Vol. 2. St. Louis, Mo: Mosby; 1999:877–955.
34. Sella EJ, Barrette C. Staging of Charcot neuroarthropathy along the medial column of the foot in the diabetic patient. *J Foot Ankle Surg.* 1999;38:34–40.
35. Lesko P, Maurer RC. Talonavicular dislocations and midfoot arthropathy in neuropathic diabetic feet: natural course and principles of treatment. *Clin Orthop.* 1989;240:226.
36. Pinzur MS, Sage R, Stuck R, et al. A treatment algorithm for neuropathic (Charcot) midfoot deformity. *Foot Ankle.* 1993;14: 189–197.
37. Myerson MS, Henderson MR, Saxby T, et al. Management of midfoot diabetic neuroarthropathy. *Foot Ankle Int.* 1994;15:233–241.
38. Mehta JA, Brown C, Sargeant N. Charcot restraint orthotic walker. *Foot Ankle Int.* 1998;19:619–623.
39. Selby PL, Young MJ, Boulton AJM. Bisphosphonates: a new treatment for diabetic Charcot neuroarthropathy? *Diabetic Med.* 1994; 11:28–31.
40. Jude EB, Selby PL, Burgess J, et al. Bisphosphonates in the treatment of Charcot neuroarthropathy: a double-blind randomised controlled trial. *Diabetologia.* 2001;44:2032–2037.
41. Hanft JR, Goggin JP, Landsman A, et al. The role of combined magnetic field bone growth stimulation as an adjunct in the treatment of neuroarthropathy/Charcot joint: an expanded pilot study. *J Foot Ankle Surg.* 1998;37:510–515.
42. Banks AS, McGlamry ED. Charcot foot. *J Am Podiatr Med Assoc.* 1989;79:213–217.
43. Fabrin J, Larsen K, Holstein PE. Long-term follow-up in diabetic Charcot feet with spontaneous onset. *Diabetes Care.* 2000; 23:796–800.
44. Pinzur MS. Benchmark analysis of diabetic patients with neuropathic (Charcot) foot deformity. *Foot Ankle Int.* 1999;20:564–567.
45. International Working Group on the Diabetic Foot. *International Consensus on the Diabetic Foot,* Amsterdam, 1999.
46. Simon SR, Tejwani SG, Wilson DL, et al. Arthrodesis as an early alternative to nonoperative management of Charcot arthropathy of the diabetic foot. *J Bone Joint Surg.* 2000;82-A:939–950.
47. Rosenblum BI, Giuini JM, Miller LB, et al. Neuropathic ulcerations plantar to the lateral column in patients with Charcot foot deformity: a flexible approach to limb salvage. *J Foot Ankle Surg.* 1997;36:360–363.
48. Schon LC, Marks RM. The management of neuroarthropathic fracture-dislocations in the diabetic patient. *Orthop Clin North Am.* 1995;26:375–392.
49. Jirkovska A, Kasalicky P, Boucek P, et al. Calcaneal Ultrasonometry in patients with Charcot osteoarthropathy and its relationship with densitometry in the lumbar spine and femoral neck and with markers of bone turnover. *Diabetic Med.* 2001;18:495–500.
50. Farber DC, Juliano PJ, Cavanagh PR, et al. Single stage correction with external fixation of the ulcerated foot in individuals with Charcot neuroarthropathy. *Foot Ankle Int.* 2002;23:130–134.
51. Jolly GP, Zgonis T, Polyzois V. External fixation in the management of Charcot neuroarthropathy. *Clin Podiatr Med Surg.* 2003; 20:741–756.
52. Cooper PS. Application of external fixators for management of Charcot deformities of the foot and ankle. *Foot Ankle Clin.* 2002; 7:207–254.
53. Wang JC, Le AW, Tsukuda RK. A new technique for Charcot's foot reconstruction. *J Am Podiatr Med Assoc.* 2002;92:429–436.
54. Papa J, Myerson M, Girard P. Salvage, with arthrodesis, in intractable diabetic neuropathic arthropy of the foot and ankle. *J Bone Joint Surg Am.* 1993;75:1056–1066.
55. Tisdel CL, Marcus RE, Heiple KG. Triple arthrodesis for diabetic peritalar neuroarthropathy. *Foot Ankle Int.* 1995;16:332–338.
56. Early JS, Hansen ST. Surgical reconstruction of the diabetic foot: a salvage approach for midfoot collapse. *Foot Ankle Int.* 1996;17: 325–330.
57. Cooper PS. Application of external fixators for management of Charcot deformities of the foot and ankle. *Semin Vasc Surg.* 2003; 16:67–78.
58. Wang JC. Use of external fixation in the reconstruction of the Charcot foot and ankle. *Clin Podiatr Med Surg.* 2003;20:97–117.
59. Prokuski LJ, Saltzman CL. External fixation for the treatment of Charcot arthropathy of the ankle: a case report. *Foot Ankle Int.* 1998;19:336–341.
60. Sella EJ, Grosser DM. Imaging modalities of the diabetic foot. *Clin Podiatr Med Surg.* 2003;20:729–740.

Anatomic Distribution of Atherosclerotic Lesions as Influenced by Diabetes and Other Risk Factors

Kendra Magee Merine   *Anton N. Sidawy*

Atherosclerosis is a significant cause of morbidity and death in the Western world. Despite the evolution of better medical therapy and the implementation of lifestyle modifications to reduce controllable risk factors, atherosclerosis continues to challenge the skills of vascular surgeons. Since there are divergent risk factors that initiate the progression of atherosclerosis, viewing it as a single disease entity is an oversimplification. It is not clear if the initial insult that these risk factors cause is similar. The initial response may take one of many forms ranging from altered endothelial cell function or altered lipid oxidation to ingress of macrophages or smooth muscle proliferation. Eventually the insults converge on a single common pathway, beginning with damage to the endothelium and culminating in plaque formation. Variations in the pattern and distribution of lesions along the arterial tree as well as the velocity of disease progression are based on patient risk factors. Clinical severity and symptom onset are also influenced by risk factors. These have important clinical implications for treatment and prognosis.

GENERAL PATTERNS

Atherosclerosis is a systemic disorder of the arteries. Large public health studies have identified the clinical risk factors associated with the development of atherosclerotic plaques.[1] These risk factors include cigarette smoking, diabetes mellitus, hypertension, elevated serum lipid levels, obesity, lack of aerobic exercise, stress, and heredity. A few of these factors have a close association with the development of atherosclerosis in specific arterial beds. The most dominant risk factor varies with anatomic location. Elevated levels of serum cholesterol and low density lipoprotein (LDL) correlate strongly with cerebrovascular and peripheral occlusive disease.[2-4] Hypertensive patients are more likely to develop cerebrovascular disease.[5] Cigarette smoking and diabetes are the principal risk factors for lower-extremity occlusive disease.[6-11]

Even within the major arteries of the leg, various segments may react differently to stressors such as smoking and diabetes. In addition to the differential influence of systemic risk factors, variability in local hemodynamic and arterial wall properties exerts effects on plaque formation.[12,13] These effects may be related to arterial diameter, vessel wall histology, and blood flow turbulence. Certain regions of each vascular bed are especially susceptible to plaque formation, while other areas are spared.[14] The coronary arteries, carotid bifurcation, infrarenal abdominal aorta, and iliofemoral arteries are examples of regions that are particularly prone to plaque formation. The thoracic aorta, common carotid, distal internal carotid, renal, mesenteric, and upper extremity arteries are relatively resistant to plaque formation. This variability has been attributed not only to the biomechanics of the vascular arcade but also to differences in the way shear and tensile stresses are applied to the arterial wall. Although plaques may occur in straight vessels away from branch points, they are usually located at bifurcation or bends, where variations in hemodynamic conditions are especially likely to occur.[15]

The arteries of the lower extremities are frequently diseased with atherosclerotic plaques, whereas vessels of similar caliber in the upper extremities are usually spared. In addition to differences in hydrostatic pressure, the arteries of the lower extremities are exposed to wide variations in flow rate, depending on the individual's level of physical activity. A sedentary lifestyle would tend to favor a low-flow state and lead to increased plaque deposition in vessels of the lower extremities.

Cigarette smoking and diabetes mellitus are the risk factors most closely associated with atherosclerotic disease of the lower extremities.[6–8,16] The manner in which these factors and special hemodynamic conditions converge to promote disease in the vessels of the lower extremities remains to be elucidated. The arterial media in the lower extremities may be thickened by the greater smooth muscle tone induced by nicotine. Such a change could interfere with the transmural transfer of materials entering the intima and favor the accumulation of atherogenic substances.[9,10]

Of the arteries of the lower extremity, the superficial femoral artery is the most common site of multiple stenotic lesions, while the profunda femoris tends to be spared. Isolated femoropopliteal lesions occur primarily in nondiabetic atherosclerosis. Disease of the profunda femoris tends to worsen with the presence of diabetes. In Haimovici's classic study of 321 atherosclerotic lesions, 9.5% of the nondiabetic subjects had a profunda lesion and 30.5% of the diabetic subjects had profunda disease.[17] Plaques in the superficial femoral artery have not been shown to occur preferentially at branching sites. Stenotic lesions tend to appear earliest at the adductor hiatus, where the vessel is straight. Increased susceptibility to plaque formation because of mechanical trauma caused by the closely associated adductor magnus tendon has been proposed to explain the selective localization of occlusive disease in this area.[18] An alternative theory is that the adductor canal segment of the superficial femoral artery is not more prone to plaque formation but rather is limited in its ability to dilate or enlarge in response to increasing intimal plaque because of anatomical constraints. Thus, an equivalent volume of intimal plaque results in more stenosis at the adductor canal.[19]

There are striking general characteristics of patients with proximal vascular disease versus patients with lesions more distal in the vascular tree. Men and women with aortoiliac disease present at a younger age than patients with more distal lesions.[20] In addition to being younger, patients with solely aortic involvement generally do not have diabetes.[20] Patients with certain patterns of vascular disease also have predictable patterns of comorbidities. They are more likely to be current smokers when they develop symptoms. Women with aortoiliac disease are more likely to have a history of ischemic heart disease and dyspnea. Men with aortoiliac disease have elevated systolic blood pressure and are more likely to have a history of chronic obstructive pulmonary disease (COPD). Both men and women with femoropopliteal lesions tend to have high blood pressure and are more likely to have a history of stroke and to be current smokers. The women with femoropopliteal disease are older than subjects without vascular disease and tend to have a diagnosis of ischemic heart disease and/or congestive heart failure.[20] Patients with tibioperoneal disease tend to be older than the control group and are more likely to have congestive heart failure. A significantly higher proportion of men with distal lesions is diabetic. Women with distal disease are more likely to have a history of stroke, hypertension, and ischemic heart disease. Lower extremity disease usually occurs with coronary and cerebral disease.[20]

The average duration of symptoms is markedly different among groups of patients with specific patterns of vascular disease. Patients with aortoiliac disease have symptoms for 4.3 years, patients with femoropopliteal disease have symptoms for 2.7 years, and patients with tibioperoneal disease have symptoms for 1.4 years before presentation. Ischemic symptoms seem to be milder and better tolerated in patients who have primarily aortic disease.[21] More rapid progression of ischemia is observed when smaller vessels of the lower extremities are principally involved.

DIABETES MELLITUS

A significant promoter of atherosclerosis is diabetes, a link which was established via the Framingham Study.[22] There are 18.2 million people with diabetes

(6.3% of the population) in the United States.[23] Eighty-four percent of them have peripheral vascular disease.[23] With 16-year follow-up, the age-adjusted risk ratio for intermittent claudication in people with diabetes is five times greater for men and four times greater for women.[24] Diabetes is an important factor for development of lower extremity arterial disease, with the occlusive process affecting the most distal vessels, namely the infrapopliteal arteries. In most studies, patients with tibial disease who are diabetic outnumber patients who do not have diabetes by two to one.[25] The percentage of patients with diabetes increases as the anatomic site of the atherosclerotic lesion becomes more distal. Diabetes accelerates the initiation and propagation of vascular disease leading to less favorable surgical outcomes, due to prolonged length of stay and elevated risk of infection. Among smokers, those with diabetes had more tissue loss and less pain at rest than nondiabetics. Although smokers presented with symptomatic disease much earlier than nonsmokers, diabetics and nondiabetics presented at comparable ages.[25]

Diabetes, like smoking, has direct effects on the arterial wall and on serum biochemistry. Causes of enhanced atherogenesis in diabetes include apoprotein and lipoprotein abnormalities, especially elevated lipoprotein (a) levels.[26] A procoagulant state coexists with the enhanced atherogenesis of diabetes. Infragenicular smooth muscle cell proliferation stimulated by fluctuating cytokine, hormone, and growth factor levels is a hallmark of diabetic atherogenesis. Increased foam cell formation attributable to the hyperinsulinemic state is unique to atherosclerosis in diabetes.[26]

It has been well described that people with diabetes have a macroangiopathy similar to atherosclerosis. There is, however, a persistent misconception about "small-vessel disease," which was felt to be an untreatable, occlusive lesion in the microcirculation.[27] This idea evolved from a study by Goldenberg et al.[28] in which periodic acid-Schiff–positive intimal material occluding the arterioles in amputated limb specimens from diabetic patients was measured. Subsequent studies have shown that diabetics do not have a distinctive form of occlusive small artery disease.[29,30] There is as much microvascular occlusion in nondiabetic as in diabetic patients. Strandness et al.[29] prospectively examined pathologic specimens from diabetic and nondiabetic patients and did not find any specific lesion of the small arteries that distinguished the diabetic patient. There is no difference in the responsiveness of the runoff bed to papaverine vasodilatation, so resistance vessel reactivity is preserved in diabetics.[31] Structural changes do exist, like thickening of the capillary basement membrane, but this does not cause narrowing of the capillary lumen, and there is no compromise of arteriolar blood flow.[31]

Some have observed that diabetics have a higher incidence of occlusive disease in the large arteries of the calf.[29] Strandness et al.[29] reported that diabetics have a higher incidence of occlusive disease in the anterior tibial, posterior tibial, and peroneal arteries. Conrad[30] studied casts made from the vascular lumina of 20 extremities amputated for gangrene and found the distribution of vascular occlusion to be similar in diabetics and nondiabetics, except that diabetics had a higher frequency of peroneal artery occlusion and somewhat less occlusion in the pedal arch.

SMOKING

Although our main focus is diabetes, so many people with diabetes smoke or have other risk factors that the distribution and the onset of atherosclerosis is also affected by those risk factors associated with diabetes. Cigarette smoking is the most powerful risk factor for atherosclerosis; 25.6 million men (25.2% of the population) and 22.6 million women (20.7% of the population) in the United States are smokers.[32] Current smokers are at higher risk for atherosclerosis than former smokers, and the number of pack-years is associated with the severity of disease. Former smokers have a sevenfold greater risk of atherosclerosis, whereas current smokers have a 16-fold increased risk.[33] Smoking greatly impacts clinical presentation. Multivariate logistic regression analysis indicates that current smoking remains the strongest independent correlate of disease in both sexes after correction for the other covariates.[20] After age-adjustment, the major characteristic associated with the presence of isolated aortoiliac and femoropopliteal disease in both men and women is smoking status.[20]

In studies of patients with peripheral vascular disease, nondiabetic nonsmokers generally constitute a small segment of the study group (<9%) and they present with symptomatic vascular disease >11 years later than smokers.[21] Aortoiliac disease occurs more commonly in younger patients who smoke than those who do not smoke (60% vs. 26.4%).[21] The association is lower in those who have stopped smoking but remains elevated compared to lifelong nonsmokers. Women with a history of smoking are particularly susceptible to aortoiliac disease. Claudication is strongly associated with smoking. In addition to the strong association with proximal disease, smokers are more likely to present with pain at rest (40%) and gangrene/ulcer (41%) than claudication (27%), indicators of more distal disease.[34] Smoking is associated with more extensive disease in the anterior/posterior tibial arteries than in the posterior tibial/peroneal distribution.[20]

In addition to being a major risk factor for atherosclerosis, current cigarette smoking also significantly affects outcomes. Sequelae of tobacco abuse referable to vascular disease include limb amputation, ischemic heart disease, and failure of bypass grafts. The exact mechanism of insult is not clear. Smoking exerts its effects in two ways. First it damages the vessel wall. Carbon monoxidemia predisposes the arterial wall to injury by inciting alterations in the vascular endothelium. These endothelial breeches make it easier for cholesterol to enter the vessel and form deposits. Smoking induces peripheral vasoconstriction. Smoking also has effects on blood components and serum biochemistry. It induces alterations in lipid metabolism, increases platelet aggregation, and increases blood viscosity.[8,21,33,34] Progression from intermittent claudication to ischemic rest pain occurs significantly more frequently in patients who use tobacco than in those who do not use tobacco. Over 5 years, 18% of patients with claudication who smoke will progress to rest pain while virtually no nonsmoking patients progress to rest pain.[35] Graft patency results (both prosthetic and vein conduits) are also significantly affected by cigarette smoking. At 1 year, the patency of a prosthetic graft in a smoker is 65%, while in a nonsmoker the patency is 85%.[35] For a vein graft the 1-year patency rate for a smoker is 70% and for a nonsmoker 90%.[35] When vein graft patency is viewed over a 3-year period, the patency rate for nonsmokers is the same 90% while the patency rate for smokers falls to 50%.[35] Amputation rates are also driven by current smoking status and are approximately two to three times those of nonsmokers. Last, patient survival is significantly worse for those who continue to smoke than for those who quit. The 5-year survival rate for smokers with peripheral vascular disease is 36%; for nonsmokers the rate is 66%.[35]

OTHER RISK FACTORS

Hypertension is a well-recognized risk factor for atherosclerotic diseases, particularly stroke and ischemic heart disease. In patients with peripheral vascular disease, hypertension increases risk approximately two to three times.[36] Hypertension has also been found to be an independent risk factor for atherosclerosis, but it is probably less important than smoking and diabetes.[37] In one major study, 55.1% of patients with peripheral vascular disease had hypertension while only 34.1% of patients without hypertension had vascular disease.[20] Both men and women with femoropopliteal lesions had high blood pressure and were more likely to have a history of stroke and to be current smokers. A history of diabetes was strongly associated with the presence of tibioperoneal lesions in men, while in women a systolic blood pressure >140 mm Hg was the most important factor. Elevated systolic blood pressure was an independent correlate of disease in each of the three arterial segments (aortoiliac, femoropopliteal, and infrapopliteal) studied in women, and of aortoiliac and femoropopliteal disease in men. The incidence of hypertension was lowest in the group of patients with femoropopliteal disease.[20]

Alterations in lipid metabolism are a major risk factor for all forms of atherosclerosis. Several large epidemiologic trials have conclusively shown that elevations in total cholesterol and in low density lipoprotein (LDL) cholesterol levels and decreases in high density lipoprotein (HDL) cholesterol levels are significantly and independently associated with cardiovascular mortality.[2] The role of triglyceride elevations has been debated, but more recent studies have conclusively shown that elevated fasting levels of triglycerides are also a strong and independent predictor of ischemic heart disease and peripheral occlusive disease.[38] In peripheral occlusive disease several lipid fractions are individually important in determining the presence and progression of peripheral atherosclerosis. Independent risk factors for peripheral occlusive disease include elevations of total cholesterol, LDL cholesterol, triglycerides, and lipoprotein (a).[39] Protective against peripheral occlusive disease are HDL cholesterol and apolipoprotein A1.[39] For every 10 mg per dL increase in total cholesterol concentration, the risk of peripheral occlusive disease increases approximately 10%.[39]

The most common lipid abnormality is type IV hyperlipoproteinemia with minimally elevated or normal serum cholesterol levels and triglyceride levels in excess of 130 mg per 100 mL.[20] Type IV hyperlipoproteinemia is most closely associated with femoropopliteal disease. Patients with primarily femoropopliteal involvement show a significantly increased incidence of type IV hyperlipoproteinemia when compared with patients who have aortic disease.[20] Hypercholesterolemia alone or type II hyperlipoproteinemia is uncommon with distal peripheral vascular disease. These patterns of dyslipidemia are seen only in patients with aortic involvement. In each group abnormal lipoprotein patterns are more frequent than elevated serum cholesterol levels. Concurrent with hypertriglyceridemia, in patients with femoropopliteal involvement the incidence of diabetes is also highest. This is significantly greater than in patients with aortic involvement alone. Type II hyperlipoproteinemia (elevation of β-lipoprotein) occurs in groups with aortic disease.[20]

All forms of vascular disease become more prevalent with age, and thus it is not surprising that peripheral occlusive disease is more frequent in the elderly population. In several studies, the risk of peripheral occlusive disease increases (1.5- to twofold) for every 10-year increase in age.[39] The youngest patients have primarily aortoiliac disease (58% vs. 66% for femoropopliteal disease).[39] The occurrence of femoropopliteal and tibioperoneal disease increases sharply with age while the more proximal disease is weakly related to increasing age. Risk factors change with age and over time. Abnormal lipid profiles decrease with age, glucose intolerance increases with age, and cigarette smoking decreases with age.[39]

Race has been described as an independent risk factor in the development of infrapopliteal peripheral vascular disease in one study that compared African-American with white American patients undergoing lower extremity arteriograms for symptomatic lower extremity peripheral vascular disease.[40] The prevalence of diabetes, smoking, and hypercholesterolemia was similar in the two groups. There was a higher prevalence of hypertension in the African-American patients. The African-American patients had more severe disease (based on an angiographic scoring system) in all three infrapopliteal arteries. When the nonhypertensive patients were considered alone, the African-American patients still had higher disease severity scores, indicating worse infrapopliteal disease in this population. And since diabetes is known to be an etiologic factor in this particular distribution of the disease, only the nonhypertensive, nondiabetic patients were analyzed; this analysis showed that the African-American group had an even worse disease pattern.[40] However, when patients with severe infrapopliteal disease and normal fasting glucose were subjected to oral glucose tolerance tests (OGTT), they were found to have positive OGTT, especially in the African-American patients (44.5%) when compared to the white patients (9%), indicating that the worse infrapopliteal disease in the African Americans is probably due to glucose intolerance rather than racial predilection in this population—again emphasizing the role that a diabetic state plays in this particular distribution of atherosclerotic disease (Dr. Sidawy's unpublished data).

SUMMARY

Atherosclerosis is a systemic vascular disease in which plaques develop at arterial bifurcations where blood flow is slow or turbulent. The atherosclerotic process in the vessels of the lower extremities usually occurs in conjunction with that in the coronary and cerebral arteries. Life expectancy is decreased by about 10 years in patients with lower extremity disease, and the majority of these patients die from cardiac disease or stroke. Lower limb atherosclerosis usually develops at several levels within the arteries but may also be restricted to a single localized region in a vessel. When stenosis is found at multiple sites, the blood flow to the lower limbs is often severely compromised, and limb ischemia may become a significant clinical problem.

Such multisegmental disease is also associated with poorer overall cardiovascular health status and higher morbidity and mortality than in localized unisegmental disease. Several studies have suggested that the etiology of the disease process in the lower extremity may vary depending on the anatomic site of the lesion. Aortoiliac disease seems to occur in younger patients who smoke, while the more distal lesions in the infrapopliteal arteries are found primarily in people with diabetes.

REFERENCES

1. Gordon T, Kannel WB. Predisposition to atherosclerosis in the head, heart, and legs: the Framingham study. *JAMA*. 1972;221:661–666.
2. Gordon DJ, Probstfield JL, Garrison RJ, et al. High-density lipoprotein cholesterol and cardiovascular disease: four prospective American studies. *Circulation*. 1989;79:8–15.
3. Martin MJ, Hulley SB, Browner WS, et al. Serum cholesterol, blood pressure, and mortality: implications from a cohort of 361,662 men. *Lancet*. 1986;2:933–936.
4. Pekkanen J, Linn S, Heiss G, et al. Ten-year mortality from cardiovascular disease in relation to cholesterol level among men with and without preexisting cardiovascular disease. *N Engl J Med*. 1990;322:1700–1707.
5. Kannel WB, McGee DL, Casteli WP. Latest perspectives on cigarette smoking and cardiovascular disease: the Framingham study. *J Cardiac Rehab*. 1984;4:267–277.
6. Kannel WB, Shurtleff D. National Heart and Lung Institute, National Institutes of Health: the Framingham study: cigarettes and the development of intermittent claudication. *Geriatrics*. 1973;28:61–68.
7. Krupski WC. The peripheral vascular consequences of smoking. *Ann Vasc Surg*. 1991;5:291–304.
8. Krupski WC, Rapp JH. Smoking and atherosclerosis. *Perspect Vasc Surg*. 1988;1:103–134.
9. Winniford MD, Wheelan KR, Kremers MS, et al. Smoking-induced coronary vasoconstriction in patients with atherosclerotic coronary artery disease: evidence for adrenergically mediated alterations in coronary artery tone. *Circulation*. 1986;73:662.
10. Caro CG, Fish PJ, Jay M, et al. Influence of vasoactive agents on arterial hemodynamics: possible relevance to atherogenesis. *Abstr Biorheol*. 1986;23:197.
11. Balaji MR, DeWeese JA. Adductor canal outlet syndrome. *JAMA*. 1981;245:167.
12. Glagov S. Hemodynamic risk factors: mechanical stress, mural architecture, medial nutrition and the vulnerability of arteries to atherosclerosis. In: Wissler RW, Geer JC, eds. *The pathogenesis of atherosclerosis*. Baltimore, Md: Williams & Wilkins; 1972:164–169.
13. Texon M. The hemodynamic concept of atherosclerosis. *Bull N Y Acad Med*. 1960;36:263.
14. Glagov S, Rowley DA, Kohut R. Atherosclerosis of human aorta and its coronary and renal arteries. *Arch Pathol Lab Med*. 1961;72:558.
15. Ravensbergen J, Ravensbergen JW, Krijger JK, et al. Localizing role of hemodynamics in atherosclerosis in several human vertebrobasilar junction geometries. *Arterioscler Thromb Vasc Biol*. 1998;18:693.
16. Kannel WB, McGee DL, Castelli WP. Latest perspectives on cigarette smoking and cardiovascular disease: the Framingham study. *J Cardiac Rehabil*. 1984;4:267–277.
17. Haimovici H. Patterns of arteriosclerotic lesions of the lower extremity. *Arch Surg*. 1967;95:918–933.

18. Balaji MR, Deweese JA. Adductor canal outlet syndrome. *JAMA.* 1981;245:167.

19. Blair JM, Glagov S, Zarins CK. Mechanism of superficial femoral artery adductor canal stenosis. *Surg Forum.* 1990;41:359.

20. Rosen AJ, DePalma RG, Victor Y. Risk factors in peripheral atherosclerosis. *Arch Surg.* 1973;107:303–308.

21. Menzoin JO, LaMorte WW, Paniszyn CC. Symptomatology and anatomic patterns of peripheral vascular disease: differing impact of smoking and diabetes. *Ann Vasc Surg.* 1989;3:224–228.

22. Kannel WB, D'Agostino RB, Wilson PW, et al. Diabetes, fibrinogen, and risk of cardiovascular disease: the Framingham experience. *Am Heart J.* 1990;120:672–676.

23. Lucas JW, Schiller JS, Benson V. Summary health statistics for U.S. adults: National Health Interview Survey, 2001. National Center for Health Statistics. *Vital Health Stat.* 2004;10(218):1–134.

24. Kannel WB, McGee DL. Update on some epidemiologic features of intermittent claudication: the Framingham study. *J Am Geriatr Soc.* 1985;33:13–18.

25. Vogt MT, Wolfson SK, Kuller LH. Segmental arterial disease in the lower extremities: correlates of disease and relationship to mortality. *J Clin Epidemiol.* 1993;46:1267–1276.

26. Ruderman NB, Haudenschild C. Diabetes as an atherogenic factor. *Prog Cardiovasc Dis.* 1984;26:373–412.

27. Akbari CM, LoGerfo FW. Diabetes and peripheral vascular disease. *J Vasc Surg.* 1999;30:373–384.

28. Goldenberg SG, Alex M, Joshi RA, et al. Nonatheromatous peripheral vascular disease of the lower extremity in diabetes mellitus. *Diabetes.* 1959;8:261–273.

29. Strandness DE, Priest RE, Gibbons GE. Combined clinical and pathologic study of diabetic and nondiabetic peripheral arterial disease. *Diabetes.* 1964;13:366–372.

30. Conrad MC. Large and small artery occlusion in diabetics and nondiabetics with severe vascular disease. *Circulation.* 1967;36:83–91.

31. Barner HB, Kaiser GC, Willman VL. Blood flow in the diabetic leg. *Circulation.* 1971;43:391–394.

32. National Health Interview Survey 2003 Faststats. Available at www.cdc.gov.

33. Fielding JE. Smoking: health effects and control. *N Engl J Med.* 1985;313(Pt 1 of 2):491–498.

34. Fielding JE. Smoking: health effects and control. *N Engl J Med.* 1985;313(Pt 2 of 2):555–561.

35. Hirsch AT, Treat-Jacobson D, Lando HA, et al. The role of tobacco cessation, antiplatelet and lipid-lowering therapies in the treatment of peripheral arterial disease. *Vasc Med.* 1997;2:243–251.

36. Safar ME, Laurent S, Asmar RE. Systolic hypertension in patients with arteriosclerosis obliterans of the lower limbs. *Angiology.* 1987;38:287–295.

37. Juergens JL, Barker NW, Hines EA. Arteriosclerosis obliterans: a review of 520 cases with special reference to pathogenic and prognostic factors. *Circulation.* 1960;21:188–195.

38. Burchfiel CM, Laws A, Benfante R, et al. Combined effects of HDL cholesterol, triglyceride, and total cholesterol concentrations on 18 year risk of atherosclerotic disease. *Circulation.* 1995;92:1430–1436.

39. Hiatt WR, Hoag S, Hamman RF. Effect of diagnostic criteria on the prevalence of peripheral arterial disease: the San Luis Valley diabetes study. *Circulation.* 1995;91:1472–1479.

40. Sidawy AN, Schweitzer EJ, Neville RF, et al. Race as a risk factor in the severity of infragenicular occlusive disease: study of an urban hospital patient population. *J Vasc Surg.* 1990;11:536–543.

Nonatherosclerotic Disease of the Tibial Vessels

Eric D. Adams   *Anton N. Sidawy*

The majority of diseases seen in tibial vessels are related to degenerative, atherosclerotic changes, particularly in the patient with diabetes. There are, however, some less common disease states that can also affect the tibial vessels and need to be considered. Prominent among these diseases is Buerger disease, otherwise known as thromboangiitis obliterans (TAO). Buerger disease is seen almost exclusively in young smokers, and has a heavy male predominance. Other systemic disease states known to affect the tibial vessels include periarteritis nodosa and Behçet disease. Specific subtypes of Ehlers-Danlos syndrome show a propensity for arterial disease and the tibial vessels are not excluded from involvement. For many of these diseases, the changes in the tibial vessels may appear at a young age and in some cases can be the presenting event leading to the diagnosis of their systemic disease. The clinician needs to be aware of these alternative diagnoses and their treatments. For many of these diseases the best treatment is avoidance of surgical intervention if at all possible. For a young patient who presents with either occlusion or aneurysmal changes of the tibial vessels, alternative diagnoses other than the usual atherosclerotic change must be entertained.

BUERGER DISEASE (THROMBOANGIITIS OBLITERANS)

Background

Buerger disease is characterized by segmental occlusion of small- and medium-sized arteries in the lower and sometimes upper extremities. It is most commonly seen in young, primarily male, smokers. Migratory thrombophlebitis is often associated with this disease.[1] Von Winiwarter[2] first described a patient with a clinical disorder called endarteritis in 1879. In 1908, Leo Buerger provided a detailed pathologic description of the pathologic findings in 11 amputated limbs and named the entity TAO.[3] Buerger disease is seen throughout the world but is more prevalent in the Middle East and Far East than in North America or western Europe. In Japan, until the 1960s, Buerger disease was more prevalent than atherosclerosis obliterans. In India, Buerger disease remains the most common type of peripheral vascular disease.[1,4] The prevalence of this disease among patients with peripheral arterial disease varies from 0.5% to 5.6% in western Europe to 16% in Japan, and as high as 66% in

India. The Mayo Clinic reported an incidence of 12.6 per 100,000 in 1986.[5]

Pathophysiology

The histologic findings of Buerger disease show progressive changes with time. Early lesions are characterized by thrombotic occlusion accompanied by prominent neutrophilic infiltration in the thrombus and all layers of the vessel wall.[6] Microabscess is seen occasionally in the thrombus. Older lesions show an organized thrombus and a change to a mononuclear infiltrate with multinucleated giant cells and epithelioid cells. The media returns to normal while the intima expands by myointimal cell proliferation. Concentric or eccentric intimal fibrous thickening, reduplication, and disruption of the internal elastic lamina are frequently seen in small arteries.[7] Analysis of the fibrinolytic activity in various parts of the arterial wall shows fibrinolytic activity along the vasa vasorum in the adventitia and the media, but not in the thickened intima.

The cause of Buerger disease remains unknown, but there is an extremely strong association between heavy use of tobacco products and development and progression of the disease.[5] Although some authors feel that Buerger disease can exist without significant tobacco exposure,[8,9] most consider it to be a requirement for the diagnosis.[9,10] A number of explanations have been advanced as to the pathogenesis of the disease. A genetic predisposition has been suggested, with one study showing a predisposition to the disease among human leukocyte antigen (HLA)-DR4 patients.[11] In a 1998 review, Tanaka[7] suggested that mechanical injury, as indicated by the frequent disruption of the internal elastic lamina, may be important. The decreased fibrinolytic activity of the thickened intima could delay thombolysis and lead to the evolution of occlusive thrombosis.[7] A Turkish study looked at the contribution of prothrombotic states in 36 patients with Buerger disease compared to 182 healthy controls. They found an increased prevalence of prothrombin 20210G to A mutation in the Buerger patients, suggesting a hypercoagulable state may promote development of the disease. Factor V Leiden (factor V 1691 G to A) and factor V 4070 A to G (His 1299 Arg) mutations were only weakly associated with increased risk.[12] These findings have not yet been replicated by other investigators.

Other mechanisms implicated in the development of Buerger disease include decreased vasoreactivity, changes in endothelial cell adhesion molecules, and presence of antiphospholipid antibodies. Various autoantibodies and cellular sensitivity to vascular components have also been demonstrated.[6] The study looking at antiphospholipid antibodies compared patients with Buerger disease, patients with premature atherosclerosis (onset prior to age 45), and healthy controls.

They found that 36% of patients with Buerger disease had a positive anticardiolipin versus 8% of the premature atherosclerosis patients and 2% of the healthy controls.[13] Vasoreactivity measurements using forearm blood flow were taken in Buerger disease patients and in healthy age-matched controls. The results revealed diminished endothelial dependent vasodilation in the nondiseased limbs of Buerger disease patients. Nonendothelial mechanisms of vasodilation remained intact.[14] A study looking at surgical arterial specimens from Buerger disease patients examined endothelial cell adhesion molecules.[6] They found increased expression of ICAM-1, VCAM-1, and E-selectin on endothelial cells in the thickened intima of all patients. They concluded that the preferential expression of inducible adhesion molecules in microvessels and mononuclear inflammatory cells suggest that angiogenesis contributes to the persistence of the inflammatory process in Buerger disease. The relative role of each of these mechanisms awaits further investigation.

Clinical Manifestations

Clinical manifestations of Buerger disease can involve the mesenteric, coronary, retinal, cerebral, pulmonary, and renal arteries.[15] By far and away, however, the most common presentations are that of claudication or cold sensation of the feet, legs, hands, or arms. One study[16] examined limbs by arteriogram and revealed universal involvement of more than one limb. As the disease progresses, patients who initially complained of foot pain may note the onset of classic calf claudication progressing to ischemic rest pain and eventual ischemic ulceration of the toes, feet, or fingers.[5,17] Not all patients follow this progression and some may present with an initial complaint of a toe or finger ulcer.[1] Superficial thrombophlebitis occurs in approximately 40% of patients.[18] While the typical patient is a young man, Lie[19] found an incidence of 11% in women in a Mayo Clinic review, and Olin found an incidence of 23% from a Cleveland Clinic review.[18] A Japanese study reported that 9% of their 850 patients were women.[8]

Diagnosis

There are no specific laboratory tests to confirm the diagnosis of Buerger disease and several diagnostic criteria have been used. The criteria used in Japan[8] include evidence of peripheral ischemia or migratory thrombophlebitis, change in temperature or pulses in the distal aspect of an extremity, age of onset before 50, appropriate findings on arteriography, and exclusion of other vascular diseases. Tobacco use is not mandatory in the Japanese criteria. In a 2000 *New England Journal of Medicine* review article, Olin[5] delineates his diagnostic criteria, which this author follows. His criteria include age at onset of symptoms of <45; current or recent tobacco use; presence of distal-extremity ischemia (indicated by claudication, pain at rest, ischemic ulcers, or gangrene); exclusion of autoimmune disease, hypercoagulable states, and diabetes by laboratory tests; exclusion of a proximal source of emboli; and consistent arteriographic findings. A biopsy is not necessary. Suggested laboratory tests to exclude other diseases include fasting blood glucose, acute phase reactants (sedimentation rate, C-reactive protein), antinuclear antibody, rheumatoid factor, complement, and markers for the *c*alcinosis, *R*aynaud phenomenon, *e*sophageal motility disorders, *s*clerodactyly, and *t*elangiectasia (CREST) syndrome and scleroderma (anticentomere antibody and Scl-70). Hypercoagulability markers should also be obtained.[5]

Angiographic findings that can suggest Buerger disease include normal proximal arteries without atherosclerotic changes and severe distal disease. The distal lesions involve the small- and medium-sized vessels such as the tibial, plantar, and digital arteries, as well as the upper extremity vessels of similar size. Segmental occlusive lesions can be seen interspersed with normal-appearing arteries. Collateralization around the areas of occlusion (corkscrew collaterals) are very common and suggestive of the diagnosis but are not pathognomonic (see Fig. 12-1).

Treatment

The only proven long-term treatment for Buerger disease is immediate and complete cessation of the use of any tobacco-containing products (including smokeless tobacco) and discontinuation of nicotine, which may also keep the disease active.[20,21] Continued smoking is strongly associated with continued symptoms. One study looked at 289 patients with Buerger disease of whom 127 did not stop smoking. Among the smokers, 48% developed ischemic ulcers, while only 9% of those who did stop smoking developed ulcers.[2] Olin suggests that the correlation between smoking and active disease is so strong that if the patient claims to have stopped smoking and continues to have active disease, measurements of urinary nicotine and conicotine (a metabolite) should be performed.

A variety of surgical methods have been advocated for the treatment of ischemic lesions in Buerger disease. Standard surgical revascularization is usually not possible because of the diffuse involvement of distal vessels, leaving no reasonable target vessel. However, in the face of severe ischemia and the presence of a target vessel, bypass with an autogenous vein can be a reasonable option. A small series of 10 patients in whom distal bypass was performed revealed a 30% occlusion rate at a mean of 41 months. Two of the three occlusions occurred in bypasses to diseased tibial targets. The

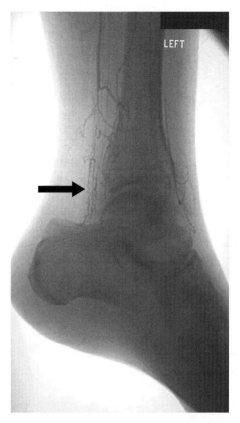

Figure 12-1 Lower extremity arteriogram from a 45-year-old, white man with a long history of heavy tobacco use. The patient had normal femoral and popliteal pulses but absent pedal pulses. He presented with a painful, gangrenous toe. The arteriogram reveals classic "corkscrew" collaterals at the level of the ankle joint (*black arrow*).

researchers concluded that a patent but diseased vessel should be avoided as a target for reconstruction.[22] A larger series of 61 patients reported overall primary patency rates of 49% and secondary patency of 62%. In those patients who continued to smoke the patency was only 35%.[23]

Another surgical technique that has been described involves pedicled omental transfer for limb salvage. This technique includes a laparotomy to mobilize a pedicle of omentum fed by the left or right gastroepiploic artery. The pedicle is brought through a subfascial tunnel on the anteriomedial thigh and down to the ankle where it is sutured to the muscle. In a series of 62 patients treated with this method,[1] one group of authors reported relief of claudication in 92%, disappearance of rest pain in 94%, and healing of ischemic ulcers in 83%. No major amputations have been required at a mean follow up of 3.5 years. Unfortunately, the authors did not have access to arteriography, so preoperative diagnoses were not confirmed with arteriograms and no follow-up images are available.

Sympathectomy has been advocated as a means of preventing amputation or treating pain. Its effectiveness remains unclear, and long-term results have been disappointing. It does not seem to exempt the patient from subsequent relapse or amputation.[24,25] A review of sympathectomy in current surgical practice found no reliable evidence to support the use of sympathectomy in Buerger disease. Any beneficial effects appear to be short lasting—especially if the patient continues to smoke.[26] A more recent article looking at the effects of sympathectomy and catecholamines in Buerger disease patients concluded that sympathectomy might be useful, but the usefulness was dependent on cessation of smoking.[27]

A variety of medications have been advocated for the treatment of Buerger disease with only limited results.[28,29] The European TAO Study Group[29] published their results with intravenous iloprost, a prostacyclin analogue. The medication is thought to stimulate blood flow and have vasodilatory and platelet inhibitory effects. Although iloprost was significantly more effective than placebo for relief of rest pain, total healing of lesions was not significantly different between treatment groups at any time point.[29] The drug must be given intravenously and is not currently available in the United States. Calcium channel-blocking agents may be useful in those patients thought to have a significant component of vasospasm associated with the disease.[30]

Case reports and small series[17,31] exist for the use of implantable spinal cord stimulators to treat the ischemic manifestations of Buerger disease when all other methods had failed. The reported results were good but the actual reason for the effect remains conjectural. It is believed that the stimulation acts as an analgesic and has an autonomic effect with consequent vasodilation. The use of gene therapy to encourage neovascularization in ischemic limbs may be another promising treatment option in the future.

Prognosis

Overall, the prognosis for a patient with Buerger disease is good—particularly if the use of all tobacco products is completely discontinued. A report from Japan followed 328 patients treated between 1968 and 1985. They found only a 3.9% major amputation rate.[2] A Cleveland Clinic study of 120 patients showed an amputation rate of only 6% in those patients who successfully stopped smoking versus a 43% incidence of amputation for those who continued to smoke.[30] Interestingly, the progression of symptoms was self-limited and recurrent ulcers occurred less frequently with ageing.[2] The overall life expectancy is thought to be nearly equal to that of healthy people and better than that of patients with atherosclerosis obliterans.[4] It is essential that the physician treating the Buerger disease patient take the time to ensure that the patient is thoroughly instructed and encouraged in tobacco cessation.

BEHÇET DISEASE

Background

In 1937, Hallushi Behçet, a Turkish dermatologist, reported three cases of oral and genital ulcerations associated with iritis. His contribution is acknowledged in the eponym for the condition he described.[32,33] The disease is a chronic, relapsing, inflammatory, multisystem disorder of uncertain etiology. It is characterized by widespread vasculitis of the large and small vessels. While the usual presenting complaint is one of the classic triad of symptoms, in a small percentage of patients the initial presentation will be that of a vascular complication. Both venous and arterial vessels can be involved leading to thrombophlebitis, deep venous thrombosis, arterial occlusion, or aneurysm.[32,34–36] Direct involvement of tibial vessels is distinctly uncommon, though they can be the site where emboli from upstream aneurysms ultimately lodge.[37] Behçet disease is most common in the "silk route" countries around the Mediterranean and Japan. The prevalence rate is extremely low in the United States at 0.13 to 0.33 per 100,000.[38,39] Onset of disease is typically in the third or fourth decade of life.[40]

Pathophysiology

The cause of Behçet disease is unknown, but it has been associated with a number of conditions. The HLA-B51 allele appears to be an important contributor to the risk of Behçet disease in areas where the disease is prevalent, but not in Western countries. Infections from both viral and bacterial causes have been suggested as causes as well. Herpes simplex virus (HSV) DNA and antibodies have been found in higher proportions in patients with Behçet disease than in controls. *Streptococcus sangis* has also been suggested as a cause.[39] However, no infectious agent has been proven to be the cause of the disease. A more widely accepted theory is that reaction to some external stimulus such as HSV or a *Streptococcal* strain may induce an immunopathologic response with activation of a heat shock protein and subsequent $\gamma\delta^+$T cell induction. Subsequently, the inflammatory cytokines stimulate neutrophils and monocytes.[35,39]

Although the underlying etiology is unclear, the histopathology produced is that of a nonspecific vasculitis of large and small vessels. Features "... include perivascular infiltrates with lymphocytes and mononuclear cells, swelling and proliferation of endothelial cells, and fibrinoid necrosis and consequent thrombosis, obstruction, and disruption of the vessel wall integrity. Obliterative endarteritis of the vasa vasorum is thought to lead to arterial dilation and aneurysm formation, or perforation with pseudoaneurysm formation."[41] Patients manifesting the disease have an increased thrombotic tendency. Kiraz et al.[34] studied their 137 patients and failed to identify any of the standard hypercoagulable states as the cause for the thrombotic tendency. They and others concluded that immunologic injury to the vascular endothelial cells themselves is the cause for the prothromotic state.[34,42]

Diagnosis

There is no one test to diagnose Behçet disease and no pathognomonic finding on biopsy to confirm the diagnosis. The pathergy reaction is highly specific for Behçet disease, although positive reactions can be seen in healthy individuals and in patients with spondyloarthropathies.[38,43] Unfortunately, pathergy is uncommon in patients with Behçet disease in the United States. Consequently, the International Study Group for Behçet disease drew up a series of criteria, which are shown in Table 12-1. For the diagnosis to be made, a patient must have recurrent oral ulceration plus at least two of the other findings in the absence of other clinical explanations.

TABLE 12-1
DIAGNOSTIC CRITERIA FOR BEHÇET DISEASE

Finding	Definition
Recurrent oral ulceration	Minor apthous, major apthous, or herpetiform observed by physician or patient, which have recurred at least 3 times over a 12-mo period
Recurrent genital ulcerations	Apthous ulceration or scarring observed by the physician or patient
Eye lesions	Anterior uveitis, posterior uveitis, or cells in the vetrious on slit-lamp examination; or retinal vasculitis detected by an ophthalmologist
Skin lesions	Erythema nodosum observed by the physician or patient, pseudofolliculits, or papulopustular lesions; or acneform nodules observed by the physician in a postadolescent patient who is not receiving corticosteroids
Positive pathergy test	Test interpreted as positive by the physician at 24 to 48 h

From International Study Group for Behçet's disease. Criteria for diagnosis of Behçet's disease. *Lancet* 1990;335:1078–80.

Clinical Manifestations

Vascular lesions develop in 7% to 38% of patient with Behçet disease.[39] The majority of these lesions are venous thrombotic episodes, but arterial occlusion and aneurysms account for much of the mortality from the disease. Although any artery may be involved,[32] the most common sites of aneurysm formation are, in order of decreasing frequency, the aorta, pulmonary arteries, femoral arteries, subclavian, popliteal, and common carotid arteries.[41] Case reports exist of primary tibial artery aneurysms.[44] The arterial lesions tend to be multiple, recurrent, and prone to rupture.[36,41,45] Flares of the disease are thought to make the arteries vulnerable to arterial wall necrosis with aneurysm and pseudoaneurysm formation. Even minor trauma can lead to significant vessel damage with several reports of late pseudoaneurysm formation after arterial puncture for arteriography.[46,47]

Treatment

Results from peripheral artery aneurysm repair have been disappointing. Kasirajan et al.[48] reviewed the results of infrainguinal arterial aneurysm repair. They found the mean time to aneurysm formation at the anastomotic site to be 3.3 months, and the longest reported patency to be 16 months.[48] Vein graft interposition was complicated by development of aneurysms at both anastomoses. Other authors have had similar experiences.[41,49]

Because the results of aneurysm repair have been so disappointing, standard surgical treatments with bypass using either autogenous or prosthetic conduit should be reserved for those patients who present with rupture and an acutely ischemic limb. First line of therapy for a nonruptured peripheral aneurysm should be medical treatment. If an aneurysm is found in a location amenable to ligation without limb loss, that aneurysm should preferentially be ligated rather than repaired. Surgical treatment should only be undertaken if there has been no significant regression detected after control of vasculitis and inflammation by medical treatment.[35] Little[50] first reported that graft occlusion is well tolerated in Behçet disease patients. Barlas,[35] in his experience with 30 peripheral aneurysms, came to the same conclusion.

Occlusive arterial disease can affect all arteries to include the tibial vessels. Claudication, rest pain, and tissue loss have all been reported.[49,51] Patients can also suffer from a Raynaud-type phenomenon.[32] If surgery is necessary to prevent limb loss, polytetrafluoroethylene (PTFE) rather than vein has been recommended as the conduit of choice because of the poor results with autogenous veins. Autogenous conduits seem prone to the development of aneurysmal changes.[37] Results of any surgical intervention are improved by aggressive medical therapy to reduce the inflammatory component.

Medical management consists of high-dose corticosteroids, immunosuppressants, or both.[36,39] Among the immunosuppressants, cyclophosphamide, cyclosporin-A, and azothioprine are the current agents of choice.[35] Colchicine acts by inhibiting neutrophil chemotaxis and has beneficial effects on the mucocutaneous symptoms. It is widely used for patients with Behçet disease, but the effect, if any, it has for vascular involvement is unclear.[39] The frequency of vascular lesions appears to decrease after 5 years from the time of diagnosis. In Koc's[36] experience with 137 patients, only one developed vascular involvement 10 years after the diagnosis was made. Long-term medical therapy seems to be beneficial in reducing new symptoms.[35]

POLYARTERITIS NODOSA

Background

Polyarteritis nodosa (PAN) was described by Kussmaul and Maier in 1866. They noted arcades of nodular arterial aneurysms visible grossly at autopsy, and noted an inflammatory process in the adventitia.[52] PAN is a collagen vascular disease exclusively involving the small- and medium-sized arteries.[53] Inflammation and necrosis lead to vessel microaneurysms, stenosis, and thrombosis. PAN is part of a heterogeneous group of disorders thought to be autoimmune related. Pathologically, they share varying degrees of vascular inflammation and vascular necrosis.[54] Histologically, the disease is characterized by necrotizing fibrinoid panarteritis with a segmental distribution leading to microaneurysms and organ infarction.[10] Clinical expression depends on the location of the affected vessels and the degree of damage. PAN is relatively rare, with a prevalence of six per 100,000 people. PAN peaks in the fourth to fifth decades of life. The male-to-female ratio is 2 to 3:1.[54]

Clinical Manifestations

The most common presentation of PAN is that of fever, weight loss, mononeuritis, and visceral manifestations.[55] The kidney is involved in up to 75% of cases with patients presenting with hematuria, hypertension, and rising serum creatinine values. Rupture of arterial aneurysms can lead to subcapsular or perinephric hematoma. Other organ systems involved include the heart, which leads to congestive failure; the gastrointestinal tract, which results in intestinal angina or bowel infarction; and the central nervous system (CNS),

which presents as seizures, strokes, and sensory changes in a stocking-glove distribution. Involvement of the peripheral vessels is seen in up to 20% of patients,[56] but symptoms from peripheral vessels are rare.

Occasionally, limited forms of the disease are reported and can involve the calf muscles or the tibial vessels, which may mimic more classic vascular diseases. Nakamura et al.[57] described one patient with acute onset of severe calf pain. Their patient developed pain and swelling over 3 days that progressed to the point of prohibiting walking. Peripheral pulses were normal. An ultrasound with subsequent magnetic resonance imaging (MRI) revealed increased signal density in the outer muscle groups, suggesting a muscular inflammatory process. The diagnosis was established with biopsy of the gastrocnemius muscle and its fascia, which revealed acute necrotising arteritis. They found an additional 11 cases in the literature with similar presentations.[57]

Case reports also exist for involvement of the tibial vessels, directly presenting as ischemia or rupture with compartment syndrome.[55,56] Digital gangrene has also been described.[58] Diagnosis in these cases was suggested by arteriography showing multiple aneurysms at the tibial vessels and remote locations.

Diagnosis and Treatment

Diagnosis of PAN is based on several factors. Arteriography can suggest the diagnosis by showing multiple aneurysms in medium and small arteries coupled with areas of stenosis and occlusion. The aneurysms have a predilection for branch points. The number of aneurysms in PAN is characteristically greater than that seen with other forms of arteritis.[52] The presence of numerous aneurysms (>30) is almost diagnostic.[59] The nature and location of symptoms should prompt appropriate biopsies. Albert et al.[60] found that a conservative approach, with one biopsy followed by angiography if the biopsy is negative, yielded a sensitivity of 90% and specificity of 96%. Hepatitis B surface antigenemia is also frequently found in classic PAN and can suggest the diagnosis in the proper clinical scenario.[58]

Untreated PAN can lead to 5-year survival rates no higher than 13%. Fortunately, with the use of immunosuppressive agents the prognosis is much improved, with up to 80% rate of 5-year survival, with the number of organs involved being one of the primary predictors of excess mortality. Steroids without other immunosuppressant agents are recommended for those patients with only one organ system involved. For those with more than one organ system, cyclophosphamide is added to the regimen. First-line treatment for PAN is medical for either visceral involvement or involvement of peripheral vessels. If surgery is necessary, for instance, for acute ischemia, the planned medical therapy should be initiated at the time of or immediately following surgery to control the disease.[61]

EHLERS-DANLOS TYPE IV

Background

In 1901, Ehlers, a Danish dermatologist, described a patient who bruised easily and had hypermobile joints and hyperextensible skin. That same year, Danlos, a French physician, described a patient with extensive scarring and hypermobile joints and skin but without bruising.[62] It took until the 1960s to recognize that some patients with the syndrome have severe vascular problems that can lead to spontaneous rupture of even nonaneurysmal arteries. There are now at least 10 subtypes of Ehlers-Danlos syndrome (EDS) described.[63] The overall incidence of EDS is one per 150,000.[62] Type IV, or vascular EDS, is the arterial or ecchymotic form and is estimated to make up only about 4% of all cases of EDS.[62,63]

Pathology

In 1975, Pope et al.[64] described the collagen defect that defines vascular EDS. Type III collagen, largely responsible for tensile strength in arteries, is reduced. The bruising seen in these patients is related not to a platelet dysfunction or clotting disorder, but rather to an inherent weakness in the capillary wall. Vascular EDS is the result of heterogeneous mutations and is transmitted as an autosomal dominant condition. Type III collagen is encoded by a single gene, COL3A1, and has been mapped to the long arm of chromosome 2 at 2q24.3-q31.[65] Pathologic examination of the arteries with simple light microscopy is often nondiagnostic, though it may show a disorganized media with fragmented elastic fibers and an irregular medial hyperplasia.[63]

Clinical Manifestations

Clinical features of vascular EDS include four primary features—distinctive facial features; thin, translucent skin; excessive bruising; and rupture of vessels or viscera. Any one of these features may be manifest to greater or lesser degrees. The facial changes include slenderness, prominent bones and sunken cheeks, bulging eyes with periorbital pigmentation, and thin lips. Unlike classic EDS, there is little skin laxity, but the skin is thin, smooth, and translucent. Minor trauma can lead to gaping wounds. Bruising can be seen with trauma

as minimal as blood pressure cuff inflation.[65] False aneurysms can be seen after only minor trauma and true aneurysms can arise spontaneously.

Because of the heterogeneity of the disease, patients may present in a variety of different ways. The development of arterial rupture or intestinal perforation may be the first sign of the disease. Arteries in the thorax and abdomen account for 50% of vascular complications. Arteries located in the extremities are the site of 25% of the complications in patients with vascular EDS. Ruptures within the anatomically closed space of the extremities can result in large hematomas.

Treatment

Because of the extreme fragility of the vessels, any invasive procedure is perilous. Angiography alone has been associated with a mortality of 17% and major morbidity of 63%.[66] Noninvasive studies such as MRI/magnetic resonance angiography (MRA), duplex examinations, or intravenous digital subtraction angiography should therefore be used preferentially. If angiography must be performed, the smallest possible catheter should be used and care should be taken to avoid intimal injury from the jet effect of injection.

Arterial reconstruction is difficult and carries a measurable mortality risk. Cikrit et al.[67] reported 19% mortality in the operating room or immediate postoperative period. Ligation is preferential to bypass whenever feasible. Ligation should be done with umbilical tape or using a Dacron or PTFE patch between the ligature and the vessel, to distribute the force and prevent the ligature from cutting through. Vascular clamps should be avoided because of their tendency to tear vessels.[68] If arterial reconstruction is felt to be absolutely necessary, prosthetic materials should be used because of the tendency of autogenous conduits to subsequently degenerate. Skin sutures should be left in for prolonged periods because of the propensity of the wounds to dehisce.

No treatment currently exists for vascular EDS. Patients should be counseled to avoid any trauma and avoid any sports that might involve contact or a risk of fall. Genetic counseling is advisable for couples. The involved vascular specialist is advised to exercise extreme caution in caring for these patients.

REFERENCES

1. Talwar S, Jain S, Porwal R, et al. Pedicled omental transfer for limb salvage in Buerger's disease. *Int J Cardiol.* 2000;72:127–132.
2. von Winiwarter F. Ueber eine eigenthumliche Form von endarteriitis und Endophlebitis mit Gangan des Fusses. *Arch Klin Chir.* 1879;23:202–226.
3. Ohta T, Shionoya S. Fate of the ischaemic limb in Buerger's disease. *Br J Surg.* 1988;75:259–262.

4. Shigematsu H, Shigematsu K. Factors affecting the long-term outcome of Buerger's disease (thromboangiitis obliterans). *Int Angiol.* 1999;18:58–64.

5. Olin JW. Thromboangiitis obliterans (Buerger's Disease). *N Engl J Med.* 2000;343:864–869.

6. Halacheva K, Gulubova MV, Manolova I, et al. Expression of ICAM-1, VCAM-1, E-selectin and TNF alpha on the endothelium of femoral and iliac arteries in thromboangiitis obliterans. *Acta Histochem.* 2002;104:177–184.

7. Tanaka K. Pathology and pathogenesis of Buerger's disease. *Int J Cardiol.* 1998;66(suppl 1):S237–S242.

8. Sasaki S, Sakuma M, Kunihara T, et al. Current trends in thromboangiitis obliterans (Buerger's Disease) in women. *Am J Surg.* 1999;177:316–320.

9. Mishima Y. Thromboangiitis obliterans (Buerger's disease). *Int J Cardiol.* 1996;54(suppl):S185–S187.

10. Mills JL, Porter JM. Buerger's disease (thromboangiitis obliterans). *Ann Vasc Surg.* 1991;5:570–572.

11. Papa M, Bass A, Adar R, et al. Autoimmune mechanism for thromboangiitis obliterans (Buerger's disease): the role of tobacco associated antigen and the major histocompatibility complex. *Surgery.* 1991;111:527–531.

12. Avcu F, Akar E, Demirkilic U, et al. The role of prothrombotic mutations in patients with Buerger's disease. *Thromb Res.* 2000; 100:143–147.

13. Maslowski L, McBane R, Alexewicz P, et al. Antiphospholipid antibodies in thromboangiitis obliterans. *Vasc Med.* 2002;7:259–264.

14. Makita S, Nakamura M, Murakami H, et al. Impaired endothelium-dependent vasorelaxation in peripheral vasculature of patients with thromboangiitis obliterans (Buerger's Disease). *Circulation.* 1996; 94:II211–II215.

15. Gore I, Burrows S. A reconsideration of pathogenesis of Buerger's disease. *Am J Clin Pathol.* 1958;29:319.

16. Rutherford RB, Shionoya S , eds. *Vascular surgery. Buerger's disease.* 3rd ed. Philadelphia, Pa: W.B. Saunders; 1989:207–217.

17. Chierichetti F, Mambrini S, Bagliani A, et al. Treatment of Buerger's disease with electrical spinal cord stimulation. *Angiology.* 2002;53:341–347.

18. Olin JW, Young JR, Graor RA, et al. The changing clinical spectrum of thromboangiitis obliterans (Buerger's disease). *Circulation.* 1990;82(suppl IV):IV3–IV8.

19. Lie JT. The rise and fall and resurgence of thromboangiitis obliterans (Buerger's disease). *Acta Pathol Jpn.* 1989;39:153–157.

20. Lie JT. Thromboangiitis obliterans (Buerger's disease) and smokeless tobacco. *Arthritis Rheum.* 1988;31:812–813.

21. Joyce JW. Buerger's disease (thromboangiitis obliterans). *Rheum Dis Clin North Am.* 1990;16:463–470.

22. Shindo S, Matsumoto H, Ogata K, et al. Arterial reconstruction in Buerger's disease: bypass to disease-free collaterals. *Int Angiol.* 2002;21:228–242.

23. Sasajima T, Kubo Y, Inaba M, et al. Role of infrainguinal bypass in Buerger's disease: an eighteen year experience. *Eur J Vasc Endovasc Surg.* 1997;13:186–192.

24. Komori K, Kawasaki K, Okazaki J, et al. Thoracoscopic sympathectomy for Buerger's disease of the upper extremities. *J Vasc Surg.* 1995;22:344–346.

25. Nakajima N. The change in concept and surgical treatment on Buerger's disease—personal experience and review. *Int J Cardiol.* 1998;66(suppl 1):S273–S280.

26. Gordon A, Zechmeister K, Collin J. The role of sympathectomy in current surgical patients. *Eur J Vasc Surg.* 1994;8:129–137.

27. Roncon-Albuquerque R, Serrao P, Vale-Pereira R, et al. Plasma catacholamines in Buerger's disease: effects of cigarette smoking and surgical sympathectomy. *Eur J Vasc Endovasc Surg.* 2002;24: 338–343.

28. Saha K, Chabra N , Gulati SM. Treatment of patients with thromboangiitis obliterans with cyclophosphamide. *Angiology.* 2001; 52:399–407.

29. The European TAO Study Group. Oral Iloprost in the treatment of thromboangiitis obliterans (Buerger's disease): a double-blind, randomised, placebo-controlled trial. *Eur J Vasc Endovasc Surg.* 1998;15:300–307.

30. Rutherford RB, Olin J, DO W, eds. Vascular surgery. In: *Thromboangiitis obliterans (Buerger's disease).* 5th ed., Philadelphia, Pa: W.B. Saunders; 2000:350–364.

31. Swigris JJ, Olin JW, Mekhail NA. Implantable spinal cord stimulator to treat the ischemic manifestations of thromboangiitis obliterans (Buerger's disease). *J Vasc Surg.* 1999;29:928–935.

32. Bradbury AW, Milne AA, Murie JA. Surgical aspects of Behcet's disease. *Br J Surg.* 1994;81:1712–1721.

33. Dhobb M, Ammar F, Bensaid Y, et al. Arterial manifestations in Behcet's disease: four new cases. *Ann Vasc Surg.* 1986;1:249–252.

34. Kiraz S, Ertenli I, Ozturk MA, et al. Pathological haemostasis and 'prothrombotic state' in Behcet's disease. *Thromb Res.* 2002;105: 125–133.

35. Barlas S. Behcet's disease an insight from a vascular surgeons point of view. *Acta Chir Belg.* 1999;99:274–281.

36. Koc Y, Gullu I, Akpek G, et al. Vascular involvement in Behcet's disease. *J Rheumatol.* 1992;19:402–410.

37. Iscan ZH, Vural KM, Bayazit M. Compelling nature of arterial manifestations in Behcet disease. *J Vasc Surg.* 2005;41:53–58.

38. Kontogiannis V, Powell RJ. Behcet's disease. *Postgrad Med J.* 2000; 76:629–637.

39. Sakane T, Takeno M, Suzuki N, et al. Behcet's disease. *N Engl J Med.* 1999;341:1284–1291.

40. Koopman WJ, Kastner DL, eds. Intermittent and periodic arthritic syndromes. In: *Arthritis and allied conditions: a textbook of rheumatology.* 13th ed. Baltimore, Md: William and Wilkins; 1997:1279–1306.

41. Sherif A, Stewart P, Mendes DM. The repetitive vascular catastrophes of Behcet's disease: a case report with review of the literature. *Ann Vasc Surg.* 1992;6:85–89.

42. Niwa Y, Miyake S, Sakane T, et al. Autooxidative damage in Behcet's disease-endothelial cell damage following the elevated oxygen radicals generated by stimulated neutrophils. *Clin Exp Immunol.* 1982;49:247–255.

43. Kaklamani V, Vaiopoulos G, Kaklamanis P. Behcet's disease. *Semin Arthritis Rheum.* 1998;27:197–217.

44. Chaillou P, Patra P, Noel SF, et al. Behcet's disease revealed by double peripheral arterial involvement. *Ann Vasc Surg.* 1992;6: 160–163.

45. Jenkins A, Macpherson AI, Nolan B, et al. Peripheral aneurysms in Behcet's disease. *Br J Surg.* 1979;63:199–202.

46. Kingston M, Ratcliffe JR, Alltree M, et al. Aneurysm after arterial puncture in Behcet's disease. *Br Med J.* 1979;1:1766–1767.

47. Freyrie A, Paragona O, Cenacchi G, et al. True and false aneurysms in Behcet's disease: case report with ultrastructural observations. *J Vasc Surg.* 1993;17:762–767.

48. Kasirajan K, Marek JM, Langsfeld M. Behcet's disease: endovascular management of a ruptured peripheral arterial aneurysm. *J Vasc Surg.* 2001;34:1127–1129.

49. Enoch BA, Castillo-Olivares JL, Khoo TC, et al. Major vascular complications in Behcet's syndrome. *Postgrad Med J.* 1968;44: 453–459.

50. Little AG, Zarins CK. Abdominal aortic aneurysm and Behcet's disease. *Am Heart J.* 1982;91:359–362.

51. Ouvry PA, Durable M. Ulceration of the toes in a young adult presenting with distal arteriopathy and recurring superficial phlebitis. Treatment using hemodilution. Apropos of a case. *Phlebologie.* 1991;44:830–832.

52. Bonsib S. Polyarteritis nodosa. *Semin Diagn Pathol.* 2001;18:14–23.

53. Jennette C, Falk RJ, Andrassy K, et al. Nomenclature of systemic vasculidities. Proposal of an international consensus conference. *Arthritis Rheum.* 1994;37:187–192.

54. LiPuma J, Sachs P, Sands M, et al. Case 4: polyarteritis nodosa (PAN). *AJR Am J Radiol.* 1997;169:264–265.

55. Heron E, Fiessinger J-N, Guillevin L. Polyarteritis nodosa presenting as acute leg ischemia. *J Rheumatol.* 2003;30:1344–1346.

56. Hasaniya N, Katzen T. Acute compartment syndrome of both lower legs caused by rupture of tibial artery aneurysm in a patient with polyarteritis nodosa: a case report and review of literature. *J Vasc Surg.* 1993;18:295–298.

57. Nakamura T, Tomoda K, Yamamura Y, et al. Polyarteritis nodosa limited to calf muscles: a case report and review of the literature. *Clin Rheumatol.* 2003;22:149–153.

58. Broussard RK, Baethge, BA. Peripheral gangrene in polyarteritis nodosa. *Cutis.* 1990;46:53–55.

59. Ha HK, Yu E. Reply and discussion—angiography in polyarteritis nodosa. *AJR Am J Radiol.* 2000;175:1747–1748.

60. Albert DA, Rimon D, Silverstein MD. The diagnosis of polyarteritis nodosa. *Arthritis Rheum.* 1988;31:1117–1127.

61. Guillevin L. Treatment of classic polyarteritis nodosa in 1999. *Nephrol Dail Transplant.* 1999;14:2077–2079.

62. Bergqvist D. Ehlers-Danlos type IV syndrome. A review from a vascular surgical point of view. *Eur J Surg.* 1996;162:163–170.

63. Lauwers G, Nevelsteen A, Daenen G, et al. Ehlers-Danlos syndrome type IV: a heterogenous disease. *Ann Vasc Surg.* 1997;11:178–182.

64. Pope FM, Martin GR, Lichtenstein JR, et al. Patients with Ehlers-Danlos type IV lack type III collagen. *Proc Natl Acad Sci USA.* 1975;72:1314–1316.

65. Germain D. Clinical and genetic features of vascular Ehlers-Danlos syndrome. *Ann Vasc Surg.* 2002;16:391–397.

66. Fann JI, Dalman RL, Harris JE, Jr. Genetic and metabolic causes of arterial disease. *Ann Vasc Surg.* 1993;7:594–604.

67. Cikrit DF, Miles JH, Silver D. Spontaneous arterial perforation: the Ehlers-Danlos specter. *J Vasc Surg.* 1987;5:248–255.

68. Wesley JR, Mahour GH, Wooley MM. Multiple surgical problems in two patients with Ehlers-Danlos syndrome. *Surgery.* 1980; 86:319–324.

Abnormalities of Microcirculation in Diabetes

Christopher J. Abularrage   **Anton N. Sidawy**   **Paul W. White**
Jonathan M. Weiswasser   **Subodh Arora**

Diabetes mellitus is caused by a metabolic derangement in glucose metabolism set off by either a lack of insulin production (type 1), or a peripheral resistance to insulin (type 2). It is characterized by a number of long-term complications, including nephropathy, retinopathy, neuropathy, peripheral and coronary vascular occlusive disease, and impaired immune response and wound healing. While these complications have multifactorial and intertwined causes, a lack of blood flow or oxygenation to the specific tissue beds caused by an impairment of the microcirculation plays a central role.

Early structural descriptions of the diabetic microcirculation were made after studying amputation specimens. In 1959, Goldenberg et al.[1] retrospectively reviewed amputation specimens from diabetic and nondiabetic patients with light microscopy. They found material within the arterioles of the diabetic specimens that stained positive with periodic acid-Schiff (PAS). This led to the misconception that diabetic ischemic lesions in the presence of palpable pedal pulses were due to arteriolar occlusive, or "small-vessel," disease in people with diabetes. With no means to improve the small-vessel disease, physicians developed a hopeless attitude regarding the treatment of these patients.[2] The theory of diabetic occlusive small-vessel disease has since been refuted. Prospective studies with blinded histologic interpretation found a similar amount of material in both diabetic and nondiabetic specimens.[3,4] Furthermore, other prospective studies have shown that there is no propensity for diabetic patients to have an increased endothelial cell proliferation in the arterioles or capillaries compared to nondiabetic patients.[5]

Some microcirculatory structural changes are unique to patients with diabetes. Reduction in capillary size and thickening of the basement membrane are some of the earliest changes found.[6,7] Quadricep muscle needle biopsies evaluated with electron microscopy have confirmed increased basement membrane thickness compared to controls.[8] Theoretically, it may impair migration of leukocytes and other inflammatory cells, making people with diabetes more susceptible to infection.[9] This basement membrane thickening is not found uniformly throughout various tissues, as skin biopsies have demonstrated similar thickness of the basement membrane between diabetics and controls.[10] Interestingly, the increase in basement membrane thickness is not accompanied by a proliferation of the microvasculature. Malik et al.[11] compared dorsal foot epidermal skin thickness and capillary density in biopsies from people with type 1 diabetes, and found no difference between diabetic and nondiabetic patients. Others have confirmed this result comparing the cutaneous capillary density in foot and forearm skin biopsies in diabetic and nondiabetic patients.[12]

Further investigation demonstrated that despite a lack of structural arteriolar occlusive disease, the diabetic microcirculation, specifically the nutritional capillaries and the subpapillary vascular plexus, is functionally impaired compared to patients without diabetes. The diabetic microcirculation is characterized by an increase in vascular permeability, impaired autoregulation, and increased arteriolar shunting compared to healthy controls.[13] It is also impaired in its ability to vasodilate in response to stress. This defect has been shown to be a key element in the characteristic complications of the disease.[14]

Symptoms associated with peripheral arterial insufficiency, specifically claudication, rest pain, and tissue loss, are caused by a lack of blood flow in the nutritional capillaries of the microcirculation that does not meet the metabolic demand of the surrounding tissues. While macrovascular occlusive disease is easily identifiable and treatable, its ultimate purpose is to restore blood flow to the microcirculation. It is because of this microcirculatory dysfunction in diabetes, mainly through its resultant neuropathy, that in some patients, even after correcting macrocirculatory occlusive disease, lower extremity ulcers may be slow to heal or recur very easily (Fig. 13-1). The findings of the central role of diabetic microcirculatory dysfunction in impaired wound healing have spawned further investigations attempting to identify methods to assess and define the microcirculation, and to devise therapies to improve it.

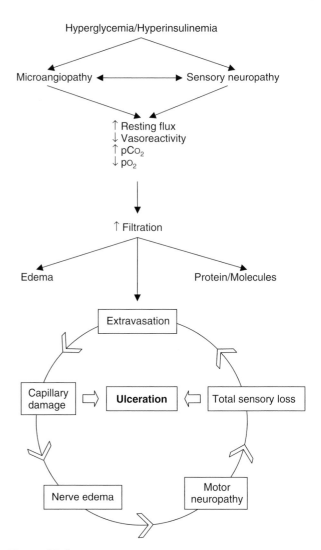

Figure 13-1   Angiopathy mechanism. Hyperglycemia and hyperinsulinemia lead to microcirculatory dysfunction, which slows healing of ulcers and allows ulceration to recur.

TECHNIQUES USED TO ASSESS THE MICROCIRCULATION

Transcutaneous Oxygen Tension

Transcutaneous oxygen tension ($TCpo_2$) is a method that has been used to assess the microcirculation of the skin since the 1970s. $TCpo_2$ quantifies oxygen molecules transferred to the skin microcirculation after heating it with a transducer above 40°C. Matsen et al.[15] showed a decrease in the foot $TCpo_2$ of patients with peripheral vascular disease compared to healthy subjects. Cina et al.[16] examined the $TCpo_2$ in patients with peripheral vascular disease and found a greater decrease in the calves of those patients with rest pain or tissue loss compared to claudicants. $TCpo_2$ measurements are decreased in diabetic patients with peripheral vascular disease, but occasionally increased in diabetic patients without macrocirculatory dysfunction. This is caused by an increase in arteriolar shunting in the microcirculation. $TCpo_2$ is limited in the fact that it is time consuming, and does not assess all

ischemic regions of the skin unless the probe is specifically placed on the tissue in question.

Iontophoresis

The recent development of noninvasive techniques that can reliably quantify endothelial function has made it possible to study factors that may lead to dysfunction or enhancement of the endothelium by measuring the vasodilatory response, or vasoreactivity. One such experimental technique is iontophoresis, which is a method that delivers medications, usually acetylcholine and sodium nitroprusside, subdermally through a chamber using a current of 200 mA. Acetylcholine causes an endothelium-dependent vasodilation through release of nitric oxide (NO) from endothelial cells (Fig. 13-2). NO then diffuses to the vascular smooth muscle cells of the media causing relaxation and vasodilation. Sodium nitroprusside acts as an NO donor

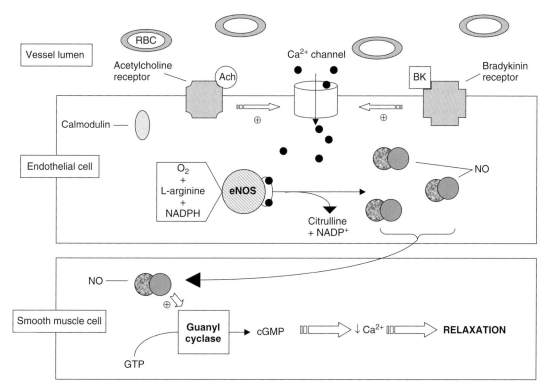

Figure 13-2   Mechanism of endothelium-dependent vasoreactivity. Acetylcholine binds its receptor, leading to an influx of calcium ions and an increase in endothelial NO synthase (eNOS) function. Nitric oxide then diffuses to the smooth muscle cell activating guanyl cyclase and causing vasodilatation. BK, bradykinin; cGMP, cyclic guanosine monophosphate; GTP, guanosine triphosphate; NADP, nicotinamide adenine dinucleotide phosphate; NO, nitric oxide; RBC, red blood cell.

causing vasodilation independent of the endothelium. After the 30 seconds, forearm microcirculatory flow can be measured using either laser Doppler fluxmetry or single-point laser probes.

Laser Doppler fluxmetry measures the flux of red blood cells through both the subpapillary vascular bed and the nutritional capillaries. It is simple to use and can be performed over a 2-cm^2 section of skin in a minimal amount of time. The flux of red blood cells causes two distinct waveforms.[17] Large waves are present in both healthy individuals and patients with peripheral vascular disease. Small waves have a frequency of 20 cycles per minute and are present in most patients with peripheral vascular disease, but in only 8% of healthy subjects. The small waves are most likely caused by respirations, present in all individuals but probably eclipsed by vasomotor activity in the microcirculation of healthy subjects. It is the appearance of small waves in ischemic tissue that identifies a dysfunctional microcirculation.

Laser Doppler fluxmetry is restricted by its inability to determine the percentage contribution of the nonnutritional subpapillary plexus and the nutritional capillaries to the total red blood cell flux. Fluxmetry results are also variable depending on skin color, temperature, and ambient light.

Single-point laser probe measurement can be used to assess endothelium-dependent microcirculatory

vasodilation in response to acetylcholine. The two single-point probes are placed within the iontophoresis delivery vehicle directly over the skin. One probe is placed within the chamber containing acetylcholine, measuring the direct response to acetylcholine iontophoresis. The second probe is placed outside but in close proximity to (5 mm) the acetylcholine-containing chamber, measuring the indirect response to acetylcholine. This indirect vasodilatory response measures the nerve axon reflex-mediated vasodilation.

Single-point laser probes have high coefficients of variation, which are much larger than those for laser scanner imagers, but are able to measure the nerve axon reflex portion of the response to acetylcholine.

Dynamic Capillaroscopy

Dynamic capillaroscopy with fluorescent dyes has been used to assess the microcirculation.[18] It can visualize both the microvascular and interstitial compartments, and assess transcapillary diffusion of fluorescein. Certain studies have shown that fluorescein diffusion is non-homogeneous in ischemic tissue beds, which improves after surgical revascularization.[19] Last, the combination of capillaroscopy with fluxmetry can be used to measure the specific contributions of the subpapillary plexus and the nutritional capillaries to the total microcirculation.

These techniques can also be performed without dyes, but require more sophisticated, computerized capillaroscopy, and are not widely available.

Hyperspectral Imaging

New innovations are being used to assess the microcirculation of the foot in patients with peripheral vascular disease. Hyperspectral imaging obtains a high-resolution image using a specialized camera, and determines the total hemoglobin, oxy- and deoxyhemoglobin, and oxygen saturation of an area of tissue based on its chemical composition and spectral profile. Obtaining the picture takes seconds, and the camera can be operated by almost any personnel. Also any portion of the picture can be analyzed, allowing assessment of a greater area of tissue without an increase in time spent.

In a pilot study of 29 patients, we showed a statistically significant decrease in all four parameters between claudicants and nonclaudicants (author's unpublished data). There were no differences found between diabetic and nondiabetic patients, but the study was not powered to answer this question. Further studies with this investigational tool, including a larger number of patients, will determine its ability to assess the diabetic microcirculation.

COMPLICATIONS CAUSED BY MICROCIRCULATORY DYSFUNCTION

Characteristic complications of diabetic microcirculatory dysfunction include nephropathy, retinopathy, and neuropathy with or without macrovascular disease. Each one of these is preceded by a loss of endothelial function, which is an early step in the development of atherosclerosis. Even if the total microcirculation appears intact, the nutritional capillaries of insulin-dependent diabetic feet are severely impaired prior to the development of macrocirculatory disease.[20]

Nephropathy is the complication associated with the greatest mortality in diabetics.[21] It develops in 20% to 45% of patients, and the incidence remains the same even as the duration of disease increases. It begins with renal hypertrophy and expansion of the glomerular basement membrane leading to proteinuria and glomerulosclerosis. Ultimately, patients develop hypertension, nephrotic syndrome, and end-stage renal disease requiring hemodialysis.

Retinopathy is a hallmark of diabetes, and is caused by microaneurysms in the terminal capillaries of the retinal microcirculation. The microaneurysms are abnormally permeable, and leak serous fluid causing hard exudates in the retina. Also, occlusion of the retinal vessels can cause ischemia of the optic nerve endings. Retinopathy ensues when new vessels proliferate in response to this ischemia. Each of these mechanisms contributes to a loss of visual acuity that worsens with duration of the disease.[22]

Peripheral neuropathy is a major contributor to the morbidity of diabetes, especially diabetic foot ulceration. In 1995, diabetic foot ulcer management cost approximately $1.5 billion in Medicare reimbursement.[23] Foot ulcers are also associated with a higher likelihood of lower extremity amputation and death.[24] Frequently, diabetic patients lack peripheral sensation and are unaware of repeated trauma to their feet. Callus formation acts like a foreign body in the patient's shoe causing further skin damage and irritation of the tissues. Hemorrhage into the callus can lead to infection and ulceration.[2] Failed wound healing of a diabetic foot ulcer is not completely due to insufficient oxygen delivery. In fact, diabetic patients are more likely to have foot ulcers in the presence of elevated TCpo$_2$ measurements compared to nondiabetic controls.[13] The pathophysiology of diabetic neuropathy and its effect on the formation of diabetic ulceration are discussed in detail in Chapter 2.

MEDIATORS OF DIABETIC MICROCIRCULATORY DYSFUNCTION

Hyperglycemia and insulin resistance in obese patients have been associated with endothelial dysfunction.[25] This dysfunction is independent of circulating insulin, as hyperinsulinemia in the presence of euglycemia potentiates endothelium-dependent vasodilation.[26] Insulin has a vasodilating effect through endothelium-dependent mechanisms caused by the muscarinic agonist methacholine chloride, while it has little effect on endothelium-independent vasoreactivity. This suggests that the endothelium is a target for insulin, and not just a passive site for transport.[27] Endothelial insulin receptors may also be a site for insulin resistance, as non–insulin-dependent type 2 diabetics have impaired endothelium-dependent vasoreactivity.[28]

Diabetes is associated with increased platelet aggregation, enhanced monocyte adhesion, increased oxidative stress, and diminished NO production.[29,30] Oxidative stress is caused by an increased production of free radicals in diabetic microangiopathy.[31] Although the exact mechanism is unclear, superoxide anions and other free radicals inactivate NO. This increase in free radicals also leads to capillary damage and microvascular complications, and may be amenable to treatment with free radical scavengers such as vitamins C and E.[32,33] Low density lipoproteins (LDL) are elevated in diabetes and are known to be another source of free radicals. LDL cholesterol impairs endothelium-dependent vasodilation in insulin-dependent diabetes, advocating tight control of hyperlipidemia with statins or other cholesterol-lowering medications.[34]

Significantly higher erythrocyte aggregation, plasma viscosity, and plasma fibrinogen levels have been found in neuropathic diabetic patients compared to non-neuropathic diabetic patients.[35] These rheologic alterations may contribute to increased capillary pressures in diabetic patients, and subsequent microvascular complications caused by endothelial damage and increased capillary transudation.

Acetylcholine causes microcirculatory vasodilation through two mechanisms, both of which are dependent on an intact endothelium. Furchgott and Zawadzki[36] described the first mechanism in 1980 when they elucidated the fact that acetylcholine directly binds muscarinic receptors on the endothelium causing release of NO (Fig. 13-2). The NO then diffuses to the media causing relaxation of the vascular smooth muscle cells and consequent vasodilation. The second mechanism is called the Lewis triple-flare response, or nerve axon reflex-mediated vasodilation, and is caused by the action of acetylcholine on C-nociceptive fibers (Fig. 13-3). Acetylcholine sensitizes the C-nociceptive fibers, augmenting the release of substance P and calcitonin gene-related peptide. Calcitonin gene-related peptide directly causes vasodilation,[37] while substance P causes a release of mast cell histamine,

indirectly leading to vasodilation and increased vascular permeability.[38]

Endothelial-derived relaxing factor was first identified as the substance that causes vasodilation in response to acetylcholine and other vasoactive compounds. This was later identified as NO.[39] Decreased NO production is a consequence of decreased endothelial NO synthase (eNOS),[40] as well as reduced availability of tetrahydrobiopterin,[41] folate,[42] and L-arginine.[43] Lack of NO impairs the ability of the microcirculation to vasodilate in response to stress, causing damage to the surrounding tissue beds. Skin biopsies from the dorsum of the foot in diabetic patients show a significant decrease in the expression of eNOS.[44,45] Decreased eNOS expression was more prevalent in diabetic patients with neuropathy than in healthy controls, suggesting that this is an early step in the dysfunction of the diabetic microcirculation and development of peripheral neuropathy. This reduction of eNOS expression in diabetic patients is associated with impaired wound healing.[44,46] Experiments with eNOS-deficient mice show impaired endothelial cell sprouting, and capillary ingrowth that directly delayed excisional wound closure and reduced tensile wound strength by 38%.[47]

Increase in NO or eNOS expression in experimental models shows improvements in wound healing. Arginine is a key element in the synthesis of NO through

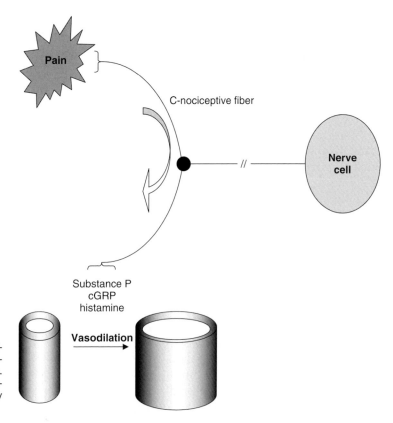

Figure 13-3 Nerve axon reflex. Acetylcholine sensitizes the C-nociceptive fibers, which then release substance P and calcitonin gene-related peptide (cGRP). Calcitonin gene-related peptide directly causes vasodilation, while substance P indirectly causes vasodilation by stimulating the release of mast cell histamine.

a deaminaselike enzymatic pathway. Arginine, when given to human subjects, increases NO, which in turn increases cyclic guanosine monophosphate, augmenting blastogenesis in lymphocytes and enhancing wound healing.[48] Inducible NOS (iNOS) is a second isoform, predominantly produced by macrophages, that leads to increased angiogenesis.[49] iNOS, and to a lesser extent eNOS, are elevated in diabetic patients with foot ulcers, but not in those without foot ulcers.[43] It is hypothesized that iNOS at the center of the ulcer increases the number of free radicals and debrides the wound, but may be detrimental to wound healing in the long run.

While it is difficult to directly measure the effect of nicotine and tobacco use on the microcirculation of people with diabetes, it has been shown that neuropathy is three times more prevalent in type 1 diabetic patients who smoke.[50] Type 2 diabetic smokers were not significantly different than controls in this study, but this group had a short duration of disease, and it was thought that they were evaluated prior to the development of worsening neuropathy. Another study found tobacco use to be an independent risk factor for progression of peripheral neuropathy in type 1 diabetic patients.[51]

ENDOTHELIAL DYSFUNCTION

Early Markers of Endothelial Dysfunction

Endothelial dysfunction is a hallmark of diabetic microvascular disease. Serum von Willebrand factor (VWF) has been used as a marker of endothelial dysfunction because of its specificity to the endothelium. Serum levels of VWF rise in type 2 diabetic patients who develop microalbuminuria, but remain normal in those who stayed normoalbuminuric. This led to the hypothesis that microalbuminuria represented a defect in vascular permeability and therefore endothelial function. Microalbuminuria also predicts cardiovascular morbidity and progression of nephropathy,[52,53] as well as insulin resistance in hypertensive diabetics.[54]

A study by Lim et al.[55] compared the microvascular reactivity, using iontophoresis, and plasma levels of various markers of endothelial activation in type 2 diabetic patients with and without microalbuminuria. They found that contrary to traditional teachings, there were other markers of endothelial dysfunction present before the appearance of microalbuminuria, specifically, elevations of soluble intercellular adhesion molecule (sICAM), soluble vascular cell adhesion molecule (sVCAM), and impaired endothelium-dependent vasodilation. Other studies have shown that sICAM was an independent predictor of myocardial infarction in healthy men,[56] and sVCAM was a marker of type 2 diabetic atherosclerotic lesions.[57]

These two molecules have also been associated with diabetic retinopathy,[58] nephropathy,[59] and neuropathy,[60] suggesting that type 2 diabetic patients are at risk for endothelial dysfunction prior to the development of microalbuminuria.

Certain studies have compared vasoreactivity between insulin-dependent and non–insulin-dependent diabetic patients. Both groups have an impaired endothelium-dependent response to acetylcholine iontophoresis,[61] while only non–insulin-dependent diabetic patients have an impaired endothelium-independent response to sodium nitroprusside.[62] Impaired vasoreactivity seen in insulin-dependent diabetes is therefore related to decreased NO synthesis and release, while impaired vascular smooth muscle cell relaxation in response to NO or increased NO inactivation is the cause in non–insulin-dependent diabetic patients.[63]

Endothelial function is impaired not only in type 2 diabetic patients, but also in healthy subjects with normal glucose metabolism who are at risk for developing the disease. Caballero et al.[64] compared the micro and macrocirculation between healthy controls, diabetic patients without peripheral vascular disease, patients with impaired glucose tolerance, and normoglycemic patients with a parental history of type 2 diabetes. Response to acetylcholine (endothelium-dependent response) and sodium nitroprusside (endothelium-independent response) iontophoresis, as well as the brachial artery vasoactivity (endothelium-dependent response in the macrocirculation), was reduced in all three groups compared to controls. The researchers concluded that abnormalities in vascular reactivity and biochemical markers of endothelial cell dysfunction were present in patients at risk for developing diabetes, and that factors other than insulin were operative in this pathology.

Poly Polymerase and Advanced Glycosylation End Products

Accumulation of advanced glycosylation end products (AGEs) has been associated with endothelial dysfunction. AGEs are increased in patients with diabetes, especially in those with peripheral neuropathy.[65] Garcia Soriano et al.[66] created a model of diabetic mice by destructing pancreatic islet cells using streptozotocin. This caused hyperglycemia, intravascular oxidant production, DNA strand breakage, poly (adenosine diphosphate [ADP]-ribose) polymerase (PARP) activation, and a selective loss of endothelium-dependent vasodilation.[66] They then treated the mice with a PARP inhibitor and found an improved vascular responsiveness despite the persistence of severe hyperglycemia. They suggested that activation of PARP, and increased AGEs, is an important factor in the pathogenesis of endothelial dysfunction in diabetes.

Szabó et al.[67] studied the expression of PARP in people with type 2 diabetes by examining forearm skin biopsies, and comparing them to microvascular vasoreactivity. They found that PARP was activated in dermal microvascular tissues in type 2 diabetic patients and in healthy patients with a parental history of type 2 diabetes. This activation was associated with a statistically significant impairment in microvascular vasoreactivity in these subjects. They concluded that the impairment in microvascular reactivity in type 2 diabetes and those at risk for developing type 2 diabetes might be caused by increased expression of PARP.

Effects of Hormone Replacement Therapy

It was originally thought that estrogen hormone replacement therapy (HRT) provided cardiovascular protection to postmenopausal women. The mechanisms through which this occurs are complex but are believed to involve improvements in lipoprotein profile, vasodilation, and inhibition of platelet aggregation and vascular smooth muscle proliferation.[68,69] In order to examine the effects of HRT on the microvascular reactivity, we used laser Doppler fluxmetry to measure forearm cutaneous vasodilation in response to iontophoresis of acetylcholine and sodium nitroprusside in healthy and type 2 diabetic women.[70] We found that both menopausal status and type 2 diabetes impaired endothelium-dependent and independent vasoreactivity compared to healthy controls. Further, HRT significantly improved microvascular vasoreactivity in healthy postmenopausal patients, but not in those with type 2 diabetes. These findings agree with other studies that have shown a positive effect of estrogens on endothelial function in postmenopausal women.[71]

NEUROPATHY AND LOSS OF NERVE AXON REFLEX-MEDIATED VASODILATION

Neuropathy is a major cause of morbidity in diabetes. While neuropathy is dealt with in Chapter 2, this section details the interrelationship of neuropathy and the microcirculation.

Hyperglycemia in diabetes causes conversion of glucose to sorbitol by aldose reductase in the nerve fibers. Intraneurial sorbitol accumulation leads to reciprocal depletion of myoinositol phosphate, altered phosphoinositide metabolism, and reduced (Na^+, K^+)-ATPase activity in nerves.[72] Nicotinamide adenine dinucleotide phosphate (NADPH) is a cofactor for both aldose reductase and NO synthase. Hyperglycemia depletes NADPH stores by preferentially shunting available NADPH down the aldose reductase pathway, causing a decrease in NO and an inability of the microvasculature to adequately vasodilate in response to stress, compounding the problem of nerve dysfunction.

Diabetic peripheral neuropathy occurs more at the level of the foot than the forearm. The exact cause of this difference is unknown, but it has been hypothesized that erect posture leads to high capillary pressures.[73] Diabetic microangiopathy is associated with a loss of the normal venoarteriolar reflex that restricts arterial inflow, increases precapillary resistance in the skin, and avoids an excessive elevation in capillary pressures upon standing.[74] We compared laser Doppler fluxmetry after iontophoresis of acetylcholine and sodium nitroprusside in the forearm and the foot.[75] We found that the endothelium-dependent and independent vasodilatory responses of the foot cutaneous microcirculation were lower than those of the forearm, and progressively worsened from healthy subjects to non-neuropathic diabetics to neuropathic diabetics. We concluded that this mechanism might also contribute to the early involvement of the foot with neuropathy compared to the forearm.

As discussed previously, acetylcholine causes microcirculatory vasodilation through two separate but synchronous mechanisms. In the Lewis triple-flare response, or nerve axon reflex, acetylcholine binds receptors on local C-nociceptive fibers that cause orthodromic conduction to the spinal cord and antidromic nerve reflex stimulation of adjacent C-nociceptive fibers. The adjacent C fibers then release vasodilatory substances such as substance P, calcitonin gene-related peptide, and bradykinin. The total response to acetylcholine is considered the sum of the two mechanisms, and is impaired in diabetic neuropathy.

Hamdy et al.[76] used single-point laser probes to measure the total vasodilation due to acetylcholine iontophoresis, and the relative contribution of the nerve axon reflex. The nerve axon reflex accounted for 36% of the total effect of acetylcholine in healthy patients and 29% in diabetic patients without neuropathy. The total acetylcholine induced neurovascular vasodilation and the portion due to the nerve axon reflex were both significantly reduced in diabetic patients with neuropathy. The percent contribution of the nerve axon response was 20% in diabetic patients with neuropathy and peripheral vascular disease, 8% in diabetic patients with neuropathy, and 5% in diabetic patients with Charcot arthropathy. They concluded that neuropathy renders the diabetic foot functionally ischemic because of its inability to increase blood flow in response to stress.

Impaired vasoreactivity in diabetes is a function of both impaired C-nociceptive fiber function and impaired reaction to the signals released by these fibers. Caselli et al.[77] delineated the role of C-nociceptive fibers in the nerve axon reflex-mediated vasodilation in diabetes.

They performed iontophoresis of acetylcholine and sodium nitroprusside on the forearms (a site not usually affected by neuropathy) and the feet of diabetics with neuropathy, diabetics without neuropathy, and healthy controls. In order to isolate the contribution of the C-nociceptive fibers they repeated these measurements after the application of a topical anesthetic, effectively causing nerve dysfunction while leaving the microcirculation intact. Blockade of the C-nociceptive fibers impaired the nerve axon reflex in healthy and non-neuropathic diabetic patients, but not in neuropathic diabetic patients. Also, the nerve axon reflex-mediated vasodilation at the foot of the two non-neuropathic groups was similar to that of the neuropathic group both before and after local anesthesia. They concluded that the C-nociceptive fibers were the main contributors to nerve axon reflex-mediated vasodilation, and impairment of these fibers is the primary cause for the decrease of nerve axon reflex-mediated vasodilation in the neuropathic diabetic foot. Furthermore, the reduction of the forearm nerve axon reflex-mediated vasodilation was similar in all three groups, suggesting that the C-nociceptive fibers contribute more to the reduced reflex than a decreased endothelial response to the vasodilators released by these fibers. Others have suggested that endothelial and vascular smooth muscle cell responses to vasodilators released by C fibers also contribute, but the percentage has not been delineated.[23,73]

Effect of Revascularization on the Neuropathic Diabetic Microcirculation

People with diabetes are prone to ischemic peripheral vascular disease by a 5:1 ratio compared to healthy subjects. This occlusive disease is typically found below the popliteal trifurcation with relative sparing of the pedal vessels.[78] Surgical revascularization plays a major role in the treatment of diabetic ischemic foot ulcers, although not all ulcers heal after surgery despite adequate restoration of blood flow.

We have examined cutaneous microvascular reactivity, using heat and iontophoresis, in neuropathic diabetic patients with peripheral ischemia before and after surgical revascularization.[14] We then compared this reactivity to that seen in neuropathic diabetic patients without peripheral vascular disease, non-neuropathic diabetic patients, and healthy controls. The maximal hyperemic response to heat and the endothelium-dependent vasodilation to acetylcholine improved after surgery but did not reach the levels of healthy controls. Endothelium-independent vasodilation to sodium nitroprusside improved to the level of non-neuropathic diabetic patients and healthy controls. Also, the nerve axon reflex-mediated vasodilation failed to improve after surgery. We concluded that successful revascularization was associated with an improvement but not a complete normalization of endothelial cell and vascular smooth muscle cell function.

While some studies have shown that peroneal nerve conduction velocity improved along with the TCp_{O_2} after surgical revascularization,[79] others have found that revascularization was associated with an arrest in the progression, but not reversal, of diabetic neuropathy if the patient had been diagnosed with diabetes for a longer period of time.[80,81] This suggests that nerve damage caused by an impaired microvasculature is cumulative and worsens over time.

SUMMARY

Diabetes is a complex disease with multiple etiologies of its characteristic complications. In the past, there was a misconception that diabetes was a small-vessel disease. Since the landmark paper by LoGerfo and Coffman, there has been a change of focus and a better understanding that diabetes is associated more with medium-vessel occlusive disease and microcirculatory dysfunction. With the use of sophisticated, noninvasive techniques, it has become apparent that the microcirculation is structurally normal, but physiologically impaired, particularly in patients with pronounced peripheral neuropathy. A better understanding of this dysfunction may allow us to target the microcirculation from a therapeutic standpoint with great implications for the treatment of diabetic foot ulcers, especially in those patients who fail to heal despite repair of the macrocirculation.

REFERENCES

1. Goldenberg SG, Alex M, Joshi RA, et al. Nonatheromatous peripheral vascular disease of the lower extremity in diabetes mellitus. *Diabetes.* 1959;8:261–273.
2. LoGerfo FW, Coffman JD. Vascular and microvascular disease of the foot in diabetes: implications for foot care. *N Engl J Med.* 1984;311:1615–1619.
3. Strandness DE, Priest RE, Gibbons GE. Combined clinical and pathologic study of diabetic and nondiabetic peripheral arterial disease. *Diabetes.* 1964;13:366–372.
4. Conrad MC. Large and small artery occlusion in diabetics and nondiabetics with severe vascular disease. *Circulation.* 1967;36:83–91.
5. Banson BB, Lacy PE. Diabetic microangiopathy in human toes: with emphasis on ultrastructural change in dermal capillaries. *Am J Pathol.* 1964;45:41–58.
6. Jaap AJ, Shore AC, Stockman AJ, et al. Skin capillary density in subjects with impaired glucose tolerance and patients with type 2 diabetes. *Diabet Med.* 1996;13:160–164.
7. Rayman G, Malik RA, Sharma AK, et al. Microvascular response to tissue injury and capillary ultrastructure in the foot skin of type I diabetic patients. *Clin Sci.* 1995;89:467–474.
8. Siperstein MD, Unger RH, Madison LL. Studies of muscle capillary basement membranes in normal subjects, diabetic, and prediabetic patients. *J Clin Invest.* 1968;47:1973–1999.

9. Flynn MD, Tooke JE. Aetiology of diabetic foot ulceration: a role for the microcirculation? *Diabet Med.* 1992;8:320–329.

10. Friederici HHR, Tucker WR, Schwartz TB. Observations on small blood vessels of skin in normal and in diabetic patients. *Diabetes.* 1960;15:233–250.

11. Malik RA, Metcalf I, Sharma AK, et al. Skin epidermal thickness and vascular density in type 1 diabetes. *Diabet Med.* 1992;9:263–267.

12. Walker D, Malik RA, Boulton AJM, et al. Structural differences in skin biopsies between the arm and foot in normal subjects and diabetic patients (Abstract). *Diabetologia.* 1996;39(S1):A266.

13. Wyss CR, Matsen FA, Simmons CW, et al. Transcutaneous oxygen tension measurements on limbs of diabetic and nondiabetic patients with peripheral vascular disease. *Surgery.* 1984;95: 339–346.

14. Arora S, Pomposelli F, LoGerfo FW, et al. Cutaneous microcirculation in the neuropathic diabetic foot improves significantly but not completely after successful lower extremity revascularization. *J Vasc Surg.* 2002;35:501–505.

15. Matsen FA, Wyss CR, Pedegana LR, et al. Transcutaneous oxygen tension measurement in peripheral vascular disease. *Surg Gynecol Obstet.* 1980;150:525–528.

16. Cina C, Katsamouris A, Megerman J, et al. Utility of transcutaneous oxygen tension measurements in peripheral arterial occlusive disease. *J Vasc Surg.* 1984;1:362–371.

17. Bongard O, Fagrell B. Discrepancies between total and nutritional skin microcirculation in patients with peripheral areterial occlusive disease (PAOD). *VASA.* 1990;19:105–111.

18. Fagrell B. Advances in microcirculation network evaluation: an update. *Int J Microcirc.* 1995;15(S1):34–40.

19. Bollinger A. Transcapillary and interstitial diffusion of Na-fluorescein in chronic venous insufficiency with white atrophy. *Int J Microcirc Clin Exp.* 1982;11:5–17.

20. Jörneskog G, Brismar K, Fagrell B. Skin capillary circulation severely impaired in toes of patients with IDDM, with and without late diabetic complications. *Diabetologia.* 1995;38:474–480.

21. Nathan DM. Long-term complications of diabetes mellitus. *N Engl J Med.* 1993;328:1676–1685.

22. Krolewski AS, Warram JH, Rand LI, et al. Risk of Proliferative diabetic retinopathy in juvenile-onset type I diabetes: a 40-yr follow-up study. *Diabetes Care.* 1986;9:443–452.

23. Harrington C, Zagari MJ, Corea J, et al. A cost analysis of diabetic lower-extremity ulcers. *Diabetes Care.* 2000;23:1333–1338.

24. Lavery LA, van Houtum WH, Harkless LB. In-hospital mortality and disposition of diabetic amputees in the Netherlands. *Diabet Med.* 1996;13:192–197.

25. Williams SB, Goldfine A, Timimi FK, et al. Acute hyperglycemia attenuates endothelium-dependent vasodilation in humans *in vivo. Circulation.* 1998;97:1695–1701.

26. Akbari CM, Saouaf R, Barnhill DF, et al. Endothelium-dependent vasodilation is impaired in both microcirculation and macrocirculation during acute hyperglycemia. *J Vasc Surg.* 1998;28:687–694.

27. Steinberg HO, Chaker H, Leaming R, et al. Obesity/insulin resistance is associated with endothelial dysfunction. *J Clin Invest.* 1996;11:2601–2610.

28. McVeigh GE, Brennan GM, Johnston GD, et al. Impaired endothelium-dependent and independent vasodilation in patients with type 2 (non-insulin-dependent) diabetes mellitus. *Diabetologia.* 1992;35:771–776.

29. Baynes JW, Thorpe SR. The role of oxidative stress in diabetic complications. *Curr Opin Endocrinol.* 1996;3:277–284.

30. Pieper GM. Review of alterations in endothelial nitric oxide production in diabetes. *Hypertension.* 1998;31:1047–1060.

31. Cesarone MR, Belcaro G, Carratelli M, et al. A simple test to monitor oxidative stress. *Int Angiol.* 1999;18:127–130.

32. Timimi FK, Ting HH, Haley EA, et al. Vitamin C improves endothelium-dependent vasodilation in patients with insulin-dependent diabetes mellitus. *J Am Coll Cardiol.* 1998;31:552–557.

33. Ruffini I, Belcaro G, Cesarone MR, et al. Evaluation of the local effects of Vitamin E (E-Mousse®) on free radicals in diabetic microangiopathy: a randomized, controlled trial. *Angiology.* 2003;54:415–421.

34. Clarkson P, Celermajer DS, Donals AE, et al. Impaired vascular reactivity in insulin-dependent diabetes mellitus is related to duration of disease and low density lipoprotein cholesterol levels. *J Am Coll Cardiol.* 1996;28:573–579.

35. Young MJ, Bennett JL, Liderth SA, et al. Rheological and microvascular parameters in diabetic peripheral neuropathy. *Clin Sci.* 1996;90:183–187.

36. Furchgott RF, Zawadzki JV. The obligatory role of endothelial cells in the relaxation of arterial smooth muscle by acetylcholine. *Nature.* 1980;288:373–376.

37. Brain SD, Grant AD. Vascular actions of calcitonin gene-related peptide and adrenomedullin. *Physiol Rev.* 2004;84:903–934.

38. Harrison S, Geppetti P. Substance p. *Int J Biochem Cell Biol.* 2001; 33:555–576.

39. Palmer RM, Ferrige AG, Moncada S. Nitric oxide release accounts for the biologic activity of endothelium-derived relaxing factor. *Nature.* 1987;327:524–526.

40. Du XL, Edelstein D, Dimmeler S, et al. Hyperglycemia inhibits endothelial nitric oxide synthase activity by posttranslational modification at the Akt site. *J Clin Invest.* 2001;108:1341–1348.

41. Stroes E, Kastelein J, Cosentino F, et al. Tetrahydrobiopterin restores endothelial function in hypercholesterolemia. *J Clin Invest.* 1997;99:41–46.

42. Stroes ES, van Faassen EE, Yo M, et al. Folic acid reverts dysfunction of endothelial nitric oxide synthase. *Circ Res.* 2000;86:1129–1134.

43. Creager MA, Gallagher SJ, Girerd XJ, et al. Arginine improves endothelium-dependent vasodilation in hypercholesterolemic humans. *J Clin Invest.* 1992;90:1248–1253.

44. Veves A, Akbari CM, Primavera J, et al. Endothelial dysfunction and the expression of endothelial nitric oxide sythetase in diabetic neuropathy, vascular disease, and foot ulceration. *Diabetes.* 1998;47:457–463.

45. Jude EB, Boulton AJM, Ferguson MW, et al. The role of nitric oxide synthase isoforms and arginase in the pathogenesis of diabetic foot ulcers: possible modulatory effects by transforming growth factor beta 1. *Diabetologia.* 1999;42:748–757.

46. Zykova SN, Jenssen TG, Berdal M, et al. Altered cytokine and nitric oxide secretion *in vitro* by macrophages from diabetic type II-like db/db mice. *Diabetes.* 2000;49:1451–1458.

47. Lee PC, Salyapongse AN, Bragdon GA, et al. Impaired wound healing and angiogenesis in eNOS-deficient mice. *Am J Physiol.* 1999;277:H1600–H1608.

48. Barbul A, Lazarou SA, Efron DT, et al. Arginine enhances wound healing and lymphocyte immune responses in humans. *Surgery.* 1990;108:331–337.

49. Leibovich SJ, Polverini PJ, Fong TW, et al. Production of angiogenic activity by human monocytes requires an L-arginine/nitric oxide-synthase-dependent effector mechanism. *Proc Natl Acad Sci USA.* 1994;91:4190–4194.

50. Mitchell BD, Hawthorne VM, Vinik AI. Cigarette smoking and neuropathy in diabetic patients. *Diabetes Care.* 1990;13:434–437.

51. Christen WG, Manson JE, Bubes V, et al, Sorbinil Retinopathy Trial Research Group. Risk factors for progression of distal symmetric polyneuropathy in type 1 diabetes mellitus. *Am J Epidemiol.* 1999;150:1142–1151.

52. Alzaid AA. Microalbuminuria in patients with NIDDM: an overview. *Diabetes.* 1996;19:79–89.

53. Mogensen CE. Microalbuminuria predicts clinical proteinuria and early mortality in maturity-onset diabetes. *N Engl J Med.* 1984;310:356–360.

54. Yip J, Mattock MB, Morocutti A, et al. Insulin resistance in insulin-dependent diabetic patients with microalbuminuria. *Lancet.* 1993;342:883–887.

55. Lim SC, Caballero AE, Smakowski P, et al. Soluble intercellular adhesion molecule, vascular cell adhesion molecule, and impaired microvascular reactivity are early markers of vasculopathy in type 2 diabetic individuals without microalbuminuria. *Diabetes Care.* 1999;22:1865–1870.

56. Ridker PM, Hennekens CH, Roitman-Johnson B, et al. Plasma concentration of soluble intercellular adhesion molecule 1 and risk of future myocardial infarction in apparently healthy men. *Lancet.* 1998;351:88–92.

57. Otsuki M, Hashimoto K, Morimoto Y, et al. Circulating vascular cell adhesion molecule-1 (VCAM-1) in atherosclerotic NIDDM patients. *Diabetes.* 1997;46:2096–2101.

58. Fasching P, Weiti M, Rohac M, et al. Elevated concentration of circulating adhesion molecules and their association with microvascular complications in insulin-dependent diabetes mellitus. *J Clin Endocrinol Metab.* 1996;81:4313–4317.

59. Koga M, Otsuki M, Kubo M, et al. Relationship between circulating vascular cell adhesion molecule-1 and microvascular complications in type 2 diabetes mellitus. *Diabet Med.* 1998;15:661–667.

60. Jude EB, Abbot CA, Young MJ, et al. The potential role of cell adhesion molecules in the pathogenesis of diabetic neuropathy. *Diabetologia.* 1998;41:330–336.

61. Johnstone MT, Creager SJ, Scales KM, et al. Impaired endothelium-dependent vasodilation in patients with insulin-dependent diabetes mellitus. *Circulation.* 1993;88:2510–2516.

62. Williams SB, Cusco JA, Roddy M, et al. Impaired nitric oxide-mediated vasodilation in patients with non-insulin dependent diabetes mellitus. *J Am Coll Cardiol.* 1996;27:567–574.

63. Akbari CM, LoGerfo FW. Diabetes and peripheral vascular disease. *J Vasc Surg.* 1999;30:373–384.

64. Caballero AE, Arora S, Saouaf R, et al. Micro and macrovascular reactivity is impaired in subjects at risk for type 2 diabetes. *Diabetes.* 1999;48:1863–1867.

65. Makita Z, Radoff S, Rayfield EJ. Advanced glycosylation end products in patients with diabetic neuropathy. *N Engl J Med.* 1991;325:836–842.

66. Garcia Soriano F, Virag L, Jagtap P, et al. Diabetic endothelial dysfunction: the role of poly (ADP-ribose) polymerase activation. *Nat Med.* 2001;7:108–113.

67. Szabó C, Zanchi A, Komjáti K, et al. Poly (ADP-ribose) polymerase is activated in subjects at risk of developing type 2 diabetes and is associated with impaired vascular reactivity. *Circulation.* 2002;106:2680–2686.

68. Lobo RA. Effects of hormonal replacement on lipids and lipoproteins in postmenopausal women. *J Clin Endocrinol Metab.* 1991;73:925–930.

69. Skafar DF, Xu R, Morales J, et al. Female sex hormones and cardiovascular disease in women. *J Clin Endocrinol Metab.* 1997;82:3913–3918.

70. Lim SC, Caballero E, Arora S, et al. The effect of hormonal replacement therapy on the vascular reactivity and endothelial function of healthy individuals and individuals with type 2 diabetes. *J Clin Endocrinol Metab.* 1999;84:4159–4164.

71. Arora S, Veves A, Caballero E, et al. Estrogen improves endothelial function. *J Vasc Surg.* 1998;27:1141–1147.

72. Stevens MJ, Dananberg J, Feldman EL, et al. The linked roles of nitric oxide, aldose reductase and (Na^+, K^+)-ATPase in the slowing of nerve conduction in the streptozotocin diabetic rat. *J Clin Invest.* 1994;94:853–919.

73. Ward JD. Upright posture and the microvasculature in human diabetic neuropathy: a hypothesis. *Diabetes.* 1997;46(S2):S94–S97.

74. Cisek PL, Eze AR, Camerota AJ, et al. Microcirculatory compensation to progressive atherosclerotic disease. *Ann Vasc Surg.* 1997;11:49–53.

75. Arora S, Smakowski P, Frykberg RG, et al. Differences in foot and forearm skin microcirculation in diabetic patients with and without neuropathy. *Diabetes Care.* 1998;21:1339–1344.

76. Hamdy O, Abou-Elenin K, LoGerfo FW, et al. Contribution of nerve-axon reflex-related vasodilation to the total skin vasodilation in diabetic patients with and without neuropathy. *Diabetes Care.* 2001;24:344–349.

77. Caselli A, Rich J, Hanane T, et al. Role of C-nociceptive fibers in the nerve axon reflex-related vasodilation in diabetes. *Neurology.* 2003;60:297–300.

78. Meijer WT, Hoes AW, Rutgers D, et al. Peripheral arterial disease in the elderly: the Rotterdam Study. *Arterioscler Thromb Vasc Biol.* 1998;18:185–192.

79. Young MJ, Veves A, Smith JV, et al. Restoring lower limb blood flow improves conduction velocity in diabetic patients. *Diabetologia.* 1995;38:1051–1054.

80. Akbari CM, Gibbons GW, Habershaw GM, et al. The effect of arterial reconstruction on the natural history of diabetic neuropathy. *Arch Surg.* 1997;132:148–152.

81. Veves A, Donaghue VM, Sarnow MR, et al. The impact of reversal of hypoxia by revascularization on the peripheral nerve function of diabetic patients. *Diabetologia.* 1996;39:344–348.

Infrapopliteal Arterial Imaging

Anil Hingorani   Enrico Ascher

Less and less invasive techniques are being explored in all fields of medicine. Advancements in robotic surgery, laparoscopic surgery, and percutaneous interventions have not only been pushed forward by technology, but by patients' demand for less invasive methods of treatment. Yet, in vascular surgery, the gold standard for evaluation of the lower extremity arterial tree, and the basic principle, techniques, and complications of contrast arteriography (CA), have remained largely unchanged since Seldinger's 1953 paper.[1] As a challenge to this widely held standard, less invasive imaging technologies that have been explored in the literature include magnetic resonance angiography (MRA), computed tomography angiogram (CTA), and duplex arteriography (DA).[2-6]

In an effort to explore these alternatives to CA, we will initially compare MRA and DA to CA as methods for defining anatomic features of patients undergoing lower extremity revascularizations. Then we will add the more recent advent of CTA to the comparison.

COMPARISON OF DUPLEX ARTERIOGRAPHY, MAGNETIC RESONANCE ANGIOGRAPHY, AND CONTRAST ARTERIOGRAPHY

From August 1, 2001, to August 1, 2002, 61 consecutive inpatients (64 procedures) with chronic lower extremity ischemia underwent CA, MRA, and DA before undergoing lower extremity revascularization procedures. Patients were excluded from the protocol if their serum creatinine was >2.0 after hydration ($n = 8$).

Cases of acute ischemia ($n = 5$) or patients who underwent outpatient preoperative evaluation only were excluded, as MR was not readily available to outpatients ($n = 161$) at our institution due to overwhelming inpatient demand. Since the magnetic resonance imaging (MRI) machine was in very high demand, it could take up to 3 to 7 days to obtain an MRA for inpatients.

The reports of these tests, images, and operative findings were collected prospectively and compared to the results of CA. The reports and exams were analyzed by a vascular surgeon blinded to the identity of the patients, but aware of the clinical information for each patient. The differences in the three segments—aortoiliac segment, femoral-popliteal segment, and infrapopliteal segment—were noted. The vessels were classified as mild disease (<50%), moderate disease (50% to 70%), severe (70% to 99%), and occluded by CA, MRA, or DA. These studies and the treatment plans based on these data were compared.

Duplex Ultrasonography

The vascular ultrasound tests were all performed on either an ATL HDI 3000 or ATL HDI 5000 duplex scanner by two registered vascular technologists. The arterial segments starting from midabdominal aorta to the pedal arteries were studied in cross-sectional and longitudinal planes using a variety of scanheads of 7-4, 10-5, 12-5, 15-2, 5-2, and 3-2 megahertz (MHz) extended operative frequency range to obtain high-quality B-mode, color, and power Doppler images as well as velocity spectra. All of these techniques were used to estimate the degree of stenosis; any discrepancies were communicated to the operating surgeon. In general, however, color and power Doppler were used primarily, and B-mode and velocity spectra were used to supplement these data, especially in the presence of long lesions or multiple lesions. The arteries were classified as normal or mildly diseased (<50%), significantly stenosed (≥50%), occluded, or not visualized. Peak systolic velocity ratios ≥2 and ≥3 as compared to the adjacent vessel were used to define hemodynamically significant stenoses ≥50% and ≥70%, respectively.[2–6] A more precise evaluation of arterial size, length, and degree of narrowing, as well as plaque characteristics, was performed for lesions suitable for balloon angioplasty and/or stent placement. At the completion of the test, a color-coded map of the entire arterial tree was drawn to help develop revascularization strategy.

Contrast Arteriography

Standard percutaneous retrograde preoperative CA with DSA was obtained. These were performed by the vascular surgery team in the operating room as a separate procedure from the revascularization. The team attempted to visualize the distal aorta to the pedal vessels. Percutaneous access was obtained through a hollow-bore single entry needle. After a metal guidewire was placed in the external iliac artery, a 4-French (Fr) sheath introducer was inserted. A 4-Fr pigtail catheter was used with a power injector with full strength Omnipaque (Sanofi Winthrop Pharmaceuticals) to obtain the angiograms using an OEC 9800 digital mobile flouroscopic unit (General Electric). Calipers and multiplanar views were used selectively. Images were obtained with and without digital subtraction. While fully appreciating the limitations of CA in the presence of multilevel disease, pseudodefects, timing, lack of detail of the vessel wall, and lack of hemodynamic information, interventions were made based upon CA.

Magnetic Resonance Angiography

MRA was performed using a 1.5 Tesla whole-body scanner (Magnatom Vision plus, Siemens Medical Systems, Iselin, NJ). Parameters for the study were a repetition time of 40 msec and an echo time of 1.6 msec. T1 weighted three-dimensional gadolinium enhanced imaging of the aortoiliac system to the level of the ankle was performed in a body array coil with a flip angle of 70 degrees. Below the ankle, two-dimensional electrocardiogram (EKG) triggered time of flight. MRA was performed using a combination of the phased array coil and the head coil with a flip angle of 30 degrees. Maximum intensity projections and source images were used in the interpretation of the study. Our stepping table was not used for this set of

data as it had not arrived yet. The timing is based upon a 1 cc test bolus during this phase. Calipers and multiplanar views were used selectively. MRA results were interpreted by MR radiologists with extensive experience who were not aware of the results of other lower extremity imaging modalities. A sample of MRA-generated images is shown in Figure 14-1.

Duplex Arteriography and Magnetic Resonance Angiography versus Contrast Arteriography

The mean age of the patients was 76 ± 10 years (SD) (range 47 to 97 years). Indications for the procedures included gangrene (43%), ischemic ulcer (28%), rest pain (19%), severe claudication (9%), and failing bypass (1%). Diabetes, hypertension, and end-stage renal disease were present in 86%, 59%, and 15% of the patients, respectively. During this time period, 41 patients could not be entered into the protocol as they could not undergo MRA (33) or angiography (eight). The reasons for patients not being able to undergo MRA included refusal or severe uncooperation (nine), pacemaker (10), recent surgery (five), acute ischemia (five), severely contracted knee and hip (one), claustrophobia (two), and morbid obesity (one). Of the total 192 arterial segments of the 64 patients (iliac, femoral-popliteal, and tibial segments), 17% could not be fully assessed by DA, and 7% could not be assessed by MRA (Table 14-1). In addition, two patients required repeat MRA to obtain more information.

TABLE 14-1

CAUSES OF INCOMPLETE EXAMS COMPARING MAGNETIC RESONANCE ANGIOGRAPHY, DUPLEX ARTERIOGRAPHY, AND CONTRAST ARTERIOGRAPHY

MRA: aortoiliac segment	Timing of dye bolus–1
MRA: femoral-popliteal segment	Contracture–1
	Knee prosthesis artifact–1
MRA: infrageniculate segment	Venous contamination–10
	Movement–1
	Contracture–1
DA: aortoiliac segment	Gas interposition–7
	Calcified iliac–1
DA: femoral-popliteal segment	Calcified–4
DA: infrageniculate segment	Severe tibial calcification–18
	Gangrene–1
	Noncooperative patient–1
CA	0

Note: MRA, 13 patients; DA, ten patients.
MRA, magnetic resonance angiography; DA, duplex arteriography; CA, contrast arteriography.

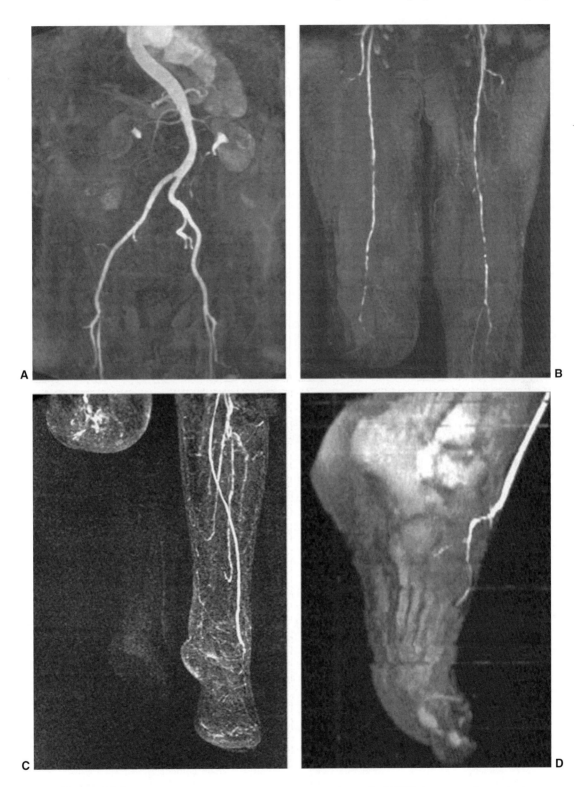

Figure 14-1 Representative magnetic resonance angiography (MRA) demonstrating patent aortoiliac system **(A)** with failing pop-dp **(C, D)** due to severe superficial artery and popliteal disease **(B)**.

Even though there were multiple arteries in each segment, any disagreement in any individual artery was counted as a disagreement in the entire segment. Disagreements with CA and DA were encountered in the iliac, femoral-popliteal, and tibial segment in 0%, 7%, and 14% of the cases, respectively, and between CA and MRA in 10%, 26%, and 42% of the segments, respectively (Tables 14-2 and 14-3). However, because some segments could not be fully evaluated with each technique and were excluded from further analysis, the

TABLE 14.2

DISAGREEMENTS BETWEEN DUPLEX ARTERIOGRAPHY AND CONTRAST ARTERIOGRAPHY WITH CLINICAL SIGNIFICANCE

DA	CA	Clinical Significance
AT open	Distal AT disease	Bypass to distal AT
Peroneal open	Peroneal stenosis	PTA of peroneal

Note: Both cases of disagreement were noted to have severely calcified tibial vessels.
DA, duplex arteriography; CA, contrast arteriography; AT, anterior tibial artery; PTA, percutaneous transluminal angioplasty.

percentage of disagreements may be underestimated. Therefore, we also calculated the data with these segments as false negatives. Clinically significant differences between DA and CA were found in two of the nine, while 28 of the 45 differences between MRA and CA were felt to be clinically significant. Clinical significance was determined if the difference would have resulted in a different procedure. The actual procedures performed included a bypass to an infrapopliteal artery (19), bypass to the popliteal artery (23), no procedure (nine), below-knee amputation (two), percutaneous balloon angioplasty (six), axillofemoral bypass (four), and an ileofemoral bypass (one). The calculated sensitivity and specificity, positive predictive and negative value, and accuracy are demonstrated in Table 14-4.

On average, the times required for DA, MRA, and CA are 30 to 60 minutes (average 46 minutes), 20 to 60 minutes, and 40 to 60 minutes, respectively. The average costs for each are $300, $2,100, and $2,200.

Limitations of Magnetic Resonance Angiography

This data set represents a continuing effort by our service to explore alternative imaging techniques. Our previous

TABLE 14-3

DISAGREEMENTS BETWEEN MAGNETIC RESONANCE ANGIOGRAPHY AND CONTRAST ARTERIOGRAPHY WITH CLINICAL SIGNIFICANCE

MRA	CA	Clinical Significance
CIA moderate disease	No CIA stenosis	CIA—No intervention needed
CFA is OK	CFA is diseased	Ileofemoral bypass
Pop peroneal stenosis	Not stenotic	Fem pop bypass
Mod disease in pop tibialis	No pop tibial disease	Fem popll bypass
Pop, peroneal mod disease	Open pop per	Fem pop bypass
Distal pop diseased	Open pop	Fem pop bypass
Pop very small	Open pop	Fem pop bypass
Pop is open	AK pop closed	Bypass to BK pop
AK pop open	AK pop closed	Bypass to BK pop
SFA pop open	SFA pop stenotic	PTA of SFA and pop
Pop open	Distal pop closed	Bypass to PT
Pop diseased	Normal pop	Fem pop bypass
Mod pop disease	Normal pop	Fem pop bypass
AK pop open	AK pop closed	Bypass to BK pop
Mod aortic and pop disease	No disease aorta and BK pop	Bypass to BK pop
Stenotic fem pop	No stenosis	No intervention needed
Pop mod disease	Pop open	Bypass to pop
TPA open	TPA closed	Bypass to peroneal
Per mod disease	Normal peroneal	Bypass to peroneal
Per diseased	Peroneal open	Fem peroneal bypass
Per closed	Per open	Fem pop bypass with runoff to per
Per diseased	Peroneal open	Fem peroneal bypass
Distal PT open	Distal PT closed	Limited runoff for bypass to PT
AT open	Stenotic AT	PTA of AT
Per closed	Per open	Bypass to peroneal
DP diseased	DP open	Fem DP bypass
DP open	DP closed	Bypass to AT with no runoff
DP closed	DP open	Bypass to DP

MRA, magnetic resonance angiography; CA, contrast arteriography; CIA, common iliac artery; CFA, common femoral artery; pop, popliteal; fem pop, femoral-popliteal; mod, moderate; per, peroneal; AK, above knee; BK, below knee; SFA, superficial femoral artery; PTA, percutaneous transluminal angioplasty; PT, posterior tibial artery; TPA, tibioperoneal artery; AT, anterior tibial artery; DP, dorsalis pedis artery.

TABLE 14-4

COMPARISON OF MAGNETIC RESONANCE ANGIOGRAPHY AND DUPLEX ARTERIOGRAPHY WITH CONTRAST ARTERIOGRAPHY

	Sensitivity	Specificity	Positive Predictive Value	Negative Predictive Value	Accuracy
MRA					
Aortoiliac	100%	81%	23%	100%	82%
Fem-pop	86%	53%	82%	60%	74%
Tibial	61%	51%	30%	79%	54%
DA					
Aortoiliac	100%	96%	67%	100%	96%
Fem-pop	97%	94%	97%	94%	96%
Tibial	81%	100%	100%	94%	95%
CA					
Aortoiliac	—	100%	—	—	100%
Fem-pop	100%	25%	80%	—	81%
Infrapopliteal	75%	50%	63%	44%	59%

Note: Table data excludes nonvisualized segments.
MRA, magnetic resonance angiography; DA, duplex arteriography; CA, contrast arteriography; fem-pop, femoral-popliteal.

work has demonstrated the use of DA in patients undergoing lower extremity revascularization.[7–11] Alongside this attempt, we have been investigating the use of MRA as a preoperative imaging tool. Our enthusiasm has been fueled by the excellent results published in the literature.[12–24] However, our initial experience combined with those published from other centers have suggested limitations in this technology in its present state.[25–30]

Due to the variety of reasons listed, a significant portion of these elderly patients with multiple comorbid conditions were not able to undergo MRA. Even with sedation, some patients simply refused to have an MRA or literally jumped off the MR table. While no one test can be used for all patients, these types of issues remain to be explored.

We have found that MRA does not yet seem able to obtain adequate data for us to perform these interventions, at least for this highly selected population at our institution. Since we have already placed >200 patients into various phases of this protocol over the last 3 years, and have a set of MRA radiologists trained at a leading center for lower extremity MRA imaging, it seems difficult to attribute these results to the early phase of a learning curve. The most common problem we encountered with MRA was assessing the degree of disease and patency of the distal vessels when it was patent and then used for the distal anastamosis. Misidentification of the distal superficial artery as the popliteal and identification of moderate aortoiliac disease with a normal contrast angiogram and pressure measurements were also issues. These issues remain despite reviewing these data on an ongoing basis with the MRA radiologists. The issues of low flow/signal dropout and venous contamination may be possible causes of the disagreements between the studies. Conversely, when severe tibial artery calcification is identified, DA may become unreliable and CA may be necessary. This case can be appreciated by the DA technologist and this information is given to the vascular team to seek alternative imaging tools. Most of the time, the areas that cannot be visualized well by DA are deemed to not have an impact on the planned procedure and the information that is obtained is adequate to perform the procedure. In this data set, if DA was solely used, we probably would have resorted to CA in 16 cases (25%), as not enough information was obtained by DA alone. Because we could not identify which segments would not be reliable by the MRA alone, the percentage that would need CA had MRA been used as the only imaging tool was not estimated.

The data presented here includes a representation of some patients with the most severe arterial diseases at a referral center for limb-threatening ischemia. This may be part of the reason why the results are suboptimal. Perhaps if more outpatients with claudication and superficial femoral artery disease were included, the results would be more favorable. The data, however, do suggest that while neither DA nor MRA may yet be able to completely replace CA at our institution, with upcoming advancements in the techniques, more centers will be able to use these imaging tools to obtain the necessary information for these complex revascularizations.

Limitations of Duplex Arteriography

Over the course of conducting 1,020 DAs, we have also explored various limitations of DA. Poor visualization of vessels with extremely calcified vessel walls and skin quality problems such as severe dermatitis, open ulcers, heavy scarring, severe lymphedema, and severe hyperkeratosis are some of the problems associated with DA, as well as rest pain, noncompliant patients, and excessive edema. Additionally, we encountered difficulty visualizing the iliac arteries due to colostomy, marked iliac tortuosity, recent abdominal surgery, ascites, morbid obesity, or gas interposition in a few of our patients.

To circumvent the problem of severe calcification, we have found increasing the gain, persistence, and sensitivity and using power Doppler and SonoCT technology quite useful. Lack of patient cooperation may be one limitation to accurate DA, particularly for the iliac and infrapopliteal segments. In fact, a small percentage of patients are uncooperative because of altered mental status, inability to position the leg, or severe ischemic pain. The inclusion of pain medications, sedation, or having a family member in the laboratory to calm the confused patient were also found to be very helpful. In certain instances, we reattempted the exam after a few days of elevation to decrease the edema, and attempted overnight fasting prior to the exam to reduce bowel gas. Often, with limited visualization of the aortoiliac segment, but with normal common femoral artery waveforms, it was elected to proceed to revascularization, realizing that an intraoperative balloon angioplasty of the inflow arteries may be needed. Nevertheless, with a small number of our patients, we could not obtain adequate information from DA, despite our attempts; these cases required preoperative contrast angiography.

Furthermore, incomplete visualization of the crural and pedal vessels by DA does not always have a major impact on the choice of the procedure. For example, if a surgeon prefers to perform a bypass to the distal anterior tibial artery rather than to the distal peroneal, and the distal peroneal was too calcified to insonate, the lack of data on the distal peroneal may have little impact on the planning of the procedure. In general, our policy of not performing femoral-distal bypasses for patients with claudication means that in the presence of severe superficial femoral artery (SFA) disease or occlusion with at least one vessel runoff and absence of significant iliac artery disease, a femoral-popliteal bypass will be planned even if the remaining two tibial arteries could not be completely evaluated.

Nevertheless, when difficulties in the evaluation of the crural and pedal vessels are encountered and the status of these vessels is necessary, additional techniques can be used. In very low-flow situations (PSV of <20 cm per second), such as in the tibial vessels in acute ischemia or cardiogenic shock, setting the pulse repetition frequency at 150 to 350 Hz and using the lowest wall filter, the highest persistence, and highest sensitivity for the color flow imaging can be beneficial. At times, distal compression can augment flow and demonstrate patency of tibial vessels.

When the tibial vessels are severely calcified, we have found power Doppler and SonoCT to be particularly useful. In addition, examining the vessels in transverse section, changing the color box angle, and increasing the gain can, at times, allow better visualization of the arterial lumen. The depth of the tibioperoneal trunk, origin of the proximal peroneal and posterior arteries, and the superficial femoral artery at Hunter's canal may necessitate the use of a lower frequency probe for visualization. However, this tends to sacrifice detail resolution and can make images of these areas difficult to interpret. In these cases, velocity spectral analysis can also be a useful adjunct. Manipulation of the leg, using multiple probes and other approaches, may be necessary for better assessment of difficult arterial segments. For example, the medial approach may help visualize the proximal peroneal artery, the medial or posterior approach may assist in visualizing the midperoneal artery, and the lateral or posterior approach may facilitate the imaging of the distal peroneal artery and its branches. Thus, the tibial vessels can be adequately evaluated by using a variety of approaches and angles.

The most difficult infrapopliteal segments to visualize in our experience were the most proximal portion of the anterior tibial artery and the bifurcation of the tibioperoneal trunk. We believe that this difficulty could be explained by the depth of these arteries. Contrary to the belief that the peroneal artery is difficult to image, we were able to visualize it using a variety of techniques. Using these techniques made possible the adequate assessment of the majority of these difficult-to-vizualize arteries.

The origin of the anterior tibial artery deserves special attention, as collaterals in this area may be mistaken for a patent proximal anterior tibial artery. Careful examination of the origin of the vessels and tracing the vessels distally often can solve some of these issues. In addition, identification of the two adjacent veins can help distinguish between large collateral and the vessel. When patency of vessels that are not visualized well despite these techniques is crucial for the revascularization procedure choice, an angiogram should be obtained before the procedure is attempted.

Advantages of Duplex Arteriography

Invasive contrast angiography remains the gold standard imaging modality in planning these revascularizations, even though this modality may not detect outflow vessels that may be more clearly visualized with duplex or MRA, as occurs in very low-flow situations with acute or severe chronic ischemia.[10,31] Conversely, DA has the capability to detect these vessels with very low flow (<20 cm per second). The visualization of these outflow vessels may result in the performance of lower extremity revascularizations that ultimately achieve limb salvage. Moreover, since biplanar arteriography is not the standard for the entire arterial tree, eccentric lesions, especially in the iliacs, may go undetected utilizing CA. Last, while MRA does have certain clear advantages over CA, we have noted that as many as 25% of patients are unable to complete their preoperative MRAs due to scheduling difficulties, claustrophobia, metal implants, or pacemakers.

The advantages of DA as compared to other imaging tools include the identification of the softest portion of the vessel wall that can be marked on the skin before the intended procedure. Skin marking of the most suitable site for outflow anastomosis, particularly for infrapopliteal segments, may limit incision size and eliminate extensive arterial dissection in search of a soft arterial segment. Identification of a noncalcified arterial segment is promptly conveyed to the surgeon, important arterial branches may be spared, and long incision-related complications reduced. While a target vessel may be patent using luminally based imaging tools, the vessel may be severely calcified in long segments, as in the diabetic and end-stage renal disease population. We have found that preoperative localization of the softest portion of the vessel by DA can accurately identify the most advantageous anastomotic site, thus decreasing the risk of damage to the artery from clamping or incomplete proximal control with a tourniquet, due to concomitant severe SFA calcification. Thus, DA can be an invaluable aid to the surgeon in determining the anastomotic site of choice.

Since DA is not just a luminal technology, it can be used to assess the actual disease of the vessel. High resolution duplex imaging can assess not only the luminal diameter, but also the thickness of the wall down to approximately 1/10 mm. While a vessel may appear to have a patent lumen with MRA and contrast angiography, the actual thickness of the wall is not evaluated via these techniques. This visualization by DA may change the site for the anastomosis. In addition, DA has the ability to more accurately assess the chronic nature of an occlusion. Therefore, it is possible to differentiate between an isolated chronic SFA occlusion and an acute embolism with little underlying disease or acute thrombosis with severe underlying atherosclerotic disease. In addition, aneurysmal vessels with partial thrombosis may have little to no luminal dilatation and may be undetectable by CA. Similarly, ulcerated and irregular plaques that may be a source of embolization are also poorly assessed with CA. High-resolution DA more clearly visualizes these plaques. Consequently, we have found this imaging modality particularly valuable in determining patient management as compared to other technologies.

Furthermore, the hemodynamic information obtained using DA may alter patient management. Volume flow and velocity measurements can help assess whether the visualized lesion is hemodynamically significant and determine whether repair of the lesion may be beneficial. For example, a poorly visualized iliac plaque with little change in the ratio of peak systolic velocities (<2) may suggest that the lesion may not be of clinical significance. On the other hand, lesions that are poorly visualized due to severe calcification with elevated ratios distal to the obscured lesion suggest a hemodynamically significant lesion. Other luminal imaging modalities do not readily furnish these details.

The portability of the duplex machine should be mentioned. Because the DA can be performed at the bedside, in the operating room, or in the holding area, time and personnel required to transport the patient are significantly reduced. Additionally, obtaining the CA or MRA and the interpretation can entail a delay in the definitive treatment of a severely ischemic limb in a debilitated patient, as well as take a toll on the operative team. With DA, once the patient is identified to need urgent revascularization, the machine and technician can be brought to any part of the hospital for an abbreviated directed exam.

The Duplex Arteriography Team

While prior studies have demonstrated the reliability of DA,[13,17,18] it is highly operator-dependent. We require an experienced technician whose capabilities are well known to the surgical staff. Our DA technicians are registered vascular technologists (RVTs) who each undergo a specialized training protocol, which includes examination of the patient by DA and angiography. The variances encountered between both modalities are then reviewed. In addition, any differences in DA and intraoperative completion angiography are analyzed by all of the surgeons and technologists, resulting in a close relationship. Prior to each procedure, the case is discussed to afford the surgeon a complete picture of the findings, rather than to have the surgeon merely review the mapping. Thus, the intricacies and nuances of the actual quality of the arteries and veins are presented to the surgeon as an adjunct to the mapping and images taken during the exam. For example, the thickness and characteristics of the target vessels can be more effectively communicated by verbal exchange than through written details or a drawing. This type of data serves to further accentuate the advantages of DA over luminally based imaging modalities, as this sort of information is not available otherwise. Areas that are not well visualized should be identified as such so the surgeon can decide if this area is crucial.

Role of Duplex Arteriography in Renal and Diabetic Patients

It has been well documented that patients with diabetes mellitus (DM) and/or chronic renal insufficiency are at an increased risk for developing contrast-induced nephropathy when subjected to CA, despite the use of nonionic contrast media.[32-35] Although the renal function in most patients with contrast-induced renal failure will return to baseline, a few patients may require hemodialysis and most will have their proposed arterial reconstruction delayed. In a modern series, up to 10% of diabetic patients will have contrast-induced renal failure and up to 12% of patients with chronic renal insufficiency will experience a significant worsening of their renal function following CA.[3,36,37] In addition, the significant osmotic load associated with dye injection poses a risk of fluid overload for the patients on hemodialysis. Yet, the gold standard imaging modality for lower limb ischemia continues to be invasive CA, even in the presence of DM and chronic renal failure.

More recently, several investigators have attempted to validate duplex arterial mapping as a reliable alternative to CA.[1,14,16,38] Although some of these studies achieved excellent correlation between DA and CA, few surgeons have actually performed infrainguinal bypasses without preoperative or prebypass CA.[3] In an effort to examine revascularization without a preoperative dye study, we will focus on our experience with DA in 145 patients who had 180 lower limb arterial bypasses and who were at risk for developing or worsening their renal failure if given nonionic contrast media.

From January 1998, to November 2000, lower extremity DAs were performed in 145 patients with DM and/or chronic renal failure prior to 180 arterial reconstructions. Among the 97 patients with diabetes alone, 121 procedures were performed, 41 procedures were done on 33 patients with diabetes and chronic renal insufficiency (CRI), and 18 procedures were done on 15 patients with CRI alone. Patient ages ranged from 45 years to 98 years (mean 73 ± 10 years). Indications for surgery were severe claudication in 20 patients (15%), rest pain in 28 (21%), nonhealing ischemic ulcers in 39 (30%), and limb gangrene in 45 (34%). Preoperative CA was performed with 16 procedures due to extremely poor runoff based on DA and limited visualization of outflow vessels. Adequacy of the inflow was confirmed by intraoperative pressure measurements. Postbypass CA or duplex imaging was obtained to verify the patency of the runoff. The DA procedure time averaged 50 ± 12 minutes (range 35 to 90 minutes). The distal anastomosis was to the popliteal artery in 65 cases (49%) and to the tibial and pedal arteries in 67 (51%). Cumulative patency rates at 1 and 3 months were 94% and 83%, respectively. Intraoperative findings confirmed the preoperative DA findings with the exception of one, where the distal anastomosis was placed proximal to a significant stenosis requiring an extension graft.

The use of high-quality arterial ultrasonography presents a safe and reliable option to preoperative lower extremity CA for many patients with diabetes or impaired kidney function. The ease of use and favorable patient outcomes achieved with this imaging modality may rival the use of CA for these patients.

This imaging modality can offer results comparable to those achieved with conventional invasive CA, while at the same time reducing associated risks. The advantages of avoiding or limiting the use of CA to decrease the incidence of postprocedure renal insufficiency for the diabetic patient and those patients with CRI are self-evident. This complication also results in substantially increased lengths of stay, additional specialty consults, and higher costs. In addition, it can also produce suffering for the patients and their family. Moreover, an analysis of natural history studies indicates that 23% to 63% of patients with diabetes will have progressive renal insufficiency, with 10% to 35% requiring dialysis.[39-43] Of the patients with CRI, up to 28% will require eventual dialysis.[44,45] It remains unclear whether the administration of intra-arterial dye may result in additional long-term complications in these high-risk patients with peripheral vascular disease.

COMPARISON OF COMPUTED TOMOGRAPHY ANGIOGRAM TO CONTRAST ARTERIOGRAPHY

Recent advances in hardware and software have made multidetector CTA an option for imaging of the lower extremity in patients undergoing lower extremity revascularization procedures. Prior authors have compared CTA and CA, and cite sensitivity and specificity levels of >93%.[46,47] Some of the advances that have lead to these improvements in CTA over prior CT technologies include increased volumetric coverage, improved z-axis resolution, better separation of different vascular phases and isotropic voxels, and the ability to obtain single image acquisition. Furthermore, in contrast to the limited projection routinely obtained during CA, a wider variety of manipulation of the volumetric data set for image display and analysis is feasible with CTA. CTA allows more postprocedure imaging processing, and one can rotate the 3-D image to any angle.

Since CTA is minimally invasive, it offers the potential to obtain the needed data to plan lower extremity revascularization procedures without the risks of CA. CTA may also offer greater patient comfort and convenience. In comparison to CA, some authors have noted shorter procedure times and less radiation exposure.[48]

In a further effort to explore newer alternatives to CA, we compared CTA to CA for defining anatomic features of patients undergoing lower extremity revascularizations.

From November 2003, to March 2004, 36 inpatients with chronic lower extremity ischemia underwent CA and CTA before undergoing lower extremity revascularization procedures. No patients included in this series had a serum creatinine >1.6 mg per dL.

Computed Tomography Angiography

A Siemens 16 slice multiplanar CT (SOMATOM Sensation 16) with bolus tracking and care dosing was used for these exams. The specifications of the CTA protocol were dye injection rate of 4 cc per second, toprogram length 1,024 mm (AP), slice thickness 3 mm, pitch 1.5 mm, KV 120, MA 180, rotation time 0.75 seconds, scan time 70 seconds, and dye bolus of Visapaque (320) 130 to 150 cc (Amersham Health). The angio runoff reconstruction was performed with 2 mm slices every 1 mm.

Contrast Arteriography

Standard percutaneous retrograde preoperative CA with DSA was obtained. These were performed by the vascular surgery team in the operating room as a separate procedure from the revascularization. Attempts were made to visualize the distal aorta to the pedal vessels. Percutaneous access was obtained through a hollow-bore single entry needle. After a metal guidewire was placed in the external iliac artery, a 4-Fr sheath introducer was inserted. A 4-Fr pigtail catheter was used with a power injector with full strength Omnipaque (Sanofi Winthrop Pharmaceuticals) to obtain the angiograms using an OEC 9800 digital mobile flouroscopic unit (General Electric). Calipers and multiplanar views were used selectively. Images were obtained with and without digital subtraction. While fully appreciating the limitations of CA in the presence of multilevel disease, pseudodefects, timing, lack of detail of the vessel wall, and lack of hemodynamic information, interventions were made based upon CA.

The reports of these tests and images were compared prospectively and the differences in the aortoiliac, femoral-popliteal, and infrapopliteal segments were noted. The vessels were classified as mild disease ($<50\%$), moderate disease (50% to 70%), severe disease (71% to 99%), and occluded. The studies and treatment plans based on these data were compared.

Both observers of the CTA and the CA were blinded to results of each study. Two patients were not able to have CTA due to severely contracted lower extremities and inability to remain still. A third patient had poor opacification of vessels, severe dense calcification of femoral and popliteal vessels, and knee prosthesis not allowing adequate imaging of the femoral-popliteal and tibial vessels. These three patients were not included in the series.

The mean age was 76 ± 12 years (SD). Indications for the procedures included gangrene (45%), ischemic ulcer (32%), rest pain (19%), and severe claudication (3%). In the group, 69% had diabetes. No complications were noted from CTA of CA in this series.

Of the disagreements between CTA and CA findings (Table 14-5), 13 of 18 (72%) resulted in a procedure

TABLE 14-5
COMPARISON OF COMPUTED TOMOGRAPHY ANGIOGRAPHY AND CONTRAST ARTERIOGRAPHY

CTA	CA	Clinical Significance
CIA diseased	Normal CIA	CIA doesn't need intervention
Diseased CIA	Normal CIA	CIA doesn't need intervention
SFA diseased	Normal SFA	No impact
Normal popliteal	Disease in above knee pop	Bypass to BK pop
Popliteal moderate disease	Normal popliteal	Bypass to pop
Popliteal closed	Popliteal open	Fem pop bypass
Popliteal diseased	Normal pop	Fem pop not failing
Popliteal disease	Normal pop	Bypass to pop
Normal tibioperoneal artery	Diseased tibioperoneal artery	Need distal bypass
Tarsal not seen	Tarsal open	Bypass to tarsal
DP not seen	DP open	No impact
DP not seen	DP open	Bypass to DP
AT open	AT closed	Bypass to peroneal
Closed plantar DP	Open plantar DP	Balloon of tibial vessels with good runoff
Closed DP	Open DP	No impact
AT open	AT diseased	No impact
Peroneal moderate disease	Normal peroneal	Bypass to peroneal
AT, DP disease	AT, DP open	No impact

CTA, computed tomography angiography; CA, contrast arteriography; CIA, common iliac artery; SFA, superficial femoral artery; pop, popliteal; BK, below knee; fem pop, femoral-popliteal; DP, dorsalis pedis artery; AT, anterior tibial artery.

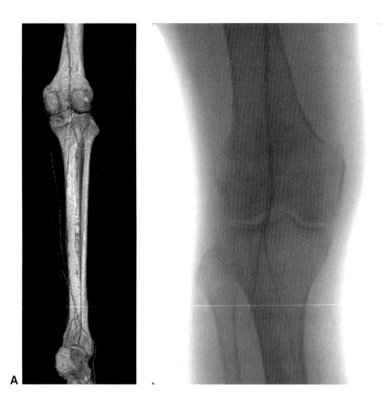

A

B

Figure 14-2 Computed tomography angiogram (CTA) **(A)** suggests severely diseased popliteal artery, but contrast angiogram does not **(B)**.

different from that suggested by CTA. Prior revascularization had been performed in 14 patients (39%). The procedures that were performed included a bypass to infrapopliteal vessels (13), angiogram alone (11), endovascular treatment (six), femoral-popliteal bypass (four), embolectomy (one), and major amputation (one). Two disagreements in CTA and CA findings are shown in Figures 14-2 and 14-3.

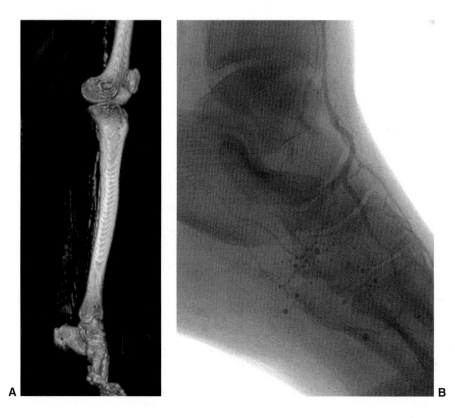

A

B

Figure 14-3 Computed tomography angiogram (CTA) **(A)** fails to demonstrate patent nondiseased lateral tarsal artery as demonstrated on contrast arteriography (CA) **(B)**.

SUMMARY

This experience represents our continuing effort to explore alternatives to invasive imaging for patients undergoing lower extremity revascularization. We have found DA to be extremely useful in the majority of patients. However, one has to fully appreciate that besides the commitment needed to overcome the learning curve, maintain the quality assurance, and establish a DA team, once severe tibial artery calcification is encountered, alternative imaging modalities may need to be acquired.

MRA has also been proposed as an alternative for evaluation of patients undergoing lower revascularization. One problem with MRA is that it is difficult to cover the large volume that needs to be imaged. Multiple protocols have been set up to solve this issue. However, even with the recent advancements in MRA, our results have been disappointing in that the imaging of the tibial and pedal vessels has had poor sensitivity and specificity. Furthermore, we found that a large percentage of our patients were unable to undergo MRA.

On the other hand, careful examination of prior reports does reveal that certain areas of difficulty have been encountered with CTA. Even in a paper by Catalano et al.,[46] the most difficult area to visualize was in the tibial area, especially the peroneal artery. This paper stated that CTA had a tendency to overestimate disease. Again, none of the prior reports have included examination of the pedal vessels.

A review of the data obtained in this series indicated that CTA does not yet seem able to obtain adequate data, at least for this highly specific population at our institution. Prior investigators have suggested that the correlation between CTA and CA was adequate.[46–49] However, other larger series have demonstrated poorer results in the infrapopliteal regions.[50–53] These discrepancies may be partially due to differences in the technologies being used as rapid advances have been made. Furthermore, there has been little correlation in prior reports in the types of interventions that would be planned based upon these data. Again because of our referral base, most of our patients were quite elderly with limb-threatening ischemia, in contrast to some of the prior series where mostly claudicants were evaluated. These data still suggest that since it is not possible to identify in which patients the data is not reliable, it seems that in this selected population, CTA does not obtain adequate results to base interventions upon. These preliminary data suggest that, with future advancements, noninvasive imaging technologies may have an important role in evaluating patients undergoing lower revascularization.

ACKNOWLEDGMENTS

Special acknowledgment to Anne Ober for editorial assistance.

REFERENCES

1. Seldinger S. Catheter replacement of the needle in percutaneous arteriography. *Acta Radiol.* 1953;39:368–376.
2. Ascher E, Markevich N, Schutzer RW, et al. Duplex arteriography prior to femoral-popliteal reconstruction in claudicants: a proposal for a new shortened protocol. *Ann Vasc Surg.* 2004;18:544–551.
3. Ascher E, Hingorani A, Markevich N, et al. Role of duplex arteriography as the sole preoperative imaging modality prior to lower extremity revascularization surgery in diabetic and renal patients. *Ann Vasc Surg.* 2004;18:433–439.
4. Hingorani A, Ascher E, Markevich N, et al. A comparison of magnetic resonance angiography, contrast arteriography, and duplex arteriography for patients undergoing lower extremity revascularization. *Ann Vasc Surg.* 2004;18:294–301.
5. Hingorani A, Ascher E, Markevich N, et al. Magnetic resonance angiography versus duplex arteriography in patients undergoing lower extremity revascularization: which is the best replacement for contrast arteriography? *J Vasc Surg.* 2004;39:717–722.
6. Ascher E, Hingorani A, Markevich N, et al. Acute lower limb ischemia: the value of duplex ultrasound arterial mapping (DUAM) as the sole preoperative imaging technique. *Ann Vasc Surg.* 2003;17:284–289.
7. Ascher E, Hingorani A, Markevich N, et al. Lower extremity revascularization without preoperative contrast arteriography: experience with duplex ultrasound arterial mapping in 485 cases. *Ann Vasc Surg.* 2002;16:108–114.
8. Mazzariol F, Ascher E, Hingorani A, et al. Lower-extremity revascularisation without preoperative contrast arteriography in 185 cases: lessons learned with duplex ultrasound arterial mapping. *Eur J Vasc Endovasc Surg.* 2000;19:509–515.
9. Ascher E, Mazzariol F, Hingorani A, et al. The use of duplex ultrasound arterial mapping as an alternative to conventional arteriography for primary and secondary infrapopliteal bypasses. *Am J Surg.* 1999;178:162–165.
10. Mazzariol F, Ascher E, Salles-Cunha SX, et al. Values and limitations of duplex ultrasonography as the sole imaging method of preoperative evaluation for popliteal and infrapopliteal bypasses. *Ann Vasc Surg.* 1999;13:1–10.
11. Hingorani A, Ascher E. Dyeless vascular surgery. *Cardiovasc Surg.* 2003;11:12–18.
12. Loewe C, Schoder M, Rand T, et al. Peripheral vascular occlusive disease: evaluation with contrast-enhanced moving-bed MR angiography versus digital subtraction angiography in 106 patients. *AJR Am J Roentgenol.* 2002;179:1013–1021.
13. Eiberg JP, Lundorf E, Thomsen C, et al. Peripheral vascular surgery and magnetic resonance arteriography—a review. *Eur J Vasc Endovasc Surg.* 2001;22:396–402.
14. Mast BA. Comparison of magnetic resonance angiography and digital subtraction angiography for visualization of lower extremity arteries. *Ann Plast Surg.* 2001;46:261–264.
15. Pellerin M, Coquille F, Hubert M, et al. Comparison between arteriography and magnetic resonance angiography in patients with leg peripheral arterial disease. *J Radiol.* 2001;82(3 Pt 1):237–243.
16. Koelemay MJ, Lijmer JG, Stoker J, et al. Magnetic resonance angiography for the evaluation of lower extremity arterial disease: a meta-analysis. *JAMA.* 2001;285:1338–1345.
17. Ruehm SG, Hany TF, Pfammatter T, et al. Pelvic and lower extremity arterial imaging: diagnostic performance of three-dimensional contrast-enhanced MR angiography. *AJR Am J Roentgenol.* 2000;174:1127–1135.

18. Kreitner KF, Kalden P, Neufang A, et al. Diabetes and peripheral arterial occlusive disease: prospective comparison of contrast-enhanced three-dimensional MR angiography with conventional digital subtraction angiography. *AJR Am J Roentgenol.* 2000;174: 171–179.

19. Sueyoshi E, Sakamoto I, Matsuoka Y, et al. Aortoiliac and lower extremity arteries: comparison of three-dimensional dynamic contrast-enhanced subtraction MR angiography and conventional angiography. *Radiology.* 1999;210:683–688.

20. Levy MM, Baum RA, Carpenter JP. Endovascular surgery based solely on noninvasive preprocedural imaging. *J Vasc Surg.* 1998; 28:995–1003.

21. Hofmann WJ, Forstner R, Kofler B, et al. Pedal artery imaging—a comparison of selective digital subtraction angiography, contrast enhanced magnetic resonance angiography and duplex ultrasound. *Eur J Vasc Endovasc Surg.* 2002;24:287–292.

22. Winchester PA, Lee HM, Khilnani NM, et al. Comparison of two-dimensional MR digital subtraction angiography of the lower extremity with x-ray angiography. *J Vasc Interv Radiol.* 1998;9: 891–899.

23. Hoch JR, Tullis MJ, Kennell TW, et al. Use of magnetic resonance angiography for the preoperative evaluation of patients with infrainguinal arterial occlusive disease. *J Vasc Surg.* 1996;23: 792–800.

24. Carpenter JP, Owen RS, Baum RA, et al. Magnetic resonance angiography of peripheral runoff vessels. *J Vasc Surg.* 1992;16:807–813.

25. Soule B, Hingorani A, Ascher E. Comparison of Magnetic Resonance Angiography (MRA) and Duplex Ultrasound Arterial Mapping (DUAM) prior to infrainguinal arterial reconstruction. *Eur J Vasc Endovasc Surg.* 2003;25:139–146.

26. Hofmann WJ, Forstner R. Pedal artery imaging using DSA, CE-MRA and duplex. *Acta Chir Belg.* 2002;102:92–96.

27. Lundin P, Svensson A, Henriksen E, et al. Imaging of aortoiliac arterial disease. Duplex ultrasound and MR angiography versus digital subtraction angiography. *Acta Radiol.* 2000;41:125–132.

28. Leyendecker JR, Elsass KD, Johnson SP, et al. The role of infrapopliteal MR angiography in patients undergoing optimal contrast angiography for chronic limb-threatening ischemia. *J Vasc Interv Radiol.* 1998;9:545–551.

29. Cambria RP, Kaufman JA, L'Italien GJ, et al. Magnetic resonance angiography in the management of lower extremity arterial occlusive disease: a prospective study. *J Vasc Surg.* 1997;25:380–389.

30. Snidow JJ, Harris VJ, Trerotola SO, et al. Interpretations and treatment decisions based on MR angiography versus conventional arteriography in symptomatic lower extremity ischemia. *J Vasc Interv Radiol.* 1995;6:595–603.

31. Carpenter JP, Owen RS, Baum RA, et al. Magnetic resonance angiography of peripheral runoff vessels. *J Vasc Surg.* 1992;16:807–813.

32. Waugh JR, Sacharias N. Arteriographic complications in the DSA era. *Radiology.* 1992;182:243–246.

33. Lautin EM, Freeman NJ, Schoenfeld AH, et al. Radiocontrast-associated renal dysfunction: incidence and risk factors. *AJR Am J Roentgenol.* 1991;157:49–58.

34. Gussenhoven MJ, Ravensbergen J, van Bockel JH, et al. Renal dysfunction after angiography; a risk factor analysis in patients with peripheral vascular disease. *J Cardiovasc Surg (Torino).* 1991;32: 81–86.

35. Martin Paredero V, Dixon SM, Baker JD, et al. Risk of renal failure after major angiography. *Arch Surg.* 1983;118:1417–1420.

36. Rudnick MR, Goldfarb S, Wexler L, et al., The Iohexol Cooperative Study. Nephrotoxicity of ionic and nonionic contrast media in 1196 patients: a randomized trial. *Kidney Int.* 1995;47:254–261.

37. Parfrey PS, Griffiths SM, Barrett BJ, et al. Contrast material-induced renal failure in patients with diabetes mellitus, renal insufficiency, or both. A prospective controlled study. *N Engl J Med.* 1989;320:143–149.

38. Wilson YG, George JK, Wilkins DC, et al. Duplex assessment of run-off before femorocrural reconstruction. *Br J Surg.* 1997;84: 1360–1363.

39. Humphreys P, McCarthy M, Tuomilehto J, et al. Chromosome 4q locus associated with insulin resistance in Pima Indians. Studies in three European NIDDM populations. *Diabetes.* 1994;43:800–804.

40. Nelson RG, Knowler WC, McCance DR, et al. Determinants of end-stage renal disease in Pima Indians with type 2 (non-insulin-dependent) diabetes mellitus and proteinuria. *Diabetologia.* 1993; 36:087–093.

41. Nelson RG, Newman JM, Knowler WC, et al. Incidence of end-stage renal disease in type 2 (non-insulin-dependent) diabetes mellitus in Pima Indians. *Diabetologia.* 1988;31:730–736.

42. Perneger TV, Brancati FL, Whelton PK, et al. End-stage renal disease attributable to diabetes mellitus. *Ann Intern Med.* 1994;121: 912–918.

43. Ismail N, Becker B, Strzelczyk P, et al. Renal disease and hypertension in non-insulin-dependent diabetes mellitus. *Kidney Int.* 1999;55:1–28.

44. Maschio G, Alberti D, Janin G, et al, for The Angiotensin-Converting-Enzyme Inhibition in Progressive Renal Insufficiency Study Group. Effect of the angiotensin-converting-enzyme inhibitor benazepril on the progression of chronic renal insufficiency. *N Engl J Med.* 1996;334:939–945.

45. Kshirsagar AV, Joy MS, Hogan SL, et al. Effect of ACE inhibitors in diabetic and nondiabetic chronic renal disease: a systematic overview of randomized placebo-controlled trials. *Am J Kidney Dis.* 2000;35:695–707.

46. Catalano C, Fraioli F, Laghi A, et al. Infrarenal aortic and lower-extremity arterial disease: diagnostic performance of multi-detector row CT angiography. *Radiology.* 2004;231:555–563.

47. Martin ML, Tay KH, Flak B, et al. Multidetector CT angiography of the aortoiliac system and lower extremities: a prospective comparison with digital subtraction angiography. *AJR Am J Roentgenol.* 2003;180:1085–1091.

48. Rubin GD, Schmidt AJ, Logan LJ, et al. Multi-detector row CT angiography of lower extremity arterial inflow and runoff: initial experience. *Radiology.* 2001;221:146–158.

49. Mesurolle B, Qanadli SD, El Hajjam M, et al. Occlusive arterial disease of abdominal aorta and lower extremities: comparison of helical CT angiography with transcatheter angiography. *Clin Imaging.* 2004;28:252–260. Jul-

50. Portugaller HR, Schoellnast H, Hausegger KA, et al. Multislice spiral CT angiography in peripheral arterial occlusive disease: a valuable tool in detecting significant arterial lumen narrowing? *Eur Radiol.* 2004;14:1681–1687.

51. Heuschmid M, Krieger A, Beierlein W, et al. Assessment of peripheral arterial occlusive disease: comparison of multislice-CT angiography (MS-CTA) and intraarterial digital subtraction angiography (IA-DSA). *Eur J Med Res.* 2003;8:389–396.

52. Ishikawa M, Morimoto N, Sasajima T, et al. Three-dimensional computed tomographic angiography in lower extremity revascularization. *Surg Today.* 1999;29:243–247.

53. Rieker O, Duber C, Schmiedt W, et al. Prospective comparison of CT angiography of the legs with intraarterial digital subtraction angiography. *AJR Am J Roentgenol.* 1996;166:269–276.

Embryology of the Arterial System to the Lower Extremities

15

Joseph Giordano

Development of the human vascular system occurs from a complicated series of events that begins with nothing more than a collection of cells. The cells unite and line up to form vascular channels, initially developing a vascular system similar to the vascular system of primitive vertebrates. These channels rearrange themselves to become the mature vascular system of the human body. The formation of the vascular system in the lower extremities is part of this system, but it is less complicated and easier to understand than formation of the vascular system in the rest of the body.

For the first 3 weeks of gestation, the embryo receives oxygen and nutrients from the yolk sac and the maternal circulation. At the end of the third week, the rapidly developing embryo needs a more complete vascular system to support its growth. The endothelial-lined channels connect to the developing heart, which, at 3 weeks, consists only of two tubes but is still capable of circulating blood.

At the beginning of the fourth week, these two tubes connect to a paired dorsal aorta that extends down the entire length of the embryo. Each dorsal aorta has 36 to 38 segmental dorsal, lateral, and ventral branches. At the level of the C7 vertebrae, the dorsal aortae fuse but maintain the segmental branches. Therefore, the fused dorsal aorta has two ventral branches, a lateral branch on each side of the aorta, and two dorsal branches.

These branches form various segments of the mature arterial system. The lateral segmental branches fuse and become single renal arteries bilaterally. The proximal ventral branches eventually coalesce to form celiac, superior mesenteric, and inferior mesenteric arteries. The dorsal branches become the vertebral arteries in the neck, the intercostal arteries in the chest, and the lumbar arteries in the abdomen. The most distal ventral arteries of the fused aorta become the common iliac artery. This connects to the most distal dorsal segmental arteries, which become internal iliac arteries. It is through these two structures that the vascular system to the lower extremities develops.

The lower extremity limbs begin to develop at the beginning of the fourth week. Small elevations or buds appear at the side of the trunk. The mesoderm pushes into the limb buds and eventually differentiates into the various components of the lower extremities. To support the developing limb bud, the embryo develops two vascular systems.[1] The initial arterial system, an axial system, courses down the center of the developing limb bud (see Fig. 15-1). This first system forms from the internal iliac artery and follows the sciatic nerve through the posterior aspect of the thigh. This developing sciatic artery ends at the level of the popliteal artery. As the sciatic artery completes its development, a second vascular system, the external iliac artery, develops

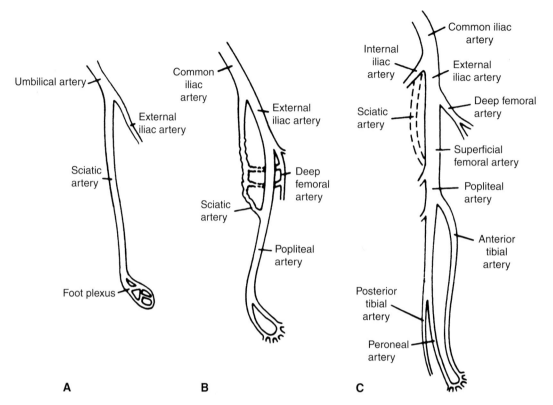

Figure 15-1   Arterial supply to the left lower extremity. **A:** Sciatic artery forming as a branch of the internal iliac artery. **B:** The sciatic artery regresses, while the external artery develops into the common femoral artery to supply the thigh. **C:** The sciatic artery disappears.

from the common iliac artery. This external iliac artery growth continues, leading to development of the common femoral, the superficial femoral, and the deep femoral arteries. Once the mature vascular system is fully developed down to the popliteal artery, the sciatic system completely regresses except for branches of the internal iliac artery and segments of the popliteal artery, tibial peroneal trunk, and the peroneal artery.

The union of the primitive sciatic system with the ileofemoral system at the level of the lower thigh produces the mature popliteal artery. The sciatic system forms a popliteal artery, but the distal segment of this popliteal artery anterior to the popliteus muscle regresses (see Fig. 15-2). The later-developing superficial popliteal artery of the ileofemoral system is posterior to the popliteus muscle, and it unites with the proximal segment of the superficial popliteal artery of the sciatic system to form the mature popliteal artery.

The development of the lower extremity vascular system proceeds perfectly in the overwhelming majority of cases. However, not surprisingly, some lower extremity vascular anomalies do develop. Although rare, they are of interest, and they highlight the importance of embryology in the development of the vascular system.

PERSISTENT SCIATIC ARTERY

The sciatic artery is the initial vascular system that supplies the developing lower extremity. This system regresses to be replaced by the ileofemoral system. However, in a very small percentage of cases, 0.05%, the sciatic system does not regress and may be the sole vascular system for the supply of blood to the lower extremity.[2] It may be complete from its origin at the internal iliac artery to its union with the popliteal artery. The artery anatomically runs with the sciatic nerve in a posterior location, entering the thigh through the sciatic notch and remaining posterior to the adductor magnus muscle as it enters the popliteal fossa to join the popliteal artery. Clinically, the patients with this condition have easily palpable popliteal and ankle pulses, but femoral artery pulses are absent.

The posterior superficial location of the artery predisposes it to traumatic injury, particularly at the sciatic notch area. This artery may occlude, become aneurysmal, or develop early atherosclerotic changes just from normal activities such as sitting.[3] The artery can also compress the sciatic nerve, causing neurologic symptoms. At times, the sciatic artery is not complete, but just segments of it remain. The incomplete artery maintains

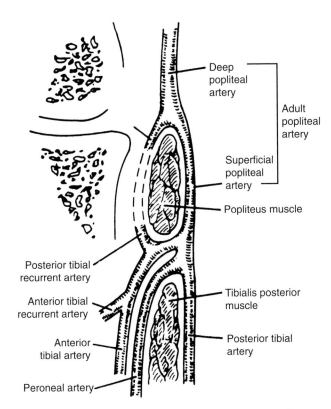

Figure 15-2 Embryologic development of the popliteal artery, as modified from Senior (*Am J Anat.* 25:55, 1919). The distal popliteal artery, part of the sciatic system, anterior to the popliteus muscle regresses, and the superficial popliteal artery, part of the ileofemoral system, unites with the proximal popliteal artery of the sciatic system to become the mature popliteal artery. (From Gibson MHL, Mills JG, Johnson GE, et al. Popliteal entrapment syndrome. *Ann Surg.* 1977;185:341, with permission.)

a connection with both the internal iliac artery and the popliteal artery through small collaterals.

POPLITEAL ENTRAPMENT SYNDROME

As the popliteal artery is developing, the gastrocnemius muscle arises from the calcaneus, migrates cephalad, and attaches to the femur. The lateral head attaches first, while the medial head attaches later. At the time of the attachment of the medial head, the popliteal artery has already formed and is in its normal anatomic location. However, if the popliteal artery develops late, or if the insertion of the medial head occurs early, the artery may be swept medially to become entrapped against the femur.[4] This is termed popliteal entrapment syndrome, an anomaly that persists throughout adulthood. The constant trauma by the gastrocnemius muscle against the medially displaced popliteal artery can cause aneurysms and occlusions. In the clinical setting, a relatively young person will develop claudication and may have reduced pulses with exercise. An arteriogram will show sweeping of the popliteal artery to the medial side due to the gastrocnemius muscle. It is quite common

for popliteal entrapment to be bilateral, so it is important that arteriography be used to investigate both legs for the syndrome. Magnetic resonance imaging (MRI) or computed tomography (CT) scan of the knee can clearly demonstrate the relationship of the popliteal artery and vein to the muscular structures of the popliteal fossa.

It is interesting to speculate why popliteal entrapment syndrome never occurs by entrapping the artery laterally instead of medially. This probably does not happen because the lateral head attaches so much earlier—well before the popliteal artery forms—and therefore cannot affect the popliteal artery.

APLASIA OR HYPOPLASIA OF ILEOFEMORAL ARTERIAL SYSTEM

The presence of persistent sciatic artery is frequently accompanied by absence of all or parts of the ileofemoral system. This is not surprising since a patent sciatic system can function as the sole blood supply to the lower extremities. However, aplasia or hypoplasia of any parts of the ileofemoral system has been described, even in the absence of a sciatic artery system.[5,6] This includes aplasia of the external iliac artery, superficial femoral artery, and deep femoral artery. Surprisingly, some of these patients can be relatively asymptomatic, although chronic lower leg ischemia can occur. Blood flow to the lower extremities in these entities is usually through collateral channels that connect to either the common femoral artery, in the case of the external iliac artery aplasia, or to the popliteal artery, in cases of superficial femoral artery aplasia. Also, anatomic anomalies of major arteries that bypass the aplastic segment have also been reported. These anomalies are usually diagnosed with complete arteriography.

In conclusion, the arterial system to the lower extremities develops from two systems: The initial sciatic system and the later-developing ileofemoral system. The merging of these two systems produces the mature arterial system to the lower extremities. Occasionally, developmental anomalies occur, but the incidence is low and rarely seen by vascular surgeons.

REFERENCES

1. Senior HD. The development of the arteries of the human lower extremity. *Am J Anat.* 1919;25:55.
2. Mayschak DT, Flye WM. Treatment of the persistent sciatic artery. *Ann Surg.* 1984;199:69.
3. McLellan GL, Morettin LB. Persistent sciatic artery: clinical, surgical, and angiographic aspects. *Arch Surg.* 1982;117:817.
4. Gibson MHL, Mills JG, Johnson GE, et al. Popliteal entrapment syndrome. *Ann Surg.* 1977;185:341.
5. Tamisier D, Melki JP, Cornier JM. Congenital anomalies of the external iliac artery. Case report and review of the literature. *Ann Vasc Surg.* 1990;4:510.
6. Schmidt J, Paety B, Allenberg ER Jr. Bilateral congenital aplasia of the deep femoral arteries. *Ann Vasc Surg.* 1990;4:498.

Labels on Figure 15-2:
- Deep popliteal artery
- Adult popliteal artery
- Superficial popliteal artery
- Popliteus muscle
- Posterior tibial recurrent artery
- Anterior tibial recurrent artery
- Tibialis posterior muscle
- Anterior tibial artery
- Posterior tibial artery
- Peroneal artery

16

Surgical Approaches, Dissection, and Control

Jamal J. Hoballah   *Christopher T. Bunch*

Lower limb revascularization in diabetic patients typically requires the construction of infrainguinal bypasses. Since the crural vessels are frequently involved in diabetic patients, lower extremity revascularization in this patient population warrants bypass to the lower leg, ankle, or foot. The success of such procedures depends on identification of an appropriate inflow source, an adequate target vessel, and the bridging of these two vessels with an autogenous vein to provide lasting uninterrupted flow to the foot. The selection of the inflow and target vessels is influenced by several factors including the length of adequate vein available, the presence of wounds or cellulitis in the lower extremity, and prior surgery. Hence, a vascular surgeon must be comfortable with exposures of all the major arteries of the lower extremity and their branches. Familiarity with alternative exposure techniques is essential to provide versatility in the construction of the bypass in challenging situations such as infection or scarring.

BLOOD VESSEL DISSECTION

Vessels are typically accessed through the shortest route possible and dissected sharply using a blunt-tipped scissors. A no.15 blade can also be used for the dissection and is especially valuable when dealing with scarred tissues in redo procedures. Self-retaining retractors are carefully placed at progressively deeper levels to avoid injury to neighboring vessels or nerves until the artery is exposed. With gentle traction applied on the adventitia and counter traction on the surrounding tissues, sharp dissection along the sidewall of the vessel will identify an avascular plane between the vessel and its surrounding tissues. This plane can be developed on each side of the vessel and followed posteriorly to achieve circumferential dissection of the vessel. Although circumferential dissection may be appealing, it is not always necessary. Anterior exposure of the tibial vessels may be all that is needed when a pneumatic external tourniquet or an internal vessel occluder is used for vascular control.

Blood vessels can be traced proximally and distally, anticipating their cylindrical shape and adjacent vascular structures. Throughout their dissection, vessels should be handled gently. Only the adventitia of arteries should be grasped with the forceps. Grasping the full thickness of the artery wall can cause intimal damage. Silastic vessel loops may be passed around a vessel and used for vessel retraction. However, only gentle traction on the vessel loop should be used to avoid damage to the vessel wall. The sites of major vascular branches can be anticipated from knowledge of surgical anatomy. Dividing arterial branches should be avoided as they may represent important collateral channels.

Vascular Control

Arterial control can be achieved using various methods. These methods include atraumatic vascular clamps, braided cotton "umbilical" tapes with Rummel tourniquets, silastic vessel loops, self-compressing clamps, internal occluders, and external pneumatic tourniquets. The size and location of the artery along with the presence or absence of plaque in its wall will influence the selection of the method used for control.

Atraumatic vascular clamps or tape with a Rummel tourniquet are typically used for control of the common femoral artery. In the absence of plaque, the vascular clamp is applied in the simplest manner that would not obscure the incision or exposure. In a diseased artery, the vascular clamp should be applied in a manner that would oppose the soft wall of the artery against the hard plaque without breaking the plaque or tearing the artery. Prior to applying a vascular clamp, it is a good habit to check the number of notches to click for complete apposition of the clamp jaws. Exceeding the number of notches may result in injury at the clamp application site even with the use of an "atraumatic" vascular clamp.

Silastic vessel loops, self-compressing clamps (such as the bulldog clamps or Yasargil intracranial aneurysm clips), internal occluders, and external pneumatic tourniquets are typically used to control smaller vessels such as the popliteal, crural, or pedal arteries.

A Silastic vessel loop can provide arterial control by encircling it around the blood vessel twice and then applying gentle tension on its ends. Excessive tension can be traumatic to the vessel wall. Vessel loops may be inadequate to control prosthetic grafts or diseased vessels the size of the common femoral artery. They can be ideal for arterial branches and may be replaced with double loops of 4-0 silk for control of small arterial branches originating from crural or pedal vessels.

Heifitz and Yasargil aneurysm clips require a special applicator for placing, which facilitates their delivery and removal in deep locations. They are less bulky than bulldog clamps, which have finger pads for pinching them open. The aneurysm clips are ideal for controlling the profunda, superficial femoral, and popliteal arteries.

Crural and pedal vessels are very prone to develop spasm during dissection and control. Furthermore, they may be very calcified, making their control challenging. The topical application of undiluted, warm papaverine solution (30 mg per mL) to crural or pedal arteries can help prevent or release the spasm. To avoid clamping such small vessels that could cause arterial damage or spasm at the clamping site, arterial control can be achieved by using internal occluders or an external pneumatic tourniquet.

Internal occluders are dumbbell-shaped devices also known as coronary occluders. They are available in sizes beginning at 1.0 mm and increasing by 0.25 mm increments to 3.0 mm. The arteriotomy is made without any clamping, and the occluder is inserted through the arteriotomy, interrupting the blood flow from within the lumen. Usually only exposure of the anterior surface of the vessel is required. Choosing the appropriate size of the internal occluder is important. A small size could result in bleeding around the occluder.

A large size could damage the intima if forced into the lumen. Occasionally, the presence of branches at the site of the arteriotomy or adjacent to the beginning or end of the arteriotomy may result in persistent bleeding. These branches need to be controlled with silk loops in order to achieve a dry field. Constructing an anastomosis with an occluder in place may be challenging at the beginning.

In the presence of heavy calcification, the arteriotomy may not allow the insertion of an internal occluder. Vascular control can be obtained by occluding the vessel from within, using two Fogarty balloon catheters, each attached to a three-way stopcock. Alternatively, an external pneumatic tourniquet can be used for control before creating the arteriotomy.

The external pneumatic tourniquet is an excellent method of controlling the infrageniculate blood vessels. The tourniquet provides arterial control without placing any intraluminal objects or any clamps that could compromise the exposure or injure the target artery. It is particularly useful in heavily calcified arteries. A sterile tourniquet is used and can be applied either above or just below the knee over a cotton roll. The leg is elevated and the venous blood is drained with the use of an Esmarch bandage firmly wrapped up the leg from the foot to the tourniquet site. The tourniquet is inflated to a pressure of 250 mm Hg and the arteriotomy is created. If there is still bleeding from the arteriotomy, the inflation pressure can be increased up to 350 mm Hg. Occluding the profunda femoris artery may also be required to provide the desired hemostasis. Prior to inflating the tourniquet, it is important to double-check the alignment of any grafts that originate proximal to it, to avoid any twists or unpleasant surprises when the tourniquet is deflated.

EXPOSURES

The Common Femoral Artery

Exposure through a Medial Infrainguinal Incision

The common femoral artery and its bifurcation are typically exposed through a vertical skin incision placed over the femoral pulse. If the femoral pulse is weak or not present, calcification in the common femoral artery may be palpable, aiding in localization of the vessel. A calcified femoral artery can often be palpated by rolling one's fingers gently over the femoral region. Alternatively, the incision is placed at a point midway between the pubic tubercle and the anterior superior iliac spine. If the saphenous vein is encountered during subcutaneous dissection, a more lateral course is sought. If nerves are encountered, the dissection is more lateral than the actual location of the femoral artery. Encountered lymphatics are ligated and divided to avoid postoperative lymph leaks. The femoral sheath is identified and incised, exposing the common femoral artery. As the common femoral artery is dissected distally, a change in the caliber of the exposed artery will mark the origin of the profunda femoris artery, and thus the transition from the common femoral to the superficial femoral artery. The superficial femoral artery can be further exposed and dissected distally by extending the incision distally (Fig. 16-1).

Exposure through a Transverse Suprainguinal Incision

An alternative approach to the common femoral artery is through a transverse suprainguinal incision placed two fingers'-breadth superior to the inguinal ligament. This incision is comparable to an inguinal hernia incision and can be used in the presence of macerated skin in the inguinal crease. The incision is deepened through the subcutaneous tissue and Scarpa's fascia until the inguinal ligament is identified. The inguinal ligament is mobilized and freed along its length to allow retraction superiorly. The femoral sheath is identified and is then incised longitudinally exposing the common femoral artery. Because exposure of the superficial and profunda femoris arteries will be limited, the potential need for extended profundaplasty or other reconstructions distal to the common femoral artery bifurcation may preclude this approach.

Exposure through a Lateral Incision

The common femoral artery can also be exposed through an incision placed lateral to its anatomic location.[1] The lateral approach is typically used in the presence of infection on the medial aspect of the groin, in the vicinity of the site where the usual vertical incision is performed. The incision can be made medial or lateral to the sartorius muscle. In the former, the skin incision is made 4 cm lateral to the femoral pulse. The incision is deepened to the level of the sartorius muscle without creating any skin flaps. The medial aspect of the sartorius muscle is mobilized and retracted laterally. The dissection is deepened medially towards the femoral vessels until the femoral sheath is identified. The femoral sheath is incised along its lateral aspect exposing the femoral arteries. In the latter exposure (Fig. 16-2), the incision is made approximately 6 to 8 cm lateral to the femoral pulse. The incision is carried down through the subcutaneous tissues until the fascia lata is identified. The fascia lata is incised and the sartorius muscle is approached from its lateral aspect. The dissection is then continued posterior to the sartorius muscle in the direction of the femoral vessels. This

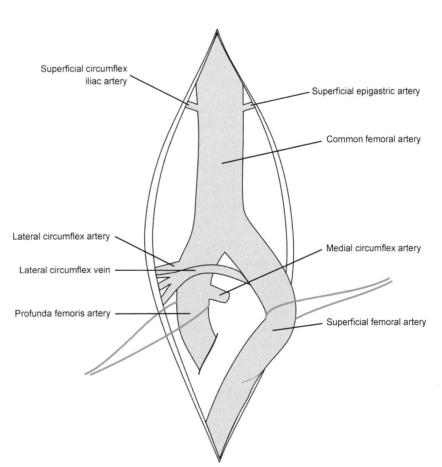

Figure 16-1 Exposure of the common femoral artery and its bifurcation. (From Hoballah JJ. *Vascular reconstructions: Anatomy, exposures, and techniques.* New York, NY: Springer-Verlag; 2000, with permission.)

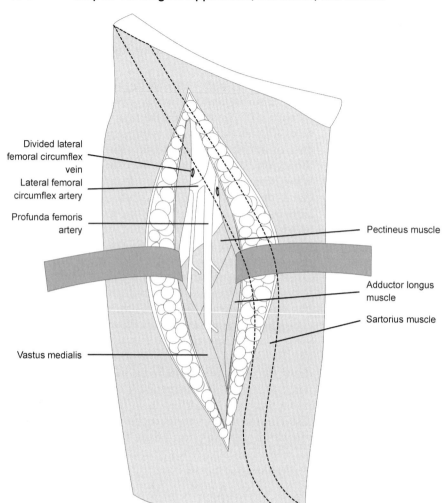

Divided lateral femoral circumflex vein

Lateral femoral circumflex artery

Profunda femoris artery

Vastus medialis

Pectineus muscle

Adductor longus muscle

Sartorius muscle

Figure 16-2 Lateral exposure of the common femoral and profunda femoris arteries. (From Hoballah JJ. *Vascular reconstructions: Anatomy, exposures, and techniques.* New York, NY: Springer-Verlag; 2000, with permission.)

usually requires mobilization of the proximal part of the sartorius muscle, which often necessitates transection of its first two segmental arterial branches. The femoral sheath is identified from beneath the sartorius muscle as the dissection is carried medially. The femoral sheath is incised along its lateral border exposing the common femoral artery. Extending the incision distally will allow for exposure of the superficial and profunda femoris arteries.

Technical Tips during Redo Procedures

After previous groin procedures, dense fibrous scarring typically surrounds the femoral vessels. Identifying and encircling the superficial femoral artery underneath the sartorius muscle a few centimeters distal to its origin, and then tracing the dissection proximally, may facilitate the exposure. The dissection begins on the medial aspect to minimize the chances of injury to the origin of the profunda femoris artery. The medial dissection is extended proximally to the level of the inguinal ligament where circumferential dissection of the common femoral or external iliac artery is performed to allow

proximal control. The dissection is then continued on the lateral aspect starting at the inguinal ligament and progressing distally to identify and control the profunda femoris artery. In the presence of dense scarring, control of the profunda femoris artery may be safer from within, using an internal occluding Fogarty catheter. Dissection with a no. 15 blade may also be necessary in dense scar tissue.

In the presence of severe calcification in the common femoral artery that does not allow the safe application of a vascular clamp, extending the dissection underneath the inguinal ligament will frequently identify a soft segment in the external iliac artery just proximal to the origin of the superficial iliac circumflex and superficial epigastric branches. The inguinal ligament may be divided to allow more proximal exposure of the external iliac artery.

The Profunda Femoris Artery

For the sake of describing surgical exposures, the profunda is divided arbitrarily into three zones. The proximal zone extends from the origin to just distal to the lateral femoral circumflex artery. The distal zone is the part distal to the femoral triangle and is usually distal to the second perforating muscle branch. The middle zone is the segment between the proximal and distal zones (Fig. 16-3).

Medial Exposure of the Proximal Profunda Femoris Artery

The profunda femoris artery can be approached by exposing the common femoral artery distally and proceeding with the dissection along its lateral and posterior aspect to expose the origin of the profunda femoris artery (Fig. 16-1). Circumferential dissection of the common femoral bifurcation to identify any posterior branches originating from the common femoral artery is important to avoid unexpected retrograde bleeding from these branches upon creating an arteriotomy.

Immediately after its origin from the common femoral artery, venous branches often cross the profunda femoris. The first large venous branch is usually the lateral femoral circumflex vein, which crosses over the profunda femoris artery to join the more medial superficial femoral vein (Fig. 16-1). Division of these veins is essential in order to expose the profunda femoris artery further distally. The dissection can continue distally, following the profunda femoris artery and its branches for 5 to 8 cm.

Medial Exposure of the Mid and Distal Zones of the Profunda Femoris Artery

Mid and distal zones of the profunda femoris artery can be exposed without exposing the common femoral bifurcation.[2] A 10- to 12-cm skin incision is performed over the medial aspect of the sartorius muscle. The superficial femoral artery and vein are noted and

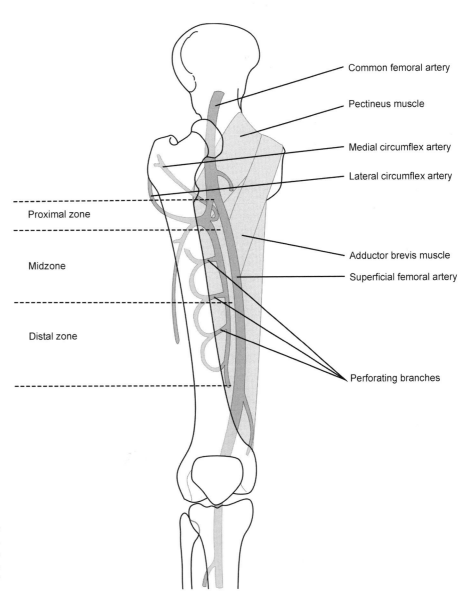

Figure 16-3 Zones of the deep femoral artery. (From Hoballah JJ. *Vascular reconstructions: Anatomy, exposures, and techniques.* New York, NY: Springer-Verlag; 2000, with permission.)

Common femoral artery

Pectineus muscle

Medial circumflex artery

Lateral circumflex artery

Adductor brevis muscle

Superficial femoral artery

Perforating branches

Proximal zone

Midzone

Distal zone

retracted without dissection along with the sartorius muscle anteriorly and laterally. The dissection is then continued posteriorly toward the femur. A fibrous layer between the adductor longus muscle and the vastus medialis muscle is incised longitudinally. The location of the profunda femoris artery underneath this layer can be identified by palpation or by using a sterile Doppler. Frequently one of the veins accompanying the profunda femoris artery is first visualized. Dissection and mobilization of the accompanying vein will expose the profunda femoris artery.

Lateral Exposure of the Profunda Femoris Artery

A 10- to 12-cm skin incision along the lateral border of the sartorius muscle is performed as described for the lateral exposure of the common femoral artery (Fig. 16-2). The sartorius muscle is mobilized medially. The superficial femoral artery is identified in a plane directly posterior and medial to the sartorius muscle. Dissecting in a deeper plane posterior to the sartorius muscle identifies the profunda femoris artery. This is achieved by incising the connective tissue membrane that extends from the adductor longus to the vastus medialis. The first vessel identified is usually the lateral femoral circumflex artery. After transecting its accompanying vein and dissecting medially toward its origin, the profunda femoris artery is exposed (Fig. 16-2).[3]

Medial Exposure of the Superficial Femoral Artery in the Upper Thigh

A longitudinal incision is performed along the course of the inferior border of the sartorius muscle. The muscular fascia is incised exposing the sartorius muscle. Care is taken to avoid injuring the greater saphenous vein. Dissection along the inferior border of the sartorius muscle is performed and the sartorius muscle is retracted laterally exposing the superficial femoral artery and its accompanying vein.

The Popliteal Artery

Medial Exposure of the Suprageniculate Popliteal Artery

A longitudinal skin incision is performed from the level of the knee joint extending 10 to 12 cm proximally (Fig. 16-4). The incision is usually placed along the anticipated location of the anterior border of the sartorius muscle when a prosthetic bypass is being used. If the ipsilateral greater saphenous vein is being utilized as a bypass, the same incision used to expose the vein can also be employed to expose the popliteal artery above the knee. The incision is deepened through the subcutaneous tissue until the adductor tendon is identified anteriorly and the upper border of the sartorius muscle is noted posteriorly. The fascia between the adductor tendon and the sartorius muscle is incised and the popliteal fossa is entered. Self-retaining retractors are placed in a deeper plane retracting the adductor tendon anteriorly and the sartorius muscle posteriorly. In order to improve the exposure, the knee is bent and a rolled towel is placed underneath the proximal thigh. Placing the rolled towel directly under the knee can compress the popliteal fossa rather than allowing it to expand for the exposure of the popliteal vessels. In patients with occlusive disease, the hardened calcified popliteal artery can be easily palpated in the popliteal fossa. The popliteal artery can be dissected proximally until it is seen exiting from the adductor canal. Care should be taken at this level to avoid injury to the

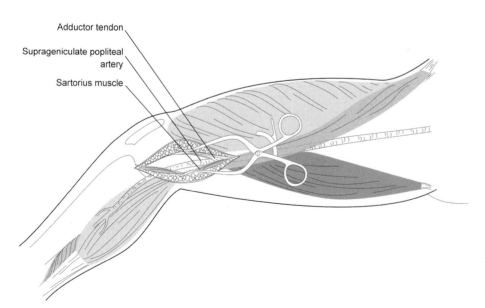

Adductor tendon

Suprageniculate popliteal artery

Sartorius muscle

Figure 16-4 Medial exposure of the suprageniculate popliteal artery: The popliteal fossa is entered. (From Hoballah JJ. *Vascular reconstructions: Anatomy, exposures, and techniques.* New York, NY: Springer-Verlag; 2000, with permission.)

greater saphenous nerve as it exits from the adductor canal and courses anteriorly to run with the greater saphenous vein. Distally, the popliteal artery can be dissected to the level of the knee joint.

Lateral Exposure of the Suprageniculate Popliteal Artery

The suprageniculate popliteal artery can also be exposed through a lateral approach.[4–6] A 10- to 12-cm, longitudinal incision is made from just above the knee joint extending proximally along the lateral aspect of the distal thigh (Fig. 16-5). The incision lies one centimeter posterior to and parallel to the iliotibial tract. Once the deep fascia is incised, the space between the iliotibial tract and biceps femoris muscle is opened, exposing the above-knee popliteal artery. The distal superficial femoral artery can be exposed by extending the incision more proximally and incising the adductor magnus muscle.

Medial Exposure of the Infrageniculate Popliteal Artery

A longitudinal skin incision is made from the level of the knee joint and extended distally for 10 to 12 cm (Fig. 16-6). The greater saphenous vein is avoided in the subcutaneous plane as the dissection continues to the underlying muscular fascia. The fascia is incised and the popliteal space is entered between the gastrocnemius and soleus muscles using a sweeping motion with the index finger. With the knee bent, self-retaining retractors are applied to retract the gastrocnemius muscle posteriorly and laterally, exposing the popliteal space further. The tendons of the semimembranosus and semitendinosus muscles are identified in the upper corner of the incision and divided. Distally, the soleus muscle typically covers the popliteal artery at the level

of its trifurcation. Dissection in the areolar tissue will identify the popliteal vascular bundle. The popliteal vein is then identified lying anterior to the popliteal artery. It is not uncommon to find two popliteal veins surrounding the popliteal artery. The popliteal vein is mobilized exposing the popliteal artery. The popliteal artery is then dissected and encircled with a Silastic vessel loop. Gentle traction on the vessel loop will assist in the extension of the dissection proximally and distally.

Exposure of the popliteal artery trifurcation typically requires dividing the overlying soleus muscle (Fig. 16-7). A right angle clamp is placed underneath the soleus muscle to guide the transection of the muscle using electrocautery. Soleal veins, if encountered, are suture ligated. The origin of the anterior tibial artery is usually first identified. Very commonly an anterior tibial vein will be seen crossing over the artery and joining the popliteal vein. The anterior tibial vein and other similar crossing veins may need to be ligated and divided in order to allow for the exposure of the origin of the anterior tibial artery, as well as the takeoff of the tibioperoneal trunk. The anterior tibial artery can be further dissected for another 1 to 2 cm by incising the interosseous membrane and the muscular fibers beneath it. This will allow for additional exposure of the anterior tibial artery from the medial aspect of the leg.

Lateral Exposure of the Infrageniculate Popliteal Artery

The more commonly used lateral approach to expose the popliteal artery involves resection of the proximal fibula.[5–9] A longitudinal incision is made starting at the head of the fibula and extending distally for 10 to 12 cm (Fig. 16-8). The incision is deepened through the subcutaneous tissue. The peroneal nerve is identified as it crosses over the neck of the fibula and is gently

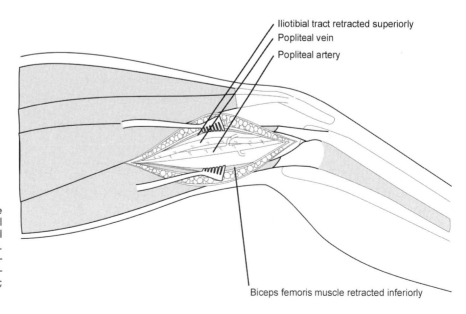

Figure 16-5 Lateral exposure of the above knee popliteal artery: The popliteal space is entered between the iliotibial tract and the biceps femoris muscle. (From Hoballah JJ. *Vascular reconstructions: Anatomy, exposures, and techniques.* New York, NY: Springer-Verlag; 2000, with permission.)

Iliotibial tract retracted superiorly
Popliteal vein
Popliteal artery

Biceps femoris muscle retracted inferiorly

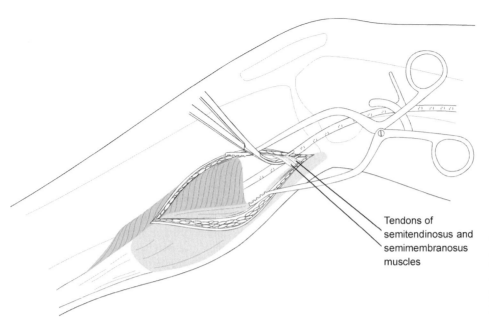

Tendons of semitendinosus and semimembranosus muscles

Figure 16-6 Exposure of the below-knee popliteal artery can be improved by dividing the tendons of the semitendinosus and semimembranosus muscles. (From Hoballah JJ. *Vascular reconstructions: Anatomy, exposures, and techniques.* New York, NY: Springer-Verlag; 2000, with permission.)

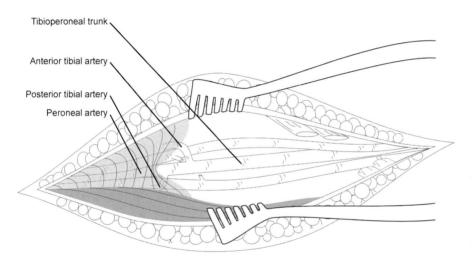

Tibioperoneal trunk

Anterior tibial artery

Posterior tibial artery

Peroneal artery

Figure 16-7 Exposure of the popliteal trifurcation: The overlying soleus muscle and the crossing tibial veins are divided to expose the origin of the tibial vessels. (From Hoballah JJ. *Vascular reconstructions: Anatomy, exposures, and techniques.* New York, NY: Springer-Verlag; 2000, with permission.)

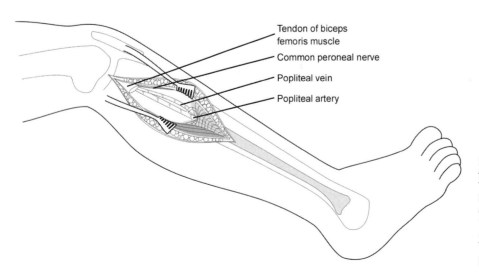

Tendon of biceps femoris muscle

Common peroneal nerve

Popliteal vein

Popliteal artery

Figure 16-8 Lateral exposure of the infrageniculate popliteal artery: The popliteal space is entered by incising the posterior periosteum of the excised fibula. (From Hoballah JJ. *Vascular reconstructions: Anatomy, exposures, and techniques.* New York, NY: Springer-Verlag; 2000, with permission.)

dissected and mobilized. The fibular periosteum is exposed, incised, and elevated off the fibula. A right angle clamp is carefully passed under the fibula and can be used to separate the fibula from its posterior attachments. The fibula is transected approximately 6 to 8 cm distal to its neck. The proximal segment is lifted with a bone grasper and the muscular and ligamentous attachment of the fibula and the biceps femoris tendon are divided. The proximal part of the fibula is removed and the popliteal fossa is entered. The popliteal artery is palpated and dissected. The tibial nerve is usually identified crossing the below-knee popliteal artery from the lateral to the medial direction and is separated from it by the popliteal vein. More distal dissection provides a very satisfactory exposure of the trifurcation vessels. Exposure of the infrageniculate popliteal artery through a lateral approach without

fibular resection has also been described. However, this exposure is usually more limited than when the proximal fibula is resected.

Posterior Exposure of the Popliteal Artery

The popliteal artery can also be exposed through a posterior approach (Fig. 16-9). This requires placing the patient in a prone position. An S-shaped incision measuring 12 to 14 cm is then performed starting along the medial aspect of the distal thigh. The incision is deepened through the subcutaneous tissues exposing the popliteal fascia. The popliteal fascia is incised and the popliteal space is entered. The first structure encountered is usually the tibial nerve, which is protected along with the common peroneal nerve. The popliteal vein is identified, dissected, and retracted, exposing the popliteal artery. This approach provides a good

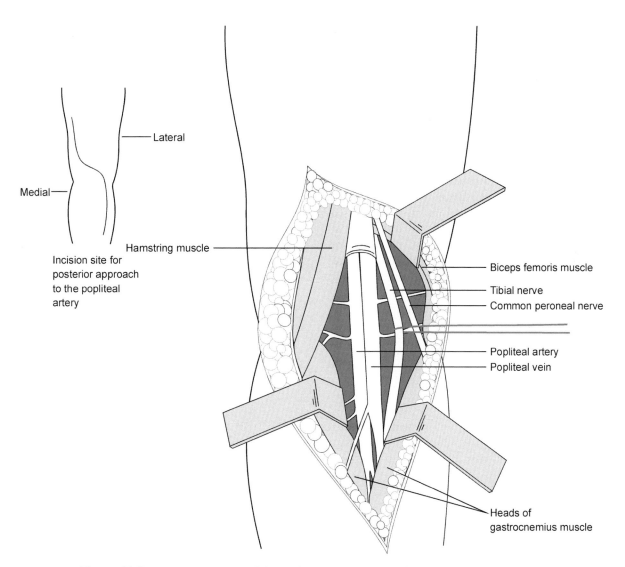

Figure 16-9 Posterior exposure of the popliteal artery. (From Hoballah JJ. *Vascular reconstructions: Anatomy, exposures, and techniques.* New York, NY: Springer-Verlag; 2000, with permission.)

exposure of the midpopliteal artery at the level of the knee joint. Proximal exposure is achieved by retracting the biceps femoris muscle laterally and the hamstring muscles medially. Dissection of the distal part of the popliteal artery is achieved by retracting the heads of the gastrocnemius muscle, exposing the origin of the anterior tibial artery as the popliteal artery dips underneath the soleus muscle. The extent of the proximal and distal dissection of the popliteal artery using this approach is limited.

The Anterior Tibial Artery

Medial Exposure of the Anterior Tibial Artery
The anterior tibial artery is usually exposed through a lateral approach (Fig. 16-10). However, the proximal few centimeters of the anterior tibial artery can be exposed from a medial approach by exposing the distal popliteal artery and incising the interosseous membrane.[10] In order to assist in the exposure of the anterior tibial artery through a medial approach, digital pressure is applied on the skin overlying the anterolateral compartment, displacing the anterior tibial artery medially. Nevertheless, the anterior tibial artery will remain in a deep location making an anastomosis from this medial approach rather challenging.

Lateral Exposure of the Anterior Tibial Artery
The lateral approach to the anterior tibial artery is achieved through a longitudinal incision performed parallel to the tibia. The incision starts 2 cm inferior to the tibial plateau and extends for 10 to 12 cm. The skin incision is deepened through the subcutaneous tissue, identifying the fascia, which is incised longitudinally. The origin of the anterior tibialis muscle is broadly attached to the tibia. The next muscle identified inferior

to the tibialis anterior muscle is the extensor hallucis muscle. The longitudinal cleft between these two muscles is entered. Using gentle blunt dissection, the interosseous membrane is approached. The anterior tibial artery and veins and peroneal nerve will be seen at the deep aspect of the incision. Positioning the self-retaining retractors deeper in the wound enhances the exposure of the vessels.

Lateral Exposure of the Anterior Tibial Artery in the Lower Leg
In the lower leg, the anterior tibial artery is more superficial and lies between the tendinous portions of the extensor muscles. A 10- to 12-cm incision is made parallel, and 2 cm inferior and lateral, to the tibia. The first tendon close to the tibia is the tendon of the tibialis anterior muscle. On the inferior aspect, the tendon of the extensor hallucis longus muscle is noted. As the anterior tibial artery progresses to become the dorsalis pedis, it continues into the foot and passes underneath the tendon of the extensor hallucis longus muscle, which crosses from lateral to medial to attach on the great toe. Just above the ankle, the anterior tibial artery is exposed by a short longitudinal incision with retraction of the extensor digitorum longus muscle laterally and the extensor hallucis longus muscle medially.

The Tibioperoneal Trunk

Medial Exposure of the Tibioperoneal Trunk
The tibioperoneal trunk is exposed by the same approach used to expose the infrageniculate popliteal artery, and then extending the dissection distally (Fig. 16-7). A right angle clamp is placed posterior to the soleus muscle and anterior to the popliteal artery. The soleus muscle is divided longitudinally exposing the tibioperoneal trunk. Care is taken to gently dissect the tibial veins

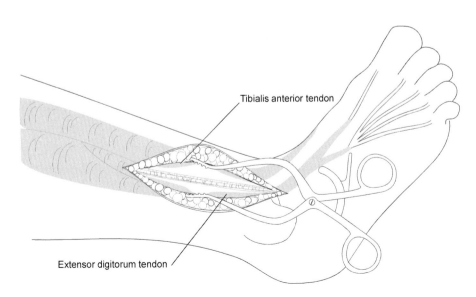

Tibialis anterior tendon

Extensor digitorum tendon

Figure 16-10 Exposure of the anterior tibial artery at the ankle. (From Hoballah JJ. *Vascular reconstructions: Anatomy, exposures, and techniques.* New York, NY: Springer-Verlag; 2000, with permission.)

crossing over the tibioperoneal trunk and the origins of the peroneal artery and posterior tibial artery. The anterior tibial and other crossing veins often cover the origin of the tibioperoneal trunk. Dissection distal to these crossing veins avoids the need to encircle and divide these vulnerable structures.

The Posterior Tibial Artery

Exposure of the Posterior Tibial Artery in the Upper Leg

A 10- to 12-cm, longitudinal skin incision is made 2 cm posterior to the edge of the tibia (Fig. 16-11). Once the incision is deepened through the subcutaneous tissue, the anterior fascia of the soleus muscle is exposed. This fascia and the soleus muscle fibers are divided along the length of the incision exposing the posterior fascia of the soleus muscle. The posterior fascia is then incised with care to avoid injury to the underlying vascular bundle.[11] After the fascia is incised, inspection at that level will reveal one muscle attached to the tibia: The flexor digitorum longus muscle (FDL). The second muscle posterior to the FDL is the flexor hallucis longus muscle (FHL). The posterior tibial artery and veins are usually lying in the groove between the FDL and the FHL muscles. The tibialis posterior muscle will be lateral to the posterior tibial vascular bundle.

The exposure of the posterior tibial artery below the middle of the leg is similar to the more proximal exposure. However, at the lower level of the leg, the soleus muscle is usually attenuated. The posterior tibial artery and veins will be seen between the tendons of the FDL muscle and the FHL muscle.

Exposure of the Posterior Tibial Artery at the Ankle

An 8- to 10-cm skin incision is performed at the ankle. The incision is deepened through the subcutaneous tissue until the flexor retinaculum is identified. The flexor retinaculum is divided and the posterior tibial artery is identified between the tendons of the FDL and the FHL.

The Peroneal Artery

Medial Exposure of the Peroneal Artery

The medial exposure of the peroneal artery in the upper leg starts by exposing the posterior tibial neurovascular bundle as described above.[12,13] The posterior tibial neurovascular bundle can be retracted anteriorly along with the FDL muscle or inferiorly along with the FHL muscle (Fig. 16-12). The former approach is preferred in the upper leg; the latter approach is often preferred in the mid and lower leg. The dissection is then continued towards the fibula in the tissue plane (intermuscular septum) between the posterior tibialis muscle and the FHL muscle. Deep in the wound, a fascial layer will be identified. Incision of this fascial layer will usually expose one of the veins surrounding the peroneal artery. Further dissection and mobilization of this vein posteriorly will expose the peroneal artery. This usually requires division of a few small and delicate venae comitantes crossing over the peroneal artery.

The exposure of the peroneal artery in the lower leg can be challenging in patients with heavy musculature and large-sized legs. In this situation, a lateral approach with resection of a fibular segment may be preferred.

Lateral Exposure of the Peroneal Artery

The lateral approach to the peroneal artery provides a more superficial access to the artery than the medial approach (Fig. 16-13). This could facilitate the exposure and the construction of an anastomosis to the peroneal artery and is ideal in redo procedures. An 8- to 10-cm, longitudinal skin incision is made over the lateral aspect of the fibula and centered over the segment

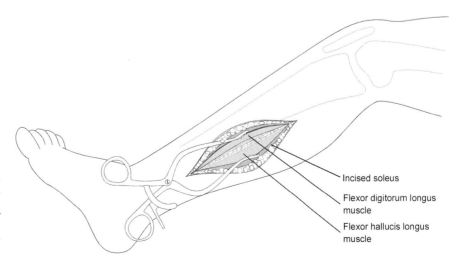

Figure 16-11 Exposure of the posterior tibial artery: The soleus muscle is incised exposing the posterior tibial vessels. (From Hoballah JJ. *Vascular reconstructions: Anatomy, exposures, and techniques.* New York, NY: Springer-Verlag; 2000, with permission.)

Incised soleus

Flexor digitorum longus muscle

Flexor hallucis longus muscle

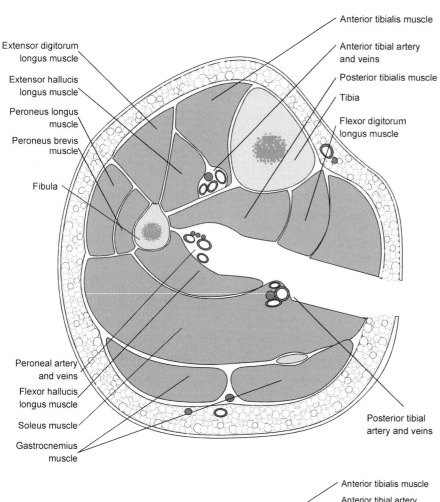

Figure 16-12 Medial approach to the peroneal artery in the mid and lower leg; cross-section view. The posterior tibial vessels are retracted inferiorly. Dissection along the intermuscular septum towards the fibula will lead to the peroneal vessels. (From Hoballah JJ. *Vascular reconstructions: Anatomy, exposures, and techniques.* New York, NY: Springer-Verlag; 2000, with permission.)

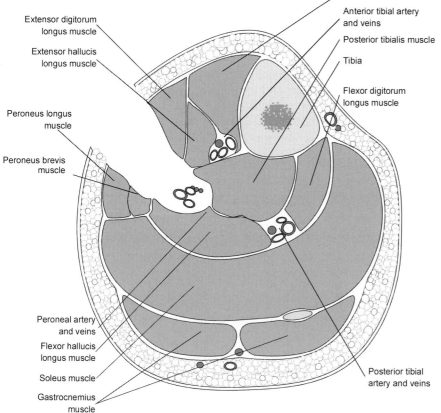

Figure 16-13 Lateral approach to the peroneal artery; cross-section view. Fibula excised. (From Hoballah JJ. *Vascular reconstructions: Anatomy, exposures, and techniques.* New York, NY: Springer-Verlag; 2000, with permission.)

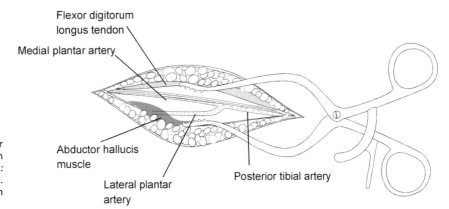

Figure 16-14 Exposure of the posterior tibial and plantar arteries at the ankle. (From Hoballah JJ. *Vascular reconstructions: Anatomy, exposures, and techniques.* New York, NY: Springer-Verlag; 2000, with permission.)

to be exposed. If the proximal part of the peroneal artery is to be exposed, care should be taken to avoid injury to the peroneal nerve as it crosses the neck of the fibula. The incision is deepened until the fibula is exposed. The periosteum is elevated circumferentially and the fibula is cleared of all tissue attachments. A right angle clamp is passed underneath the fibula to engage one end of a Gigli saw. The Gigli saw will be used to transect the fibula at the proximal and distal end of the incision. It is important to completely clear the tissues from the fibula before passing the right angle clamp below it to avoid injury to the underlying peroneal vessels. The exposed segment of fibula is carefully excised. The medial periosteum of the resected fibula is then incised exposing the peroneal artery and venae comitantes, which lie just beneath it. This approach provides an excellent exposure of the peroneal artery down to its terminal branches especially in redo procedures.

The Plantar Arteries

A 6- to 8-cm skin incision is performed between the medial malleolus and the calcaneus bone. After deepening the incision through the subcutaneous tissue, the flexor retinaculum is identified. The flexor retinaculum is incised exposing the posterior tibial artery, which is usually surrounded by the tendinous sheath of the FDL superiorly and the FHL inferiorly. The posterior tibial artery is followed distally until it bifurcates into the medial and lateral plantar arteries.[14] The lateral plantar artery can be further exposed by dividing the overlying muscles, mainly the abductor hallucis and the flexor digitorum brevis muscles (Fig. 16-14).

The Dorsalis Pedis Artery

Exposure of the dorsalis pedis artery is usually performed through a longitudinal incision placed directly over the vessel (Fig. 16-15). The location of the dorsalis

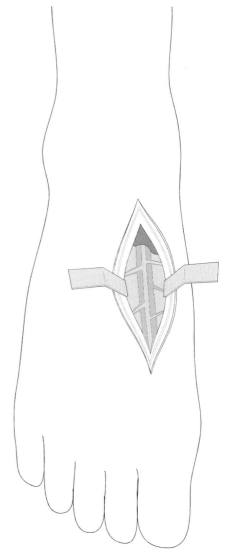

Figure 16-15 Exposure of the dorsalis pedis artery. (From Hoballah JJ. *Vascular reconstructions: Anatomy, exposures, and techniques.* New York, NY: Springer-Verlag; 2000, with permission.)

pedis can also be mapped preoperatively using duplex ultrasonography to avoid flap creation. However, some surgeons prefer to create a curved incision placed medial to the vessel and then create a skin flap. This technique is proposed to avoid having the graft and the anastomosis directly under the skin suture line, which can be prone to nonhealing problems that could result in graft exposure at the anastomotic site. The retinaculum is identified and incised exposing the dorsalis pedis artery and its surrounding veins. Alternatively, the dorsalis pedis artery can be exposed beyond the flexor retinaculum in the first metatarsal space.

REFERENCES

1. Bridges R, Gewertz BL. Lateral incision for exposure of femoral vessels. *Surg Gynecol Obstet.* 1980;150:733.
2. Nunez AA, Veith FJ, Collier P, et al. Direct approaches to the distal portions of the deep femoral artery for limb salvage. *J Vasc Surg.* 1988;8:576–581.
3. Naraysingh V, Karmody AM, Leather RP, et al. Lateral approach to the profunda femoris artery. *Am J Surg.* 1984;147:813–814.
4. Padberg FT Jr. Lateral approach to the popliteal artery. *Ann Vasc Surg.* 1998;2:397–401.
5. Hoballah JJ, Chalmers RT, Sharp WJ, et al. Lateral approach to the popliteal and crural vessels for limb salvage. *Cardiovasc Surg.* 1996;4:165–168.
6. Veith FJ, Ascer E, Gupta SK, et al. Lateral approach to the popliteal artery. *J Vasc Surg.* 1987;6:119–123.
7. Danese CA, Singer A. Lateral approach to the trifurcation popliteal artery. *Surgery.* 1968;63:588–590.
8. Dardik H, Dardik I, Veith FJ. Exposure of the tibioperoneal arteries by a single lateral approach. *Surgery.* 1974;75:377–382.
9. Usatoff V, Grigg M. A lateral approach to the below-knee popliteal artery without resection of the fibula [Letter to the Editor]. *J Vasc Surg.* 1997;26:168–170.
10. Dardik H, Elias S, Miller N, et al. Medial approach to the anterior tibial artery. *J Vasc Surg.* 1985;2:743.
11. Imparato AM, Kim GE, Chu DS. Surgical exposure for reconstruction of the proximal part of the tibial artery. *Surg Gynecol Obstet.* 1973;136:453–455.
12. Dardik H, Ibrahim IM, Dardik II. The role of the peroneal artery for limb salvage. *Ann Surg.* 1979;189:189–198.
13. Minken SL, May AG. Use of the peroneal artery for revascularization of the lower extremity. *Arch Surg.* 1969;99:594–597.
14. Ascer E, Veith F, Gupta S. Bypasses to plantar arteries and other tibial branches: an extended approach to limb salvage. *J Vasc Surg.* 1985;8:434.

Choice of Inflow Vessel for Distal Arterial Bypass

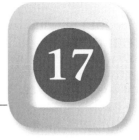

Paul W. White   **Anton N. Sidawy**   **Christopher J. Abularrage**
Jonathan M. Weiswasser   **Subodh Arora**

Although the common femoral artery has been the inflow vessel usually used for infrapopliteal bypasses, other inflow arteries are sometimes preferred because of anatomical necessity, unavailability of a patent common femoral artery, or the superior patency rates provided by other arteries. Over the past 20 years, the common femoral artery has been supplanted as the inflow source of choice by the distal superficial femoral artery or the popliteal artery when no significant atherosclerotic disease exists proximal to these arteries. Distal inflow vessels provide higher patency rates and the advantage of requiring shorter segments of autogenous vein for bypass. Arteries proximal to the common femoral artery have been used when the common femoral artery is occluded or when prior procedures make it more dangerous and more difficult to redissect the common femoral. Such proximal arteries include the external iliac artery, the common iliac artery and, in very rare occasions, the aorta itself. Additional inflow arteries include the profunda femoris artery and the tibial arteries.

The choice of inflow vessel for distal bypass in patients with diabetes is dependent on the distribution of atherosclerotic disease and the availability of sufficient autologous vein to be used for conduit. With the frequency of repeat revascularization procedures in patients with distal peripheral vascular disease and the fact that these patients often undergo coronary artery bypass grafting, which requires autologous vein, the need for procedures that minimize the length of

vein required for conduit has become paramount. Additionally, the restoration of pulsatile blood flow to the foot is essential for achieving rapid and durable healing of tissue loss and gangrene. Whereas a bypass to an isolated segment of the popliteal artery may be sufficient to relieve rest pain, it will not reliably provide adequate blood flow for wound healing.[1] The tibial arteries, therefore, are often the target outflow vessel in diabetic patients.

COMMON FEMORAL ARTERY

The traditional source for distal bypass has been the common femoral artery. Patency rates reported in the literature have varied from 50% to 70%. The common femoral artery was viewed as the inflow source of choice because it was thought that atherosclerosis of the superficial femoral artery (SFA) would threaten grafts originating from more distal arteries. In other words, stenotic lesions would develop more proximally to the inflow of the bypass graft causing graft failure.

In 1969, Noon et al.[2] published a series of 91 patients who underwent arterial reconstruction with a distal anastomosis in the tibial arteries. A majority of these grafts arose from the common femoral artery. The patency rate at 4 years was 56.8% for all grafts and 58% for those originating at the common femoral artery. Auer et al.[3] reported a patency rate of 59% for vein grafts originating at the common femoral artery and terminating in the tibial vessels. Berkowitz et al.[4] reported a primary patency rate of 47% and a secondary patency rate of 70% utilizing reversed saphenous vein. Taylor et al.[5] reported primary and secondary patency rates of 69% and 77% with reversed saphenous or other autogenous veins. Belkin[6] found a similar primary patency of 64% and a secondary patency of 75% when using *in situ* saphenous vein, as well as a primary patency of 69% and secondary patency of 77% for nonreversed saphenous vein. Veith et al.[7] reported a primary patency of 49% at 2 years using autologous vein for bypass to the infrapopliteal arteries in a multicenter, prospective, randomized trial comparing autologous vein to prosthetic conduit. Dardik et al.[8] demonstrated a cumulative patency rate of 50% at 12 months when performing femoral-peroneal bypasses in diabetic patients. In comparing *in situ* to reversed saphenous long vein grafts to the tibial or peroneal arteries, Harris[9] reported a primary patency of 77% for *in situ* grafts and a primary patency of 64% for reversed grafts. Secondary patency rates (66%, 68%) and limb salvage rates (78%, 87%) were equivalent in the two groups.

The patency rates for tibial bypass in diabetic patients are equivalent to those obtained in nondiabetic patients.[10] Shah et al.,[11] in a series of 2,058 *in situ* saphenous vein bypasses, of which 1,023 terminated in an infrapopliteal artery, showed no difference in the patency rates of diabetic patients when compared to nondiabetic patients at 1, 5, or 10 years. Rosenblatt et al.[12] showed equivalent patency rates for diabetic patients (95% at 1 year, 85% at 4 years) and nondiabetic

patients (89% at 1 year, 80% at 4 years) despite the fact that a greater percentage of the bypasses in diabetic patients ended below the popliteal artery (52% vs. 34%).

DISTAL SUPERFICIAL FEMORAL AND POPLITEAL ARTERIES

Since diabetic patients often undergo coronary artery bypass grafting and multiple revascularization surgeries, all of which require autologous vein, the need to minimize the length of vein required for conduit is essential. Several attributes of the pathophysiology of atherosclerosis in diabetic patients play a role in the choice of an inflow artery. The anatomic pattern of atherosclerosis in diabetics is concentrated in the infragenicular arteries, especially at the popliteal trifurcation; this distribution of occlusive disease often requires that the outflow target is a distal tibial artery, peroneal, or pedal artery. Additionally, since a distal inflow site minimizes the length of vein needed, the surgeon can choose from the entire length of the vein that segment of vein that will be most suitable as a conduit. A distal inflow site also avoids dissections in obese or reoperative hostile groins, and decreases the extent and length of incisions and dissections needed to harvest vein in the remainder of the leg[13] (Fig. 17-1).

Veith et al.[14] first presented arguments for using the distal superficial femoral artery or popliteal arteries as an inflow source. They reported a 6-year patency rate of 58% for grafts originating at the superficial femoral

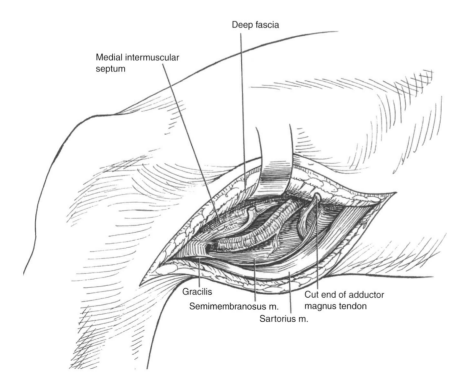

Deep fascia

Medial intermuscular septum

Gracilis

Semimembranosus m.

Sartorius m.

Cut end of adductor magnus tendon

Figure 17-1   Exposure of the proximal popliteal artery. (From Wind GG, Valentine RJ, eds. *Anatomic exposures in vascular surgery.* Baltimore, Md: Williams and Wilkins; 1991:387, with permission.)

artery or popliteal arteries, and terminating in the infrapopliteal arteries. The 6-year patency rate for similar reconstructions originating at the common femoral artery was 50%. Diabetic patients may present with a palpable popliteal pulse and an ischemic foot. Cantelmo et al.[15] performed arterial reconstructions arising from the superficial femoral artery or popliteal artery in 30 patients with a palpable popliteal pulse, of whom 77% were diabetic. Their patency rate of 79% at 1 and 3 years compares favorably with patency rates for grafts beginning at the common femoral artery. In a retrospective analysis, we compared tibial bypasses originating in the common femoral artery (group I) to those originating in the SFA or popliteal arteries (group II). All patients in group II had palpable popliteal pulses, and 74% were diabetic as opposed to 35% in group I. Patency rates at 6 years were 81% in group II and 65% in group I.[16] The use of *in situ* saphenous vein has yielded excellent results as well. In a series of 26 patients, of whom all but one were diabetic, patency rates and limb salvage rates at 30 months were 95%.[17] Some investigators reported that bypass grafts off the SFA and popliteal artery have a higher patency rate in diabetic patients as opposed to nondiabetic patients.[18] Patency rates of 60% to 90% for grafts arising from distal sites have additional support in published literature.[19–22]

In examining the role of atherosclerosis proximal to a graft originating from the SFA or popliteal artery, Rosenbloom et al.,[23] in reviewing all patients with these grafts at three hospitals, found that a stenosis >20% in the SFA preoperatively was a significant risk factor for graft failure. The overall patency rates (41% primary and 42% secondary) in this study were substantially lower at 5 years than in other studies. In part to assess the frequency of proximal arterial disease progression, Ballard et al.[24,25] reviewed 23 patients who underwent arterial reconstruction with grafts originating at the popliteal artery. They did not find disease progression in any patients. A similar review by Mills et al.[26] found proximal disease progression requiring balloon angioplasty in a single patient of a series of 53 in whom 56 (1.8%) grafts arising from the popliteal artery were placed. Treiman et al.[27] reported 159 grafts originating below the common femoral artery. Inflow source was chosen as the most distal site possible with no stenosis >50% more proximal. Graft surveillance was performed with duplex ultrasound. The patency rate (91% at 5 years) and the fact that only one graft appeared to have thrombosed due to proximal stenosis led them to argue that graft surveillance was in fact unnecessary and that graft patency was not affected by more proximal disease. The preferential use of the distal SFA or popliteal arteries as an inflow source when no stenosis >30% existed proximal to these sites resulted in a patency rate of 88% at 36 months. Patients with a proximal stenosis underwent bypasses arising from the common femoral artery and had a patency rate of 89% at 3 years.[28]

Wengerter et al.[29] also addressed the issue of proximal disease progression. Reviewing 153 nonsequential popliteal-to-distal artery bypasses for limb salvage, they found primary and secondary patency rates at 5 years of 55% and 60%. Bypasses distal to stenosis of 20% or less had a 2-year patency rate of 77%; those distal to a 21% to 35% stenosis had a 70% 2-year patency rate; and those distal to a 35% or greater stenosis had a 53% 2-year patency rate. In fact, the superiority in some circumstances of short vein grafts arising from the superficial femoral, popliteal, or tibial arteries has been argued by Ascher and Veith.[30] They compared bypasses utilizing vein grafts of <40 cm to those using vein grafts of >40 cm. The patency rate for short vein grafts was 63% at 3 years compared to a patency rate of 45% for long grafts. The difference was even greater when outflow was impaired (53% to 22%). The proposed reasons for the improved patency rates of short bypasses are that since vein graft stenosis takes place along the length of the bypass, the longer the bypass the greater the chance of developing a stenosis, and, more important, that since only a short segment of vein is needed, the surgeon is more likely to use the best segment of vein available and is able to intraoperatively discard those segments of vein that are not satisfactory.

ILIAC ARTERIES

Since an aggressive approach to critical ischemia has been shown to reduce the rate of amputation, the incidence of repeat operations after graft thrombosis or infection is significant. The increased risk of infection, lymphorrhea, and neurovascular injury in reoperations of the groin has prompted surgeons to explore more proximal arteries as inflow sites. Ascher et al.[31] reported two series using the iliac arteries as inflow sources in distal bypasses. In the first, the external iliac artery was used as the inflow vessel. An incision above the inguinal ligament and lateral to the rectus sheath, and a retroperitoneal dissection were used to expose the external iliac. A patency rate of 87% at 2 years using ringed polytetrafluoroethylene (PTFE) as conduit was reported. In a later retrospective study, Ascher et al.[32] compared suprainguinal and infrainguinal inflow sites in patients undergoing distal bypass to the infrapopliteal arteries. The suprainguinal group had ringed PTFE grafts arising from the common or external iliac; the infrainguinal group had ringed PTFE grafts originating at the common femoral artery. The patency rates were equivalent. The rate of local wound complications, however, was higher in the common femoral artery group with the groin incision. Since the distance between the iliac arteries and distal tibial outflow targets is significant, and because grafts originating at the iliacs must cross two joints, the common femoral artery (or a more distal artery) should be chosen as the inflow source for tibial bypasses when possible. The use of the iliac arteries as inflow should be reserved for cases when a hostile groin or femoral artery occlusion make its use or the use of more distal arteries for inflow impossible.

PROFUNDA FEMORIS ARTERY

The profunda femoris artery is often spared by atherosclerosis and is often used as an outflow vessel for proximal bypasses for aortoiliac disease. An advantage of the profunda femoris artery is its accessibility through several approaches that obviate the need for dissection in an infected or hostile groin.[33,34] Using the distal portions of the profunda femoris artery as an inflow site for distal grafts has the advantage of decreasing the length of vein conduit needed for a bypass.[35] Anatomically, the profunda femoris artery is divided into three parts (Fig. 17-2). The portion of the artery from its origin off the posterolateral aspect of the common femoral artery to the lateral circumflex femoral artery is termed the proximal profunda femoris artery. The middle portion extends from the lateral circumflex femoral artery to the second perforating branch and lies posterior to the adductor longus muscle. The final portion extends distal to the second perforating branch until the main trunk separates into branches at the fourth perforator.

The indication for using the profunda femoris artery, whether a hostile groin or need for a short bypass, will dictate which surgical approach is used to dissect the artery. The proximal profunda femoris artery can be accessed through a typical groin incision and the femoral sheath. An anterolateral approach has been described with an incision along the lateral border of the sartorius muscle, approximately 6 cm lateral to the femoral pulse. The sartorius is then retracted medially. Dissection along the medial border of the rectus femoris muscle will reveal the lateral circumflex femoral vessels, which can be followed medially to the main trunk of the profunda femoris artery.[32] Access to the distal profunda femoris artery can be obtained by incising the fascia between the adductor longus and the vastus medialis muscle. A posteromedial approach with an incision along the medial border of the sartorius and dissection confined to the plane posterior to the adductor longus can also be used. This approach can be especially helpful in isolating an infected groin from the surgical field.[34] A posterior approach to the middle and distal profunda femoris artery with the patient prone has also been described. An incision is made lateral to the hamstring muscle group above and below the gluteal crease. The gluteus maximus muscle is dissected along its inferomedial border and is retracted superolaterally. The sciatic nerve and superior portions of the hamstring are now visible. The hamstring group is retracted medially exposing the adductor magnus. This muscle is incised longitudinally using the perforating branches as a guide to the location of the profunda femoris artery (Fig. 17-3).[33]

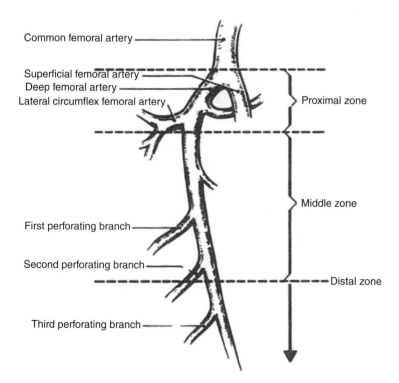

Common femoral artery

Superficial femoral artery
Deep femoral artery
Lateral circumflex femoral artery

Proximal zone

Middle zone

First perforating branch

Second perforating branch

Distal zone

Third perforating branch

Figure 17-2 Zones of the profunda femoris artery. (From Nunez AA, Veith FJ, Collier P, et al. Portions of the deep femoral artery for limb salvage bypasses. *J Vasc Surg.* 1988;8(5):576–581, with permission.)

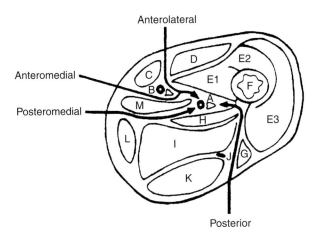

Figure 17-3 Approaches to the profunda femoris artery. (From Bertucci WR, Marin ML, Veith FJ, et al. Posterior approach to the deep femoral artery. *J Vasc Surg.* 1999;29(4):741–744, with permission.)

A retrospective review of cases by Darling et al.[36] revealed the use of the profunda femoris in 20% of distal bypasses. Of these, >60% used an infragenicular artery as the outflow vessel. Patency rates for all grafts were excellent, with a primary patency of 75% at 2 years and 63% at 5 years, and compared favorably with rates for bypasses originating at the common femoral (65% at 5 years) and superficial femoral (71% at 5 years) arteries. Patency for grafts terminating in the peroneal, anterior tibial, and posterior tibial had primary patency rates of 71%, 65%, and 51%, respectively. In comparison, grafts terminating in the below-knee popliteal and above-knee popliteal had patency rates of 63% and 81%, respectively. Mills et al.[37] reported similar patency rates in a smaller series in which only 40% of the procedures terminated in a tibial vessel. Primary and secondary patency rates for grafts arising from the profunda femoris artery at 3 years were 78% and 96%. No significant difference existed between these rates and those of grafts arising from the common femoral artery (66% and 89%), the SFA (69% and 87%), or the popliteal arteries (66% and 87%). The authors noted that 22 of the 56 operations used the profunda femoris artery because of inadequate vein length, and 20 others used the profunda femoris artery to avoid a groin scarred by previous operations or infection.

TIBIAL AND PERONEAL ARTERIES

In patients with a severe shortage of autologous vein, tibiotibial bypasses have been used with success. Veith et al.[38] reported a series of 14 patients without longer segments of vein who underwent tibiotibial bypasses as a last resort before amputation. Of the 14 patients, 11 (79%) had patent grafts and a functional limb at 6 to 50 months after surgery. Quinones-Baldrich et al.[39] reported a 2-year patency rate of 72% for tibiotibial

bypasses, identical to the patency rate for bypasses with a femoral or popliteal takeoff. In a small series of popliteotibial and tibiotibial bypasses, Moñux Ducajù et al.[40] reported a 2-year primary patency rate of 71%, with no difference attributable to inflow source. Lyon et al.[41] reported a larger series of 42 grafts originating from infrapopliteal arteries (28 arising from the anterior tibial artery, nine from the posterior tibial, three from the peroneal, and two from tibioperoneal trunk). The primary patency rate was 77% at 1 year and 62% at 5 years. Tibiotibial bypass appears to have similar patency rates to more traditional bypasses, but experience is limited.

PROXIMAL BYPASS GRAFT

The use of a prior prosthetic bypass graft as an inflow source has also been described to address several clinical situations. First, in patients who have had a prior aortobifemoral graft, distal grafts arising from the groin have used the prior conduit as an inflow source. Second, bypasses to tibial vessels in patients with inadequate vein or a prior popliteal bypass have been performed with jump grafts. In other words, a femoropopliteal bypass is performed with synthetic conduit from which a short vein bypass takes off to a tibial target.

Bliss and Fonseka[42] described such a "hitch-hike" graft in 1976, and reported that 11 of 16 grafts remained functional at 1 year. Alexander et al.[43] reported a 2-year primary patency rate of 35% in patients with sequential composite grafts to the tibial arteries. McCarthy et al.[44] reported primary patencies of 72% at 1 year, 64% at 2 years, and 48% at 3 years, with a limb salvage rate at 4 years of 70% in a series of 62 patients, of whom 51% had diabetes. Flinn et al.[45] reported a limb salvage rate of 76%, and indicated that an important additional benefit of sequential bypasses may be improved outflow, allowing the proximal portion of the bypass to remain open until healing has occurred and limb salvage affected. Verta[46] achieved patency rates of 81.4% at 2 years and 72.4% at 4 years in a series of composite sequential grafts, of which 31 terminated in tibial vessels and 23 in pedal vessels.

Although not as typical as isolated infragenicular arteriosclerosis, aortoiliac inflow disease does occur in diabetic patients. The combination of inflow disease and distal disease is not uncommon as well. The treatment of inflow disease has reliably and effectively been treated with aortobifemoral bypass with prosthetic graft for many years. In patients with multilevel occlusive disease, combinations of inflow and outflow procedures have been used. The common femoral artery is most often the site of the distal anastomosis in this surgery. Dardik et al.[47] found a patency rate of 76% when comparing simultaneous inflow and outflow procedures.

Eidt and Charlesworth[48] found a patency of 80% at 4 years in 153 patients undergoing simultaneous aorto-bifemoral and femoropopliteal bypasses. The common femoral artery is most often the site of the distal anastomosis in this surgery. The concurrent or sequential treatment of outflow disease can utilize as the inflow source either the common femoral artery, if enough distance exists below the proximal graft's distal anastomosis, or the limbs of the prosthetic graft. Lam et al.[49] compared the efficacy of grafts originating from the native common femoral artery to the efficacy of grafts originating from a prosthetic limb of a proximal graft. They found a 5-year primary patency rate of 75% for grafts off a native artery and a 5-year primary patency rate of 50% for grafts off a prosthetic limb. Similar differences existed in survival (69% vs. 56%) and limb salvage (90% vs. 78%).

SUMMARY

When treating diabetic patients, the choice of an inflow source for infragenicular bypasses is affected by several factors including length of autologous vein available for conduit, the anatomic pattern of atherosclerotic occlusive disease, prior operations or infections causing a hostile groin, patient body habitus, and the ease with which the chosen artery can be exposed. If no significant proximal disease exists, the use of the most distal site available is optimal. In comparing the patency rates in the literature, it seems that the popliteal artery and distal SFA appear to be ideal inflow sources for many diabetic patients. This being said, the principles of treatment should be applied specifically to the unique disease presentation and circumstances of each individual patient.

REFERENCES

1. Gibbons GW. Lower extremity bypass patients with diabetic foot ulcers. *Surg Clin North Am.* 2003;83:659–669.
2. Noon GP, Diethrich EB, Richardson WP, et al. Distal tibial arterial bypass. Analysis of 91 cases. *Arch Surg.* 1969;99:770–775.
3. Auer AI, Hurley JJ, Binnington HB, et al. Distal tibial vein grafts for limb salvage. *Arch Surg.* 1987;118:597–602.
4. Berkowitz H, Greenstein S. Improved patency in reversed femoral-infrapopliteal autogenous vein grafts by early detection and treatment of the failing graft. *J Vasc Surg.* 1987;5:755–761.
5. Taylor LM Jr, Edwards JM, Porter JM. Present status of reversed vein bypass grafting: five-year results of a modern series. *J Vasc Surg.* 1990;11:193–206.
6. Belkin M, Knox J, Donaldson MC, et al. Infrainguinal arterial reconstruction with nonreversed greater saphenous vein. *J Vasc Surg.* 1996;24:957–962.
7. Veith FJ, Gupta SK, Ascer E, et al. Six-year prospective multicenter comparison of autologous saphenous vein and expanded polytetrafluoroethylene grafts in infrainguinal arterial reconstructions. *J Vasc Surg.* 1986;3:104–114.
8. Dardik H, Ibrahim IM, Dardik II. The role of the peroneal artery for limb salvage. *Ann Surg.* 1979;189:189–198.
9. Harris PL. Prospective randomized comparison of *in situ* and reversed infrapopliteal vein grafts. *Br J Surg.* 1993;80:173–176.
10. Akbari CM, Pomposelli FB Jr, Gibbons GW, et al. Lower extremity revascularization in Diabetes: late observations. *Arch Surg.* 2000; 135:452–456.
11. Shah DM, Darling RCR, Chang BB, et al. Longterm results of *in situ* saphenous vein bypass: analysis of 2058 cases. *Ann Surg.* 1995;222:438–448.
12. Rosenblatt MS, Quist WC, Sidawy AN, et al. Results of vein Graft reconstruction of the lower extremity in diabetic and nondiabetic patients. *Surg Gynecol Obstet.* 1990;171:331–335.
13. Pomposelli FB, Kansal N, Hamdan AD, et al. A decade of experience with dorsalis pedis artery bypass: analysis of outcome in more than 1000 cases. *J Vasc Surg.* 2003;37:307–315.
14. Veith FJ, Gupta SK, Samson RH, et al. Superficial femoral and popliteal arteries as inflow sites for distal bypass. *Surgery.* 1981; 90:980–990.
15. Cantelmo NL, Snow JR, Menzoian JO, et al. Successful vein bypass in patients with an ischemic limb and a palpable popliteal pulse. *Arch Surg.* 1986;121:217–220.
16. Sidawy AN, Menzolan JO, Cantelmo NL, et al. Effect of inflow and outflow sites on the results of tibioperoneal vein grafts. *Am J Surg.* 1986;152:211–214.
17. Rhodes GR, Rollins D, Sidawy AN, et al. Popliteal-to-tibial *in situ* vein bypasses for limb salvage in diabetic patients. *Am J Surg.* 1987;154:245–247.
18. Reed AB, Conte MS, Belkin M, et al. Usefulness of autogenous bypass grafts originating distal to the groin. *J Vasc Surg.* 2002; 35:48–55.
19. Stonebridge PA, Tsoukas AI, Pomposelli FB, et al. Popliteal-to-distal bypass for limb salvage in diabetic patients. *Eur J Vasc Surg.* 1991;5:265–269.
20. Najmaldin A, Clifford PC, Chant AD, et al. Inflow site: its effect on femoropopliteal and distal graft patency. *Br J Surg.* 1988;75: 434–435.
21. Brown PS Jr, McCarthy WJ, Yao JST, et al. The popliteal artery as inflow for distal bypass grafting. *Arch Surg.* 1994;129:596–602.
22. Marks J, King TA, Baele H, et al. Popliteal-to-distal bypass for limb-threatening ischemia. *J Vasc Surg.* 1992;15:755–759.
23. Rosenbloom MS, Walsh JJ, Schuler JJ, et al. Long-term results of infragenicular bypasses with autogenous vein originating from the distal superficial femoral and popliteal arteries. *J Vasc Surg.* 1988;7:691–696.
24. Ballard JL, Killeen JD, Smith LL. Popliteal-tibial bypass grafts of limb-threatening ischemia. *Arch Surg.* 1993;128:976–980.
25. Ballard JL, Killeen DJ, Blunt TJ, et al. Autologous saphenous vein popliteal-tibial artery bypass for limb threatening ischemia: a reassessment. *Am J Surg.* 1995;170:251–255.
26. Mills JL, Gahtan V, Fujitani RM, et al. The utility and durability of vein bypass grafts originating from the popliteal artery for limb salvage. *Am J Surg.* 1994;168:646–651.
27. Treiman GS, Ashfari A, Lawrence PF. Incidentally detected stenoses proximal to grafts originating below the common femoral artery: do they affect graft patency in asymptomatic patients? *J Vasc Surg.* 2000;32:1180–1189.
28. Pomposelli FB, Jepsen SJ, Gibbons GW, et al. A flexible approach to infrapopliteal vein grafts in patients with diabetes mellitus. *Arch Surg.* 1991;126:724–729.
29. Wengerter KR, Yang PM, Veith FJ, et al. A twelve-year experience with the popliteal-to-distal bypass: the significance and management of proximal disease. *J Vasc Surg.* 1992;15:143–149.
30. Ascer E, Veith FJ, Gupta SK, et al. Short vein grafts: a superior option for arterial reconstructions to poor or compromised outflow tracts. *J Vasc Surg.* 1988;7:370–378.
31. Ascer E, Kirwin J, Mohan C, et al. The preferential use of the external iliac artery as an inflow source for redo femoropopliteal and infrapopliteal bypass. *J Vasc Surg.* 1993;18:234–241.

32. Ascher E, Scheinman M, Mazzariol F, et al. Comparison between Supra- and infrainguinal inflow sites for infrapopliteal PTFE bypasses with complementary arteriovenous fistula and vein interposition. *Eur J Vasc Endovasc Surg.* 2000;19:138–142.

33. Naraynsingh V, Karmody AM, Leather RP, et al. Lateral approach to the profunda femoris artery. *Am J Surg.* 1984;147:813–814.

34. Bertucci WR, Marin ML, Veith FJ, et al. Posterior approach to the deep femoral artery. *J Vasc Surg.* 1999;29:741–744.

35. Nunez AA, Veith FJ, Collier P, et al. Direct approaches to the distal portions of the deep femoral artery for limb salvage bypasses. *J Vasc Surg.* 1988;8:576–581.

36. Darling RC, Shah DM, Chang BB, et al. Can the deep femoral artery be used reliably as an inflow source for infrainguinal reconstruction? Long term results in 563 procedures. *J Vasc Surg.* 1994;20:889–895.

37. Mills JL, Taylor SM, Fujitani RM. The role of the deep femoral artery as an inflow site for infrainguinal revascularization. *J Vasc Surg.* 1993;18:416–423.

38. Veith FJ, Ascer E, Gupta SK, et al. Tibiotibial vein bypass grafts: a new operation for limb salvage. *J Vasc Surg.* 1985;2:552–557.

39. Quinones-Baldrich WJ, Colburn MD, Ahn SS, et al. A very distal bypass for salvage of the severely ischemic extremity. *Am J Surg.* 1993;166:117–123.

40. Moñux Ducajù G, Serrano Hernando FJ, Sanchez Hervàs L. Popliteo-distal and tibiotibial bypasses: a viable alternative for the revascularization of the critically ischaemic limb. *J Cardiovasc Surg.* 2001;42:651–656.

41. Lyon RT, Veith FJ, Marson BU, et al. Eleven-year experience with tibiotibial bypass: an unusual but effective solution to distal tibial artery occlusive disease and limited autologous vein. *J Vasc Surg.* 1994;20:61–69.

42. Bliss BP, Fonseka N. "Hitch-hike" grafts for limb salvage in peripheral arterial disease. *Br J Surg.* 1976;63:562–564.

43. Alexander JJ, Wells KE, Yuhas JP, et al. The role of composite sequential bypass in the treatment of multilevel infrainguinal arterial occlusive disease. *Am J Surg.* 1996;172:118–122.

44. McCarthy WJ, Pearce WH, Flinn WR, et al. Long-term evaluation of composite sequential bypass for limb threatening ischemia. *J Vasc Surg.* 1992;15:761–770.

45. Flinn WR, Flanigan DP, Verta MJ, et al. Sequential femoral-tibial bypass for severe limb ischemia. *Surgery.* 1980;88:357–365.

46. Verta MJ Jr. Composite sequential bypass to the ankle and beyond for limb salvage. *J Vasc Surg.* 1984;1:381–386.

47. Dardik H, Ibrahim IM, Jarrah M, et al. Synchronous aortofemoral or iliofemoral bypass with revascularization of the lower extremity. *Surg Gynecol Obstet.* 1979;149:676–680.

48. Eidt J, Charlesworth D. Combined aortobifemoral and femoropopliteal bypass in the management of patients with extensive atherosclerosis. *Ann Vasc Surg.* 1987;1:453–460.

49. Lam EY, Landry GJ, Edwards JM, et al. Risk factors for autogenous infrainguinal bypass occlusion in patients with prosthetic inflow grafts. *J Vasc Surg.* 2004;39:336–342.

Choice of Outflow Infragenicular Artery

18

Joseph D. Raffetto   James O. Menzoian

The arterial supply to the leg can be anatomically divided into tibial vessels and inframalleolar or pedal vessels. The tibial vessels that are accessible to the vascular surgeon include the anterior tibial, posterior tibial, and peroneal arteries. Inframalleolar vessels include the medial and lateral plantar arteries from the posterior tibial artery, the dorsalis pedis artery, and the lateral tarsal artery. In patients with diabetes and atherosclerosis of the lower limb, one or more of the tibial arteries can develop stenosis or partial or complete occlusion.[1,2] In a recent study, it was demonstrated that diabetes was a strong predictor for tibial revascularization in patients with critical limb ischemia compared with patients presenting with claudication.[3] Atherosclerosis can also affect the pedal vessels resulting in arterial arch disease and limited runoff. However, it has been demonstrated that patients with diabetes and atherosclerosis have sparing of the inframalleolar arteries, and if disease is present, it is no different than those patients with atherosclerosis and no diabetes.[4]

The goal of revascularization is restoration of arterial perfusion to enable tissue healing, limb salvage, and return of function. The underlying principle of revascularization of leg arteries is to bypass distal to any proximal disease so that the end result is continuity of the runoff vessel to the inframalleolar and digital arteries. In certain cases no tibial artery offers continuity and an inframalleolar vessel is chosen to re-establish arterial flow and tissue perfusion.

It is well accepted that important determinants of graft patency and favorable outcomes of limb salvage and ulcer healing require an adequate conduit, good inflow, a suitable distal target, modification of risk factors especially smoking, and aggressive medical risk factor control.[5,6] However, there exists controversy in the literature as to which is the best suitable artery to bypass to when there are two tibial arteries patent or both a peroneal and inframalleolar vessels available for anastomosis.[7-10] A significant discrepancy in results may be due to variations of reporting standards, indications for surgery, patient selection and characteristics, surgical technique, and adjuvant therapy employed. Furthermore, it is unclear which is the best artery to revascularize when patients present with tissue loss in the forefoot versus midfoot versus heel.

In this chapter we will discuss the literature pertaining to successful or failed infrapopliteal bypass, with specific attention to the choice of tibial artery (peroneal versus anterior or posterior tibial), tibial vessels versus pedal artery revascularization, peroneal artery revascularization compared to inframalleolar bypass, and the choice of tibial or inframalleolar vessel with respect to location of tissue loss on the foot.

PERONEAL VERSUS ANTERIOR OR POSTERIOR TIBIAL

In an earlier retrospective review by Karmody et al.,[11] the authors compared results in patients undergoing anterior tibial, posterior tibial, and peroneal revascularization for rest pain and tissue loss. Peroneal revascularization resulted in increased ankle-brachial indices, a cumulative limb salvage rate at 3 years of 81%, and only 11 major amputations. The authors concluded that peroneal revascularization had comparable results to anterior or posterior tibial bypass. Another retrospective study by Sidawy et al.[12] evaluated two groups of patients based on the proximal anastomosis to the common femoral artery or superficial femoral-popliteal artery. The study found that peroneal, anterior tibial, and posterior tibial artery bypasses had comparable patency rates at 5 years.

Evaluation of angiographic patterns of the peroneal artery and pedal branches may be helpful in determining whether successful revascularization is possible via the peroneal vessel. A retrospective study by Elliott et al.[8] evaluated 34 peroneal bypasses and 194 tibial and pedal bypasses, performed for limb salvage. The study demonstrated similar patency rates at 48 months; however, the limb salvage rates were significantly worse for peroneal bypass (55%) than for the remaining tibial and pedal artery bypasses (67%). The authors identified four anatomic characteristics of the peroneal artery that were significant predictors of limb loss following peroneal artery grafting. These characteristics are:

1. peroneal length <10 cm
2. peroneal artery diameter <2 mm
3. absence of collaterals visualized
4. lack of pedal arch visualization.

Of interest, renal failure, diabetes, smoking, and male gender did not affect limb loss following peroneal bypass. Although this study had a small number of patients undergoing peroneal revascularization compared to patients with tibial and pedal bypasses, the authors recommended that alternatives to peroneal artery bypass should be considered when less favorable anatomic patterns of the peroneal artery are encountered.

Although the peroneal artery may be inferior as a target, especially in the presence of unfavorable anatomic parameters (diameter, length, collaterals), other authors report that the peroneal bypass has excellent hemodynamic qualities as compared to anterior or posterior tibial revascularization. In a retrospective study by Raftery et al.,[9] the authors compared 36 peroneal bypasses to 82 tibial and popliteal bypasses. Hemodynamics of the peroneal bypasses, as measured by ankle-brachial index, transmetatarsal pulse volume recording, graft peak systolic velocity by ultrasound, and intraoperative outflow resistance, were no different when compared to the other tibial and popliteal bypasses. In addition, all patients with peroneal artery revascularization healed their wounds at a mean follow-up period of 17 months. In a large retrospective series reported by Darling et al.,[13] 157 bypasses to the peroneal artery, all done for limb salvage, were assessed for durability. In the analysis, 65% of patients were diabetic; autogenous vein was used in 96% of cases; and the average age was 72.6 years. The secondary patency rate of peroneal reconstructions at 5 years was 75%, with limb salvage of 87%. These results were not different from other perimalleolar reconstructions.

Recommendation

Although no prospective randomized studies are available and may never be performed, the current literature suggests that the peroneal artery is an acceptable vessel for revascularization with patency, limb salvage, and healing rates that are comparable to anterior tibial and posterior tibial artery reconstructions. However, if the peroneal artery is small with only a short patent segment and poor visualization of collaterals through the posterior and anterior branches perfusing the foot, an alternative tibial or inframalleolar bypass is recommended.

PERONEAL, ANTERIOR TIBIAL, AND POSTERIOR TIBIAL VERSUS INFRAMALLEOLAR

Revascularization to tibial vessels has been demonstrated to be feasible and to have excellent long-term results. There is skepticism for inframalleolar bypass due to the location and size of the target artery, mandatory non–weight bearing status for healing to occur, and the notion that runoff in a single foot vessel (such as in the lateral plantar branch of the posterior tibial) may have inferior results. In a study by Schneider et al.,[14] the authors retrospectively reviewed their experience with 53 pedal (inframalleolar) bypasses with 203 supramalleolar bypasses. All patients underwent surgery for limb salvage and had autogenous conduit used for revascularization. There were significant differences in the patients undergoing pedal bypass due to associated increased incidence of diabetes (85%), congestive heart failure (49%), and a higher perioperative mortality (9%), compared to tibial bypass patients with only 47% having diabetes, 30% with heart failure, and an operative mortality of only 2%. The 3-year primary graft patency and limb salvage rates for pedal versus tibial bypass were, respectively, 58% versus 61% and 92% versus 87%, neither of which were statistically different. The authors concluded that pedal bypasses had comparable results to more proximal tibial bypasses, and that the observed increased mortality of patients requiring pedal arterial reconstructions may reflect the associated comorbidities, specifically diabetes and congestive heart failure.

A significant amount of controversy exists when the only tibial vessel remaining in the leg is the peroneal artery, and there is a concomitant inframalleolar vessel available for bypass. There is concern that the ability for healing foot wounds and improving hemodynamics will be compromised, and that limb salvage and graft patency rates will be inferior with a peroneal bypass than with an inframalleolar bypass. In a retrospective review of 77 consecutive peroneal bypasses, Plecha et al.[7] evaluated the influence of peroneal bypass patency with respect to patent inframalleolar runoff (dorsalis pedis and posterior tibial at the ankle) and a patent pedal arch. The 5-year primary and secondary patency rates for peroneal bypasses were 61% and 92%, respectively, and the presence of patent inframalleolar vessels and a pedal arch did not influence the peroneal patency. The authors recommended that the peroneal artery should be selected as the target artery for revascularization when the anterior or posterior tibial arteries are occluded, and the peroneal artery is more preferable to bypass to than inframalleolar arteries are.

Other authors have investigated the patency and outcomes of peroneal versus pedal revascularization with attention to runoff score (see "Predicting Results of Bypass Procedures"), conduit availability, adjacent tissue planes that are infected or necrotic, and time to healing. In a retrospective review by Bergamini et al.[10] the authors compared 175 pedal to 77 peroneal vein bypasses. All patients had critical limb ischemia, and in 152 of the 252 bypasses, both the peroneal and pedal arteries were patent by angiography. Of these 152 bypasses, there were 99 pedal and 53 peroneal bypasses. The primary and secondary 2-year patency rates evaluated in patients with equivalent runoff scores for pedal versus peroneal were 70% versus 60% and 77% versus 72%, respectively; the differences were not statistically significant. Furthermore, the limb salvage for pedal and peroneal bypasses for all patients during the same interval was similar (74% vs. 73%), and was not different in patients who had both the pedal and peroneal arteries patent (83% vs. 72%). In patients with diabetes the limb salvage rate was also similar for pedal or peroneal bypass (76% vs. 66%).

In a retrospective review by Darling et al.,[15] the authors compared 732 peroneal artery reconstructions with 238 inframalleolar (dorsalis pedis artery) reconstructions in patients with critical limb ischemia. The secondary patency and limb salvage rates at 5 years for dorsalis pedis bypass were 67% and 86%, respectively, and for peroneal bypass were 78% and 93%, respectively, with no statistical difference between dorsal pedal and peroneal bypass. The authors concluded that either the dorsalis pedis or peroneal artery is an acceptable outflow tract, and that the determination should depend on conduit limitations and areas of tissue compromise that may affect conduit tunneling. In a follow-up report by Darling et al.[16] that included 885 peroneal and 291 dorsalis pedis reconstructions for patients with critical limb ischemia, the results indicated no difference in patency or limb salvage. The authors concluded

that both targets are satisfactory and the decision of which artery to revascularize should be based on conduit availability and the location of tissue planes that are infected or necrotic, which may jeopardize graft placement.

In a prospective review by Abou-Zamzam et al.,[17] patients undergoing peroneal or inframalleolar vein bypasses were investigated with attention to healing of pedal gangrene, graft patency, and limb salvage. There were 83 peroneal and 46 pedal bypasses performed, and the groups were matched for diabetes, gender, coronary disease, renal failure, prior bypass, smoking, and preoperative hemodynamics. Patients who had an inframalleolar bypass were significantly younger (63.9 years vs. 71.6 years) and had a significantly higher postoperative ankle-brachial index (1.02 vs. 0.91). However, despite these differences, comparison of inframalleolar with peroneal bypass showed 3-year survival rates of 69.1% versus 60%, 2-year limb salvage rates of 70.3% versus 85.8%, and time to wound healing of 19.7 weeks versus 21.6 weeks, respectively. None of the differences were significant. The authors concluded that peroneal bypass offers equivalent results to a pedal bypass, and in the presence of ischemic foot gangrene, the peroneal artery is an appropriate target for revascularization.

A subgroup analysis by Schneider et al.[14] that evaluated pedal versus peroneal bypass determined that there was no difference in primary, assisted primary, or secondary 3-year graft patency rates (58% vs. 65%; 80% vs. 78%; 82% vs. 78%, respectively). The authors concluded that an inframalleolar graft is as durable as a peroneal bypass.

Recommendation

Despite the lack of randomized prospective studies evaluating tibial versus inframalleolar vessels, the available data supports the use of either outflow tract when available with essentially equivalent results. In addition, the peroneal artery should not be considered inferior to inframalleolar targets with respect to patency, limb salvage, and hemodynamics. In patients who present with critical limb ischemia and have both a patent peroneal and inframalleolar vessel to revascularize, the decision of which vessel to bypass should be based on consideration of conduit availability and regional tissue necrosis that may hinder conduit placement.

TIBIAL VERSUS INFRAMALLEOLAR AND LOCATION OF FOOT TISSUE LOSS

Patients presenting with either heel gangrene or forefoot gangrene present a challenging clinical problem for healing and return to ambulatory status. Investigators have tried to determine which tibial vessel or inframalle-olar vessel is best to revascularize in order to maximize tissue perfusion to the anatomic location of the foot wound. In a multi-institutional retrospective review by Treiman et al.,[18] the authors investigated factors that would predict healing of heel ulcer or gangrene. The study consisted of 91 patients with nonhealing heel wounds, with 70% having diabetes, 24% on dialysis, and 64% smoking. In the cohort, 81 patients underwent infrainguinal revascularization to the popliteal artery (34 patients), tibial artery (40 patients), and pedal vessels (seven patients). The mean follow-up for the entire group was 21 months. In 73% of patients, the heel wound healed in a mean time of 3 months; 11% of patients underwent amputation. During the follow-up period, 91% of bypasses were patent, and at 3 years the primary assisted patency rate was 87% and limb salvage rate was 86%. The significant variables that were predictive of heel ulcer healing were a patent posterior tibial artery beyond the ankle, normal renal function, a palpable pedal pulse, and the number of patent tibial arteries beyond the bypass in continuity to the ankle. Factors that did not influence outcome were diabetes, perioperative ankle-brachial index, or other cardiovascular risk factors. No patient with a failed graft experienced healing of the heel ulcer.

In a retrospective study by Berceli et al.,[19] the authors reviewed the efficacy of revascularizing the dorsal pedal artery for limb salvage in patients with ischemic heel ulcer or gangrene compared with patients having forefoot ulcer or gangrene. More than 90% of patients in both groups had diabetes and the majority of patients had autogenous conduit available for revascularization. Complete healing rates were similar for both forefoot and heel wounds (90.5% vs. 86.5%), with no difference in amputation rates (9.8% vs. 9.3%). Of interest, only 48.8% of patients with heel ulcers had an intact pedal arch despite the dorsalis pedis artery being the outflow target that was revascularized. Healing, as well as graft patency, was independent of the presence of an intact pedal arch. The authors concluded that patients with heel wounds who have had the dorsalis pedis revascularized have adequate heel perfusion irrespective of a patent pedal arch, and healing and limb salvage rates were equivalent to patients with forefoot wounds.

In a retrospective review by Roddy et al.,[20] the authors identified 18 patients that underwent 19 bypasses for pedal gangrene and had the plantar artery as their only runoff vessel (no tibial vessels). None of the patients had an intact pedal arch, and 84% had diabetes. All patients had autogenous venous conduit and the targets chosen were lateral plantar (42%), common plantar (37%), and medial plantar (21%). The 30-day bypass failure rate was 26% in patients who lost their limb. Of the patients with a patent graft at 30 days, the

patency and limb salvage rates at a mean follow-up of 15 months was 74%. The authors concluded that plantar artery bypass is a reasonable alternative to amputation, and acceptable results can be anticipated if the bypass remains patent for the first 30 days.

As previously mentioned, Abou-Zamzam et al.[17] reviewed patients undergoing peroneal or inframalleolar vein bypasses with attention to healing of pedal gangrene. There were no differences between inframalleolar and peroneal bypass (3-year survival rates of 69.1% vs. 60%, 2-year limb salvage rates of 70.3% vs. 85.8%, and time to wound healing of 19.7 weeks vs. 21.6 weeks, respectively).

However, because the peroneal artery is a terminal vessel at the ankle with collateral branches to pedal vessels, its anatomic characteristics may affect foot healing. In the study by Elliott et al.,[8] patients having had a peroneal bypass who had forefoot necrosis had significant limb loss when they had any of the following angiographic findings: Absence of collateral vessels perfusing the foot; peroneal artery <10 cm in length; or peroneal artery <2 mm in diameter.

Recommendation

The current literature (retrospective reviews, nonrandomized) strongly supports revascularization to either peroneal or inframalleolar vessels to achieve pedal wound healing with outcomes that are comparable. Patients with renal failure on dialysis have worse outcomes with limb salvage despite patent grafts; however, they should not be denied revascularization. Although an intact pedal arch intuitively should be predictive of foot wound healing following revascularization, revascularization should not be precluded if the pedal arch is partially patent. Caution should be exercised in choosing the peroneal artery as the target vessel when it has a paucity of collaterals to the foot or is small and patent only for a short distance.

PREDICTING RESULTS OF BYPASS PROCEDURES

Once a surgical bypass procedure is done, it would be helpful if some expectation of success was possible. It is usually felt that there are three factors that contribute to a successful bypass: Inflow, outflow, and the nature and quality of the bypass conduit. It is usually easy to assess the quality of the inflow. For example, a good clinical femoral artery pulse along with some type of noninvasive assessment of the inflow is usually adequate. In those patients undergoing some type of arteriogram or duplex ultrasound imaging, the presence of any suspect lesions limiting the inflow is easily determined. A complete discussion of various conduits is presented in Chapters 19, 20, and 22. We will limit our subsequent discussion to methods of assessing outflow and how helpful they are in predicting results of bypass surgery to the tibial vessels.

Outflow Assessment

Traditional methods of assessing outflow have been based on the quality of the tibial vessels on a preoperative arteriogram. Outflow or runoff has been described as poor or good, or is sometimes graded according to the number of tibial vessels that were patent on the arteriogram, such as grade 0, 1, 2, or 3. We have demonstrated[21] that this scoring method correlates poorly with actual measurements of peripheral resistance in patients undergoing bypass grafting. The failure of this method of scoring appears to result from imprecise criteria for grading a vessel as present or absent, an inability to distinguish poor vessels from good-quality vessels, and the assumption that each of the tibial vessels contributes equally to the runoff. We have developed a scoring system that does correlate well with a measured intraoperative assessment of runoff resistance.[22] The study included 80 patients undergoing bypass surgery at the popliteal and tibial level. We could not find a correlation between measured runoff resistance and bypass graft patency at 3, 6, or 12 months. Some patients with measured poor runoff resistance had successful bypass graft patency. Others have reported a good correlation with measured runoff resistance and bypass graft patency.[23] Our only explanation of the difference is that in our study all the bypass grafts were autogenous vein, which we believe will remain patent in spite of diminished runoff. Graft patency is most likely a multifactorial process in which graft material, runoff resistance, and other factors play a role.

Society for Vascular Surgery and the International Society for Cardiovascular Surgery Scoring System

As previously mentioned, techniques for scoring the preoperative arteriogram prior to bypass surgery have suffered from vagueness in the scoring system, failure to correlate with measured runoff resistance, and lack of universal acceptance. The Committee on Reporting Standards of the Society for Vascular Surgery (SVS) and the International Society for Cardiovascular Surgery (ISCVS), the predecessors of the current SVS, introduced the SVS/ISCVS scoring system, a system of grading of peripheral runoff based on the preoperative arteriogram.[24] In addition to choosing which vessels are important to the runoff bed, the scoring system attempts to assign relative importance to each runoff vessel. Using multiple linear regression, we identified angiographic components that correlated best with

measured runoff resistance and applied a weighting of the various components of the SVS/ISCVS score, thus improving the prediction of the runoff score.[25] We were able to demonstrate that the pedal arch was an important contributor to runoff. In addition, in a bypass to the peroneal artery, the score of the peroneal artery was more important than the pedal arch score.

Runoff Assessment and Bypass Graft Patency

Although we were not able to make a correlation between runoff and bypass graft patency,[22] others have made this association. Wengerter et al.[26] reported a correlation between good runoff and bypass graft patency to the tibial vessels. They defined good outflow as continuity of outflow vessels with the foot, or for the peroneal artery, a direct communication between one of the terminal branches and a pedal vessel. For the foot vessels, good outflow was defined as continuity with a patent pedal arch. The 2-year primary patency rate with good outflow was 72% and for poor outflow was 54% ($p <0.05$).

Blankensteijn et al.[27] reported that none of the intraoperative tests, continuous wave Doppler, pulse volume recording, ultrasonic volume flowmetry, intraoperative arteriogram, or a palpable pulse, was predictive of bypass graft patency at 12 months, but that the SVS/ISCVS score was predictive.

In 77 bypass grafts to crural vessels for critical limb ischemia, Biancari et al.[28] was able to show a predictive correlation between the SVS/ISCVS revised score and bypass graft patency and limb salvage.

In contradistinction to the above report, Alback et al.[29] reported that the SVS/ISCVS score had no impact on femorocrural graft patency. They also showed that an occluded pedal arch was associated with a poor outcome. Graft flow and maximal flow capacity following an injection of papaverin were good predictors of 1-year graft patency.

In a report by Ulus et al.,[30] patency rates in limbs with good runoff were better than those in limbs with fair or poor runoff (88%, 70%, and 21%, respectively, $p <0.01$). These authors defined good runoff as patency of two or three lower leg arteries or patency of one lower leg artery in continuity with an intact anterior or posterior foot arch. Poor runoff was defined as no patent lower leg artery or one patent lower leg artery with deficient or occluded foot arches. In this study they also made comparisons with the traditional SVS/ISCVS score, the modified SVS/ISCVS score, the traditional scoring of 1, 2, or 3 tibial vessels, and their new score. The best correlation with bypass graft patency was with their new scoring system.

In a recent study, Heise et al.[31] reports a significant correlation between SVS/ISCVS score and the recipient vessel diameter. The angiographic score did not correlate with peripheral resistance or impedance, as measured by an extracorporeal bypass flow method or bypass graft patency rates. They suggest that patients with angiographically poor outflow should not be denied peripheral reconstructions.

Foot Scoring System

In a study by Toursarkissian et al.,[32] the severity and distribution of atherosclerotic disease in the foot and calf vessels of diabetics with critical limb ischemia was studied. In addition, they assessed whether the severity of the occlusive disease present in the foot was predictive of bypass graft patency, limb salvage, or both. Each vessel was assigned a score from 0 to 3 on the basis of the tightest degree of stenosis present in the vessel, according to the SVS/ISCVS scoring system. The foot score was the sum of the dorsalis pedis, medial plantar, and lateral plantar scores plus one. Patency of bypass grafts correlated with the foot score and the medial plantar score. Bypass grafts with a foot score >7 had a 30% failure rate. Foot scores <7 and a medial plantar score <2 had only a 2% failure rate. The authors, however, point out that although better results were obtained with favorable foot scores, bypass grafts in patients with foot scores ≥7 did have a 70% success rate, and thus foot scores are unable to predict which patients will benefit from bypass grafting surgery.

Foot Arterial Anatomy and Bypass Graft Patency

The impact of the arterial foot anatomy on bypass graft patency and limb salvage has been considered for some time. The patency of foot vessels and the presence of branches of the peroneal artery that connect with foot vessels seem to be predictive of results. O'Mara et al.,[33] using operative arteriography, defined arterial foot anatomy in 56 patients after the completion of a distal bypass. Foot vessel anatomy was classified into primary and secondary pedal arches, analogous to the superficial and deep volar arches of the hand. For peroneal bypass, special attention was given to perforating branches and their communications with these two pedal arches. In femoral-to-anterior tibial or femoral-to-posterior tibial bypasses there was excellent patency when either a primary or secondary arch was present. When neither arch was present there was a high graft failure rate. Bypass grafts to the peroneal artery were successful when a primary or secondary arch was reconstituted via either the anterior or posterior perforating branches. When both arches were occluded, there were no grafts patent at 6 months.

In a study of bypass graft patency in diabetic patients <50 years old, the success of limb salvage in patients undergoing infrainguinal bypass procedures

was greatly influenced by the presence of severe stenoses in all three major foot vessels. The presence of a stenosis >70% in the dorsalis pedis, medial plantar, and lateral plantar arteries was associated with a high likelihood of limb loss despite a patent bypass graft.[34] No other factors could be identified that were predictive of graft thrombosis or amputation. Again it was pointed out that bypass grafts can be successful in this population, but that patients need to be made aware that in the presence of severe foot vessel occlusive disease, amputation is still possible in spite of a patent bypass graft.

Recommendation

Predicting results of bypass procedures is difficult at best. Many factors can predict good results or poor results in groups of patients. Predicting results for a particular patient is difficult and runoff scores can only serve as a guide. Denying a patient a bypass due to poor runoff is not recommended because of the wide variability of published results.

REFERENCES

1. Strandness DE Jr, Priest RE, Gibbons GE. Combined clinical and pathologic study of diabetic and nondiabetic peripheral arterial disease. *Diabetes.* 1964;13:366–372.
2. Haimovici H. Patterns of arteriosclerotic lesions of the lower extremity. *Arch Surg.* 1967;95:918–933.
3. Raffetto JD, Chen MN, LaMorte WW, et al. Factors that predict site of outflow target artery anastomosis in infrainguinal revascularization. *J Vasc Surg.* 2002;35:1093–1099.
4. Menzoian JO, LaMorte WW, Paniszyn CC, et al. Symptomatology and anatomic patterns of peripheral vascular disease: differing impact of smoking and diabetes. *Ann Vasc Surg.* 1989;3:224–228.
5. Weitz JI, Byrne J, Clagett GP, et al. Diagnosis and treatment of chronic arterial insufficiency of the lower extremities: a critical review. *Circulation.* 1996;94:3026–3049.
6. Johnson WC, Lee KK. A comparative evaluation of polytetrafluoroethylene, umbilical vein, and saphenous vein bypass grafts for femoral-popliteal above-knee revascularization: a prospective randomized Department of Veterans Affairs cooperative study. *J Vasc Surg.* 2000;32:268–277.
7. Plecha EJ, Seabrook GR, Bandyk DF, et al. Determinants of successful peroneal artery bypass. *J Vasc Surg.* 1993;17:97–105; discussion 105–106.
8. Elliott BM, Robison JG, Brothers TE, et al. Limitations of peroneal artery bypass grafting for limb salvage. *J Vasc Surg.* 1993;18:881–888.
9. Raftery KB, Belkin M, Mackey WC, et al. Are peroneal artery bypass grafts hemodynamically inferior to other tibial artery bypass grafts? *J Vasc Surg.* 1994;19:964–968; discussion 968–969.
10. Bergamini TM, George SM Jr, Massey HT, et al. Pedal or peroneal bypass: which is better when both are patent? *J Vasc Surg.* 1994;20:347–355; discussion 355–346.
11. Karmody AM, Leather RP, Shah DM, et al. Peroneal artery bypass: a reappraisal of its value in limb salvage. *J Vasc Surg.* 1984;1:809–816.
12. Sidawy AN, Menzoian JO, Cantelmo NL, et al. Effect of inflow and outflow sites on the results of tibioperoneal vein grafts. *Am J Surg.* 1986;152:211–214.

13. Darling RC III, Shah DM, Chang BB, et al. Arterial reconstruction for limb salvage: is the terminal peroneal artery a disadvantaged outflow tract? *Surgery.* 1995;118:763–767.

14. Schneider JR, Walsh DB, McDaniel MD, et al. Pedal bypass versus tibial bypass with autogenous vein: a comparison of outcome and hemodynamic results. *J Vasc Surg.* 1993;17:1029–1038; discussion 1038–1040.

15. Darling RC III, Chang BB, Paty PS, et al. Choice of peroneal or dorsalis pedis artery bypass for limb salvage. *Am J Surg.* 1995; 170:109–112.

16. Darling RC III, Chang BB, Shah DM, et al. Choice of peroneal or dorsalis pedis artery bypass for limb salvage. *Semin Vasc Surg.* 1997;10:17–22.

17. Abou-Zamzam AM Jr, Moneta GL, Lee RW, et al. Peroneal bypass is equivalent to inframalleolar bypass for ischemic pedal gangrene. *Arch Surg.* 1996;131:894–898; discussion 898–899.

18. Treiman GS, Oderich GS, Ashrafi A, et al. Management of ischemic heel ulceration and gangrene: an evaluation of factors associated with successful healing. *J Vasc Surg.* 2000;31:1110–1118.

19. Berceli SA, Chan AK, Pomposelli FB Jr, et al. Efficacy of dorsal pedal artery bypass in limb salvage for ischemic heel ulcers. *J Vasc Surg.* 1999;30:499–508.

20. Roddy SP, Darling RC III, Chang BB, et al. Outcomes with plantar bypass for limb-threatening ischemia. *Ann Vasc Surg.* 2001;15:79–83.

21. Menzoian JO, La Morte WW, Cantelmo NL, et al. The preoperative angiogram as a predictor of peripheral vascular runoff. *Am J Surg.* 1985;150:346–352.

22. LaMorte WW, Menzoian JO, Sidawy A, et al. A new method for the prediction of peripheral vascular resistance from the preoperative angiogram. *J Vasc Surg.* 1985;2:703–708.

23. Peterkin GA, LaMorte WW, Menzoian JO. Runoff resistance and early graft failure in infrainguinal bypass surgery. *Arch Surg.* 1988;123:1199–1201.

24. Rutherford RB, Flanigan DP, Gupta SK, et al. Suggested standards for reports dealing with lower extremity ischemia. Prepared by the Ad Hoc Committee on Reporting Standards, Society for Vascular Surgery/North American Chapter, International Society for Cardiovascular Surgery. *J Vasc Surg.* 1986;4:80–94.

25. Peterkin GA, Manabe S, LaMorte WW, et al. Evaluation of a proposed standard reporting system for preoperative angiograms in infrainguinal bypass procedures: angiographic correlates of measured runoff resistance. *J Vasc Surg.* 1988;7:379–385.

26. Wengerter KR, Yang PM, Veith FJ, et al. A twelve-year experience with the popliteal-to-distal artery bypass: the significance and management of proximal disease. *J Vasc Surg.* 1992;15:143–149; discussion 150–141.

27. Blankensteijn JD, Gertler JP, Brewster DC, et al. Intraoperative determinants of infrainguinal bypass graft patency: a prospective study. *Eur J Vasc Endovasc Surg.* 1995;9:375–382.

28. Biancari F, Alback A, Ihlberg L, et al. Angiographic run-off score as a predictor of outcome following femorocrural bypass surgery. *Eur J Vasc Endovasc Surg.* 1999;17:480–485.

29. Alback A, Roth WD, Ihlberg L, et al. Preoperative angiographic score and intraoperative flow as predictors of the mid-term patency of infrapopliteal bypass grafts. *Eur J Vasc Endovasc Surg.* 2000;20:447–453.

30. Ulus AT, Ljungman C, Almgren B, et al. The influence of distal runoff on patency of infrainguinal vein bypass grafts. *Vasc Surg.* 2001;35:31–35.

31. Heise M, Kruger U, Ruckert R, et al. Correlation between angiographic runoff and intraoperative hydraulic impedance with regard to graft patency. *Ann Vasc Surg.* 2003;17:509–515.

32. Toursarkissian B, D'Ayala M, Stefanidis D, et al. Angiographic scoring of vascular occlusive disease in the diabetic foot: relevance to bypass graft patency and limb salvage. *J Vasc Surg.* 2002; 35:494–500.

33. O'Mara CS, Flinn WR, Neiman HL, et al. Correlation of foot arterial anatomy with early tibial bypass patency. *Surgery.* 1981; 89:743–752.

34. Toursarkissian B, Hassoun HT, Smilanich RP, et al. Efficacy of infrainguinal bypass for limb salvage in young diabetic patients. *J Diabetes Complications.* 2000;14:255–258.

Autogenous Venous Options and Preparation of Veins Using Angioscopy

19

Sherry D. Scovell   Frank W. LoGerfo

Arterial reconstruction of the lower extremity circulation is one of the most common surgical procedures for the patient with diabetes. In these patients, tibial arterial occlusive disease often predominates. Because of this distribution of disease, bypass grafting in the case of nonhealing ulceration or rest pain often requires the distal anastomosis to be created at the dorsalis pedis artery, the peroneal artery, or the distal posterior tibial artery at the ankle. It has been clearly demonstrated through numerous studies that autogenous conduits have superior results with respect to long-term patency in bypass grafts that extend below the knee.[1,2] Preferentially, the ipsilateral greater saphenous vein is utilized if it is available. However, in around 40% to 45% of patients, and up to 80% of patients requiring lower extremity revascularization, the ipsilateral greater saphenous vein has already been partially or completely harvested for either coronary reconstruction or a previous lower extremity bypass graft.[3] Therefore, alternate options for conduits are often required. The options include the contralateral greater saphenous vein, the lesser saphenous veins, and the upper extremity veins, including the cephalic and basilic veins. With respect to the contralateral greater

saphenous vein, it is usually of adequate caliber and length for bypass grafting; however, there is often distal disease in the vessels of the contralateral leg, making it attractive to retain that saphenous vein for *in situ* revascularization if and when needed in the future. In the previous work, we have shown that the likelihood of contralateral revascularization is about 60% at 3 years.[4] On the basis of the need for contralateral revascularization, the diminished success with redo procedures, and our good results with arm veins, we consider arm veins the first alternative when ipsilateral saphenous vein is unavailable. Either the basilic or cephalic veins may be utilized for this purpose. Another potential option is the lesser saphenous vein.

These alternate sources of vein are not as ideal as the greater saphenous vein to harvest and prepare, secondary to a number of factors. The lesser saphenous veins are considerably shorter in overall length and often require harvest of another segment of vein with a venovenostomy to reach a distal target. Arm veins, especially the central end of the cephalic vein, may have extremely thin walls, requiring meticulous dissection. The basilic and cephalic arm veins may provide an adequate length of vein. However, these veins are commonly used for venopuncture; the repeated trauma of venopuncture often leads to the development of sclerotic segments as well as focal webs and bands within the lumen. These less than ideal segments of arm veins, left undetected, may be a source of early bypass graft failure. For this reason, angioscopic evaluation of the venous lumen was introduced as a means to identify these segments during the bypass procedure and to allow correction of these abnormalities under direct vision, in an attempt to secure a more ideal conduit and therefore a graft with better long-term patency.

Bypass grafting may be performed with the venous conduit in a reversed configuration, an *in situ* manner, or a nonreversed, transposed arrangement called the "flexible approach."[5] With respect to the latter two methods, valve lysis is required. When valvulotomy is performed blindly, it may lead to injury of the vein, especially if the valvulotome becomes caught in the lumen of a small side branch. Blind valve lysis does not allow for the detection and correction of intraluminal webs that are often present in these arm veins. Additionally, incomplete valve lysis is a significant etiology of early graft thrombosis. Angioscopy in conjunction with valvulotomy allows for complete valve lysis under direct visualization.

Angioscopy allows the intraoperative evaluation of the venous conduit, the identification of factors that may lead to early graft thrombosis, and a means by which to correct these factors under direct vision. It has been shown to be an advantageous adjunct to the bypass procedure without adding significant morbidity or time in the operating room (OR).[6] Through the identification of the above-mentioned issues, angioscopy may increase the patency of the bypass graft by allowing the identification and correction of technical errors prior to leaving the operating theater, especially with the use of alternate conduits such as arm veins. Our choice of arm vein as the first alternative to ipsilateral saphenous vein is contingent upon the high quality of the arm vein, as confirmed with angioscopy. If resection of a segment of vein is necessary, we have not found it to affect patency.[7]

This chapter will examine the options for autogenous conduit in lower extremity bypass grafting. It will also discuss the preparation of these conduits and the utility of intraoperative angioscopy in attempt to assure that each vein utilized is in the most optimal condition at the time of surgery.

AUTOGENOUS CONDUITS

Greater Saphenous Vein

The greater saphenous vein is preferentially utilized for bypass grafting in the lower extremity. This is primarily because of its length, its proximity to the operative site, and its ease of harvest. It is infrequently insulted for venopuncture and has provided excellent results for lower extremity bypass grafting. However, it is also often used for coronary artery bypass grafting. For this and other reasons, the ipsilateral saphenous vein is unavailable in roughly 30% of our patients.[4]

Anatomically, the greater or long saphenous vein originates on the medial aspect of the dorsum of the foot, ascends along the medial aspect of the thigh, and joins the deep venous system at the fossa ovalis where it joins the common femoral vein (Fig. 19-1). It is the longest vein in the body and is accompanied by the saphenous nerve below the knee. It arises from the dorsal venous arch, which becomes the medial marginal vein of the foot. The vein then ascends along the anterior aspect of the medial malleolus. It travels posterior to the medial border of the tibia and posterior to the medial condyle of the tibia as it ascends to the medial aspect of the thigh, before diving deep to join the deep venous system. It is located deep in the subcutaneous tissue, just superficial to the muscular fascia.

Although this is the typical course of the greater saphenous vein, there are many variations in its anatomy. Shah et al.[8] prospectively examined the greater saphenous venous system in 331 patients through the use of prebypass phlebography. There was a single continuous trunk in both the calf and the thigh in only 38.2% of patients. In the remaining 61.8% of patients,

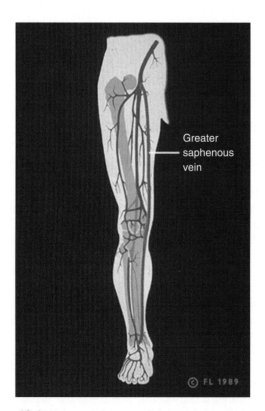

Figure 19-1 Anatomic location of the greater saphenous vein.

there was a variant of a double venous system. With respect to the distal portion of the greater saphenous vein in the thigh, there was a single trunk in 65% of patients. For the 35% of patients who had a double system with both medial and lateral branches, they could be further characterized as medial dominant, lateral dominant, or equal. These double trunks rejoined each other within 10 cm of the knee joint in the majority of cases. Only 15% rejoined in the middle third of the thigh. In 11% of patients, the double trunks extended the entire length of the thigh without connecting. Only in a minority of cases (4%) were there triple trunks or multiple branching systems. In the calf, there was a single trunk in only 45% of cases. These double branches are in either anterior or posterior positions. However, in the majority of cases, the anterior branch was dominant. In 94% of cases, the saphenous vein bifurcated within 5 cm of the knee joint.

The valves in the saphenous vein are usually bicuspid, with the cusps oriented parallel to the skin surface. Occasionally, single cusp or tricuspid valves may be seen. Typically, the greater saphenous vein has 6.3 valves with a range from 1 to 13.

There are several approaches to harvesting the saphenous vein. The dissection may begin in the groin and is usually done at a 45-degree angle bisecting a line drawn along the groin crease and a line drawn over the femoral pulse. The dissection is carried out by identifying the insertion of the greater saphenous vein into the common femoral vein at the saphenofemoral junction. An alternate option is to identify the greater saphenous vein distally along the anterior aspect of the medial malleolus where it is quite superficial. If so, the vein can be cannulated with a Horsley needle and irrigated with a solution of heparin 4,000 U and papaverine 120 mg in 1,000 cc of Normosol or Plasmalyte (not Ringer lactate). These steps help in identifying branches and preventing venospasm.[9]

Lesser Saphenous Vein

Another choice for a venous conduit is the lesser or short saphenous vein. It is a less favorable option because it is usually less than half the length of the greater saphenous vein. Harvest of this vein for a bypass extending from the femoral region to the tibial region may require that multiple segments of vein be harvested to create a composite vein graft. It is also less easily accessible during surgery, as it travels along the posterior aspect of the calf. For this reason, dissection is often preferred with the patient initially in the prone position or in a frog-legged position. In most circumstances, utilization of this vein also requires another incision along the posterior aspect of the calf. Alternatively, a flap may be created from a medial approach to expose this vein, although this method

may lead to flap necrosis and large areas of dead space if meticulous technique is not utilized.

This vein begins distally at the level of the foot and extends up the posterior aspect of the calf, joining the deep venous system in the popliteal fossa. This vein originates as the dorsal venous arch of the foot as well. It extends along the lateral aspect of the foot, running just posterior to the lateral malleolus. It crosses the Achilles tendon and ascends up the posterior aspect of the calf. It travels close to the sural nerve. Last, at the level of the popliteal fossa, it dives into the deep fascia and joins the popliteal vein. The level that the lesser saphenous vein penetrates the fascia may be quite variable.

In addition, the length of the lesser saphenous vein is considerably shorter than the greater saphenous vein. Rutherford et al.[10] reported the average useable length of the vein to be approximately 37.4 cm, although it has been reported to be shorter in other series. Often this conduit will only reach from the femoral to the above-knee popliteal region or from the below-knee region to the distal tibial vessels. Occasionally, two full-length veins may be used as a composite for a femoral to distal tibial vessel bypass graft.

Cephalic and Basilic Veins

As mentioned previously, arm veins are becoming an increasingly more common conduit used for bypass grafting, especially in patients without saphenous vein as an option, or in the case of a failed previous bypass graft. Arm veins as conduits are typically thinner walled than the saphenous veins, especially the central end of the cephalic vein. They require extra care in their harvest and preparation. In addition, they have frequently been insulted by venopuncture, leading to regions with webs and thrombotic segments, which requires diligence when evaluating these conduits for use in a bypass graft. These damaged segments of arm vein are not often apparent on gross external inspection, even when the gentle distention technique is utilized. In spite of these features, arm veins are usually of considerable length since both the cephalic and basilic veins extend the length of the entire arm.

Anatomically, the cephalic vein begins at the wrist, running on the lateral aspect of the radius up to the level of the antecubital fossa (Fig. 19-2). In the antecubital fossa, the median cubital vein connects the cephalic and basilic veins. The cephalic vein then extends along the lateral aspect of the biceps muscle, where it travels in the deltopectoral groove to join the axillary vein.

The basilic vein begins on the ulnar aspect of the wrist and extends up the forearm on that side. Similarly, near the antecubital fossa, it is joined by the median cubital vein. The basilic vein ascends along the medial aspect of the biceps muscle. It terminates by

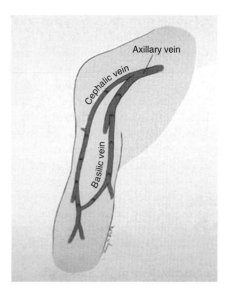

Figure 19-2 Anatomy of upper extremity veins.

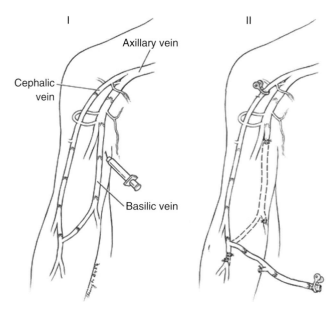

Figure 19-3 Method to harvest cephalic-basilic vein loop.

emptying into the deep system in the mid upper arm, where it penetrates the deep fascia and joins the brachial vein.

There are several choices of vein configuration that may be used. These include the following:

1. The entire cephalic vein from the wrist to the deltopectoral groove
2. The entire basilic vein from the posterior aspect of the wrist to the axilla
3. Cephalic-basilic upper arm vein loop connected via the median cubital vein, as forearm veins are often of poorer quality when compared to upper arm veins[11] (Figs. 19-3 and 19-4)
4. Cephalic vein in the forearm connected to the median cubital vein in the antecubital fossa and then crossing over to the basilic vein up to the axilla.

There may be regions of poor arm vein conduit secondary to sclerotic segments or webs throughout these veins. Therefore, several segments of arm vein may be harvested and joined together in end-to-end venovenostomies. These venovenostomies are typically performed in an end-to-end manner using 7-0 proline sutures (Ethicon, Sommerville, NJ).

ANGIOSCOPY

The concept of angioscopy was introduced nearly 70 years ago as a technique used to visualize the luminal surface of blood vessels.[12] Initially, the angioscopes were quite rigid and could only be used in large vessels. In addition, they were traumatic to the endothelial surface of the blood vessels. However, due to advances in fiberoptics, smaller, more flexible angioscopes have been developed. Now scopes with diameters of <2 mm may be utilized in the evaluation of vein graft conduits and smaller caliber vessels. Better fiberoptic technology has improved the visualization of the luminal surfaces.

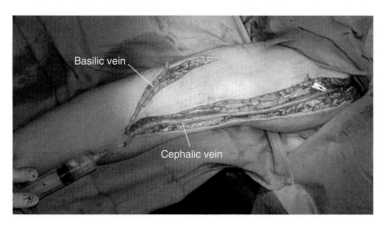

Figure 19-4 Cephalic-basilic vein loop harvest.

Angioscopy has become a useful adjunct in vascular surgery. Following a bypass graft, it allows the detection of technical errors, defines the exact location of the problem, and allows for immediate correction under direct vision. It is especially useful in the preparation of venous conduits for arterial bypass surgery. It accurately detects unsuspected regions of intraluminal pathology that might otherwise cause a graft to fail. Angioscopy allows not only the identification of these lesions, but correction with angioscopic-directed lysis of webs and intraluminal bands. It also assists in the selection of optimal-quality vein segments in composite situations. Again, this is particularly helpful with sclerotic segments of arm vein, which may be promptly detected and excluded. In addition, angioscopy allows for direct visualization of valvulotomy during vein preparation, to ensure accurate and complete valve lysis in both *in situ* and nonreversed vein grafts. It may also be utilized in patients following thrombectomy to ensure that all thrombus has been removed.[13]

There are numerous angioscopes available today (Fig. 19-5). Some are disposable and others are reusable. They are also characterized by the outer diameter of the body of the scope, the length of the scope, and the diameter of the working channel. Angioscopes that are utilized in vascular surgery have body diameters that range from 0.8 mm to 2.8 mm. The size of the scope is usually tailored to the size of the vessel to be examined. The lengths of the scopes vary as well, from 30 to 100 cm in length. Most angioscopes have a working channel that is coaxial with the body of the scope and used for irrigation. The diameter of this working channel varies as well.

For inspection of venous conduits, the smaller angioscopes are utilized, with a 1.8 mm diameter being typical. The scope is introduced through the distal vein and

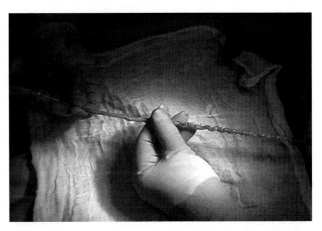

Figure 19-6   Arm vein conduit with angioscopically directed valve lysis.

passed retrograde in the vein until a valve is encountered (Fig. 19-6). A modified Mills valvulotome for transposed, nonreversed bypass grafts or the Olympus valvulotome for *in situ* bypass grafts is then introduced either through the proximal end of the vein or through a side branch. The vein is gently dilated with a heparinized, papaverine solution by hand injection or pump. Both leaflets of each valve are lysed under direct vision using the angioscope (Figs. 19-7 and 19-8). The process is repeated until all valves are lysed. The angioscope is then withdrawn slowly, and the luminal surfaces are inspected to identify incompletely lysed valves, webs, or sclerotic segments (Fig. 19-9).

The angioscope may be used while the vein is still *in situ*. If utilized in this manner, the angioscope may be inserted into the vein at the level of the wrist, and the vein followed proximally prior to division of the median cubital vein. This technique is often useful,

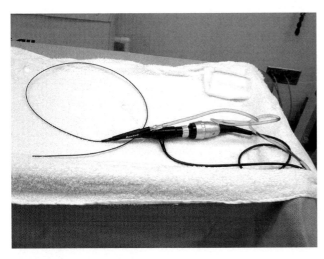

Figure 19-5   Angioscope with separate channel for continuous irrigation.

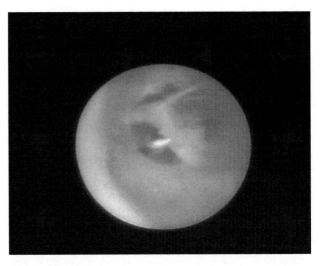

Figure 19-7   Angioscopically visualized valvulotome prior to lysis of valve cusp.

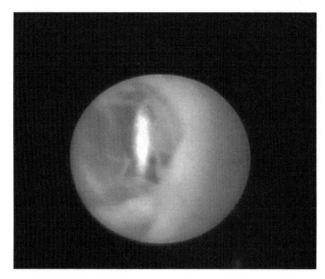

Figure 19-8 Angioscopically visualized valve following lysis with gentle distention.

especially as previous studies have noted a high incidence of intraluminal disease in arm vein harvest.[14] Using angioscopy in an *in situ* manner allows for the immediate identification of a markedly diseased vein or unusable conduit, which may be left intact while vein harvest is directed to another region. This technique may be accomplished through limited incisions on the forearm. It avoids unnecessary vein dissection and skin incisions.

Angioscopy and the Use of Greater Saphenous Vein Bypass Grafting

Angioscopy is not only useful in the arm vein conduit, but may also be beneficial in the evaluation of other venous conduits. In one study, 101 patients were assigned to one of two groups: One in which the vein conduit was evaluated with angioscopy, and the other in which angioscopic evaluation was not done.[15] Ultimately, the

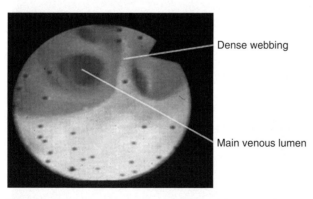

Dense webbing

Main venous lumen

Figure 19-9 Angioscopically visualized webbing noted in arm vein conduit. The small black objects represent fiberoptics that are not transmitting appropriately.

1-year primary patency rate was better in the group with angioscopic evaluation of the conduit when compared to the control group. The primary assisted and secondary patency rates did not differ between the groups. It is intuitive that inspection of the vein with determination of the vein quality prior to using it as a conduit should ensure longer intervention-free patency.

Angioscopy and the Use of Arm Vein Bypass Grafting

The largest series of patients with arm vein conduits in lower extremity revascularization was done at Beth Israel Deaconess Medical Center.[7] Over an 8-year period, 520 lower extremity revascularization procedures were performed, with many using arm vein conduits and intraoperative angioscopy for valve lysis and identification of luminal abnormalities. At this institution, arm vein for bypass grafts is utilized as the initial alternate conduit when ipsilateral greater saphenous vein is not available or is inadequate. Arm vein harvest, although tedious, has been found to result in minimal morbidity, usually <2%.

In a separate study of 109 infrainguinal arm vein bypasses, angioscopy was found to be an extremely sensitive method of detecting intraluminal disease that is often so prevalent in arm veins.[3] It was also found to be an excellent technique to aid in the direct visualization of endoluminal interventions that may be undertaken to upgrade the quality of the conduit.

Angioscopy Compared to Angiography

Angioscopy has been compared to intraoperative angiography in a prospective, randomized trial for infrainguinal bypass grafts.[13] In this single-center study, 250 patients were randomized. There was no statistically significant difference in the early (<30 days) patency between the two methods of evaluation in this patient population. Angioscopy, however, led to more vein conduit interventions, such as web lysis or exclusion of sclerotic vein segments. Arteriography was more likely to define technical problems associated with the anastomoses or the runoff vessels than to evaluate the quality of the conduit.

Criticism surrounding angioscopy stems from the added expense; the theoretic increase in operative time and cost; the learning curve initially associated with angioscopy, including both the technique as well as the interpretation of the results; and the potential injury to the venous conduits. In addition, when done in conjunction with *in situ* arterial or venous conduits, there may be problems with fluid overload associated with large irrigation volumes. Such factors have all been evaluated, and these concerns all found to be theoretic.

CONCLUSIONS

With arterial reconstruction to distal tibial arteries, autogenous venous conduit is important, if not essential, to success. Surprisingly, there is little difference in patency of tibial reconstructions as a function of the length of the vein graft. Rather the patency of vein grafts seems to be most dependent upon the quality of the conduit. It is the availability of high-quality autogenous venous conduits that drives much of the decision-making in distal tibial reconstruction. The vascular surgeon must have in mind several options for each operation—alternative targets, alternative inflow, alternative conduit—and be able to make the risk–benefit decisions surrounding each of these alternatives to achieve the necessary goal in a given patient. It is a creative process built around the limitations of quality conduit.

REFERENCES

1. Bergamini TM, Towne JB, Bandyk DF, et al. Experiences with *in situ* saphenous vein bypasses during 1981–1989: determinant factors of long-term patency. *J Vasc Surg.* 1991;13:137–149.
2. Veith FJ, Gupta SK, Ascer E, et al. Six-year prospective multicenter randomized comparison of autogenous saphenous vein and expanded PTFE grafts in infrainguinal arterial reconstructions. *J Vasc Surg.* 1986;3:104–114.
3. Marcaccio EJ, Miller A, Tannenbaum GA, et al. Angioscopically directed interventions improve arm vein bypass grafts. *J Vasc Surg.* 1993;17:994–1004.
4. Holzenbein TJ, Pomposelli FB Jr, Miller A, et al. Results of a policy with arm veins used as the first alternative to an unavailable ipsilateral greater saphenous vein for infrainguinal bypass. *J Vasc Surg.* 1996;23:130–140.
5. Pomposelli FB Jr, Jepsen SJ, Gibbons GW, et al. A flexible approach to infrapopliteal vein graft in patients with diabetes mellitus. *Arch Surg.* 1991;126:724–729.
6. Gilbertson JJ, Walsh DB, Zwolak RM, et al. A blinded comparison of angiography, angioscopy, and duplex scanning in the intraoperative evaluation of *in situ* saphenous vein bypass grafts. *J Vasc Surg.* 1992;15:121–129.
7. Faries PL, Arora S, Pomposelli FB Jr, et al. The use of arm vein in lower-extremity revascularization: results of 520 procedures performed in eight years. *J Vasc Surg.* 2000;31:50–59.
8. Shah DM, Chang BB, Leopold PW, et al. The anatomy of the greater saphenous venous system. *J Vasc Surg.* 1986;3:273–283.
9. LoGerfo FW, Haudenschild CC, Quist WC. A clinical technique for prevention of spasm and preservation of endothelium in saphenous vein grafts. *Arch Surg.* 1984;119:1212–1214.
10. Rutherford RB, Sawyer JD, Jones DN. The fate of residual saphenous vein after partial removal of ligation. *J Vasc Surg.* 1990;12:422–426.
11. Holzenbein TJ, Pomposelli FB Jr, Miller A, et al. The upper arm basilic-cephalic loop for distal bypass grafting: technical considerations and follow-up. *J Vasc Surg.* 1995;21:586–594.
12. Cutler EC, Levine A, Beck CS. The surgical treatment of mitral stenosis: experimental and clinical studies. *Arch Surg.* 1924;9:689–821.
13. Miller A, Marcaccio EJ, Tannenbaum GA, et al. Comparison of angioscopy and angiography for monitoring infrainguinal bypass vein grafts: results of a prospective randomized trial. *J Vasc Surg.* 1993;17:382–396.
14. Stonebridge P, Miller A, Tsoukas A, et al. Angioscopy of arm vein infrainguinal bypass grafts. *Ann Vasc Surg.* 1991;5:170–175.
15. Thorne J, Danielsson G, Danielsson P, et al. Intraoperative angioscopy may improve the outcome of *in situ* saphenous vein bypass grafting: a prospective study. *J Vasc Surg.* 2002;35:759–765.

20

Tibial Bypasses with Autogenous Tissue

R. Clement Darling, III   *Benjamin B. Chang*   *Sean P. Roddy*

The development of tibial artery bypasses over the past several decades has proven to be one of the more remarkable success stories for modern vascular surgery. When one considers that bypasses below the knee were unusual in the 1950s and 1960s, whereas bypasses today are constructed routinely to pedal arteries with a high expectation of success, the scope of the improvement in this area should seem nothing less than breathtaking.

However, this is not to say that these operations are the favorite of vascular surgeons worldwide. In fact, a large number of surgeons regard these procedures as difficult, tedious, and fraught with failure. Many surgeons would prefer to perform a carotid endarterectomy or an aortic aneurysm repair rather than undertake a femorotibial bypass. The current research in infrainguinal reconstruction for limb salvage centers on alternatives to autogenous bypass, utilizing either prosthetic conduits or catheter-based therapies.[1-3] In fact, many of these alternative therapies are promoted not because of superior results but rather because of the relative ease in performing the procedures. This implies that many surgeons would do just about anything rather than perform an infrapopliteal bypass with autogenous vein. This situation is analogous to those investigators who advocate carotid stenting in lieu of endarterectomy even though the complication rate of stenting still appears to be higher than the complication rate of surgery.

The purpose of this chapter is to provide a general overview of the various types of autogenous bypass available to the operating surgeon with a brief discussion of methodologies and results. The conduit discussed in this chapter is almost exclusively cutaneous vein, while recognizing that radial artery and superficial femoral vein can be successfully used in some limited circumstances.[4,5] These latter conduits are inherently limited in length and are therefore not typically useful for the large majority of infrapopliteal bypasses.

PREOPERATIVE PREPARATION

As with most operations, a degree of preoperative preparation is necessary to ensure the successful completion of the procedure. This is especially important in complex reconstructive procedures such as femorotibial bypass. Some form of arterial imaging is desirable to aid in the selection of proper inflow and outflow vessels; these topics are addressed in preceding chapters of this book. Noninvasive testing, including pulse volume recordings (PVRs), is useful in demonstrating the degree of preoperative hypoperfusion, the adequacy of inflow, and, if repeated postoperatively, the relative improvement in distal tissue perfusion.

An adjunctive measure that has proven to be of inestimable benefit to us is preoperative ultrasound vein mapping.[6,7] Because superficial veins are rife with anatomic variations and prone to acquired defects such as superficial phlebitis, preoperative imaging allows the surgeon to plan the procedure in a more efficient manner, while helping to avoid problems with the vein that can result in time-consuming delays, unnecessary added incisions, or even bypass failure. While the same knowledge may be gained by preoperative venography, the noninvasive nature of ultrasonography has its obvious advantages.

That being said, mapping does require special training and methodologies for its use. A probe of >5 MHz is recommended to obtain sufficient resolution. Leg veins are best mapped in a heated environment with the limb dependent to promote maximal dilatation. The ultrasonographer ideally should have a working knowledge of the anatomic variations of the veins as they pertain to operative surgery.[8] This knowledge is not easily acquired, and continual feedback to the ultrasonographer can only aid in developing this knowledge base. Mapping can be performed with the probe primarily in the transverse plane. It is usually helpful to the surgeon to have the vein location marked on the skin preoperatively with a relatively indelible marker in order to aid in the appropriate placement of incisions. However, the marked line can only be used as a general guide and is more inaccurate as the girth of the leg and the redundancy of excessive skin increases.

As the probe is advanced along the limb, major branch points can be marked. The diameter can also be assessed and marked at several places along the course of the vein. The diameter measured is a minimum diameter and may well underestimate the size of the vein when distended at the time of operation. Thus, vein size is the least accurately assessed feature of vein morphology as defined by ultrasonography. Conversely, ultrasonography is quite useful in determining the absolute presence and absence of the vein in question.

Other information that may be gleaned from preoperative ultrasonography are evidence of recent or old phlebitis, wall calcification, varices, and increased wall thickness suggestive of recanalization. Webs and synechia from previous injury or thrombosis (very commonly seen in arm veins at the antecubital fossa or wrist) are not well identified by ultrasonography, as the flow in these veins is insufficient to generate an accurate spectral pattern.

If an adequate vein is identified for the purposes of the operation, so much the better. If there is a question about vein length or adequacy, alternative sources of vein may be mapped at the same time in order to maximize the options available to the surgeon in the operating room. While it is certainly true that this information could also be gained in the operating room by making further incisions and exploring veins,

obtaining this information preoperatively allows one to have options planned in advance and therefore limit operative time considerably.

COMMONLY USED VEINS

Autogenous conduits for femorotibial bypass, as mentioned previously, are almost without exception a superficial vein from a limb. The most ideal vein for this type of reconstruction is certainly the greater saphenous vein, which possesses both the length and diameter to complete a bypass with one continuous segment. This vein may have a number of important anatomic variations that should be familiar to the operating surgeon, many of which have been reported previously.[8] The most important of these include what has been termed the lateral dominant saphenous vein in the thigh. With this variation, the largest vein starts from what is usually the lateral accessory vein at the saphenofemoral junction and runs somewhat more anterior and lateral to the usual saphenous vein course. This vein runs in a subcutaneous (not subfascial) plane and is generally thinner walled with a large number of small branches than the usual thigh saphenous vein. It typically rejoins the usual saphenous vein course within 2 or 3 in. of the knee, but in some circumstances may run down the length of the leg in parallel to the usual saphenous vein (full double system) (Fig. 20-1). The most common major anatomic variant of the saphenous vein below the knee has been called the posterior dominant vein, which merely means that the posterior

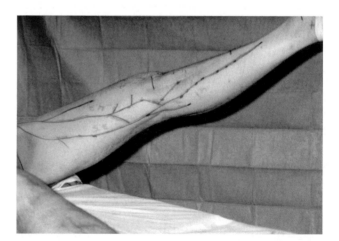

Figure 20-1 Duplex "vein map" illustrating a double saphenous system. It is important to note that the diameter measured by duplex is an internal dimension (ID) under relatively low venous pressure, whereas surgeons are accustomed to gauging its attributes as a conduit in terms of outside diameter (OD) when under arterial pressure. (From Leather RP, Shah DM, Darling RC, et al. *In situ* saphenous vein arterial bypass. In: Hobson RW and Wilson SE, eds. *Vascular surgery: Principles and practice*, 3rd ed. London: Taylor & Francis; 2004:485–494, with permission.)

arch vein, at or just below the knee joint, is the largest vein. This posterior vein also runs in a subcutaneous plane, is thinner walled, and has more small branches. It is prone to spasm, is relatively difficult to harvest, and typically rejoins the usual course of the greater saphenous vein at the junction of the calf and ankle. There are multiple variations in saphenous vein anatomy that are less common, often involving loops or parallel systems with unexpected communications. Preoperative imaging can help the surgeon lessen time sorting out this issue in the operating room.

Last, frequently overlooked are major segments of saphenous vein present even if the patient has had previous surgery utilizing the saphenous vein. The lower portion of this vein from the upper ankle to the foot is usually spared following a femoropopliteal bypass and is often of excellent quality. Preoperative mapping of previously operated limbs can reveal vein where none was thought available.

The lesser saphenous vein is also a useful autogenous conduit. Its anatomy and methods of harvest have also been described elsewhere.[9,10] Harvest can be done with a stocking-seam incision along the back of the leg. Some surgeons place the patient prone, harvest the vein, close the wounds, reposition the patient in a supine position, and redrape the patient. This is the easiest way to access the vein, but inherently causes the greatest delay between harvest and arterialization, and therefore maximizes ischemic injury to the vein. Alternatively, the lesser saphenous vein may be harvested through a posterior incision with the patient prone. This requires the leg to be held up to get the portion of the vein in the lower ankle and is therefore more awkward. However, this allows one to have the arteries dissected prior to vein harvest, and the length of conduit necessary for bypass more precisely determined.

Another method of lesser saphenous vein harvest involves the elevation of a full-thickness fascial-cutaneous flap raised through the usual greater saphenous vein harvest incision.[10] The surgeon can then look downward on the lesser saphenous vein. This exposure is most useful when a short segment of the lesser saphenous is needed, as exposure is limited to the upper three fourths of the vein. The flap raised is somewhat vulnerable to ischemia, especially if the flap is not drained and a hematoma develops.

The quality of the lesser saphenous vein is somewhat more variable than that of the greater saphenous in that the wall is more likely to be overly thick. The length of the vein is capable of performing a femoropopliteal bypass or a bypass to the most proximal portions of the tibial arteries only if the entire length of the vein is harvested. More frequently, the lesser saphenous is utilized as a portion of a composite (spliced) vein bypass. The most notable anatomic variation of the lesser saphenous

vein is its extension cephalic past the popliteal fossa up the thigh. This so-called vein of Giacomimi can be of good quality, and when present, can provide the surgeon with an unexpected source of autogenous conduit.

Veins of the arms are also commonly employed for autogenous femorotibial bypass.[11,12] They are easily accessible and require no special techniques for harvest. They are often large in diameter, especially in the upper arm. The largest diameter vein is more often the basilic, which has rarely been damaged by previous venipunctures, but tends to be short and somewhat more difficult to dissect due to its close proximity to nerves. At the elbow, the basilic vein is confluent with the antecubital vein leading into the cephalic vein, such that these two veins can be used as one segment. Alternatively, the basilic vein can continue along the medial posterior aspect of the forearm or more deeply down the center of the volar surface of the forearm. The cephalic vein runs from the wrist to the deltopectoral groove in the shoulder, and therefore is the second longest segment of autogenous vein available for use. This vein is easily harvested and often of usable diameter.

Arm veins have several limitations (besides insufficient length) as autogenous bypass conduit. First, arm veins typically have a very thin wall, which makes working with them more difficult during anastomosis. A venovenostomy of two small arm veins may be the most problematic anastomosis in leg bypass surgery. Second, arm veins have almost always been injured to a greater or lesser extent by venipuncture and intravenous infusions. The resultant vein may have near-obstructing webs and synechia that are inapparent from external examination of the vein. In fact, this happens so often with the antecubital vein that some surgeons routinely discard this segment. Use of arm veins is improved by assessing patency in the operating room, whether by angiography, endoscopy, or instrumentation with a valvulotome.

Last, the cephalic vein is often quite tapered from the shoulder portion to the forearm portion. Use as a reversed vein is somewhat more problematic in that one is attaching the small end of the vein to a large artery and the large end to a small artery. Such an arrangement automatically results in a relative stenosis of the bypass.

TYPES OF AUTOGENOUS RECONSTRUCTIONS

Given an adequate length of vein to perform the desired reconstruction, there are three general methods of employing this conduit: Reversed excised vein, nonreversed excised vein, and *in situ* vein. In addition, any of the general methods may be used in combination with others to prepare shorter segments of vein that can be spliced together with venovenostomies to form a composite vein bypass.

Vein Harvest

For all types of vein bypass, the conduit is by necessity isolated and dissected to a greater or lesser extent. What is often overlooked is that the method of vein harvest is an important factor in preserving the physiologic functions of the vein. The following discussion will describe some methods and considerations that we regard as important.

First, every effort should be given to harvesting the vein as if it were any other mesenchymal organ (such as a kidney or liver), with an eye to minimizing injury (especially ischemic injury). The endothelium of the vein is uniquely able to resist and counteract the blood's tendency to thrombose. This is due in part to the more passive barrier function of the endothelium (shielding the blood from the subendothelium) as well as to the more active nature of the endothelium in counteracting thrombosis (prostacyclin secretion, for instance). Without a living vein, the conduit is little better than a collagen tube.

Like all complex organs, veins require oxygenation. Oxygenated blood is usually delivered to the vein wall via the vasa vasorum; interruption of this network of vessels will cause a relative ischemia. Interestingly, the physiologic function of the vein wall may be preserved by the installation of oxygenated, arterialized blood within the lumen of the vein.[13] Therefore, the vasa vasorum of the vein should be interrupted at the last minute, only after the inflow and outflow arteries are exposed and ready for clamping. In addition, branches of the vein are divided with the bulk of the vein being left in place under the investing fascia through which the vasa vasorum traverses. The practice of dissecting the vein out from its bed to be put in saline on the back table for an indefinite time should be assiduously avoided. While such a practice might seem extreme, certainly the harvest of other complex organs is centered on minimizing the ischemic insult engendered by the harvest procedure. The vein should ideally be treated with the same care and respect.

Other factors that are known to cause vein injury during harvest include the pressure to which the vein is dilated and the pH of the dilating solution.[14,15] Dilatation of the vein is almost always necessary to counteract the spasm caused by dissection; unfortunately, dilatation with a hand-held syringe can generate pressures in the range of 1,000 Torr and can be injurious. Restriction of the dilatation pressure by the use of a pressure bag inflated to no more than 250 to 300 Torr that encloses the dilating solution, which in turn is connected to the dilating cannula by means of intravenous tubing, removes this potential source of injury.

Use of such a method takes a little time longer but is ultimately quite effective.

Heparinized normal saline is not an ideal dilatation medium, as it is relatively acidic and not oxygenated. While some experimental studies have used oxygenated tissue culture medium, this is not practical. Cold gelatinized arterial blood may in many ways be the most physiologic for the vein, but is somewhat more difficult to employ due to its opaque nature. As a compromise, we use a solution of low-molecular-weight Dextran (500 mL) to which is added 1,000 U of heparin and 60 mg of papaverine (to counteract vein spasm). While this is a relatively neutral solution, it is not oxygenated. The transparent nature of this solution makes it easy to rinse away accumulated blood and helps prevent the formation of intraluminal thrombus in the vein and artery.

Reversed Vein Bypass

This method has two major advantages over other techniques of autogenous femorotibial bypass: The technique is simple and is almost universally applicable. Any surgeon of even modest training should be capable of harvesting the vein, turning it around, and performing two anastomoses. Any suitable vein can be used and occlusions of any length and location can be bridged.

Given these advantages, why would one try to use any other technique? First, if there is marked taper in the vein, sewing the smaller end to the larger vein is more difficult, and sewing the larger end to the tibial artery requires a much larger anastomosis than necessary. In addition, harvest of a long segment, unless done very carefully, will tend to accrue more injury from ischemia simply because of the duration of time necessary to isolate a longer length of vein. This may well explain the differences in patency seen by some investigators when comparing long *in situ* versus reversed vein bypasses.[16] In spite of these reservations, reversed vein bypass remains a cornerstone in femorotibial bypass and must be used by all vascular surgeons at least some of the time, if not exclusively.

Excised Nonreversed Orthograde Bypass

In order to counteract the effect of vein taper while using an excised vein, some surgeons employ what may be termed an excised but nonreversed conduit (orthograde excised vein bypass). In doing so, an anastomosis is created between the ostensibly larger end of the vein and the inflow artery, following which the vein is distended and the valves incised with the modified Mills valvulotome.[17,18] This has the advantage of improved size matching and may be used in any tapered vein segment. Furthermore, division of the valves is easier than in most *in situ* procedures in that the vein is entirely mobile during valvulotomy and the valves are more easily seen for division.

This technique has two limitations: First, instrumentation of the vein is necessary to perform valvulotomy with the possibility for injury from poor technique; second, the vein is completely dissected with its attendant risks of ischemic injury as previously discussed. In general, if the excised vein is not tapered (usually shorter segments of vein) there is no general advantage to using the vein in a nonreversed configuration. If the vein taper approaches 2:1 or greater, use of this technique is to be favored. In addition, this allows for improved matching of vein sizes when performing venovenostomy for a composite vein bypass.

In Situ Bypass

The primary alternative method of vein utilization in femorotibial bypass is the *in situ* bypass. This procedure has been described in great detail by multiple investigators.[19-23] The principal advantages of this procedure are that the vein is minimally dissected with the large majority of vasa vasorum being preserved, minimizing ischemia caused by dissection; there is improved size-matching at the vein to artery anastomoses; and the antithrombogenic physiologic properties of the vein are more likely to be preserved.

Its limitations for use as a femorotibial bypass are that it requires the presence of a usable ipsilateral greater saphenous vein, and it is not particularly useful when short lengths of arterial occlusion need to be bypassed. This method, therefore, cannot be used in all cases, and the surgeon who employs an *in situ* technique must also be well versed with excised vein bypass techniques.

The simplest method of performing an *in situ* bypass is the so-called open method, solely employing the modified Mills valvulotome to perform valve incision. Schematically, the arteries and the length of the greater saphenous are exposed through appropriate incisions. The vein is unroofed, but the investing fascia with its vasa vasorum is not divided in order to keep the tissue perfused. Branches of the vein are ligated in continuity with the larger ones. The proximal anastomosis is constructed after mobilizing the minimal amount of vein necessary to reach the artery (Fig. 20-2). After unclamping, the vein is dilated through a nearby side branch under controlled pressure. The retrograde valvulotome is then introduced into the side branch and passed up the vein. The valvulotome is used to catch and divide each cusp, first the anterior and then the posterior. This process is performed serially down the length of vein needed for the particular operation. A Doppler is used to detect the presence of arteriovenous fistulae, which are then ligated or clipped. As the end of the vein is

approached distally, the vein can be divided and dilated, and the remaining valves can be addressed through the open end. The distal anastomosis is then performed.

The advantage of this approach over other *in situ* techniques is that the vein is exposed and thereby visualized by the surgeon as the valves are rendered incompetent. It is the simplest method of dividing the valves and the least likely to cause injury to the vein; in this sense, if one is to have a single technique for the *in situ* bypass, this is the safest. It can be used on the smallest of usable veins and the most complicated of vein systems.

The downside of the open technique is that the skin incision must expose the entire vein used; complications with wound healing can lead to prolonged hospitalization, need for secondary wound procedures, and at worst, loss of the bypass.

Various methods of valve division with an intraluminal "cutter" have been developed by multiple investigators with spotty results in many cases. Use of these devices allows the operator to divide a majority of the valves without necessarily making an incision along the entire length of the vein (Fig. 20-3). However, this means an important portion of the procedure is done blind (unless an endoscope is used, which is both cumbersome and potentially damaging to the vein). These techniques are generally not effective in the hands of the occasional user, but function best when one commits to learning how to use a particular device and realizes that there will be a learning curve for its effective use.

The device with which we are most familiar is the cutter developed by Leather, which has been used by our group for decades. There have been reports that the newer LeMaitre cutter is also able to produce satisfactory results.[24] It is important to note that intraluminal cutters are safely used in the upper (above-knee) portion of the vein, as this segment tends to be larger. Use through the upper calf segment has a higher likelihood of causing vein injury. The vein is generally smaller in this area and the multiple branches and perforating veins arising from the saphenous in this section make dilatation difficult. In general, we strongly recommend that the below-knee portion of the greater saphenous vein be prepared open with the modified Mills valvulotome.

The complexity of using a closed or semiclosed technique makes it less attractive to many surgeons. The main advantage of these methodologies is the minimization of skin incisions. These techniques may also make an *in situ* bypass somewhat quicker in some circumstances. Careful selection and preparation of the patient is mandatory. Preoperative imaging of the saphenous vein is necessary to exclude those patients with smaller saphenous veins or with anatomic variations; these cases are best managed with an open technique and the modified Mills valvulotome.

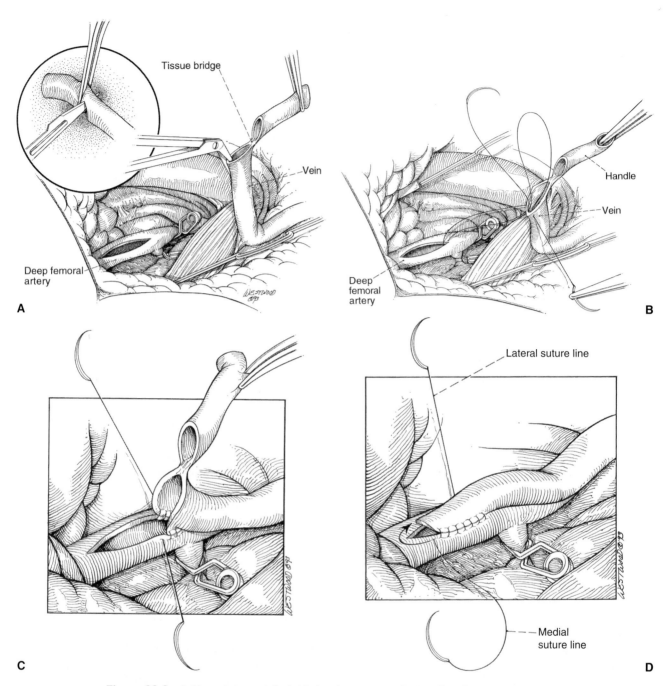

Figure 20-2   A: The vein is partially divided with a no. 11 scalpel. A "handle" is retained to allow traction on the vein. **B:** Proximal anastomosis of the bypass vein to the deep femoral artery is carried out by the "open parachute" technique, which allows for accurate and atraumatic placement of each individual suture in the heel portion of the anastomosis. A single, double-needle suture of 7-0 prolene is used. **C:** After placement of as many sutures as the length of suture material allows, the vein is drawn down to the artery. The "handle" will be excised. **D:** Arterialization of the saphenous vein is completed by continuing the medial suture line clockwise around the end of the arteriotomy to meet the lateral suture line at the midpoint of the arteriotomy. (Illustrations © 1993 Wm. B. Westwood, with permission.)

Composite Vein Bypass

When the length of arterial occlusion is greater than that of any one available vein, several options are available to the surgeon. Prosthetic bypass, often with a boot, cuff, or arteriovenous fistula has been employed frequently, but with mediocre results. A composite bypass made up of prosthetic sewn end-to-end to a segment of vein appears to behave much in the same fashion as a bypass made strictly from prosthetic, so there is little to

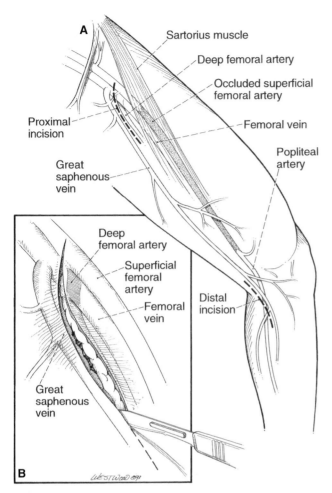

A

Sartorius muscle

Deep femoral artery

Occluded superficial femoral artery

Femoral vein

Proximal incision

Popliteal artery

Great saphenous vein

Deep femoral artery

Superficial femoral artery

Femoral vein

Distal incision

Great saphenous vein

B

WESTWOOD '93

Figure 20-3 Proximal and distal incisions will be used for the *in situ* bypass. The proximal incision **(inset)** will start approximately at the level of the femoral-artery bifurcation and will continue directly over the medial course of the great saphenous vein. The distal incision will be made later in the operation. (Illustrations © 1993 Wm. B. Westwood, with permission.)

vein. The lesser saphenous vein is rarely the largest vein available.

The second special consideration given to constructing these bypasses involves trying as best as possible to perform venovenostomies between veins of similar diameters. This means that very tapered veins may need to be used in an orthograde fashion requiring that the valves be divided with the modified Mills valvulotome.

In order to minimize vein ischemia, only one segment of vein should be excised at a time. The other veins may be unroofed in order to verify their suitability, but their blood supply should be interrupted only when the segment is ready for anastomosis to the more proximal vein segments.

After the largest vein is sewn to the inflow artery, the vein is dilated with the arterialized blood; the oxygen in this blood is now available to the vein wall. The second segment is then excised and a venovenostomy to the first segment is created. Sewing two pieces of vein together in an end-to-end fashion can range from easy to difficult. Large veins (>4 mm) can be joined end-to-end with continuous 7-0 polypropylene using little or no beveling of the vein ends. Small veins may benefit from the use of 8-0 polypropylene and more frequent beveling before anastomosis. Arm veins have little form of their own, so the use of two or three separate sutures can triangulate the vein to allow for easier placement of properly spaced sutures. Use of an interrupted technique can be helpful, especially with the smallest veins, but this is obviously very tedious to perform. If there is a profound size mismatch between the two veins, it is easier to close the end of the larger (proximal) vein with sutures and to make a venotomy into the side of the vein. The smaller (distal) vein can then be sewn in what is effectively an end-to-side fashion. Particular care is given to avoid handling the intima of the vein. This may lessen injury and therefore future development of anastomotic strictures. Last, the continuous suture is tied with the proximal vein partially unclamped, allowing pressure distention of the vein, which may avoid purse-stringing of the anastomosis. If the venovenostomy does not appear ideal, it should be cut out and performed again.

Veins used for composite bypasses should be the best available veins; failure is often related to the use of questionable segments of vein. For instance, use of the antecubital vein should be looked at very critically. These procedures are usually the last autogenous option available in a given limb and require a great deal of work, so taking questionable shortcuts by using mediocre vein can only lead to disappointment for the patient and surgeon. It is better to perform an extra venovenostomy than take an unnecessary chance. Given the tedious nature of this kind of bypass, having multiple surgeons is usually helpful.

recommend this practice. If there is an isolated popliteal segment that is patent, then the so-called composite sequential bypass constructed from a prosthetic femoropopliteal bypass coupled with a popliteal to tibial bypass with vein actually functions quite credibly.[25] In these difficult circumstances, the use of a composite vein bypass is an effective method of performing an autogenous femorotibial bypass. As with all femorotibial bypasses, there are advantages and disadvantages as well as special considerations attached to the use of this technique.

Preoperative imaging of all available veins allows the surgeon to have some idea of which veins will be used and in what order they will be employed. Generally, these bypasses are easier to perform if they are constructed using the largest diameter veins more proximally and the smallest more distally. The basilic vein is often the largest available as is the proximal cephalic

The advantages of these bypasses are that the operation is completely autogenous, and if the vein segments used are of good quality, they perform well; conversely, if the vein used is marginal, this is probably worse than using a prosthetic conduit. These decisions are clearly subjective. A prosthetic bypass to a proximal tibial artery may well be a good first choice when compared to a three-piece (or more) composite vein bypass, especially if the option to perform this vein bypass is still available to the patient if the prosthetic fails.[26]

Conversely, prosthetic bypasses to arteries at the ankle or foot rarely perform well and greater consideration should be given to performing a composite vein bypass as the initial procedure. The role of nonvascular techniques in these situations remains to be defined clearly, but short stenotic lesions would probably better be managed with angioplasty initially, rather than a complicated bypass.

These procedures are almost always lengthy, even with multiple surgeons, and require an unusual amount of commitment to perform well. High-risk patients might well be treated with a different approach.

RESULTS

During the past 30 years (1973 to 2003), our group at several different hospitals has performed 4,946 bypasses to tibial arteries. The large majority (4,713, 95%) have utilized an autogenous vein conduit. A smaller number (233, 5%) have been performed with prosthetic, almost always when no autogenous option existed or if the option was deemed inappropriate because of patient comorbidities.

Within the group of autogenous bypasses, 2,796 (59%) were performed with an *in situ* technique, which clearly was preferred when the option was available. Single segment excised vein bypasses (reversed or orthograde) were used in 1,325 (28%). The remaining 591 (13%) were composite vein bypasses, which were themselves composed of segments of vein prepared using *in situ*, reversed, or retrograde techniques. The demographics of this group reveal a mean age of 70, a majority of men, and over half of the patients with diabetes. Chronic critical limb ischemia was by far the most common indication in our femorotibial bypass group. Claudication was an indication in 253 cases (5.3%). Some of these procedures were planned, but many were cases in which a femoropopliteal bypass were converted at the time of surgery to a femorotibial bypass due to the amount of disease in the popliteal artery. The location of the distal anastomosis is spread relatively evenly among all three tibial vessels. Adjunctive inflow operations performed at the same sitting were most commonly a local reconstruction of the common femoral artery, usually by endarterectomy. Distal reconstructions were linked to an aortic or axillary-based operation concomitantly only if the affected limb was marginal and had no obvious improvement after unclamping the inflow.

Primary patency at 5 years for *in situ*, excised vein, and spliced vein bypasses was 68.7%, 59.2%, and 45.1%, respectively. The spliced vein patency was significantly less than the other two. Similarly, the secondary patency at 5 years for *in situ*, excised vein, and spliced vein bypasses to tibial vessels was 80.3%, 69.1%, and 59.8%, respectively. The secondary patency of spliced vein bypasses to a tibial level was significantly less than those performed with an *in situ* technique. Limb salvage did not differ among the three groups and at 5 years in the *in situ*, excised vein, and spliced vein groups was 94.2%, 89.7%, and 87.0%, respectively.

SURVEILLANCE

The primary reason for optimizing our results in infrainguinal reconstruction using autogenous tissue is a surveillance protocol, which consists of duplex ultrasound of the entire graft. The ultrasound examination begins at the level of the groin using a transverse orientation, the proximal anastomosis is located, and the probe is rotated onto a sagittal plane. Using simultaneous B-mode imaging and Doppler spectral analysis, the inflow artery is studied and a Doppler spectrum is recorded. The examination continues with a transducer slowly being moved down the limb, following the course of the bypass. A stenosis >50% diameter reduction is manifested by doubling of the peak systolic velocity along the conduit. Most lesions are confirmed by angiography. However, angiography is not always performed when a single lesion is seen and was obviously hemodynamically significant. An example of this would be an identified valve leaflet.

Postoperatively, patients are evaluated on at least 3-month intervals for 1 year, and then every 6 months thereafter. The postoperative evaluation includes clinical examination, postoperative pulse volume recordings, and duplex ultrasound scanning. Any deterioration in the clinical status of the lower extremity in question or a change in the pulse volume recordings at any measured level prompted further investigation.

In our experience, long-term surveillance has demonstrated a significant number of hemodynamically significant lesions. Most of these lesions may require surgical intervention to prolong the life of the bypass graft. About 9% of all patients undergoing *in situ* bypass will need a revision. This percentage goes up as one goes to excised veins, which is minimal, at 11% in our experience. Spliced composite vein bypasses require revision in approximately 15% of our series. Intuitively, it is much better to intervene in a failing bypass than to replace the entire bypass because of thrombosis.

CONCLUSION

Excellent results for limb salvage can be achieved with arterial bypass to the tibial level. We preferentially use the *in situ* technique especially for long femoral to tibial reconstructions. However, we have had acceptable success with long-term patency in limb salvage for patients who do not have an ipsilateral greater saphenous vein. Reversed vein and composite spliced vein reconstructions are much more preferable than prosthetic bypass or, at worst, amputation. A system of objective preoperative vein mapping, adequate visualization of inflow and outflow vessels, optimization of arterial inflow, meticulous surgical technique, and rigorous postoperative duplex follow-up will provide optimal results.

REFERENCES

1. Neville RF, Tempesta B, Sidawy AN. Tibial bypass for limb salvage using polytetrafluoroethylene and a distal vein patch. *J Vasc Surg.* 2001;33:266–271.
2. Bolia A, Miles KA, Brennan J, et al. Percutaneous transluminal angioplasty of occlusions of the femoral and popliteal arteries by subintimal dissection. *Cardiovasc Int Radiol.* 1990;13: 357–363.
3. London NJM, Srinivassan R, Naylor AR, et al. Subintimal angioplasty and femoropopliteal occlusion. Longterm results. *Eur J Vasc Surg.* 1994;8:148–155.
4. Fearn SJ, Parkinson E, Nott DM. Radial artery as a conduit for diabetic crural bypass. *Br J Surg.* 2003;90:57–58.
5. Wozniak G, Gortz H, Akinturk H, et al. Superficial femoral vein in arterial reconstruction for limb salvage: outcome and fate of venous circulation. *J Cardiovasc Surg.* 1998;39:405–411.
6. Kupinski AM, Evans SM, Khan AM, et al. Ultrasonic characterization of the saphenous vein. *Cardiovasc Surg.* 1999;1:513–517.
7. Chang BB, Kupinski AM, Darling RC III. Preoperative saphenous vein mapping. In: AbuRahma AF, Bergan JJ, eds. *Noninvasive vascular diagnosis.* Godalming: Springer-Verlag London LTD;1999: 335–344.
8. Shah DM, Chang BB, Leopold PW, et al. The anatomy of the greater saphenous venous system. *J Vasc Surg.* 1986;3:273–283.
9. Rutherford RB, Sawyer JD, Jones DN. The fate of residual saphenous vein after partial removal or ligation. *J Vasc Surg.* 1990;12: 422–426.
10. Chang BB, Paty PSK, Shah DM, et al. The lesser saphenous vein: an underappreciated source of autogenous vein. *J Vasc Surg.* 1992;15:214–217.
11. Faries PL, Logerfo FW, Arora S, et al. Arm vein conduit is superior to composite prosthetic-autogenous grafts in lower extremity revascularization. *J Vasc Surg.* 2000;31:1119–1127.
12. Holzenbein TJ, Pomposelli FB Jr., Miller A, et al. The upper arm basilic-cephalic loop for distal bypass grafting: technical considerations and follow-up. *J Vasc Surg.* 1995;21:586–592.
13. Corson JD, Leather RP, Naraynsingh V, et al. *The role of vasa vasorum in maintaining endothelial integrity in vein bypasses. International symposium on vascular prostheses, Nijmegen, Netherlands.* London, UK: Avebury Publishing Company, Ltd; 1984.
14. LoGerfo FW, Quist WC, Cantelmo NL, et al. Integrity of vein grafts as a function of initial intimal and medial preservation. *Circulation.* 1983;68(3 Pt2):II117–II124.
15. Haudenschild C, Gould KE, Quist WC, et al. Protection of endothelium in vessel segments excised for grafting. *Circulation.* 1981;64 (2 Pt2):II101–II107.
16. Wengerter KR, Veith FJ, Gupta SK, et al. Prospective randomized multicenter comparison in *in situ* and reversed vein infrapopliteal bypasses. *J Vasc Surg.* 1991;13:189–197.
17. Sottiurai VS. Nonreversed translocated vein bypass. *Semin Vasc Surg.* 1993;6:180–184.
18. Belkin M, Knox J, Donaldson MC, et al. Infrainguinal arterial reconstruction with nonreversed greater saphenous vein. *J Vasc Surg.* 1996;24:957–962.
19. Leather RP, Karmody AM. A reappraisal of the *in situ* bypass: its use in limb salvage. *Surgery.* 1979;86:453–460.
20. Leather RP, Shah DM, Buchbinder D, et al. Further experience with the saphenous vein used *in situ* for arterial bypass. *Am J Surg.* 1981;142:506–510.
21. Leather RP, Shah DM, Corson JD, et al. Instrumental evolution of the valve incision method of *in situ* saphenous vein bypass. *J Vasc Surg.* 1984;1:113–123.
22. Leather RP, Chang BB. Femorotibial bypass—preferred techniques and site of distal anastomosis. In: Brewster DC, ed. *Common problems in vascular surgery.* Chicago, Ill: Year Book Medical Publishers; 1988:244–252.
23. Leather RP, Shah DM, Chang BB. *In situ* saphenous vein arterial bypass. In: Bergan JJ, Yao JST, eds. *Techniques in arterial surgery.* Philadelphia, Pa: WB Saunders; 1990:123–133.
24. Gangadharan SP, Reed AB, Chew DKW, et al. Initial experience with minimally invasive *in situ* bypass procedure with blind valvulotomy. *J Vasc Surg.* 2002;35:1100–1106.
25. Roddy SP, Darling RC III, Ozsvath KJ, et al. Composite sequential arterial reconstruction for limb salvage. *J Vasc Surg.* 2002;36: 325–329.
26. Kreienberg PB, Darling RC III, Chang BB, et al. Early results of a prospective randomized trial of spliced vein versus PTFE with a distal vein cuff for limb threatening ischemia. *J Vasc Surg.* 2002; 35:299–306.

Distal Bypasses to Inframalleolar Vessels

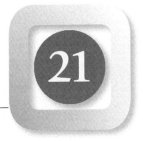

Manju Kalra *Peter Gloviczki*

Bypass grafting to inframalleolar vessels has become an accepted form of treatment for patients with severe distal arterial occlusive disease with critical limb ischemia, tissue loss, or gangrene, regardless of age or diabetic status.[1-3] The safety and durability of these procedures with excellent limb salvage rates has been demonstrated in several surgical series over the last 2 decades.[4-11]

PERIPHERAL ARTERIAL DISEASE IN DIABETES

Fifteen percent of all people with diabetes will have a foot ulcer during their lifetime, and nearly half of all nontraumatic lower extremity amputations in the United States are performed in diabetic patients.[12] Lower extremity arterial disease in people with diabetes is secondary to accelerated atherosclerosis with significant medial calcification. Although the aortoiliac and femoral segments can be involved in the disease process, characteristically, the infrapopliteal, tibial, and crural arteries are the site of maximal occlusive disease in diabetics. Several authors have confirmed this preferential infrageniculate pattern of arterial disease in diabetics, although the reasons for this remain unknown (Figs. 21-1 and 21-2).[13] Patients with diabetes were also thought to have "small-vessel disease" based on evidence of arteriolar occlusion on histopathology of amputated limbs. This distal pattern of arterial occlusive disease rendered these patients "unsuitable" for vascular reconstruction for many decades, with primary amputation being the only treatment offered in the face of

ischemic foot ulceration. Subsequent prospective pathologic studies by Strandness,[13] Conrad,[14] and LoGerfo[15] demonstrated the absence of structural microvascular arteriolar occlusive disease in the diabetic foot. These, along with angiographic studies by Menzoian et al.[16] confirming relative sparing of the pedal vessels, especially the dorsalis pedis artery, finally dispelled the notion of "small-vessel disease" making these patients candidates for arterial bypass grafting to the inframalleolar vessels. On the basis of this data, Ascer et al.,[4] Andros et al.,[17] and Pomposelli et al.[18] independently explored the possibility of distal bypass grafts to the plantar, dorsalis pedis, and other pedal arteries, thereby increasing the potential for limb salvage in diabetic patients.

PREOPERATIVE EVALUATION

The indications for a distal bypass to inframalleolar vessels are similar to those for infrainguinal vascular reconstruction in general—critical foot ischemia with rest pain, nonhealing ulcer, or gangrene. The absence of palpable pedal pulses in such a patient should prompt further evaluation. Noninvasive vascular evaluation is often not very contributory in diabetic patients, as the significant medial calcification frequently causes falsely elevated ankle-brachial indices (ABI) due to noncompressibility of the tibial vessels at the ankle. Transcutaneous oxygen measurements ($TcPO_2$) have been used to predict healing potential of foot ulcers, but drawbacks include sampling errors away from toe/heel ulceration sites and presence of edema. Anatomic evaluation of the lower

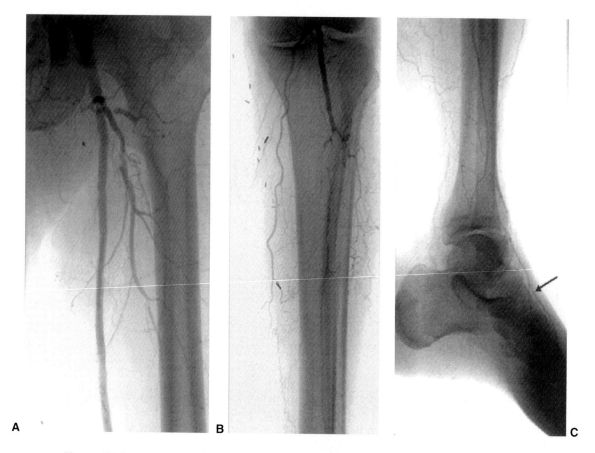

Figure 21-1 Left lower extremity angiogram demonstrating pattern of lower extremity vascular disease in diabetics. Patent common, superficial, and profunda femoral arteries **(A)**, occlusion of the infragenicular popliteal artery **(B)**, and reconstitution of the dorsalis pedis artery **(C,** *arrow***)**.

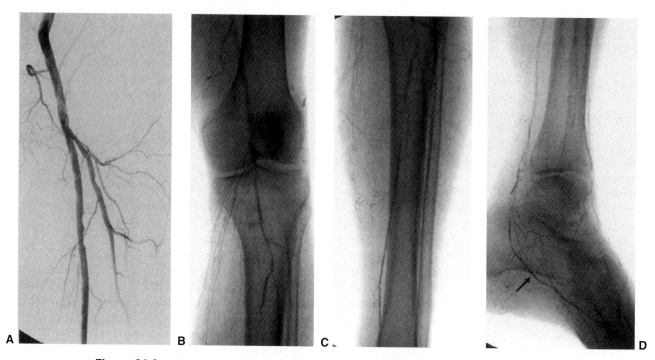

Figure 21-2 Left lower extremity angiogram demonstrating pattern of lower extremity vascular disease in diabetics. Patent common, superficial, and profunda femoral arteries **(A)**, occlusion of the tibioperoneal arteries **(B** and **C)**, and reconstitution of the lateral plantar artery **(D,** *arrow***)**.

extremity arterial circulation with a digital subtraction arteriogram (DSA), including biplanar foot views with magnification if necessary, is the next step and has been considered the gold standard (Fig. 21-3A). In patients with no opacification of a runoff vessel, exploration of the foot vessels based on the presence of a Doppler signal over a pedal artery has been reported. Increasing sophistication of magnetic resonance angiography (MRA) over the last few years has revealed its ability to unmask reliable target vessels for pedal bypass grafting (Fig. 21-3B). Dorweiler et al.[19] reported successful pedal bypass to 10 dorsalis pedis and five plantar arteries following identification of the target vessel with MRA. This is attributable to the ability of MRA to image blood flow at velocities slower than 2 cm per second, whereas with DSA, passage through multisegmental occlusions leads to dilution of the contrast to such an extent that patent pedal vessels may not be visualized. The addition of a contrast enhancement phase in the MRA can potentially improve upon this capability.[20] Recently, preoperative duplex scanning of potential pedal target vessels with evaluation of the diameter, calcification, and resistive index has been evaluated to predict success of inframalleolar bypass grafting. Duplex scanning identified significantly more pedal vascular segments than DSA or MRA, and may prove to be a helpful ancillary tool.[21] Resistive index, however, could not be correlated to the runoff, as assessed by intraoperative angiography. Last, preoperative angiographic scoring of the extent of occlusive disease in the foot vessels in patients with diabetes can be used to predict graft patency; however, the high patency rates even in the presence of high scores (poor runoff) precludes this being used as a means of denying patients a bypass procedure.[22]

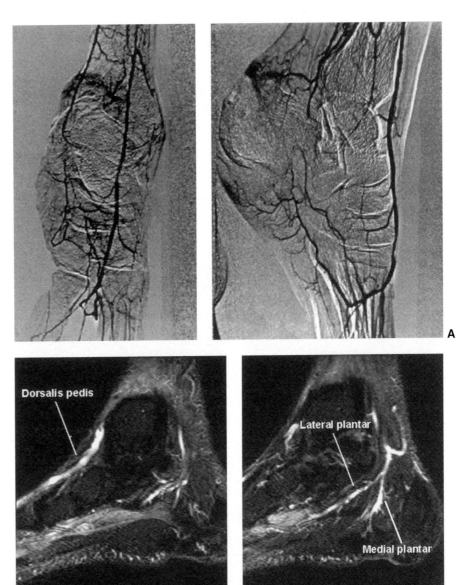

Figure 21-3 **A:** Digital subtraction angiogram (DSA) with reconstitution of the dorsalis pedis artery (*AP view*) and visualization of the pedal arch (*lateral view*). **B:** Magnetic resonance angiogram (MRA) showing opacification of the dorsalis pedis and plantar arteries.

SELECTION OF INFLOW AND OUTFLOW

The goal of distal revascularization to promote healing in a diabetic foot is to provide inline pulsatile flow with restoration of a pedal pulse. A pedal bypass is indicated only if no other proximal vessel is in direct continuity with the foot. Controversy exists regarding the choice of distal target for bypass grafting between the peroneal and a pedal artery in a patient with tissue loss in the foot. Comparable long-term graft patency and limb salvage rates have been reported in patients with equivalent angiogram scores.[23,24] However, in patients with absence of collaterals perfusing the foot and poor, or no, visualization of the pedal arch, results of peroneal artery bypass have been disappointing.[25] Selection of a peroneal or pedal distal target may depend on availability of adequate suitable vein for use as a conduit.

The common femoral artery (CFA) has been traditionally considered a reliable inflow vessel for infrainguinal reconstruction because of fear of progression of atherosclerosis in the superficial femoral artery (SFA). However, the length of conduit required to reach the foot can be a limiting factor, and use of more distal vessels for inflow has been met with equal success. Veith et al.[26] reported early experience with bypasses using the SFA and popliteal artery for inflow over two decades ago with encouraging results. The pattern of preferential infrageniculate occlusive disease in diabetics especially lends itself to successful use of the distal SFA or popliteal artery as an adequate inflow vessel. In a retrospective study comparing common femoral to superficial femoral/popliteal inflow, Sidawy et al.[27] found superior 72-month patency in the latter group (89% vs. 65%), 74% of which comprised people with diabetes. Biancari et al.[28] found short grafts to be a predictor of improved long-term patency in a series of 162 pedal bypass grafts (Table 21-1). Balloon angioplasty/stenting of localized SFA lesions to improve inflow along with a shorter bypass from popliteal inflow is a viable option, especially in patients with limited availability of autogenous vein. Schneider et al.[29] reported equivalent 2-year primary patency rates in three groups of diabetic patients treated with femoral-distal, popliteal-distal bypasses, and focal SFA angioplasty with distal bypass arising from the popliteal artery, 72%, 82%, and 76%, respectively.

Selection of a distal target vessel for outflow is guided by preoperative imaging. The dorsalis pedis artery is the dominant artery of the foot, and if patent, is the vessel of choice (Table 21-2). Bypass to the dorsalis pedis artery is associated with excellent patency and durable limb salvage with equivalent healing rates of forefoot and heel ischemic lesions.[8,11,30] Intuitively, however, if the posterior tibial/plantar artery is patent, it should be the outflow vessel of choice in patients with heel ulceration.

TABLE 21-1

SITES OF PROXIMAL ANASTOMOSIS OF INFRAMALLEOLAR VEIN GRAFTS IN TWO SERIES

Artery	Number (%) Kalra et al.[a]	Number (%) Pomposelli et al.[b]
Long grafts	**130 (46.4%)**	**414 (40.1%)**
External iliac	1 (0.4%)	6 (0.6%)
Common femoral	51 (18.2%)	294 (28.5%)
Superficial femoral	78 (27.9%)	114 (11.0%)
Deep femoral	—	6 (0.6%)
Short grafts	**150 (53.6%)**	—
Popliteal	139 (49.6%)	550 (53.3%)
Tibioperoneal trunk	1 (0.4%)	—
Peroneal	2 (0.7%)	—
Posterior tibial	3 (1.1%)	6 (0.6%)
Dorsalis pedis	1 (0.4%)	—
Other artery	4 (1.4%)	—
Previous graft	—	56 (5.4%)
TOTAL	**280**	**1,032**

[a]From Kalra M, Gloviczki P, Bower TC, et al. Limb salvage after successful pedal bypass grafting is associated with improved long-term survival. *J Vasc Surg.* 2001;33:6–16, with permission.
[b]From Pomposelli FB, Kansal N, Hamdan AD, et al. A decade of experience with dorsalis pedis artery bypass: analysis of outcome in more than 1000 cases. *J Vasc Surg.* 2003;37:307–315, with permission.

TABLE 21-2

SITES OF DISTAL ANASTOMOSIS IN 280 PEDAL BYPASSES

Artery	Number (%)
Anterior pedal	**203 (72.5%)**
Dorsalis pedis	193 (68.9%)
Lateral tarsal	8 (2.9%)
Deep plantar	1 (0.4%)
First dorsal metatarsal	1 (0.4%)
Posterior pedal	**79 (28.2%)**
Posterior tibial	9 (3.2%)
Common plantar	37 (13.2%)
Lateral plantar	23 (8.2%)
Medial plantar	10 (3.6%)
TOTAL	**282**[a]

[a]Two bifurcated grafts.
From Kalra M, Gloviczki P, Bower TC, et al. Limb salvage after successful pedal bypass grafting is associated with improved long-term survival. *J Vasc Surg.* 2001;33:6–16, with permission.

CONDUIT

Autogenous vein is the conduit that has been used extensively for bypasses to inframalleolar vessels. Prosthetic (polytetrafluoroethylene [PTFE]) bypasses to infrageniculate arteries have a significantly higher incidence of thrombosis than vein grafts because of the higher flow rate required to maintain patency. Although prosthetic and composite prosthetic/vein bypasses have been occasionally performed to inframalleolar targets, experience with them has been uniformly discouraging.[10,11]

Ipsilateral great saphenous vein used *in situ,* nonreversed translocated, or reversed is the conduit of choice (Table 21-3). A nonreversed configuration is preferred for bypass grafts to the inframalleolar vessels to provide a better match of graft to distal outflow artery and allow bidirectional flow, which may reduce stasis in the low-flow graft.[31] In the absence of ipsilateral vein, contralateral great saphenous vein may be used, provided the contralateral limb is not threatened. Arm veins (cephalic and basilic) are a good second choice conduit in the absence of the great saphenous vein.[32] In fact, arm vein harvest has been proposed as a first alternative if ipsilateral vein is unavailable and has been reported to be associated with superior results when compared to composite prosthetic/vein conduits.[32,33] The small saphenous vein remains a final option for an autogenous conduit. Bifurcated vein grafts have been used on occasion. A branch of the *in situ* great saphenous vein may be used to revascularize an isolated popliteal segment. In the event of absent arterial communications in the foot and extensive ulceration, a bifurcated great saphenous vein graft may be anastomosed to both the anterior and posterior inframalleolar vessels.

SURGICAL TECHNIQUE

The technique of performing a distal bypass to inframalleolar vessels is, for the most part, similar to that of any infrainguinal reconstruction. The artery selected to provide inflow is exposed, and the venous conduit procured in a standard manner. If the bypass is long, with inflow from the common femoral artery, the

TABLE 21-3

CONDUITS USED FOR INFRAMALLEOLAR BYPASSES IN TWO SERIES

Conduit	Number (%) Kalra et al.[a]	Number (%) Pomposelli et al.[b]
Translocated saphenous vein	183 (65.4%)	327 (31.6%)
In situ saphenous vein	35 (12.5%)	273 (26.4%)
Reversed saphenous vein	17 (6.1%)	235 (22.8%)
Arm vein	—	170 (16.5%)
PTFE	—	2 (0.2%)
Composite vein	**45 (16.1%)**	**25 (2.4%)**
Bilateral leg veins	18 (40.0%)	—
Ipsilateral leg veins	14 (31.1%)	—
Leg plus arm veins	8 (17.8%)	—
Arm veins alone	4 (8.9%)	—
PTFE plus leg vein	1 (2.2%)	—
TOTAL	**280**	**1,032**

PTFE, polytetrafluoroethylene.
[a]From Kalra M, Gloviczki P, Bower TC, et al. Limb salvage after successful pedal bypass grafting is associated with improved long-term survival. *J Vasc Surg.* 2001;33:6–16, with permission.
[b]From Pomposelli FB, Kansal N, Hamdan AD, et al. A decade of experience with dorsalis pedis artery bypass: analysis of outcome in more than 1000 cases. *J Vasc Surg.* 2003;37:307–315, with permission.

entire length of the ipsilateral great saphenous vein is exposed and left in its bed for an *in situ* bypass, or harvested and used in a translocated manner. The valves are incised with a Karmody scissor or Mills valvulotome. For bypass to the dorsalis pedis artery and its branches, the translocated technique is preferable as it avoids parallel incisions at the ankle and tension on the vein graft. If a short bypass is planned, with inflow from the superficial femoral or popliteal artery, the great saphenous vein is harvested from the thigh and translocated distally so as to use the larger caliber vein and also to avoid multiple parallel incisions in the leg. When translocated, the vein is usually oriented in a nonreversed manner so as to avoid a significant size mismatch at the distal anastomosis. Angioscopic examination of the vein, especially when used *in situ*, along with division of valves under vision has been recommended by some authors.[11] The vein may be tunneled in a subcutaneous plane from the groin to the ankle, or in an anatomical plane to below the knee and from thereon subcutaneously. It is important to leave a skin bridge in the distal leg between the vein harvest wound and the site of the distal target vessel in the foot, under which the vein graft is finally tunneled. Prior to making the skin incision for exposure of the inframalleolar vessels, it is useful to locate them precisely with Doppler ultrasonography so as to make the incision directly over the vessel and avoid undermining the skin.

Exposure of the Dorsalis Pedis Artery

The dorsalis pedis artery is exposed through a 3- to 4-cm incision on the dorsum of the foot, directly over the patent segment of the vessel (Fig. 21-4A). The inferior extensor retinaculum is divided to expose the artery in the proximal foot between the extensor hallucis longus tendon medially and the extensor digitorum longus tendon laterally. The extensor hallucis longus tendon crosses the artery at the ankle, and the anastomosis needs to be situated such that the graft will not be compressed by the tendon. Occasionally, if the patient has great toe gangrene that will require amputation, the tendon may be divided.

Exposure of the Lateral Tarsal Artery

The lateral tarsal artery originates from the dorsalis pedis artery at the level of the navicular bone and runs laterally across the dorsum of the foot, deep to the extensor digitorum brevis muscle toward the fifth metatarsal bone. It supplies the dorsal aspect of the foot and anastomoses with the arcuate artery, which also arises from the dorsalis pedis artery further distally and courses across the dorsal aspect of the midfoot. Distal dissection of the dorsal pedis artery exposes the origin of the lateral tarsal artery. Further exposure is facilitated by retraction of the extensor digitorum longus tendon and partial excision of the extensor digitorum brevis muscle. If further exposure is required for performance of the distal anastomosis, the first and second extensor digitorum longus tendons may be divided.

Exposure of the Deep Plantar Artery

The deep plantar artery is the main continuation of the dorsalis pedis artery. It arises at the proximal metatarsal level and dives deep between the bases of the first and second metatarsal bones to connect with the lateral plantar artery to form the deep plantar arch. A 3- to 4-cm incision is made over the dorsum of the midfoot to expose the distal dorsalis pedis artery and its bifurcation into the deep plantar and first dorsal metatarsal arteries. The extensor hallucis brevis muscle is retracted laterally or divided, and the dorsal interosseous muscle is split to expose the proximal segment of the deep plantar artery. Further exposure is facilitated by subperiosteal resection of the proximal portion of the second metatarsal bone.

Exposure of the Plantar Arteries

The posterior tibial artery becomes the common plantar artery at the level of the ankle joint, which soon divides into the medial and lateral plantar arteries (Fig. 21-4B). The lateral plantar artery is the larger of the two and forms the plantar arch, which runs medially across the plantar aspect of the foot finally communicating with the deep plantar branch of the dorsalis pedis artery. The medial plantar branch provides blood supply to the intrinsic muscles of the first, second, and third toes through small branches. In the eventuality of lateral plantar occlusion, it may enlarge significantly and communicate with the plantar arch through collaterals. Exposure of the plantar arteries commences with exposure of the retromalleolar posterior tibial artery between the medial malleolus and the Achilles tendon, followed by progressive distal dissection towards the sole of the foot. This technique ensures distal incision placement precisely over the plantar arteries with minimal retraction in the region of the sole where the skin is usually tough. The flexor retinaculum is incised to expose the common plantar artery, and the abductor hallucis muscle is divided to expose its bifurcation as well as the proximal 2 to 3 cm of the medial and lateral plantar arteries. The lateral plantar is the larger of the two and is located more inferiorly. Further distal exposure of these vessels is facilitated by division of the plantar aponeurosis and the flexor digitorum brevis muscle, if required.

After performance of the proximal anastomosis and confirmation of satisfactory flow through the distal end of the vein graft after valve division, the graft is

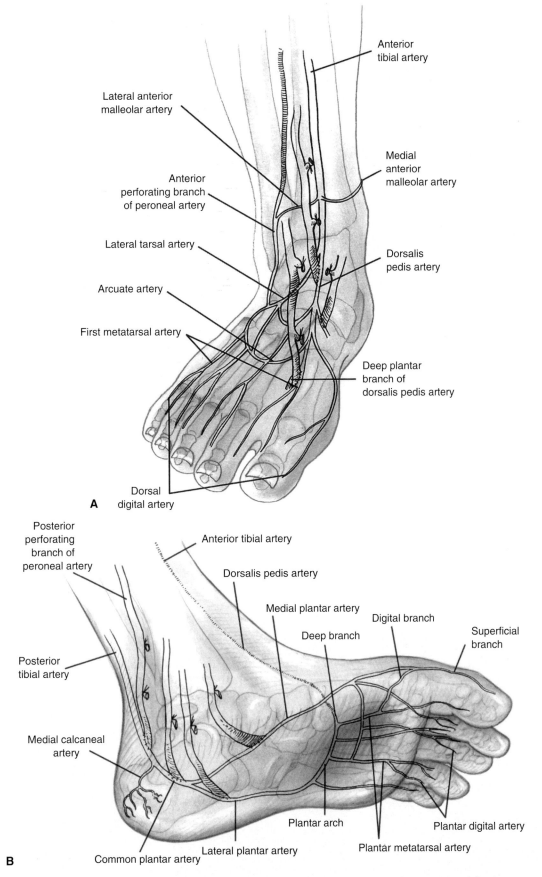

Figure 21-4 **A:** Sites of distal outflow arteries of the anterior circulation in the foot. **B:** Sites of distal outflow arteries of the posterior circulation in the foot. (From Kalra M, Gloviczki P, Bower TC, et al. Limb salvage after successful pedal bypass grafting is associated with improved long-term survival. *J Vasc Surg.* 2001;33:6–16, with permission.)

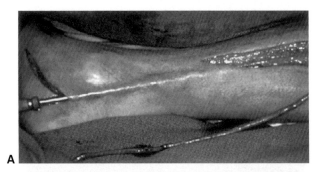

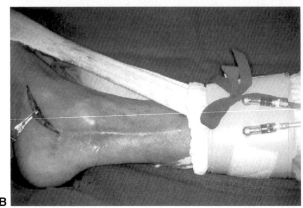

Figure 21-5 A: Intraoperative photograph demonstrating translocation of saphenous vein from the thigh to the leg with preservation of a skin bridge at the ankle. **B:** Use of a tourniquet inflated to 300 mm Hg to create a bloodless field for the distal anastomosis.

tunneled to the site of the target vessel (Fig. 21-5A). An above-knee or below-knee tourniquet is applied and inflated to 300 mm Hg to create a bloodless field at the distal anastomosis site and avoid clamping the delicate pedal artery (Fig. 21-5B). Sometimes, however, the

tourniquet will not adequately control bleeding in circumferentially calcified arteries, in which situation intraluminal occluders or Fogarty balloon catheters are preferable to clamping the vessel. A second tourniquet at a different level can also be placed. The distal anastomosis is performed in a standard fashion with 7-0 or 8-0 nonabsorbable monofilament suture material, using a running or rarely interrupted technique based on the size of the recipient vessel. High-power loupe magnification or operating microscope and good operating room lighting are essential adjuncts to performing a technically perfect distal anastomosis. Frequently, the outflow vessel is circumferentially calcified and use of a taper-cut needle or fracture technique is necessary for performance of the anastomosis. Originally described by Ascer et al.,[34] this technique involves partially fracturing the artery with a hemostat at 3- to 4-mm intervals, thereby rendering it suitable for clamping and suturing. Significant medial arterial calcification does not preclude successful bypass to these vessels and is not a predictor of graft failure or limb loss. Blood flow through the bypass graft measured with an electromagnetic flow meter is a good indicator of the runoff. A completion arteriogram is routinely performed to exclude technical problems (Fig. 21-6). Meticulous technique as well as recognition and correction of any technical defects intraoperatively are fundamental to the success of a distal bypass to inframalleolar vessels. Distal foot wounds are usually closed in a single layer with an interrupted monofilament suture technique or rarely with a subcuticular suture. Tension at the suture line must be strictly avoided and occasionally multiple, small release incisions on either side may be used in the "pie-crusting" method.

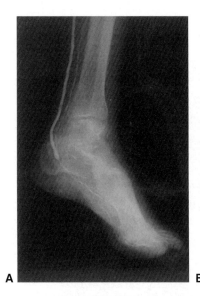
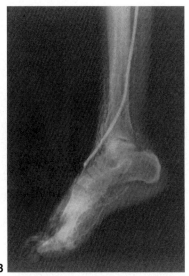
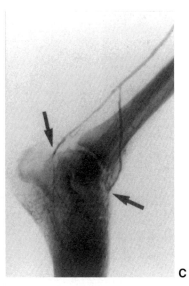

Figure 21-6 Intraoperative completion angiograms demonstrating patent bypass grafts to the lateral plantar artery **(A)**, dorsalis pedis artery **(B)**, and bifurcated nonreversed translocated saphenous vein **(C)**, with posterior arch vein graft to the dorsalis pedis and common plantar arteries.

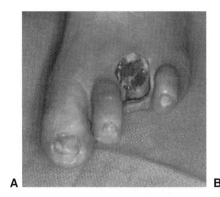
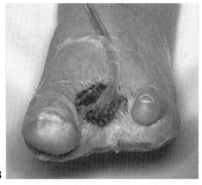
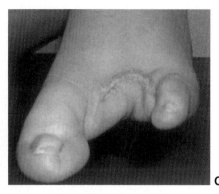

Figure 21-7 Accelerated healing of the open forefoot wound **(A)**, following second, third, and fourth toes amputation with use of a wound vacuum device **(B** and **C)**.

POSTOPERATIVE MANAGEMENT

All patients receive aspirin therapy postoperatively, the first dose being in the form of a suppository in the recovery room. On the basis of our experience, patients with an intraoperative flow rate <50 mL per minute are started on low-dose heparin sodium infusion (200 to 500 U per hour) 4 hours postoperatively. The heparinization is increased slowly to a therapeutic level by 48 hours, and these patients are discharged home on oral anticoagulation with warfarin sodium to keep the International Normalized Ration (INR) between 2 and 3. Patients are kept in bed with the extremity elevated for 48 hours. Ambulation is commenced thereafter, with customized cushioned footwear to prevent compression of the graft as well as avoid weight bearing on gangrenous/ulcerated areas of the foot.

ADJUNCTIVE PROCEDURES

Incision and drainage of deep-space infections or abscesses, or debridement/open toe or forefoot amputation for wet gangrene should be performed as a separate operation a few days prior to the distal bypass procedure. Distal bypass to the foot can be performed safely in the presence of an open wound as long as the infection is controlled first and the site of the distal anastomosis is away from the open wound.[5] A clean, closed-toe amputation may be performed concomitantly at the end of the bypass procedure. A significant number of patients will require additional wound management with wound vacuum devices, split skin graft, or myocutaneous graft cover (Figs. 21-7–21-9).

POSTOPERATIVE SURVEILLANCE

Postoperative graft surveillance with duplex ultrasound is recommended as it is for other infrainguinal bypass grafts at 3- to 6-month intervals for the first year, and every 6 months thereafter. The importance of recognizing and correcting graft stenoses in a timely fashion cannot be overemphasized. Long-term results of interventions to maintain graft patency are significantly better than those of interventions following graft

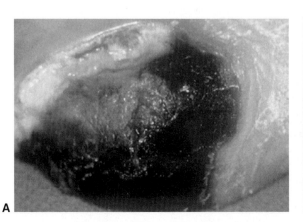
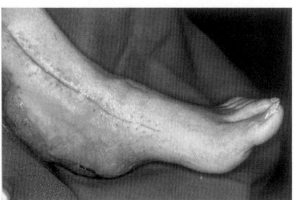

Figure 21-8 Eventual healing of heel ulcer **(A)** obtained with split-thickness skin grafting **(B)** following pedal bypass to the lateral plantar artery.

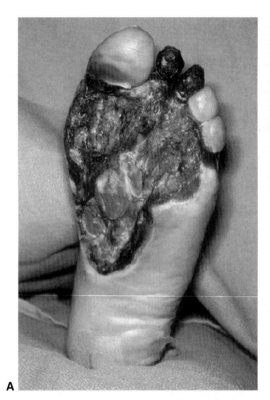
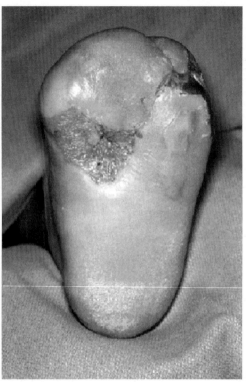

Figure 21-9   Successful salvage of extensive foot gangrene **(A)** with pedal bypass graft, forefoot amputation, and skin coverage with local flap from the dorsum of the foot **(B)**.

thrombosis. Rhodes et al.[35] reported a 2-year patency rate of 81% and limb salvage rate of 77% following revision of failing pedal bypass grafts, compared to 7% and 44%, respectively, for failed grafts using both endovascular and surgical techniques.

RESULTS

Distal bypass grafting to inframalleolar vessels using autologous vein is safe, effective, and durable, as demonstrated by several published studies.[4,6–8,18,28,36–39] Operative mortality has been decreasing with increasing experience, from 10% in 1989 to 1% in 2003.[11,36] Patency rates of 41% to 84% and limb salvage rates of 54% to 89% have been reported following pedal bypass grafting (Table 21-4). In our series of 280 pedal bypass grafts in 256 patients, the 5-year secondary patency rate was 71% and the limb salvage rate was 78%.[10] Recently, Pomposelli et al.[11] reported on the results of 1,032 bypasses to the dorsalis pedis artery over a decade with 5- and 10-year secondary

TABLE 21-4
LONG-TERM RESULTS OF PEDAL BYPASS GRAFTS

First Author, Year	No. of Bypasses	Primary Patency (%)	Secondary Patency (%)	Limb Salvage (%)	Survival (%)	Follow-up Year
Ascer, 1988[4]	20	81	—	85	—	2
Andros, 1989[36]	20	85	73	89	—	0.25
Tannenbaum, 1992[5]	56	—	92	98	—	3
Schneider, 1993[40]	41	58	82	92	61	3
Quinones-Baldrich, 1993[6]	35	—	72	89	—	2
Isaksson, 1994[3]	33	76	89	89	82	1
Eckstein, 1996[38]	56	55	62	66	52	4
Biancari, 1999[28]	162	34	41	60	55	3
Kalra, 2001[10]	280	58	71	78	60	5
Pomposelli, 2003[11]	1,032	57 (38%)	63 (42%)	78 (58%)	47 (24%)	5 (10 y)

patency rates of 63% and 42%, and limb salvage rates of 78% and 58%, respectively.

The disease pattern in diabetic patients with atherosclerosis of the infrageniculate arteries and relative sparing of the pedal vessels lends itself to successful pedal bypass, with limb loss often occurring because of uncontrolled sepsis.[16] In fact, diabetic patients fare significantly better in terms of primary and secondary graft patency than nondiabetics (Fig. 21-10).[10,11] However, in our experience, ultimate limb salvage was not significantly different from nondiabetics (80% vs. 77%), with nearly 40% of all amputations being performed in the presence of patent grafts. Unlike other reports,[41,42] we failed to confirm poorer long-term survival in diabetic patients with critical limb ischemia compared to nondiabetics, 64% versus 50% at 5 years.[9,10] Akbari et al.[1] also reported similar long-term survival of 58% at 5 years in diabetic and nondiabetic patients following lower extremity revascularization. Long-term survival in these patients is, however, significantly less than in age- and sex-matched cohorts (60% vs. 87% at 5 years, respectively) (Fig. 21-11).

Diabetic patients with end-stage renal disease (ESRD) present a challenge to the vascular surgeon. Patients with ESRD traditionally fare significantly worse in all respects following infrainguinal reconstruction—limb salvage and patient survival—and the wisdom of revascularization in these patients is questioned, with dismal results reported by several authors.[43] Hakaim et al.[44] evaluated early outcome of 83 tibial bypass grafts in 53 diabetic patients and 23 diabetic patients with ESRD. They reported significantly poorer patency at 1 year in patients with diabetes and ESRD compared to diabetes alone (53% vs. 82%), a trend toward lower limb salvage (63% vs. 84%), as well as significantly worse survival (52% vs. 90%). In our series of 23 pedal bypasses in 19 patients with ESRD, patients with a renal transplant fared slightly better than those on hemodialysis, although the numbers were too small to make any firm conclusions. These observations were confirmed by McArthur et al.[45] in infrainguinal revascularization of 60 successful renal transplant patients. They reported graft patency rates of 78% and 44% at 1 and 5 years, and limb salvage

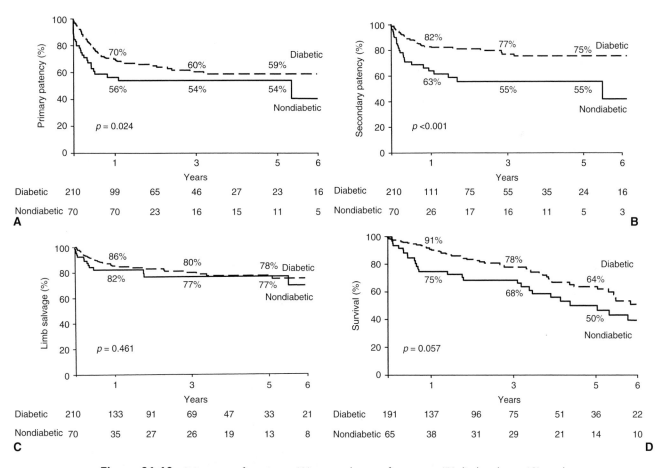

Figure 21-10 Primary graft patency (**A**), secondary graft patency (**B**), limb salvage (**C**), and patient survival (**D**) following 210 pedal bypasses in 191 diabetic patients compared to 70 bypasses in 65 nondiabetic patients. SEM <10% for all time points. (From Kalra M, Gloviczki P, Bower TC, et al. Limb salvage after successful pedal bypass grafting is associated with improved long-term survival. *J Vasc Surg.* 2001;33:6–16, with permission.)

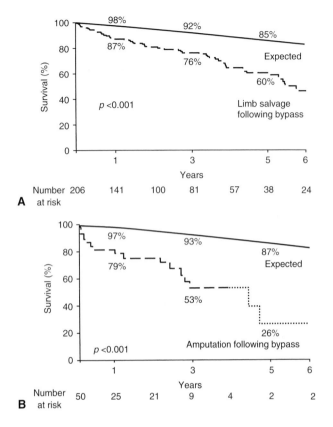

Figure 21-11 Cumulative survival rates in 206 patients with limb salvage **(A)** and 50 patients with amputation **(B)** following pedal bypasses, compared to expected survival in an age- and sex-matched cohort. Dotted line represents SEM >10%. (From Kalra M, Gloviczki P, Bower TC, et al. Limb salvage after successful pedal bypass grafting is associated with improved long-term survival. *J Vasc Surg.* 2001;33:6–16, with permission.)

rates of 87% and 78%, respectively. In addition, survival was significantly improved (73% vs. 38%) in patients with a well-functioning allograft and a serum creatinine level <2 mg per dL.

The quality of the conduit used for distal bypass to inframalleolar vessels has a significant impact on graft patency and limb salvage. Single-length great saphenous vein is the ideal conduit followed by arm vein and finally small saphenous vein.[31] Composite vein grafts were used as a conduit to bypass to the pedal arteries in 16% of patients without single-length vein in our series,[10] and 2.5% by Pomposelli et al.[11] They were associated with significantly worse results in terms of graft patency and limb salvage compared to single-length vein, in spite of long-term anticoagulation with warfarin sodium. Other authors have also observed inferior results following infrainguinal revascularization with composite vein grafts.[32] However, these results are still superior to those obtained with prosthetic grafts in this location, and their use seems justified.[46] In addition, long-term foot salvage following pedal bypass is 10% to 15% higher than graft patency, endorsing the fact that late failure of a bypass graft does

not always result in limb loss if foot ulceration has healed prior to graft occlusion.[10,11]

The decision between revascularization and primary amputation in an elderly patient with multiple comorbidities and limited life expectancy is still a challenging and soul-searching exercise. Published series of lower extremity revascularization in the elderly report limb salvage rates comparable to younger patients with satisfactory functional results in terms of preservation of ambulation and residential status at the cost of a modest increase in operative mortality (2.2% vs. 6.7%).[2,47] In our experience with pedal bypasses, octogenarians fared well with no significant difference in graft patency or limb salvage compared to their younger counterparts.[10] Long-term patient survival was, understandably, worse in these elderly patients. However, mortality following primary amputation is also higher in this age group (14.7% vs. 9.8%), with a considerably decreased chance of rehabilitation following amputation.[48,49]

Does failed distal revascularization result in a higher level of amputation? This question remains unanswered with several reports in the literature on either side of the argument.[50,51] Preservation of the knee in 88% of secondary amputees following failed pedal bypass is in concordance with the successful healing rate of primary below-knee amputations (85% to 92%).[10,50] The cumulative probability at 5 years of having a below-knee amputation was not significantly different in diabetics compared to nondiabetics (21% vs. 17%,); nor was the probability of an above-knee amputation (2% vs. 6%).

The presence of an additional functional microvascular disease in diabetics is responsible for continued tissue loss and amputation of the foot, despite successful revascularization to the pedal vessels.[52] In our experience, as well as that reported by other authors, >50% of patients require multiple operative procedures resulting in prolonged or repeated hospitalization to achieve complete foot healing (Table 21-5).[5,10] The microvascular disease is characterized by nonocclusive thickening of the basement membrane that adversely affects blood-flow regulation and vascular permeability. Decreased endothelial nitric oxide production causes reduced vasodilatation and neuropathy secondary to ischemia of the nerves. Inability to mount a hyperemic response to injury as well as impaired leukocyte migration and diffusion of nutrients play a significant role in the susceptibility of the diabetic foot to infection.[53,54] Arora et al.[55] evaluated the cutaneous microvascular reactivity of the foot in patients with diabetic neuropathy before and after successful revascularization and found improvement with successful treatment of macrovascular disease, but not complete reversal of dysfunction to levels comparable to diabetics without neuropathy and normal controls. Therefore, the diabetic foot remains at increased risk of nonhealing as well as new ulceration in spite of successful pedal bypass.

TABLE 21-5

ADJUNCTIVE PROCEDURES FOLLOWING 280 PEDAL BYPASSES

Procedures	Number of Limbs (%)
Within 30 days	**97 (34.6%)**
Wound debridement	49 (17.5%)
Minor amputation	37 (13.2%)
Graft thrombectomy	10 (3.6%)
Graft revision	9 (3.2%)
Hematoma evacuation	8 (2.9%)
Myocutaneous flap	8 (2.9%)
Skin grafting	7 (2.5%)
Major amputation	9 (3.2%)
Inflow procedure	3 (1.1%)
During follow-up	**97 (34.6%)**
Major amputation	42 (15.0%)
Minor amputation	34 (12.4%)
Wound debridement	27 (9.6%)
Graft revision	23 (8.2%)
Graft thrombectomy	8 (2.9%)
Inflow procedure	1 (0.4%)
New graft	1 (0.4%)
Skin grafting	1 (0.4%)
Sympathectomy	1 (0.4%)

From Kalra M, Gloviczki P, Bower TC, et al. Limb salvage after successful pedal bypass grafting is associated with improved long-term survival. *J Vasc Surg.* 2001;33:6–16, with permission.

Immense commitment through multidisciplinary care is necessary to achieve final healing. Efforts to correct mechanical pressure points surgically or with appropriate footwear, further wound debridements or forefoot amputations, as well as plastic surgical procedures to provide skin and soft-tissue cover continue well into the late postoperative period.

Disappointing functional results have been reported following infrainguinal revascularization for limb salvage, with only 45% of patients reporting feeling "back to normal" at 6 months, and 54% requiring reintervention.[56] Successful outcome following pedal bypass is often at the cost and morbidity of repeated interventions to salvage the graft and limb.[5,10] However, in an assessment of residential and ambulatory status together at 1 year following lower extremity revascularization in elderly patients, Pomposelli et al.[2] reported encouraging results with improvement in 78% and maintenance in 88% of patients. They and other authors identified preoperative baseline functional status as a predictor of good functional outcome following revascularization.[56] In our experience following successful pedal bypass, 78% of limbs were being used for ambulation at last follow-up or death.[10] Return to an ambulatory and independent functional status is the ultimate goal of aggressive distal revascularization to the inframalleolar vessels. We observed that patients with failed pedal revascularization and resultant amputation had worse long-term

survival compared to our entire patient cohort, and amputation was a significant risk factor predicting higher long-term mortality.[10] Panayiotopoulos et al.[51] reported better survival in 70 patients with successful femorocrural/pedal grafts compared to 82 amputees (62% vs. 39% at 3 years), which included both primary and secondary amputations.

Revascularization of ischemic lower extremities in diabetic patients with distal bypasses to inframalleolar vessels results in good long-term limb salvage and functional ability for ambulation. It should be attempted in all anatomically suitable patients, even high-risk ones, who are deemed capable of ambulation or transfer with the affected extremity. Successful limb salvage may improve functional status of these patients with a potential benefit on long-term survival.

REFERENCES

1. Akbari CM, Pomposelli FB Jr, Gibbons GW, et al. Lower extremity revascularization in diabetes. *Arch Surg.* 2000;135:452–456.
2. Pomposelli FB Jr, Arora S, Gibbons GW, et al. Lower extremity arterial reconstruction in the very elderly: successful outcome preserves not only the limb but also residential status and ambulatory function. *J Vasc Surg.* 1998;28:215–225.
3. Isaksson L, Lundgren F. Vein bypass surgery to the foot in patients with diabetes and critical ischaemia. *Br J Surg.* 1994;81:517–520.
4. Ascer E, Veith FJ, Gupta SK. Bypasses to plantar arteries and other tibial branches: an extended approach to limb salvage. *J Vasc Surg.* 1988;8:434–441.
5. Tannenbaum GA, Pomposelli FB Jr, Marcaccio EJ, et al. Safety of vein bypass grafting to the dorsal pedal artery in diabetic patients with foot infections. *J Vasc Surg.* 1992;15:982–988.
6. Quinones-Baldrich WJ, Colburn MD, Ahn SS, et al. Very distal bypass for salvage of the severely ischemic extremity. *Am J Surg.* 1993;166:117–123.
7. Gloviczki P, Bower TC, Toomey BJ, et al. Microscope-aided pedal bypass is an effective and low-risk operation to salvage the ischemic foot [Review]. *Am J Surg.* 1994;168:76–84.
8. Pomposelli FB Jr, Marcaccio EJ, Gibbons GW, et al. Dorsalis pedis arterial bypass: durable limb salvage for foot ischemia in patients with diabetes mellitus. *J Vasc Surg.* 1995;21:375–384.
9. Panneton JM, Gloviczki P, Bower TC, et al. Pedal bypass for limb salvage: impact of diabetes on long-term outcome. *Ann Vasc Surg.* 2000;14:640–647.
10. Kalra M, Gloviczki P, Bower TC, et al. Limb salvage after successful pedal bypass grafting is associated with improved long-term survival. *J Vasc Surg.* 2001;33:6–16.
11. Pomposelli FB, Kansal N, Hamdan AD, et al. A decade of experience with dorsalis pedis artery bypass: analysis of outcome in more than 1000 cases. *J Vasc Surg.* 2003;37:307–315.
12. Reiber GE, Pecoraro RE, Koepsell TD. Risk factors for amputation in patients with diabetes mellitus. A case-control study. *Ann Intern Med.* 1992;117:97–105.
13. Strandness DE, Priest RE, Gibbons GE. Combined clinical and pathological study of diabetic and non-diabetic peripheral arterial disease. *Diabetes.* 1964;13:366–372.
14. Conrad M. Large and small artery occlusion in diabetics and non-diabetics with severe vascular disease. *Circulation.* 1967;36:83–91.
15. LoGerfo FW, Coffman JD. Current concepts. Vascular and microvascular disease of the foot in diabetes. Implications for foot care. *N Engl J Med.* 1984;311:1615–1619.

16. Menzoian JO, LaMorte WW, Paniszyn CC, et al. Symptomatology and anatomic patterns of peripheral vascular disease: differing impact of smoking and diabetes. *Ann Vasc Surg.* 1989;224–228.

17. Andros G, Harris RW, Salles-Cunha SX, et al. Bypass grafts to the ankle and foot. *J Vasc Surg.* 1988;7:785–794.

18. Pomposelli FB Jr, Jepsen SJ, Gibbons GW, et al. Efficacy of the dorsal pedal bypass for limb salvage in diabetic patients: short-term observations [see comments]. *J Vasc Surg.* 1990;11: 745–751.

19. Dorweiler B, Neufang A, Kreitner KF, et al. Magnetic resonance angiography unmasks reliable target vessels for pedal bypass grafting in patients with diabetes mellitus. *J Vasc Surg.* 2002;35: 766–772.

20. Kreitner KF, Kalden P, Neufang A, et al. Diabetes and peripheral arterial occlusive disease: prospective comparison of contrast-enhanced three-dimensional MR angiography with conventional digital subtraction angiography. *AJR Am J Roentgenol.* 2000;174: 171–179.

21. Hofmann WJ, Walter J, Ugurluoglu A, et al. Preoperative high-frequency duplex scanning of potential pedal target vessels. *J Vasc Surg.* 2004;39:169–175.

22. Toursarkissian B, D'Ayala M, Stefanidis D, et al. Angiographic scoring of vascular occlusive disease in the diabetic foot: relevance to bypass graft patency and limb salvage. *J Vasc Surg.* 2002; 35:494–500.

23. Darling RC III, Chang BB, Paty PS, et al. Choice of peroneal or dorsalis pedis artery bypass for limb salvage. *Am J Surg.* 1995;170: 109–112.

24. Abou-Zamzam AM Jr, Moneta GM, Lee RW, et al. Peroneal bypass is equivalent to inframalleolar bypass for ischemic pedal gangrene. *Arch Surg.* 1996;131:894–899.

25. Elliott BM, Robison JG, Brothers TE, et al. Limitations of peroneal artery bypass grafting for limb salvage. *J Vasc Surg.* 1993;18: 881–888.

26. Veith FJ, Gupta SK, Samson RH, et al. Superficial femoral and popliteal arteries as inflow sites for distal bypasses. *Surgery.* 1981; 90:980–990.

27. Sidawy AN, Menzoian JO, Cantelmo NL, et al. Effect of inflow and outflow sites on the results of tibioperoneal vein grafts. *Am J Surg.* 1986;152:211–214.

28. Biancari F, Alback A, Kantonen I, et al. Predictive factors for adverse outcome of pedal bypasses. *Eur J Vasc Endovasc Surg.* 1999;18:138–143.

29. Schneider PA, Caps MT, Ogawa DY, et al. Intraoperative superficial femoral artery balloon angioplasty and popliteal to distal bypass graft: an option for combined open and endovascular treatment of diabetic gangrene. *J Vasc Surg.* 2001;33:955–962.

30. Berceli SA, Chan AK, Pomposelli FB Jr, et al. Efficacy of dorsal pedal artery bypass in limb salvage for ischemic heel ulcers. *J Vasc Surg.* 1999;30:499–508.

31. Andros G. Bypass grafts to the ankle and foot. A personal perspective. [Review]. *Surg Clin North Am.* 1995;75:715–729.

32. Holzenbein TJ, Pomposelli FB Jr, Miller A, et al. Results of a policy with arm veins used as the first alternative to an unavailable ipsilateral greater saphenous vein for infrainguinal bypass. *J Vasc Surg.* 1996;23:130–140.

33. Faries PL, Logerfo FW, Arora S, et al. Arm vein conduit is superior to composite prosthetic-autogenous grafts in lower extremity revascularization. *J Vasc Surg.* 2000;31:1119–1127.

34. Ascer E, Veith FJ, Flores SA. Infrapopliteal bypasses to heavily calcified rock-like arteries. Management and results. *Am J Surg.* 1986;152:220–223.

35. Rhodes JM, Gloviczki P, Bower TC, et al. The benefits of secondary interventions in patients with failing or failed pedal bypass grafts. *Am J Surg.* 1999;178:151–155.

36. Andros G, Harris RW, Salles-Cunha SX, et al. Lateral plantar artery bypass grafting: defining the limits of foot revascularization. *J Vasc Surg.* 1989;10:511–519; discussion 520–521.

37. Gloviczki P, Morris SM, Bower TC, et al. Microvascular pedal bypass for salvage of the severely ischemic limb [see comments]. *Mayo Clin Proc.* 1991;66:243–253.

38. Eckstein HH, Schumacher H, Maeder N, et al. Pedal bypass for limb-threatening ischaemia: an 11-year review. *Br J Surg.* 1996; 83:1554–1557.

39. Panayiotopoulos YP, Tyrrell MR, Owen SE, et al. Outcome and cost analysis after femorocrural and femoropedal grafting for critical limb ischaemia. *Br J Surg.* 1997;84:207–212.

40. Schneider JR, Walsh DB, McDaniel MD, et al. Pedal bypass versus tibial bypass with autogenous vein: a comparison of outcome and hemodynamic results. *J Vasc Surg.* 1993;17:1029–1038.

41. Kalman PG, Johnston KW. Predictors of long-term patient survival after *in situ* vein leg bypass. *J Vasc Surg.* 1997;25:899–904.

42. Luther M, Lepantalo M. Femorotibial reconstructions for chronic critical leg ischaemia: influence on outcome by diabetes, gender and age. *Eur J Vasc Endovasc Surg.* 1997;13:569–577.

43. Leers SA, Reifsnyder T, Delmonte R, et al. Realistic expectations for pedal bypass grafts in patients with end-stage renal disease. *J Vasc Surg.* 1998;28:976–980.

44. Hakaim AG, Gordon JK, Scott TE. Early outcome of *in situ* femorotibial reconstruction among patients with diabetes alone versus diabetes and end-stage renal failure: analysis of 83 limbs. *J Vasc Surg.* 1998;27:1049–1054.

45. McArthur CS, Sheahan MG, Pomposelli FB Jr, et al. Infrainguinal revascularization after renal transplantation. *J Vasc Surg.* 2003;37: 1181–1185.

46. Calligaro KD, Syrek JR, Dougherty MJ, et al. Use of arm and lesser saphenous vein compared with prosthetic grafts for infrapopliteal arterial bypass: are they worth the effort? *J Vasc Surg.* 1997;26: 919–924.

47. Nehler MR, Moneta GL, Edwards JM, et al. Surgery for chronic lower extremity ischemia in patients eighty or more years of age: operative results and assessment of postoperative independence. *J Vasc Surg.* 1993;18:618–624.

48. Frykberg RG, Arora S, Pomposelli FB, et al. Functional outcome in the elderly following lower extremity amputation. *J Foot Ankle Surg.* 1998;37:181–185.

49. Andrews KL. Rehabilitation in limb deficiency. 3. The geriatric amputee. [Review]. *Arch Phys Med Rehabil.* 1996;77(3 Suppl): S14–S17.

50. Evans WE, Hayes JP, Vermilion BD. Effect of a failed distal reconstruction on the level of amputation. *Am J Surg.* 1990;160:217–220.

51. Panayiotopoulos YP, Reidy JF, Taylor PR. The concept of knee salvage: why does a failed femorocrural/pedal arterial bypass not affect the amputation level? [see comments]. *Eur J Vasc Endovascu Surg.* 1997;13:477–485.

52. Carsten CG III, Taylor SM, Langan EM III, Crane MM. Factors associated with limb loss despite a patent infrainguinal bypass graft. *Am Surg.* 1998;64:33–37; discussion 37–38.

53. Rayman G, Williams SA, Spencer PD, et al. Impaired microvascular hyperaemic response to minor skin trauma in type I diabetes. *Br Med J (Clin Res Ed).* 1986;292:1295–1298.

54. Flynn MD, Tooke JE. Aetiology of diabetic foot ulceration: a role for the microcirculation? *Diabet Med.* 1992;9:320–329.

55. Arora S, Pomposelli F, LoGerfo FW, et al. Cutaneous microcirculation in the neuropathic diabetic foot improves significantly but not completely after successful lower extremity revascularization. *J Vasc Surg.* 2002;35:501–505.

56. Gibbons GW, Burgess AM, Guadagnoli E, et al. Return to well-being and function after infrainguinal revascularization. *J Vasc Surg.* 1995;21:35–44.

Prosthetic Infrapopliteal Bypasses

22

Evan C. Lipsitz   Frank J. Veith   Tejas R. Shah

Although the conduit of choice for tibial bypasses is autologous saphenous vein, the availability of prosthetic grafts has offered a ray of hope for many diabetic and nondiabetic patients with absent or inadequate autologous vein. A full 15% of all diabetics will develop some form of foot injury during their lifetime and 85% of these patients will be forced to have their foot amputated due to advanced necrosis and gangrene.[1] Since diabetic patients with peripheral vascular disease (PVD) are set apart from nondiabetic patients with PVD by their predilection for extensive disease within the tibial and peroneal arteries, tibial bypass takes on a heightened importance. Several alternatives to the use of greater saphenous vein have been proposed, including use of lesser saphenous vein; arm vein; spliced vein; composite grafts that use prosthetic, usually polytetrafluoroethylene (PTFE) plus autologous vein; and prosthetic grafts, usually PTFE alone with or without surgical adjuncts such as vein cuffs and arteriovenous fistulas. However, when used for tibial bypass grafts, the reduction in patency and limb salvage rates for these alternative conduits compared to good-quality autologous saphenous vein is greater than is seen for femoropopliteal and more proximal bypasses.[2] For this reason, some clinicians have advocated primary amputation rather than prosthetic tibial revascularization and attempt at limb salvage.[3] On the other hand, many surgeons favor a more aggressive approach since reported limb salvage rates are typically much greater than reported graft patency rates.[2,4,5]

This chapter presents some of the advances, developments, and complications of prosthetic bypasses to crural arteries. The specific features, physical properties, and biologic reactions to various synthetic materials are examined. Particular emphasis is placed on PTFE vascular grafts and their advantages in tibial bypasses. We also present developments that have increased prosthetic infrapopliteal bypass patency through antiplatelet and antithrombotic therapy. Last, issues of graft surveillance are reviewed as well as the treatment of failed or failing prosthetic grafts.

PROSTHETIC GRAFTS: BACKGROUND AND PHYSICAL CHARACTERISTICS

In many patients with diabetes, the preferred conduit for tibial bypass procedures—autologous greater saphenous vein—may not be of suitable quality or may not be available. In these cases, prosthetic grafts remain a viable alternative for patients requiring bypass procedures with the goal of achieving limb salvage. The available synthetic grafts are generally satisfactory for large-vessel reconstruction but have several limitations and produce inferior results compared to autologous vein when used for medium and small-vessel reconstructions below the knee. Two major categories of synthetic grafts are utilized for the performance of tibial bypasses. These include textile synthetic grafts, which are polymer yarns that are knitted or weaved into grafts, and nontextile synthetic grafts made by expanding polymers from sheets of material.

Textile Synthetic Grafts

Textile polyester grafts, such as Dacron, are made into prosthetics by weaving, knitting, or braiding yarn that shapes the graft into an elastic tube. In woven grafts, the fibers of yarn are interlaced with each other. The advantages of this particular graft are that it reduces bleeding through the interstitial region compared to knitted grafts, and it has less of a tendency to undergo dilatation and deformation over time. Knitted Dacron grafts are constructed by looping yarn around a needle and forming continuous interlocking chains of fibers. Knitted grafts have greater porosity, and produce more stretch in all directions than woven grafts.

Historically, knitted Dacron grafts required preclotting before implantation in order to seal the porous fabric and limit bleeding. Higher-porosity knitted grafts were often more difficult to preclot than lower-porosity woven grafts. However, from a healing perspective, higher-porosity grafts had some advantage.[6] In addition to rendering the graft impervious to bleeding, proper preclotting also created a less thrombogenic flow surface by depositing a compacted nonthrombogenic fibrin layer.[7] Currently, these grafts are coated with collagen or other substances that eliminate the need for preclotting.

Fabric grafts are generally manufactured with crimps or waves in the material. While crimping imparts some amount of flexibility, elasticity, and retention of shape even while being bent, it has a number of disadvantages. Crimping increases the thickness of a graft and reduces the relative internal diameter of the prosthetic material. In addition, it creates a turbulent flow as the unevenness of the inner graft surface interferes with blood movement. Turbulent flow invariably leads to increased fibrin deposition and increased surface thrombogenicity.[7,8] Although such factors may not be a problem for large-diameter grafts, the consequences may be significant when dealing with smaller-caliber grafts. Crimping is particularly disadvantageous for tibial bypasses due to the propensity for kinking at the knee. Dacron has also been shown to have a relative increased frequency of thrombosis due to low flow rates and dilated conduits.[9]

Despite some of the known disadvantages of Dacron, a recent study by Johansen et al.[10] found that there was no significant difference in primary or secondary patency between PTFE and Dacron inserted in a highly selected group of patients with favorable features known to increase the likelihood of prosthetic graft patency. Conclusions from this study, however, are limited as femoropopliteal bypasses were performed on low-risk patients with claudication.

Nontextile Synthetic Grafts

Nontextile synthetic grafts or expanded PTFE (Teflon) grafts have become the preferred prosthetic graft of many surgeons for the performance of crural bypasses because of their ease of use, favorable handling characteristics, and ready availability. Successfully developed in 1972 by Soyer and associates, PTFE grafts were initially evaluated to replace the vena cava in experimental animals.[11] This expanded Teflon was modified for vascular prosthesis by making it chemically inert, highly electronegative, and hydrophobic. In 1973, Matsumoto et al.[12] extended the use of PTFE as an arterial substitute in a canine model achieving patency rates comparable to vein grafts. In the first clinical use of PTFE for arterial circulation, Campbell et al.[13] performed femoropopliteal and femorotibial bypasses in 15 patients who did not have adequate saphenous veins. They were able to salvage limbs in 13 of these patients. PTFE has shown the ability to achieve acceptable patency rates extending 4 to 5 years for infrainguinal and infragenicular bypasses.[14-17]

PTFE is manufactured by heating and mechanically stretching a Teflon polymer. This produces a porous material with solid bands of nodes and interconnecting fibers (Fig. 22-1). Although the graft becomes incorporated by surrounding tissue, very little tissue grows into the PTFE.[18] Kohler et al.[19] suspect that this is due to the microporous nature of the material and the reinforcing tissue around the PTFE. Consequently, expanded PTFE grafts usually have a maximum of 1 to 2 cm of endothelial ingrowth at the ends of the graft.

A variety of modified expanded PTFE grafts have come into common use. These grafts have a thinner wall construction, which allows for easier handling, greater conformability, and increased compliance. Another variety based on processing alterations has allowed for increased elasticity of PTFE that was not present in previous types. This "stretch" feature was created by giving

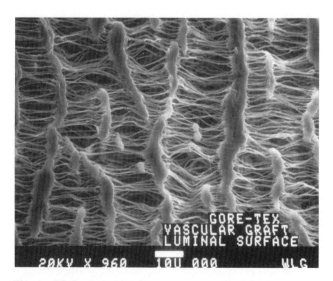

Figure 22-1 Scanning electron micrograph of the luminal surface of a PTFE graft showing porosity with nodes and interconnected fibers. (From W. L. Gore, Inc.)

the fibrils of the PTFE tube microcrimps. Because this crimping occurs on a microscopic level, the luminal surface remains smooth. Stretch PTFE grafts provide improved handling and greater ease of implantation without a negative impact on graft patency.

Although PTFE is less likely to kink due to its overall inflexibility, it is still susceptible to bends and kinks, especially at certain anatomic locations, such as across the knee joint. This prompted investigators to accommodate for graft bending by adding external supports, or rings, to the PTFE. It is thought that such supports would decrease mechanical compression, especially in subcutaneous grafts. More importantly, external rings help reduce the possibility of kinking across joints by allowing the graft to take a more gradual curve rather than to kink. The addition of these removable rings improved both the flow rate and patency of prosthetic tibial and below-knee popliteal artery bypasses.[20-23] More recently, these rings have been incorporated into the graft itself and are comprised of a modified PTFE. In this setting, the rings are integral to the graft and are not removable.

In an ongoing effort to improve patency of PTFE grafts, a relatively new PTFE design was introduced to mimic some of the effects of vein cuffs and patches that are often added to the distal anastomoses of small-vessel bypasses. Vein cuffs have the theoretic advantages of reducing the narrowing due to neointimal hyperplasia by widening the anastomoses, improving compliance, and providing biologic material at the distal anastomosis. The new precuffed PTFE grafts, found under the brand name Distaflo (C. R. Bard, Murray Hill, New Jersey), seek to optimize flow dynamics and improve bypass patency with the addition of a preshaped hood at the distal end. In a recent study by Panneton et al.,[24] the 1-year and 2-year limb salvage rates for patients using these grafts were 72% and 65%, respectively, while for a vein cuffed group of patients the limb salvages rates were 75% and 62%, respectively. The authors concluded that not only do PTFE precuffed grafts serve as a reasonable alternative in infrageniculate arterial reconstruction, but also that the benefit of vein cuffs does not lie in the material (biologic vs. synthetic), but rather the shape of the graft.

There are several advantages to the use of expanded PTFE grafts as prosthetic bypasses. PTFE is known to have fewer leaks, greater resistance to dilatation, and greater biocompatibility than Dacron. A few studies have also pointed to the idea that, compared to Dacron, PTFE grafts are more resistant to infection.[25-27] In addition, PTFE has been shown to have a greater potential for endothelial cell growth and thus a less thrombogenic flow surface.[28]

The major disadvantage of PTFE grafts is their less compliant nature compared to other prosthetic grafts as well as autogenous veins. This decreased compliance has been found to play an important role in anastomotic healing abnormalities, the development of neointimal hyperplasia, and an increased rate of distal arteriosclerosis, which may lead to graft failure.[29-31] PTFE also seems to be particularly prone to bleeding through needle holes at sutured anastomoses. This problem can be alleviated by choosing a needle and suture material combination with minimal diameter discrepancy and/or by applying hemostatic agents such as powdered collagen, oxidized cellulose, and/or fibrin glue. Last, PTFE grafts may be more expensive.

POLYURETHANE

Another type of graft synthesized from polymer extraction is polyurethane, which gained popularity as a vascular reconstructive material in the mid-1980s due to its elasticity, compliance, and exceptional biocompatibility.[32,33] Recent work by Jeschke et al.[34] showed that polycarbonate polyurethane also promotes faster endothelialization, forms a thinner neointima, and induces less chronic intimal proliferation than expanded PTFE. In addition, Park et al.[35] concluded that polyurethane is less likely to become calcified than PTFE, resulting in greater function and long-term durability. Despite these promises of low thrombogenicity and relatively high compliance, polyurethanes have been found to have poor patency rates when tested in vivo.[36,37] Polyurethanes have also been shown to degenerate and form aneurysms quite easily when compared to other prosthetic grafts.[38] Recently, a newly manufactured polyurethane material containing hydrolytically and oxidatively stable polycarbonate polyols with high hydrolase resistance was introduced and has been shown to be more resistant to biodegradation.[28] However, its effects in vivo have yet to be established, especially for small-diameter infrageniculate arteries.

MODIFICATIONS TO PROSTHETIC GRAFTS

Although the currently available prosthetic grafts have provided some great success, there is still much room for improvement regarding long-term patency. Theoretically, maximal patency is achieved by creating a graft with the least thrombogenic flow surface and with a very thin, stable neointimal layer. Certain modifications that attempt to address this goal include carbon and heparin coating, and endothelial seeding.

Carbon and Heparin Coating

Carbon and heparin have been known to decrease thrombogenicity by different mechanisms.[9] Thus it was a natural progression to use either or both materials to modify prosthetic grafts, and thus decrease the overall thrombogenicity of the entire graft. Sawyer and Pate[39] first looked at the electronegativity of luminal surfaces and suggested that knowledge of this property may help prevent graft thrombosis. With negatively charged circulating platelets, a second negatively charged material lining the luminal surface of the prosthetic graft would repel platelet attachment. Consequently, carbon, with its negative charge, was considered a likely candidate both because of its thromboresistance and its ability to repel platelets. Carbon promotes thromboresistance by delaying the accumulation of coagulant proteins, such as thrombin and factor Xa, on the luminal surface after graft implantation.[40] A thin layer of isotopic carbon is deposited on expandable PTFE at ultra-low temperatures to prevent the carbon from making the graft material more stiff and noncompliant. In one study by Akers et al.,[41] after coating PTFE with isotopic carbon using ultra-low temperatures, patency of >85% was achieved in dog models for >2 months, as compared to 42.9% during the same time with standard PTFE. In addition, a greater percentage of thrombus-free surface area was also achieved with these carbon coated grafts.

Heparin serves a dual role when coated on prosthetic grafts. An inhibitor of certain thrombus-inducing factors, heparin reduces thrombin formation and consequently prevents platelets from aggregating on luminal surfaces. In addition, heparin has also been proven to have a very strong antiproliferative effect on vascular smooth muscle,[42,43] thus theoretically reducing the incidence of neointimal hyperplasia. Its significant inhibitory effect is mediated in part through interactions with cell receptors, growth factors, adhesion molecules, and proteinase inhibitors.[44] A recent study by Lin et al.[45] showed that platelet deposition in baboon models decreased by 75% to 84% over 4 hours. In addition, neointimal cell proliferation in and adjacent to heparin-coated grafts was significantly reduced compared to noncoated grafts. In a multicenter clinical trial of heparin-bonded Dacron grafts, Devine et al.[46] concluded that the heparin-coated grafts resulted in greater patency rates and fewer amputations than uncoated PTFE grafts when used for femoropopliteal bypasses.

A biologically active analog of heparin, silyl-heparin, was recently studied by Laredo et al.[47] to improve the performance of carbon-coated expanded PTFE grafts. Their results showed that based on canine aortoiliac artery models, this analog improves patency, increases *in vivo* graft thromboresistance, and decreases intraluminal graft thrombus. Thus, the dual effects of carbon and heparin coating provided better patency and thromboresistance in this model than coating with simply one material. Although these results appear promising, the efficacy of carbon and heparin coating have yet to be proven clinically. More important, the durability of these grafts remains to be tested both in the animal model and in clinical trials.

Endothelial Cell Seeding

One of the contributing causes to thrombosis and decreased patency of prosthetic grafts is the lack of an endothelial cell layer lining the luminal surface, as is the case with vein grafts. This cell layer is a major factor that gives autologous saphenous veins a comparative advantage over prosthetic bypasses. PTFE, at best, allows for endothelial regeneration at sites of anastomosis with autogenous vessels. Hence, investigators have gone to great lengths in an attempt to directly "seed" prosthetic grafts with mechanically or enzymatically derived endothelial cells at the time of graft placement, with the hope that further attachments would create a continuous layer of living endothelial cells that will cover the entire graft flow surface and decrease thrombogenicity.

Mansfield[48] first introduced the concept of endothelial cell seeding in 1970 by placing a combination of endothelial cells, fibroblasts, and macrophages on Dacron patches placed in dog hearts. After 3 weeks, all of the patches that were seeded were free of thrombus. In 1978, Herring et al.[49] were able to mechanically scrape off endothelial cells and plant them in Dacron grafts in dog models. Prosthetic grafts that were thrombus-free were also achieved. However, mechanical removal of endothelial cells is inefficient and difficult. Thus, enzymatically derived methods were created by Graham et al.[50] that were far more efficient.

The significance of these promising developments in endothelial cell seeding would be especially helpful in infrageniculate grafts. Seeding in animal models has resulted in fewer platelet depositions, greater early patency, better tolerance to low-flow states, and prostacyclin-generating capacity.[51–53] Seeded grafts have also shown to be more resistant to bacterial infection due to decreased bacterial adherence.[54]

Despite all of these positive laboratory results, endothelial cell seeding has not been duplicated in clinical practice. Not only has it been difficult to harvest the right type of cells for seeding, investigators have also been challenged by the difficulty of having the cells adhere to the prosthetic material. In a study by Rosenman et al.,[55] a full 30% of seeded cells were detached within the first 30 minutes, and further detachment occurred at the rate of 2% per hour for the next 24 hours. However, Seeger[56] showed that coating expandable PTFE grafts with fibronectin significantly improves adherence of endothelial cells.

PATIENT EVALUATION AND SELECTION

Although noninvasive vascular laboratory evaluation should be the initial step in the evaluation of patients being considered for lower extremity revascularization, these exams may be misleading in diabetic patients. The waveform obtained on pulse volume recordings (PVRs) provides useful information regarding the overall status of the circulation to the extremity. Ankle-brachial indices (ABIs) are likely to be falsely elevated in the majority of diabetic patients due to their propensity for extensive calcific disease of the arteries. As such, they may not be useful for preoperative evaluation and/or follow-up surveillance of bypass procedures. Duplex arterial mapping has been shown to have value in the preoperative planning of bypass procedures, but again, in this group of patients who generally have extensive calcific disease of the tibial vessels, results are likely to be suboptimal. Other new imaging methods such as magnetic resonance angiography (MRA) and computed tomography angiography (CTA) may also provide useful information, but because of the limitations listed above these studies have not yet been uniformly definitive. Additionally, CTA has the disadvantage of contrast requirement and MRA is costly. The definitive preprocedural evaluation in most centers is still contrast angiography done with digital subtraction. Both the inflow and outflow should be thoroughly evaluated for the presence of lesions and the quality of the vessels. Calcification at all levels can be evaluated on scout films prior to the injection of contrast material. It should also be kept in mind that many diabetic patients will have concomitant renal dysfunction and may require hydration and/or other pretreatment prior to any contrast studies. Patients on metformin should discontinue this medication during the immediate periprocedural period. Because of the relatively low long-term patency rates associated with prosthetic tibial bypasses, these procedures should only be performed for limb salvage in the setting of rest pain, nonhealing ulcers, or ischemic gangrene. There is no suggestion to perform these procedures in patients with intermittent claudication.

SURGICAL APPROACHES

Standard surgical approaches are used for the performance of prosthetic tibial bypasses. Since the length of the graft (as opposed to cases when only limited vein may be available) is not a primary issue, the best possible inflow site should be used. In general, the common femoral artery will be the inflow vessel of choice. In cases where there is an uncompromised proximal portion of superficial femoral artery (SFA), this vessel may be used in order to avoid groin dissection and resulting wound problems. If the common femoral artery has been dissected for a previous bypass, and if the deep femoral artery is of good quality, this vessel may be used for inflow in order to avoid a reoperative groin dissection. Last, if the common femoral artery is not adequate the external iliac or common iliac artery may be used for inflow and exposed via a retroperitoneal approach. Any of the three tibial vessels may be used

for outflow. If more than one vessel is available, in general, the vessel with the best runoff to the foot should be chosen. It is important to try to identify a noncalcified or only minimally calcified portion of the artery for the distal anastomosis, as this will facilitate its technical performance. We prefer a lateral approach with lateral subcutaneous tunneling for bypasses to the anterior tibial or mid to distal peroneal arteries. In cases of a peroneal bypass, a partial fibulectomy is performed to expose this vessel (Fig. 22-2). For bypasses to the posterior tibial artery, tibioperoneal trunk, and proximal-most peroneal artery we prefer a medial approach with either anatomic or subcutaneous tunneling depending on the location of the distal anastomosis and whether

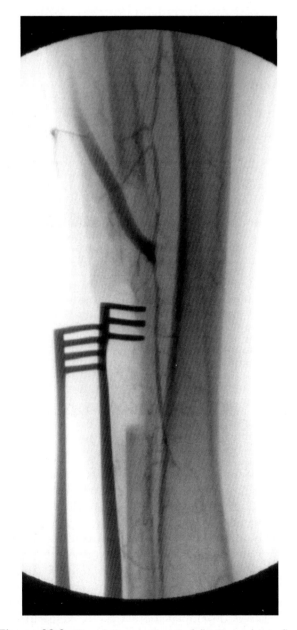

Figure 22-2 Completion angiogram following polytetrafluoroethylene (PTFE) peroneal bypass graft done via a lateral approach with partial fibulectomy.

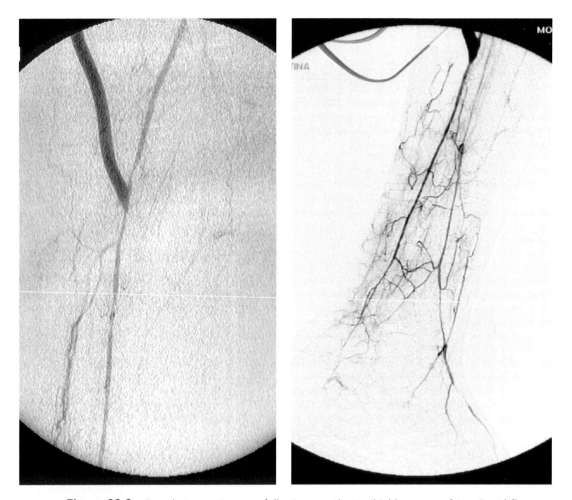

Figure 22-3 Completion angiograms following prosthetic tibial bypass grafting. Rapid flow through the anastomosis without evidence of stenosis is seen.

or not previous anatomic tunnels have been made. Some form of evaluation following completion of the bypass is imperative, either with completion angiography or duplex (Fig. 22-3). Any true defects identified at that time should be corrected.

SURGICAL ADJUNCTS AND THEIR LEVEL OF IMPORTANCE

Because of the relatively low patency rates achieved when performing PTFE bypasses to tibial vessels, many surgeons favor the addition of surgical adjuncts. Such surgical adjuncts include arteriovenous fistulas (AVFs), vein cuffs, and/or vein patches. The concept of AVFs to improve the patency of bypass operations dates back to 1902.[57] The proposed mechanism of function for AVFs is decreased vascular resistance of the distal arterial bed, which increases flow through the prosthetic graft, improving patency. The concept behind vein cuffs and patches was developed more recently. Vein cuffs or patches are believed to exert their effect because of an

improved compliance profile at the distal anastomosis, the presence of autologous vein at the distal anastomosis, or both. Vein cuffs have also been shown to inhibit juxta-anastomotic neointimal hyperplasia in animal models.[58] Details of these procedures are discussed elsewhere in this volume.

Despite several studies that have suggested the advantages of adjunctive cuffs, patches, or AVFs, no large, randomized, prospective trials have been performed that unequivocally prove the benefits of these adjuncts. Moreover, Parsons et al.,[59] over the course of a 9-year study, were able to obtain 3- and 5-year cumulative primary patency rates of 39% and 28%, respectively, without the use of patches, cuffs, or fistulas. They were also able to achieve secondary patency rates at 3 and 5 years of 55% and 43%, respectively. The limb salvage rate at 3 years was 71% and at 5 years was 66%. These results are very similar to the patencies achieved by PTFE grafts with surgical adjuncts added to the tibial bypass grafts. The addition of patches, cuffs, or fistulas also increases operative and anesthesia time, both significant considerations especially for elderly patients with multiple comorbidities. The use of these adjuncts also increases the complexity of the operation by generally necessitating a greater number and larger size of incisions, thereby increasing the chances of wound infection. Another consideration that is often overlooked is that vein cuffs and patches require viable veins for such procedures to be successful. However, in many of these patients suffering from peripheral vascular disease, the veins are inadequate or simply not available for use due to previous operations. Last, the addition of a vein patch may make the performance of the distal anastomosis somewhat easier. This should not, however, be a substitute for meticulous surgical technique. Until patches, cuffs, and other adjuncts have proven value in infrageniculate bypasses, many authors, including our own group, do not perform them routinely as part of tibial PTFE grafts.

ANTIPLATELET AND THROMBOTIC THERAPY

Over the last 15 years, primary patency for below-knee PTFE grafts has significantly improved from the initial 12% 4-year patency rate reported by Veith et al.[2] Because vascular prostheses lack an endothelial lining, they are more susceptible to thrombosis and failure. Studies with indium-111–labeled platelets in humans have shown a marked uptake of labeled platelets on femoropopliteal bypass grafts made of Dacron or PTFE, but little or no uptake on vein bypasses.[60,61] In addition, during the early postoperative period in distal bypasses, patients develop greater than normal coagulability, with increased platelet reactivity and factor VIII–related antigen and decreased activity of antithrombin III.[62] Bandyk et al.[63] and Sauvage et al.[64] have also noted the importance of maintaining a baseline level of blood flow in prosthetic grafts, below which thrombus formation is more likely to occur. All of these observations suggested that antithrombotic therapy may be a useful way to improve patency in prosthetic grafts.

In one of the first studies to propose antithrombotic therapy after infrageniculate prosthetic bypasses, Flinn et al.[65] administered heparin both intraoperatively and postoperatively up to 24 hours in patients. After 24 or 48 hours, oral warfarin was administered to maintain a prothrombin time twice that of control subjects. The results of this study showed a 2-year patency rate of 45% and 4-year patency rate of 37%. During the observation period, 15 of the patients were noted to have subtherapeutic levels of anticoagulation therapy, which resulted in graft occlusion. If these patients were not included, 2-year patency rates would increase to 58% and 4-year patency rates would be as high as 50%, further emphasizing the potentially important contribution of antithrombotic therapy. However, historical controls were used in this study and patient selection may have played a role in the improved graft patencies.

Antiplatelet therapy has been known to decrease platelet aggregation but it has no effect on initial platelet deposition. Clinically, aspirin, an antiplatelet agent, has been shown to decrease platelet adherence to prosthetic vascular grafts, thus resulting in increased patency rates.[66] The efficacy of dipyridamole added to aspirin therapy has not yet been proven. However, because animal studies have demonstrated that dipyridamole increases the antithrombotic effects of aspirin on artificial material, dipyridamole has been used in conjunction with aspirin in patients with vascular prosthetics.[67]

With anticoagulating agents retarding thrombin generation and antiplatelet agents lowering platelet adherence, theoretically a combination of both agents would result in a very attractive antithrombotic therapy. This idea was promoted by Jackson et al.[68] in a study that showed fewer femoropopliteal bypass occlusions after a combination of warfarin and aspirin therapy, as opposed to administration of aspirin alone. Vein grafts have also been evaluated with the combination therapy with excellent 4-year primary patency rates of 74%.[69] Low doses of these combined agents might possibly offer better antithrombotic effectiveness while limiting hemorrhagic side effects.

Clopidogrel (Plavix) has recently been introduced as a potent antiplatelet agent. It exhibits its effects by irreversibly interfering with activation of the platelet glycoprotein IIb/IIIa complex, thus inhibiting platelet aggregation. Because it exerts its effect at a different place in the platelet activation cycle than aspirin, it may act synergistically with aspirin and has been shown to potentiate the effect of aspirin on collagen-induced platelet aggregation. However, as yet no convincing data exists to show that this medication improves distal graft patency.

GRAFT SURVEILLANCE

Duplex surveillance of lower extremity vein bypass grafts is widely accepted based largely on the benefit of preserving the patient's autologous conduit by detecting and fixing lesions before they can cause graft thrombosis. Duplex surveillance for prosthetic grafts has not been as widely accepted because of the rare occurrence of inherent lesions within the conduit itself, and the fact that prosthetic material can be more easily replaced.[70] In a study by Lalak et al.,[71] the authors concluded that the low yield of detecting lesions is not worth the cost of duplex surveillance in infrainguinal prosthetic bypass grafts. However, in addition to the cost and morbidity of reoperation, thrombosis of the graft will often be complicated by thrombosis within the outflow tract, which may be extensive and which may significantly alter the outcome of subsequent procedures. With our group's aggressive approach to limb salvage, we find duplex scans highly effective in early detection of stenosis of prosthetic grafts. In a study by Calligaro et al.,[72] it was shown that routine use of duplex scans serves to accurately diagnose failing femorotibial prosthetic grafts. According to this study, stenosis in a failing graft can be identified by the following: a) Elevations of peak systolic velocity >300 cm per second at anastomoses or at inflow and outflow arteries; b) peak systolic velocity of <45 cm per second in the remainder of the graft distal to the stenosis; or c) monophasic signals throughout the graft. The authors advocated that duplex scans should be carried out regularly; every 3 months for the first year after operation and 6 months thereafter.

Graft surveillance can also be assisted by plethysmography and pressure measurements. Within 48 hours after bypass graft surgery, an increase in the ABI of 0.15 should be noted. Subsequently, an equal drop in pressure or decrease in air plethysmography amplitude of 5 mm may be indicative of a failed or failing graft requiring further investigation by duplex scan or arteriography.[73] While ABI is often suggestive of stenosis, this index is functional and not anatomic. Thus, such tests cannot distinguish between inflow, outflow, and the conduit problems. Additionally, these measurements must be viewed with caution given the degree of arterial calcification seen in these patients as mentioned above.

RESULTS: PATENCY AND LIMB SALVAGE

With PTFE as the graft of choice for distal limb bypasses, its efficacy has been extensively studied and compared with other materials. A study performed by Veith et al.[2] was one of the first large-scale, multicenter studies that compared autogenous saphenous veins with PTFE grafts infrainguinally, both above and below the knee. Among the results of this study, the 4-year primary patency rate of infrapopliteal PTFE grafts was 12%, with the sharpest drop in patency during the first 6 months. However, the 4-year limb salvage rate in this study was 61%. These poor long-term patency results led many investigators to search for mechanisms to improve these results. In a subsequent study by Schweiger et al.[74] of tibial bypasses with ringed PTFE grafts, primary patency rates of 37% and 23% were achieved 2 years and 5 years after the operation. Further studies by Eagleton et al.[75] obtained 2-year primary patency rates of 46% after altering the conformation of the distal anastomosis with AVFs and vein patches. Nevertheless, the limb salvage rate remained relatively the same at 64% after 2 years.

PATIENTS REQUIRING REPEAT BYPASSES

Many patients requiring a prosthetic bypass to a tibial vessel will have failed one or more previous attempts at lower extremity revascularization. These previous bypasses may have been performed with vein, prosthetic, or composite grafts. The optimal treatment of these patients, many of whom are facing imminent amputation, is not well known. Many authors believe that in this setting a primary amputation is better than performing another bypass, while other reports have supported the role of multiple bypass attempts for limb salvage after the failure of one or more previous bypass grafts.[76-78] It is reasonable to expect that patients undergoing a lower extremity bypass after previous failures would have a poorer outcome on the basis of disease severity and progression alone, in addition to the difficulties associated with reoperation. Such difficulties include the frequent need for complicated redo dissections, an increased risk of subsequent graft and/or wound infection, the lack of a suitable autogenous conduit, and the need to choose more proximal inflow sites and/or more distal outflow sites. Our own policy has been to attempt to avoid amputation in patients with imminent limb threat and to proceed with further attempts at limb revascularization even when patients have failed two or more previous bypasses.[79,80]

We have performed 105 surgical revascularization procedures in 55 limbs of 54 patients for imminently limb-threatening lower extremity ischemia after failure of two or more prior ipsilateral infrainguinal bypasses. The overwhelming majority of these cases were performed to tibial or pedal vessels in diabetics with PTFE. These patients underwent between three and nine ipsilateral arterial reconstructions. We found no negative impact on patency or limb salvage rates in this group of patients. Interestingly, both we and others also found that the overall morbidity and mortality in this specific cohort of patients with greatly advanced PVD was surprisingly low, with a 3-year mortality of 62% in patients undergoing three reconstructions and 73% in patients undergoing four or more reconstructions.[81,82] Additionally, there was no significant increase in operative or late mortality in the group having four or more bypasses. Thus, the likelihood of success of repetitive limb revascularization was unrelated to the number of previous failures, and the expected incremental failure rate with each successive bypass was not found. These results, coupled with the 3-year limb salvage rate of >50% in patients who otherwise would have required amputation, support the aggressive use of limb revascularization even after two or more failed bypasses.

COMPLICATIONS

The most common complications of PTFE grafts are the development of thrombosis, infection, and aneurysms. Aneurysms in the body of PTFE grafts have become relatively rare in the absence of graft injury or infection, since the introduction of an extra reinforcing outer layer. False aneurysms may occur when there is breakdown of the suture line between the graft and artery, usually due to infection.[83] Prophylactic antibiotics are administered prior to the start of all bypass procedures in order to reduce the chances of graft infection.

Although several investigators have researched the relative susceptibility of PTFE to bacterial infection, conclusive results have not been produced. Moore et al.,[84] in experiments with dogs, found that PTFE grafts may actually be more susceptible to infection than Dacron grafts. However, Schmitt et al.[85] found the exact opposite with bacteria adhering more to Dacron than to PTFE. Bleeding from the site of an infection at a PTFE anastomosis may necessitate graft removal and ligation of the involved artery proximally and distally. A new bypass in a clean field may be required to salvage the limb. If, however, a wound infection is noted early enough and there is no significant graft involvement, debridement of infected regions and necrotic tissue followed by daily wound packing with dilute betadine solution and high-dose antibiotic administration is recommended. This has been shown in several instances to be a viable alternative to graft removal, even in cases where there is exposed prosthetic material.[71,86] Patients need to be closely observed in a monitored setting within the hospital until the graft is covered with healthy tissue.

Thrombosis is, by far, the most common complication with PTFE grafts. Thrombosis can be categorized based on time of occurrence—early or late. Early thrombosis (<2 months) is typically due to technical errors or compromised inflow or outflow. Late thrombosis (>2 months) is caused by intimal hyperplasia or progression of disease either proximally or distally. Both early and late thrombosis in PTFE grafts are markedly different than that seen with vein grafts in that PTFE grafts can be thrombectomized at any time after initial failure.[65,87] These thrombectomies are best carried out under fluoroscopic guidance for a variety of reasons.[88] For late thrombosis it is important to evaluate the inflow and outflow by repeat angiography. In cases of intimal hyperplasia, patch angioplasty or graft extension may be performed. Completion angiography is mandatory to assure adequacy of repair and patency of the conduit and the outflow.

TREATMENT OF FAILED OR FAILING GRAFTS

In many cases, a failed bypass will require no treatment, particularly when a patient remains asymptomatic, i.e., when a gangrenous lesion has healed. Several studies have shown that graft occlusion, even when the graft was done for limb salvage, does not necessarily lead to a threatened limb. In one study by Ascher et al.,[89] approximately 50% of the patients with infrapopliteal limb salvage bypass failure of either PTFE or vein grafts had few or no symptoms if the graft failed even after the third postoperative month. In these circumstances, a nonoperative approach to the management of their ischemia is often best.

CONCLUSION

With tibial bypasses, the graft material of choice is autogenous saphenous veins. However, if such veins are inadequate or unavailable, as is often the case in diabetic patients, PTFE bypasses serve as an acceptable alternative. Several modifications have been made to PTFE grafts to improve patency rates. Carbon and heparin coating may decrease thrombogenicity and decrease proliferation of smooth muscle cells. Aggressive antithrombotic therapy and graft surveillance have almost certainly increased long-term patency and limb salvage rates. Despite all of the improvements, complications and graft failure remain an imminent reality in prosthetic tibial procedures. We advocate an aggressive approach and appropriate reoperations for failed or failing grafts to improve overall results and provide limb salvage rates that are almost comparable to autogenous vein bypasses. Last, the surgeon must not forget that graft failure does not necessarily equal overall failure, and that limb salvage may be achieved even in the setting of a failed graft.

REFERENCES

1. Pecoraro RE, Reiber GE, Burgess EM. Pathways to diabetic limb amputation: basis for prevention. *Diabetes Care.* 1990;13:513–521.
2. Veith FJ, Gupta SK, Ascher E, et al. Six year prospective multicenter randomized comparison of autologous saphenous vein and expanded polytetrafluoroethylene grafts in infrainguinal arterial reconstructions. *J Vasc Surg.* 1986;3:104–114.
3. Bell PR. Are distal vascular procedures worthwhile? *Br J Surg.* 1996;23:130–140.
4. Brewster DC, LaSalle AJ, Robinson JG, et al. Femoropopliteal graft failure. Clinical consequences and success of secondary reconstructions. *Arch Surg.* 1983;118:1043.
5. DeWeese JA, Rob CG. Autogenous venous grafts ten years later. *Surgery.* 1977;82:775.
6. Weslowski SA, Fries CC, Karlson KE, et al. Porosity: primary determinant of ultimate fate of synthetic vascular grafts. *Surgery.* 1961;50:91.

7. Sauvage LR. Biologic behavior of grafts in arterial system. In: Haimovici H, ed. *Vascular surgery: Principles and techniques*. 3rd ed. Norwalk, Conn: Appleton & Lange; 1989:136–160.

8. Lindenauer SM. The fabric vascular prosthesis. In: Rutherford RB, ed. *Vascular surgery*. 3rd ed. Philadelphia, Pa: WB Saunders; 1989: 450–460.

9. Rutherford R. Prosthetic grafts. *Vascular surgery*. Philadelphia, Pa: WB Saunders; 2000:559–584.

10. Johansen K, Watson J. Dacron femoral-popliteal bypass grafts in good-risk claudicant patients. *Am J Surg*. 2004;187:5.

11. Soyer T, Lempinen M, Cooper P, et al. A new venous prosthesis. *Surgery*. 1972;72:864.

12. Matsumoto H, Hasegawa T, Fuse K, et al. A new vascular prosthesis for small caliber artery. *Surgery*. 1973;74:519.

13. Campbell CD, Goldfarb D, Roe R. A small arterial substitute: expanded microporous polytetrafluoroethylene: patency versus porosity. *Ann Surg*. 1975;182:138.

14. De Frang RD, Edwards JM, Moneta GL, et al. Repeat leg bypass after multiple prior bypass failures. *J Vasc Surg*. 1994;19:268–276; discussion 276–277.

15. Charlesworth PM, Brewster DC, Darling RC, et al. The fate of polytetrafluoroethylene grafts in lower limb bypass surgery: a six year follow-up. *Br J Surg*. 1985;72:896.

16. Christenson JT, Broome A, Norgren L, et al. Revascularization of popliteal and below knee arteries with polytetrafluoroethylene. *Surgery*. 1985;97:141.

17. Cranley JJ, Hafner CD. Revascularization of femoropopliteal arteries using saphenous vein, polytetrafluoroethylene, and umbilical vein graft. Five- and six year results. *Arch Surg*. 1982; 117:1543.

18. Mathisen SR, Wu HD, Sauvage LR, et al. An experimental study of eight current arterial prostheses. *J Vasc Surg*. 1986;4:33.

19. Kohler TR, Stratton JR, Kirkman TR, et al. Conventional versus high-porosity polytetrafluoroethylene grafts: clinical evaluation. *Surgery*. 1992;112:901.

20. Kenney DA, Sauvage LR, Wood SJ, et al. Comparison of non-crimped, externally supported (EXS) and crimped, non-supported Dacron prostheses for axillo-femoral and above-knee femoropopliteal bypass. *Surgery*. 1982;92:931.

21. Kempczinski RF. Physical characteristics of implanted polytetrafluoroethylene grafts: a preliminary report. *Arch Surg*. 1979;114:917.

22. Burnham SJ, Flanigan DP, Goodreau JJ, et al. Ankle pressure changes in distal bypass grafts during knee flexion. *Surgery*. 1980;87:652.

23. Dunn MM, Robinette DR, Peoples JB. Comparison between externally stented and unstented PTFE vascular grafts. *Am Surg*. 1988;54:324.

24. Panneton JM, Hollier LH, Hofer JM. Multicenter randomized prospective trial comparing a precuffed polytetrafluoroethylene graft to a vein cuffed polytetrafluoroethylene graft for infragenicular arterial bypass. *Ann Vasc Surg*. 2004;18:199–206.

25. Bergamini TM, Bandyk DF, Govostis D, et al. Infection of vascular prostheses caused by bacterial biofilms. *J Vasc Surg*. 1988;7:21.

26. Bandyk DF, Bergamini TM, Kinney EV, et al. *In situ* replacement of vascular prostheses infected by bacterial biofilms. *J Vasc Surg*. 1991;13:575.

27. Shah PM, Ito K, Clauss RH, et al. Expanded microporous polytetrafluoroethylene grafts in contaminated wounds: experimental and clinical study. *J Trauma*. 1983;23:1030.

28. Shepard AD, Gelfand JA, Callow AD, et al. Complement activation of synthetic vascular prostheses. *J Vasc Surg*. 1984;1:829.

29. Echave V, Koornick AR, Haimov M, et al. Intimal hyperplasia as a complication of the use of the polytetrafluoroethylene graft for femoropopliteal bypass. *Surgery*. 1979;86:791.

30. Sottiurai VS, Yao JS, Flinn WR, et al. Intimal hyperplasia and neointimal: an ultrastructural analysis of thrombosed grafts in humans. *Surgery*. 1983;93:809.

31. Sladen JG, Maxwell TM. Experience with 130 polytetrafluoroethylene grafts. *Am J Surg*. 1981;141:546.

32. Zdrahala RJ. Small caliber vascular grafts. Part II: polyurethane revisited. *J Biomater Appl*. 1996;11:37–61.

33. Tiwari A, Salacinski H, Seifalian AM, et al. New prostheses for use in bypass grafts with special emphasis on polyurethanes. *Cardiovasc Surg*. 2002;10:191–197.

34. Jeschke M, Hermanutz V, Wolf S, et al. Polyurethane vascular prostheses decreases neointimal formation compared with expanded polytetrafluoroethylene. *J Vasc Surg*. 1999;29:168–176.

35. Park J, Song M, Hwang Y, et al. Calcification comparisons of polymers for vascular grafts. *Yonsei Med J*. 2001;42:304–310.

36. Geeraert AJ, Callaghan JC. Experimental study of selected small caliber arterial grafts. *J Cardiovasc Surg*. 1977;18:155.

37. Cronenwett JL, Zelenock GB. Alternative small arterial grafts. In: Stanly JC, ed. *Biologic and synthetic vascular prostheses*. New York, NY: Grune & Stratton; 1982:595–620.

38. Yeager A, Callow AD. New graft materials and current approaches to an acceptable small diameter vascular graft. *Trans Am Soc Artif Intern Organs*. 1988;34:88.

39. Sawyer PN, Pate JW. Bio-electric phenomena as an etiologic factor in intravascular thrombosis. *Am J Physiology*. 1953;175: 103–107.

40. Toursarkissian B, Eisenberg PR, Abendschein DR, et al. Thrombogenicity of small-diameter prosthetic grafts, relative contributions of graft-associated thrombin and factor Xa. *J Vasc Surg*. 1997;25:730–735.

41. Akers D, Du YH, Kempczinski RF. The effect of carbon coating and porosity on early patency of expanded polytetrafluoroethylene grafts: an experimental study. *J Vasc Surg*. 1993;18:1.

42. Guyton JR, Rosenberg RD, Clowes AW, et al. Inhibition of rat arterial smooth muscle cell proliferation by heparin: *in vivo* studies with anticoagulant and nonanticoagulant heparin. *Circ Res*. 1980;46:625–634.

43. Clowes AW, Karnovsky MJ. Suppression by heparin of smooth muscle cell proliferation in injured arteries. *Nature*. 1977;265: 625–626.

44. Letourneur D, Caleb BL, Castellot JJ Jr. Heparin binding, internalization, and metabolism in vascular smooth muscle cells. I: upregulation of heparin binding correlates with antiproliferative activity. *J Cell Physiol*. 1995;165:676–686.

45. Lin P, Chen C, Ruth B, et al. Small-caliber heparin-coated ePTFE grafts reduce platelet deposition and neointimal hyperplasia in a baboon model. *J Vasc Surg*. 2004;39:1322–1328.

46. Devine C, Hons BA, McCollum C. Heparin-bonded Dacron or polytetrafluoroethylene for femoropopliteal bypass grafting: a multicenter trial. *J Vasc Surg*. 2001;33:533–539.

47. Laredo J, Lian X, Vicki H, et al. Silyl-heparin bonding improves the patency and *in vivo* thromboresistance of carbon-coated polytetrafluoroethylene vascular grafts. *J Vasc Surg*. 2004;39: 1059–1065.

48. Mansfield PB. Tissue cultured endothelium for vascular prosthetic devices. *Rev Surg*. 1970;27:291.

49. Herring MB, Gardiner A, Glover JL. A single-staged technique for seeding vascular grafts with autogenous endothelium. *Surgery*. 1978;84:498.

50. Graham LM, Vinter DW, Ford JW, et al. Endothelial seeding of Dacron and polytetrafluoroethylene grafts: the cellular events of healing. *Surgery*. 1984;96:745.

51. Stanley JC, Burkel WE, Ford JW, et al. Enhanced patency of small-diameter externally supported Dacron iliofemoral grafts seeded with endothelial cells. *Surgery*. 1982;92:994.

52. Clagett GP, Burkel WE, Sharefkin JB, et al. Platelet reactivity *in vivo* in dogs with arterial prostheses seeded with endothelial cells. *Circulation*. 1984;69:632.

53. Budd JS, Allen K, Hartley J, et al. Prostacyclin production from seeded prosthetic vascular grafts. *Br J Surg*. 1992;79:1151.

54. Birinyi LK, Douville EC, Lewis SA, et al. Increased resistance to bacteremic graft infection after endothelial cell seeding. *J Vasc Surg.* 1987;5:193–197.

55. Rosenman JE, Kempczinski RF, Pearce WH, et al. Kinetics of endothelial cell seeding. *J Vasc Surg.* 1985;2:778.

56. Seeger JM. Improved endothelial cell seeding density after flow exposure in fibronectin-coated grafts. *Surg Forum.* 1985;36:450.

57. San Martin YYY, Satrustegui A. Anastomose arterio-veneuse pot remedier a obliteration desarteres des members. *Bull Med.* 1902;16:451.

58. Suggs WD, Henriques HF, DePalma RG. Vein cuff interposition prevents juxta-anastomotic neointimal hyperplasia. *Ann Surg.* 1988;207:717–723.

59. Parsons R, Suggs WD, Veith FJ, et al. Polytetrafluoroethylene bypasses to infrapopliteal arteries without cuffs or patches: a better option than amputation in patients without autologous vein. *J Vasc Surg.* 1996;23:347–356.

60. Pumphrey CW, Chesebro JH, Dewanjee MK, et al. *In vivo* quantitation of platelet deposition on human peripheral arterial bypass grafts using indium-111-labeled platelets: effects of dipyridamole aspirin. *Am J Cardiol.* 1983;51:796–801.

61. Stratton JR, Ritchie JL. Failure of ticlopidine to inhibit deposition of indium-111-labeled platelets on Dacron prosthetic surfaces in humans. *Circulation.* 1984;69:677–683.

62. McDaniel MD, Pearce WH, Yao JST, et al. Sequential changes in coagulation and platelet function following femorotibial bypass. *J Vasc Surg.* 1984;1:261–268.

63. Bandyk DF, Cato RF, Towne JB. A low flow velocity predicts failure of femoropopliteal and femorotibial bypass grafts. *Surgery.* 1985;98:799–807.

64. Sauvage LR, Walker MW, Berger KG, et al. Current arterial prostheses. *Arch Surg.* 1979;114:687–691.

65. Flinn WR, Harris JP, Rudo ND, et al. Results of repetitive distal revascularization. *Surgery.* 1982;91:566.

66. Zammit M, Kaplan S, Sauvage L, et al. Aspirin therapy in small-caliber arterial prostheses: long-term experimental observations. *J Vasc Surg.* 1984;1:839–851.

67. Hanson SR, Harker LA. Effects of platelet-modifying drugs on arterial thromboembolism in baboons. *J Clin Invest.* 1985;75:1591–1599.

68. Jackson MR, Johnson WC, Williford WO. The effect of anticoagulation therapy and graft selection on the ischemic consequences of femoropopliteal bypass graft occlusion results from a multicenter randomized clinical trail. *J Vasc Surg.* 2002;35:292–298.

69. Johnson WC, Blebea J, Cantelmo NL, et al. Does oral anticoagulation improve patency of vein bypasses? A prospective randomized study. Paper presented at: *51st Annual Meeting of Society of Vascular Surgery*, Boston, Mass, June 1–2, 1997.

70. Hobollah JJ, Nassal MM, Ryan SM, et al. Is color duplex surveillance of infrainguinal polytetrafluoroethylene grafts worthwhile? *Am J Surg.* 1997;174:133–135.

71. Lalak NJ, Hanel KC, Hunt J, et al. Duplex scan surveillance of infrainguinal prosthetic bypass grafts. *J Vasc Surg.* 1994;20:637–641.

72. Calligaro K, Doerr K, McAfee-Bennett S, et al. Should duplex ultrasonography be performed for surveillance of femoropopliteal and femorotibial arterial prosthetic bypasses? *Ann Vasc Surg.* 2001;15:520–524.

73. Wengerter K, Berdejo G. Noninvasive Studies. In: *Handbook of vascular surgery*. St. Louis, Mo: Quality Medical Publishing Inc; 1994:29–60.

74. Schweiger H, Klein P, Lang W. Tibial bypass grafting for limb salvage with ringed polytetrafluoroethylene prostheses: results of primary and secondary procedures. *J Vasc Surg.* 1993;18:867–874.

75. Eagleton M, Ouriel K, Shortell C, et al. Femoral-infrapopliteal bypass with prosthetic grafts. *Surgery.* 1999;126:759–765.

76. Bartlett ST, Olinde AJ, Flinn WR, et al. The reoperative potential of infrainguinal bypass: long-term limb and patient survival. *J Vasc Surg.* 1987;5:170–179.

77. George SM Jr, Klamer TW, Lambert GE Jr. Value of continued efforts at limb salvage despite multiple graft failures. *Ann Vasc Surg.* 1994;8:332–336.

78. Veith FJ, Gupta SK, Samson RH, et al. Progress in limb salvage by reconstructive arterial surgery combined with new or improved adjunctive procedures. *Ann Surg.* 1981;194:386–401.

79. Veith FJ, Gupta SK, Wengerter KR, et al. Changing atherosclerotic disease patterns and management strategies in lower-limb-threatening ischemia. *Ann Surg.* 1990;212:402–414.

80. Rutherford RB, Baker JD, Ernst C, et al. Recommended standards for reports dealing with lower extremity ischemia: revised version. *J Vasc Surg.* 1997;26:517–538.

81. Kalra M, Gloviczki P, Bower TC, et al. Limb salvage after successful pedal bypass grafting is associated with improved long-term survival. *J Vasc Surg.* 2001;33:6–16.

82. Belkin M, Conte MS, Donaldson MC, et al. Preferred strategies for secondary infrainguinal bypass: lessons learned from 300 consecutive reoperations. *J Vasc Surg.* 1995;21:282–293; discussion 293–295.

83. Bhat DJ, Tellis VA, Kohlberg WI, et al. Management of sepsis involving expanded polytetrafluoroethylene grafts for hemodialysis access. *Surgery.* 1980;87:445.

84. Moore WS, Malone JM, Keown K. Prosthetic arterial graft material. Influence of neointimal healing and bacteremic infectibility. *Arch Surg.* 1980;115:1379.

85. Schmitt DD, Bandyk DF, Pequet AJ, et al. Bacterial adherence to vascular prostheses. *J Vasc Surg.* 1986;3:732.

86. Veith FJ. Surgery of the infected aortic graft. In: Bergan JJ Yao JST, eds. *Surgery of aorta and its body branches*. Orlando, Fla: Grune and Stratton; 1979:521.

87. Veith FJ, Gupta SK, Samson RH, et al. Progress in limb salvage by reconstructive arterial surgery combined with new or improved adjunctive procedures. *Ann Surg.* 1981;194:386.

88. Lipsitz EC, Veith FJ. Fluoroscopically assisted thromboembolectomy: should it be routine? *Semin Vasc Surg.* 2001;14:100–106.

89. Ascher E, Veith FJ, Lesser ML, et al. Collateral back pressure–Is it a valid predictor of infrainguinal bypass graft patency? *J Surg Res.* 1985;38:453.

Distal Arteriovenous Fistulas in Prosthetic Distal Bypasses

Herbert Dardik **Theresa M. Impeduglia**

23

Restoration and maintenance of distal lower extremity perfusion for relief of critical ischemia is generally accomplished by inserting a new vascular conduit around the arterial obstruction. Over the past 5 decades, a number of advances have established various means of augmenting perfusion to an ischemic limb. A major challenge facing vascular surgeons today is to accomplish this goal despite severely compromised distal runoff, since continued graft patency is inversely related to outflow resistance. The combination of a high-resistance and a low-flow distal runoff circuit will result in predictable thrombosis of a bypass graft. This is particularly true of prosthetics that are employed for bypass because the critical thrombotic threshold for these materials is much lower than that for autologous vein. Factors contributing to increased resistance include both graft length and inadequate runoff vessels in the leg and pedal circulation. The results of crural vascular reconstruction are significantly inferior to those performed at more proximal levels. This has been attributed to a wide variety of factors, including kinking of the graft as it crosses the knee, technical considerations including graft material, and, more recently, to a variety of biochemical and physical imbalances, such as compliance mismatch and myointimal proliferation. However impressive the progress in peripheral vascular surgical techniques in providing pulsatile flow to the ischemic lower extremity, the limiting factor remains the capacity of the distal arterial circuit to accept adequate inflow to nourish the extremity.[1]

HISTORY

The adjunctive distal arteriovenous fistula (dAVF) is a unique means to ensure durable graft patency in the crural circulation. It is particularly important with the use of prosthetics in this site and in the face of a compromised runoff circulation. Although there has been a resurgence of interest in this approach, its historical basis dates back to the late 19th century (Table 23-1). In 1881, Francois-Franck[2] first anastomosed the femoral artery and vein in dogs. Lack of clinical utility for this procedure was reinforced by the first attempts to apply it to patients with extremity gangrene. In 1902, San Martín y Satrústegui performed arteriovenous reversal in one case and arteriovenous fistula in a second. Although the first case terminated in thigh amputation and death, the second case appears to have remained stable following forefoot amputation. By 1912, 58 arteriovenous fistulas had been performed in humans for limb salvage. Halstead and Vaughan[4] summarized this experience and concluded that the procedure lacked merit as a means of treating gangrene of the extremities. This view was strongly supported by Szylagi, et al.[5] in 1951 despite the interest generated by several favorable reports.[6,7] However, during this time, several important experimental observations were made. Zweifach[8] demonstrated molecular exchange in the microcirculation following reversed venous perfusion. Confirmation of tissue oxygenation via reversed

TABLE 23-1

LANDMARKS FOR LIMB SALVAGE ARTERIOVENOUS FISTULA

Year	Author(s)	History
1881	Francois-Franck[2]	Experimental femoral AVF No apparent value
1902	San Martín[3]	First clinical attempts for limb salvage
1912	Halstead and Vaughan[4]	Review of 58 AVFs Procedure condemned
1951	Szylagi[5]	Failure of nine of nine femoral AVFs Procedure ineffective
1965	Root and Cruz[11]	Experimental RVF
1966	Amir-Jahed[15]	Sympathectomy and RVF
1966	Blaisdell[13]	Closure of three of four popliteal AVFs Amputations: Two of four "Promising procedure"
1970	Kistner and Vermeulen[14]	Clinical efficacy
1979	Johansen and Bernstein[17]	Staged procedures to establish AVR

AVF, arteriovenous fistula; RVF, reversed venous flow; AVR, arteriovenous reversal.

or retrograde flow of arterial blood into the venous circulation then followed.[9-12] In 1966, Blaisdell et al.[13] renewed interest in the clinical application of arteriovenous fistula as an adjunct to bypass procedures where runoff was severely compromised. In fact, they suggested that "this technique may permit reconstruction of almost any peripheral artery." Despite this optimism and the experience reported by Kistner and Vermeulen in 1970,[14] the only major advances in this field were in the laboratory. Amir-Jahed[15] reconfirmed the feasibility of reversing venous flow, even

in the presence of intact venous valves, provided sympathectomy had been performed. Matolo et al.[16] showed that the creation of a popliteal arteriovenous fistula in the ischemic limb of a turkey could reverse the ischemia by retrograde venous perfusion and the development of collateral flow. Johansen and Bernstein[17] demonstrated in the canine model that by staging a side-to-side arteriovenous fistula prior to ligation of the central venous limb, they could achieve arteriovenous reversal and salvage in otherwise irreversibly ischemic limbs.

The modern era for creating distal fistulas may well have begun on November 7, 1979, when the senior author decided to use a concomitant vein for decompression in a patient sustaining multiple intraoperative thromboses in a peroneal bypass graft. Appreciation at that time of there being a high runoff resistance prompted the creation of a decompressing fistula between the graft and the adjacent peroneal vein. That fistula was constructed end-to-side, cephalad segment of vein to the umbilical graft, thereby permitting steady flow in the graft, flow in the fistula as well as distally into the runoff circulation. Graft patency with limb salvage in this first case was maintained until the patient's death from a stroke 4 years later (Fig. 23-1). This model is the one proposed by Jacobs et al.,[18] who advocated ligation of the cephalad segment of the fistula with the hope that perfusion through the caudad segment would result not only in increased microcirculatory flow, but also improved graft patency and limb salvage rates. Subsequent experience has confirmed the need to maintain the cephalad component of the dAVF in order to achieve maximal benefit.

Our early experience with 13 patients was reported in 1979.[19] This was subsequently corroborated by the report of Sauvage et al.,[20] Hinshaw et al.,[21] and Harris et al.[22] One of the requirements for securing success of the

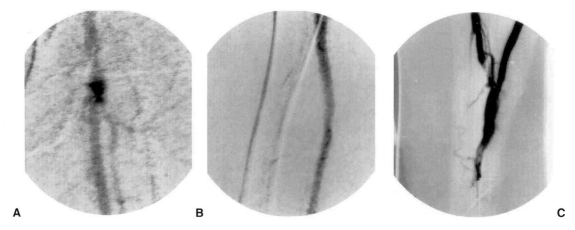

Figure 23-1 Angiogram at 3.5 years of first distal arteriovenous fistula (dAVF) (1979) with a femoral peroneal bypass using an umbilical vein graft. **A:** Proximal anastomosis. **B:** Subcutaneous midportion of graft. **C:** Distal anastomosis with peroneal artery runoff and significant flow into the venous component of the fistula.

dAVF is that its use be restricted to bypasses in the crural circulation, generally the middle and lower third levels. The experience of previous investigators was limited to femoral and popliteal sites, which are clearly not conducive to a successful outcome, particularly when the resistance is high in the distal leg and foot.

PHYSIOLOGIC CONSIDERATIONS

The success of lower extremity vascular bypasses, and particularly crural reconstructions, depends on many factors including size and quality of the arteries; integrity of the runoff, including the pedal arch; and the nature of the graft material employed. Operative technique is critical as well as a thorough assessment of the adequacy of the arterial inflow, which may be deceptive on routine biplane angiography. Assuming an adequate inflow, durable patency of crural bypass becomes less likely with an increasing peripheral resistance, an absent or deficient pedal arch, and decreasing arterial caliber and quality.[23–25] Although these features can be assessed by preoperative arteriography and sonography, direct operative inspection, including the tactile response to fluid injected directly into distal artery, is much simpler. Precise measurement of vascular resistance $(R = P/Q)$ is difficult. Pressure-to-flow ratios can be calculated to suggest a level of resistance for an individual case, but are often imprecise. We previously deployed a method to measure resistance by observing the pressure responses to controlled rates of fluid infusion. This was performed intraoperatively using a manometer and a variable flow rate pump.[26] Computer-derived curves can be calculated and recorded as slope measurements that suggest alternative modes of therapy (Fig. 23-2). Increasing slopes indicate higher resistances. On this basis, a planned bypass might be either abandoned or complemented by adjunctive procedures such as remote angioplasty, sequential bypass, or arteriovenous fistula. Vein bypasses

may tolerate higher runoff resistance than prosthetic grafts, but they too must ultimately face the problem of sustained high peripheral resistance and subsequent graft closure.

Theoretically, an adjunctive dAVF might be necessary whenever the velocity of blood flow in a distal bypass graft is critically limited by high peripheral resistance due to extensive atherosclerosis obliterans. Normally, blood velocity decreases from the central circulation to the periphery (Fig. 23-3). This occurs because of the increase in total cross-sectional area of the distal vascular bed in the face of a constant cardiac output. For example, peak aortic blood flow velocity is approximately 100 cm per second, while major limb arterial velocity is 50 cm per second.[27] Similarly, volume flow decreases from approximately 150 mL per minute in the superficial femoral artery to 100 mL per minute in the popliteal artery and 10 mL per minute in each of the tibial arteries. If a long femoral-to–distal crural artery bypass is constructed, a potentially unphysiologic situation is created. When outflow resistance is high, as might occur in patients with an inadequate pedal arch or severely diseased distal crural artery, the volume of blood flow that can be accommodated by these limited runoff vessels is small, but nonetheless often sufficient to lead to a remarkable amelioration of distal ischemia. The resulting velocity of flow in a large-diameter, unbranched vascular bypass may be quite low. If this fails to exceed the critical thrombotic threshold velocity specific to that conduit, a cascade of events that generally culminates in graft thromboses ensues. If the resistance of the runoff is fixed, increasing blood flow velocity in the graft involves creation of a low-resistance runoff bed. This can be accomplished by a second sequential anastomosis, if possible, or by fashioning a dAVF.

Studies have shown increased volumetric and velocity flow in umbilical vein (UV) grafts in the crural position with adjunctive dAVFs, attributed to the low resistance and high capacitance of the venous system (Figs. 23-4

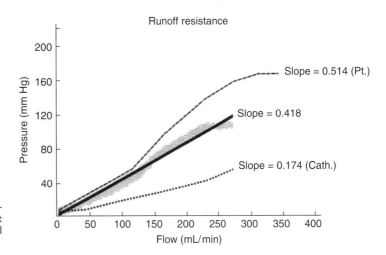

Figure 23-2 Computer-derived resistance curves. A rising slope indicates increased resistance suggesting that bypass procedures, without some adjunct, such as distal arteriovenous fistula (dAVF), will fail.

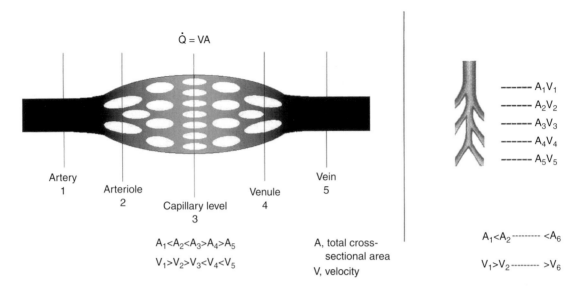

$\dot{Q} = VA$

Artery 1
Arteriole 2
Capillary level 3
Venule 4
Vein 5

$A_1 < A_2 < A_3 > A_4 > A_5$

$V_1 > V_2 > V_3 < V_4 < V_5$

A, total cross-sectional area

V, velocity

$------ A_1V_1$
$------ A_2V_2$
$------ A_3V_3$
$------ A_4V_4$
$------ A_5V_5$

$A_1 < A_2 -------- < A_6$

$V_1 > V_2 -------- > V_6$

Figure 23-3 Velocity decreases from the central circulation to the periphery. With a constant flow (Q), velocity flow (V) is inversely related to total cross-sectional area (A). The largest cross-sectional area of the circulatory system is at the capillary level (A3, **left panel**). This corresponds to the slowest velocity (V3). The **right panel** is a schema for the limb circulation, again emphasizing the increased total cross-section area of the arterial system as one proceeds distally (A5), with corresponding decreased velocity flow (V5). These relationships, in addition to the hemodynamic phenomena described in Figures 14-4 and 14-5, dictate the need for a modulating system such as the distal arteriovenous fistula (dAVF).

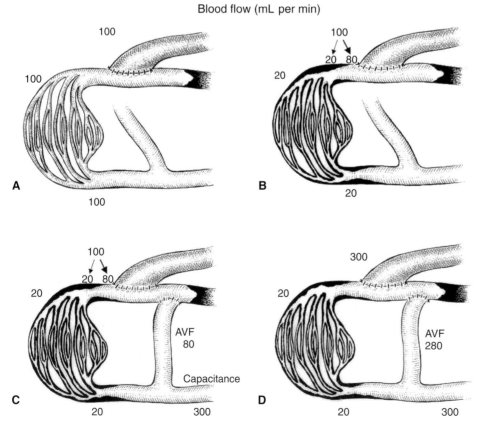

Blood flow (mL per min)

Figure 23-4 Hemodynamics of distal arteriovenous fistula (dAVF). **A:** Theoretical flow (100 mL per minute) in bypass and runoff with excellent runoff. **B:** With increased resistance, only 20 mL per minute can flow through, resulting in graft stasis and thrombosis. **C:** Diversion of 80 mL per minute through an arteriovenous bridge should result in continued graft patency and distal flow. **D:** In reality, flow increasing graft and venous return via the fistula; flow also continues distally into arterial circuit albeit at a lower but definitely increased quantity compared to preoperative baseline values.

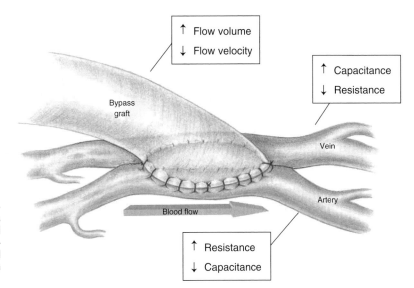

Figure 23-5 Illustration of the basic hemodynamics of a bypass to a common ostium arteriovenous fistula. The increased resistance and decreased capacitance of the arterial component is compensated by the increased capacitance and decreased resistance of the venous system. This results in increased volume velocity flow in the graft.

and 23-5).[28] Although the flow into the distal arteries constitutes only a small part of the total graft flow, remarkably, it is capable of reversing even advanced ischemia. The role of reversed flow in the distal veins communicating with the dAVF is uncertain. Valvular competency prevents early reversal but continued venous hypertension will result in valvular incompetence and flow reversal. Certain patients demonstrate variable hemodynamic responses during the early weeks of dAVF function, which we presume to represent variations in flow through the fistula and distal veins. Eventual flow stabilization is the rule.

Concern regarding "stealing" of blood from the foot does not appear justified. Unlike the hemodynamics of reversed flow and steal that can be demonstrated with

experimental models and in patients with arteriovenous fistulas for access or congenital or traumatic fistulas, the adjunctive dAVF is only established in patients with extensive and diffuse atherosclerosis obliterans. With a gradient between the proximal inflow and the distal runoff that is high, coupled with no alternative pressurized inflow, reversal of flow in the distal circulation cannot occur (Fig. 23-6). On the other hand, and often confused with steal, maldistribution of flow can occur as a function of the conduit material or concomitant vein diameter. Use of an incompliant conduit, such as polytetrafluoroethylene (PTFE), results in a fixed quantity of blood that can be delivered per unit time. In the face time of high peripheral arterial resistance, most of the blood will enter the high-capacitance, low-resistance

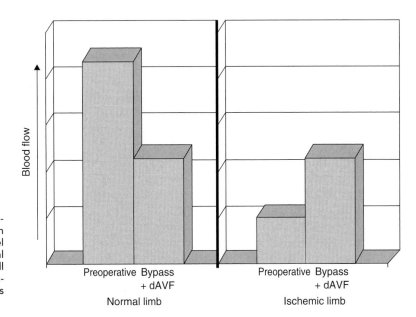

Figure 23-6 Steal occurs if a distal fistula is constructed in a normal flow situation **(left panel)**. When critical ischemia exists, the starting blood flow level is low and flow established with bypass plus distal arteriovenous fistula (dAVF), though minimal, is still an increase over baseline **(right panel)**. Note comparable final levels for both left and right panels of this illustration.

venous circulation of the fistula, creating what would appear to be a steal, but correctable by increasing the resistance in the venous circuit with a stenosing ligature, forcing more blood into the distal circuit. By using a more compliant conduit such as the UV graft, higher volumes of blood can be delivered to the periphery that will supply the requisite quantity for both outflow areas, namely the low-resistant venous circulation and the high-resistant arterial bed. Ascher et al.,[29] a leading proponent for the use of dAVF, has demonstrated the value of increasing the resistance in the venous circuit to effect better distal perfusion when deploying a PTFE graft. Our data with the UV graft has shown a remarkable augmentation of volume flow to match the requirements for both runoff areas—the venous bed of the fistula and the runoff arterial and nutritional circulatory bed.

Experimental support for the deployment of dAVF in crural revascularization has recently been provided by Qin et al.[30] Using the rat model, arteriovenous fistulas were established at the femoral level and flow dynamics assessed both acutely and longitudinally. Histopathologic analysis confirmed decreased myointimal hyperplasia, which was felt to be secondary to the decreased shear stress associated with the creation of an arteriovenous fistula. Additional studies by these authors also implicated the overexpression of von Willebrand factor in relation to the myointimal response associated with experimental fistula.[31]

TECHNIQUE

Most arteriovenous fistulas are constructed by a side-to-side technique employing 7-0 polypropylene suture. This procedure is enormously facilitated by using a tourniquet, which permits minimal dissection and obviates need for control of branches of the artery and particularly the vein.[32] The anterior surfaces of the artery and vein are dissected and cleared of all tissue for a distance of 3 cm. This portion of the dissection is performed in standard manner using the medial and anterolateral approaches for the posterior and anterior tibial arteries, respectively, and the lateral approach with fibulectomy for the peroneal artery.[33] The vein is marked with methylene blue at this time to facilitate subsequent identification when it is often collapsed following application of the tourniquet. Topical papaverine is also helpful in the early dissection phase when spasm of noncalcified crural vessels is common.

Once vascular control has been secured with the tourniquet, parallel arteriotomy and venotomy incisions (2.5 cm) are established and the opposing walls sutured to create a common ostium. The bypass graft is then sutured directly onto this common ostium (Fig. 23-7). A single running 7.0 polypropylene suture is used to

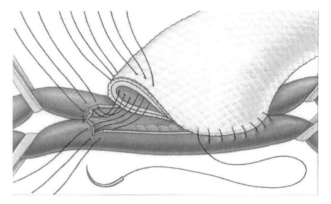

Figure 23-7 Common ostium is established with 7-0 polypropylene suture. The graft is then sutured end-to-side to the ostium using interrupted suture in each proximal and distal quadrant. Continuous suture techniques complete the anastomosis along the lateral margins.

create the fistula but is not tied until each end is tied to one of the mid-interrupted sutures placed at the heel and toe. We place three interrupted sutures in each quadrant of the heel and toe for a total of 12. All these sutures are then tied in place, and the one closest to the fistula suture at either end is also tied. These maneuvers are facilitated by having one individual hold the graft in place to allow accurate placement of all sutures and to provide counter pressure to the operator tying the sutures in place. Our sequence is usually to deploy the first six sutures (V1,2,3; A1,2,3) at the heel and then run the V3 and A3 sutures toward the midpoint. The process is reversed at the toe and the anastomosis completed with running sutures on either side of the fistula. The most common variation of this technique has been developed by Ascher et al.[29] in which the proximal end of the divided concomitant vein is sutured directly end-to-side to the runoff artery, and the bypass graft then piggybacked end-to-side to this vein. Other variations include placement of the fistula proximal or distal to the distal anastomosis, and use of a segment of the saphenous vein. Loupe magnification ($\times2$ to $\times3$) is essential. Completion sonography is routine, as well as arteriography in most instances, the exception being patients with azotemia and a clearly satisfactory sonogram. With completion of the distal anastomosis, the tourniquet is released and back bleeding permitted into the graft. Retrograde tunneling is the next step in preparation for performing the proximal anastomosis. Integrity of the anastomosis is assessed with sequential release of all occluding clamps. On occasion, bleeding points are noted and controlled with pressure or placement of additional sutures. This is particularly true if the artery is densely calcified or if inadequate suture bites were taken through the venous component of the fistula. Favorable prognostic signs are palpation of a

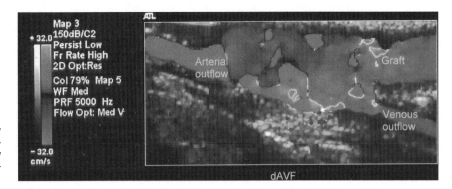

Figure 23-8 Completion duplex study illustrates distal anastomosis, runoff via peroneal artery (no steal), and cephalad flow into the vein component of distal arteriovenous fistula (dAVF).

thrill overlying the fistula, increased diastolic flow by duplex sonography, and suffusion of contrast into the venous circuit as well as the runoff artery on arteriography (Figs. 23-8 and 23-9).

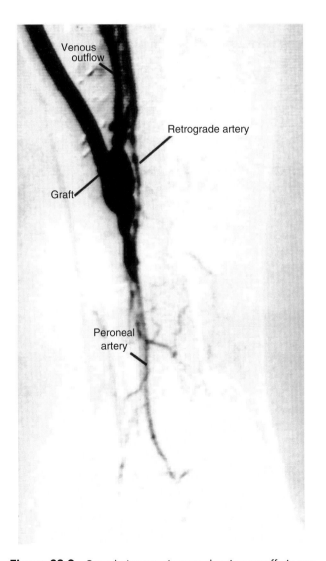

Figure 23-9 Completion arteriogram showing runoff via peroneal artery and retrograde suffusion of contrast into venous system—a favorable observation for predicting a successful outcome when employing a distal arteriovenous fistula (dAVF).

CLINICAL EXPERIENCE

Since 1979, the senior author and his associates have performed >400 dAVFs as adjuncts to distal crural bypasses. The first 61 cases, reported in 1983, helped define the indications for this procedure and improve patient selection. General indications for use of the dAVF include the following: a) Revascularization is for critical limb ischemia; b) standard revascularization techniques with autologous vein are not possible or appropriate; c) a potentially useful limb can be salvaged with successful bypass; and d) the dAVF can be performed in the mid or lower third of the leg.

In our earlier experience, we required that the pedal arch be deficient or absent. With our increasing experience we now deploy a dAVF in *all* of our prosthetic (UV) reconstructions to the crural arteries. From a technical perspective, the only contraindication to performing a dAVF includes a virtual absence of some arterial vasculature in the foot, inadequacy of the venous system (small size, sclerosis, thromboses), and extensive gangrene or infection with major tissue loss that would preclude limb salvage even with a successful revascularization procedure. Primary amputation should be considered in these circumstances.

There has been no significant morbidity directly attributable to the use of the dAVF. Cardiac output measurements performed after construction of the fistula were unchanged from preoperative baseline determinations. Postoperative leg and foot edema did occur but was not unlike that which occurs after any standard bypass for advanced ischemia. Patient concern regarding the swelling is easily allayed by simple explanation of the temporal and benign nature of this condition. Failure of a bypass with dAVF does not raise the level of amputation.[28,34]

Early failure of dAVF reconstruction is related to operative technique, total inadequacy of the arterial runoff, or venous disease. Many of our early failures were caused by using veins that were small (<2 mm), sclerotic, or occluded at a more proximal level. The decreased compliance and capacitance of such systems precludes an adequate runoff for the graft as evidenced by the lack of a thrill overlying the fistula at the conclusion of the operation, an ominous sign that is predictive of failure. The presence of some demonstrable flow into the distal arterial bed is essential if a successful clinical outcome is to be expected. Reliance on the dAVF alone in the hope of early distal tissue perfusion by retrograde flow via the caudad venous component of the dAVF will result in failure. The development of such flow depends on venous valvular incompetence and is time dependent.[17] Attempts to make the valves incompetent at surgery are usually ineffective and potentially dangerous in these small and fragile veins. If no distal arterial flow is present, then efforts to construct a dAVF should be abandoned.

Late failure of dAVF reconstruction is generally caused by myointimal hyperplasia or by progression of distal arterial disease. Avoiding small or diseased veins may decrease the incidence of these phenomena, but the ultimate solution lies in the ability to suppress or prevent myointimal hyperplasia pharmacologically or by genetic manipulation.

Documentation of efficacy of dAVF has been provided.[35-37] The most recent data confirmed improved patency rates and impressive decreased perioperative thrombotic events for crural reconstructions when composed to historic controls. Comparative cumulative graft patency rates for the 1975 to 1985 and 1990 to 2000 decades are depicted in Figure 23-10.

CONCLUSION

The goal of achieving durable graft patency and limb salvage with prosthetic reconstructions of the crural vessels is a challenge for all vascular surgeons, as is the maintenance of distal lower extremity perfusion with restricted runoff. This goal can be achieved in selected cases with judicious application of the dAVF. The actual

numbers of patients requiring dAVF have decreased over the past few years in direct relationship to the recognition of autologous vein as the conduit of choice for crural bypass. Furthermore, the renaissance of the *in situ* method has expanded the ability to use autologous vein where prosthetics might have otherwise been required as a desperate measure to secure limb salvage. Nevertheless, a patient population does exist where a prosthetic and dAVF should be considered but, in the absence of specific criteria and indications, recognizing that primary amputation might, in fact, be the wisest course of action.

On the basis of our laboratory clinical experience, we have concluded that:

1. dAVF has a definite role as an adjunct to lower limb distal revascularization procedures, particularly if the required graft material is a prosthetic. Its role with autologous vein conduits is limited to instances of poor runoff.
2. Indications for the procedures should be limited to patients who suffer critical ischemia and might require major amputation if no reconstruction were to be performed.
3. Additional criteria for case selection should be based on objective data, including preoperative and intraoperative arteriography, sonographic data, and intraoperative observations of vessel size, quality, runoff, and resistance.
4. dAVF construction should be limited to the middle or distal third of the leg.
5. Arterial runoff must be present, even if limited.
6. Adequate venous system based on caliber (>2 mm) and quality (no sclerosis or obstruction) is essential.
7. The use of a tourniquet is *imperative*. Dissection time is decreased, clamp trauma is avoided, and the procedure is enormously facilitated.
8. dAVF construction should be performed with loupe magnification.

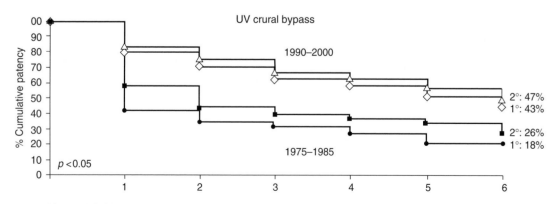

Figure 23-10 Comparative cumulative graft patency rates for crural reconstruction performed during the 1975 to 1985 and 1990 to 2000 decades. The difference between the curves, which is statistically significant, is associated with the use of distal arteriovenous fistula (dAVF) during the latter decade.

9. A palpable thrill should be present intraoperatively overlying the dAVF to be adequate technical construction and to suggest a favorable prognosis with regard to early graft patency. Completion duplex sonography should be routine. Completion angiography might also be considered in most cases in the absence of decreased renal function.

10. There is a need for continued laboratory experimentation to simulate the clinical setting in which dAVF has already been demonstrated to be advantageous.

The theoretical basis for using dAVFs as adjuncts to crucial reconstructions is based on the need to keep graft flow over the critical thrombotic threshold level. This results in increased velocity and volume flow with most being directed into the high-capacitance, low-resistance venous circulation. The amount of blood that can be accepted by the arterial runoff, albeit limited, will perfuse distally and reverse the ischemic state. Minimal increments of blood are required to affect this change. There are differences in the hemodynamics of the dAVF and the alternative adjuncts that include cuffs, boots, patches, and flow-through flaps. Further effort is essential to define these processes and thereby enable precise clinical deployment. What is clear is that a severely compromised runoff requires something more than routine bypass. Rather, a method that will alter the hemodynamics and biologic response to the graft. This challenge can be met in part by creating an arteriovenous fistula at the distal anastomosis to divert the circulatory overload normally delivered to the highly resistant arterial runoff into the high-capacitance, low-resistance venous circulation. Though not universally understood or accepted, the concept of the dAVF is basically simple but requires serious attention and evaluation under controlled circumstances. Based on personal experience with >400 such procedures, we have become convinced of the importance of adding a distal fistula to crural reconstruction when prosthetic material is employed or when runoff is compromised if autologous vein is being deployed as the conduit.

REFERENCES

1. Dardik H. The threatened limb. *Science & Medicine*. 1997;4:44–53.
2. Francois-Franck: Note a propos de la communication de raymond petit sur la suture arterio-veineuse. *Compt Rend Soc Biol*. 1896;10:150.
3. San Martín y Satrústegui AF. Anastomose. *Deutsche Ztschr Chir*. 1912;119:515.
4. Halstead AE, Vaughan RT. Arteriovenous anastomosis in the treatment of gangrene of the extremities. *Surg Gynecol Obstet*. 1912;14:1.
5. Szylagi DE, Jay GD, Munnel ED. Femoral arteriovenous anastomosis in the treatment of occlusive arterial disease. *Arch. Surg*. 1951;68:435.
6. Bernheim BM. Arteriovenous anastomosis. *JAMA*. 1931;96:1296.
7. Johnson CG, Jordan P Jr., Cloud T. Arteriovenous anastomosis in traumatic vascular lesions. *Am J Surg*. 1950;80:809.
8. Zweifach BW. The structural basis of permeability and other functions of blood capillaries. *Cold Spr Harb Symp Quant Biol*. 1940; 18:216.
9. Heimbecker T, Thomas V, Blalock A. Experimental reversal of capillary blood flow. *Circulation*. 1951;4:116.
10. Ingebrigtsen R, Krog J, Kerand S. Circulation distal to experimental arterio-venous fistulas of the extremities. *Acta Chir Scand*. 1963;125:308.
11. Root HD, Cruz AB Jr. Effects of an arteriovenous fistula on the devascularized limb. *JAMA*. 1965;191:109.
12. Vetto RM, Belzer FO. Use of an arterio-bone fistula in advanced ischemia. *Surg Forum*. 1965;16:131.
13. Blaisdell FW, Lim RC Jr, Hall AD, et al. Revascularization of severely ischemic extremities with an arteriovenous fistula. *Am J Surg*. 1966;112:166.
14. Kistner RL, Vermeulen WJ. Therapeutic arteriovenous fistula in management of severe ischemia of the extremities. *Surg Clin N Am*. 1970;50:291.
15. Amir-Jahed AK. Revascularization of lower extremities by reversal of blood flow with and without lumbar sympathectomy: an experimental study. *Surgery*. 1966;59:243.
16. Matolo NM, Cohen SE, Wolfman EF Jr. Use of an arteriovenous fistula for treatment of the severely ischemic extremity. *Ann Surg*. 1976;184:622.
17. Johansen K, Bernstein EF. Revascularization of the ischemic canine hind limb by arteriovenous reversal. *Ann Surg*. 1979;190:243.
18. Jacobs MJHM, Reul GJ, Gregoric ID, et al. Creation of a distal arteriovenous fistula improves microcirculatory hemodynamics of prosthetic graft bypass in secondary limb salvage procedures. *J Vasc Surg*. 1993;18:1–9.
19. Ibrahim IM, Sussman D, Dardik I, et al. Adjunctive arteriovenous fistula with tibial and peroneal reconstruction for limb salvage. *Am J Surg*. 1980;140:246.
20. Sauvage L, Berger K, Davis C, et al. Composite biosynthetic prosthesis of fibrin and filamentous knitted Dacron for abdominal and lower extremity arterial surgery. In: Stanley J, Burke W, Lindenauer SM, et al., eds. *Biologic and prosthetic grafts*. New York, NY: Grune and Stratton; 1982:553.
21. Hinshaw DB, Schmidt CA, Hinshaw DB, et al. Arteriovenous fistula in arterial reconstruction of the ischemic limb. *Arch Surg*. 1983;118:589.
22. Harris PL, Campbell H. Adjuvant distal arteriovenous shunt with femorotibial bypass for criteria ischaemia. *Br J Surg*. 1983;70:377.
23. Dardik H, Ibrahim IM, Koslow A, et al. Evaluation of intraoperative arteriography as a routine for vascular reconstructions. *Surg Gynecol Obstet*. 1978;147:853.
24. Dardik H, Ibrahim IM, Sussman B, et al. Morphologic structure of the pedal arch and its relationship to patency of crural vascular reconstruction. *Surg Gynecol Obstet*. 1981;152:645.
25. O'Mara CS, Flinn WR, Neiman HL. Correlation of foot arterial anatomy with early tibial bypass patency. *Surgery*. 1981;89:743.
26. Svoboda JJ, Dardik H. *A method of quantitating peripheral arterial runoff for vascular surgery by measurement of regional vascular resistance with saline perfusion*. Data on file.
27. McGrath MA. Dynamics of the peripheral circulation. *Int Angiol*. 1984;3:3–15.
28. Dardik H, Sussman B, Ibrahim IM. Distal arteriovenous fistula as an adjunct to maintaining arterial and graft patency for limb salvage. *Surgery*. 1983;94:478.
29. Ascher E, Gennaro M, Pollina RM, et al. Complimentary distal arteriovenous fistula and deep vein interposition: a five year experience with a new technique to improve infrapopliteal prosthetic bypass patency. *J Vasc Surg*. 1996;24:134–143.
30. Qin F, Dardik H, Pangilinan A, et al. Remodeling and suppression of intimal hyperplasia of vascular grafts in a rat model. *J Vasc Surg*. 2001;34:701–706.

31. Qin F, Impeduglia T, Schaffer P, et al. Overexpression of von Willebrand factor is an independent risk factor for pathogenesis of intimal hyperplasia. Preliminary studies. *J Vasc Surg.* 2003;37: 433–439.

32. Ciervo A, Dardik H, Qin F, et al. The tourniquet revisited as an adjunct to lower limb revascularization. *J Vasc Surg.* 2000;31: 436–442.

33. Dardik H, Dardik I, Veith FJ. Exposure of the tibial peroneal arteries by a single lateral approach. *Surgery.* 1974;75:377–382.

34. Dardik H, Kahn M, Dardik I, et al. Influence of failed vascular bypass procedures on conversion of below knee to above knee amputation levels. *Surgery.* 1982;91:64.

35. Dardik H, Pecoraro J, Ibrahim IM, et al. Infrapopliteal prosthetic graft patency by use of the distal adjunctive arteriovenous fistula. *J Vasc Surg.* 1991;13:685–691.

36. Dardik H, Silvestri F, Alasio T, et al. Improved method to create the common ostium variant of the distal arteriovenous fistula for enhancing crural prosthetic graft patency. *J Vasc Surg.* 1996;23: 240–248.

37. Dardik H, Wengerter K, Qin F, et al. Comparative decades of experience with glutaraldehyde-tanned human umbilical cord vein graft for lower limb revascularization: An analysis of 1,275 cases. *J Vasc Surg.* 2002;35:64–71.

24

Vein Cuffs, Patches, and Boots in Prosthetic Distal Bypasses

Richard F. Neville

There is little question that autologous saphenous vein is the ideal conduit for lower extremity revascularization, especially to a tibial artery. Excellent patency and limb salvage rates have been reported for tibial artery bypass when saphenous vein is used as the bypass conduit. The use of autogenous vein as the conduit can result in a durable reconstruction no matter which configuration is favored by the surgeon: *In situ*, reversed, or translocated. However, the lack of an adequate saphenous vein can present a major challenge in the care of those patients in need of tibial revascularization for limb salvage. An increasing number of patients in need of tibial bypass do not have adequate saphenous vein due to previous procedures, thrombophlebitis, or inadequate vein. Alternative conduits have been proposed including lesser saphenous vein, arm vein, composite veins, composite vein with polytetrafluoroethylene (PTFE), and PTFE with or without a distal arteriovenous fistula (dAVF). Unfortunately, these alternative conduits have not resulted in equivalent results when used for distal bypass to tibial arteries.[1–4] Because of these poor results, consideration is given to primary amputation with no attempt at limb salvage in certain patient subgroups without a vein.[5] Conversely, several authors have reported on the use of venous tissue at the distal anastomosis in the form of cuffs, collars, and boots to improve the results of prosthetic grafts in this challenging patient population.[6–8] These techniques have been proposed as an option for revascularization in patients without adequate saphenous vein in an attempt to obtain limb salvage. This chapter will examine some of those techniques and their results, as well as corresponding advantages and disadvantages.

BACKGROUND

Increased longevity and the aging of the population have led to an increase in the number of patients in need of lower extremity revascularization. Additionally, improved surgical and anesthetic techniques have led to an increasingly aggressive approach to limb salvage that can be offered to older and sicker patients. Therefore, lower extremity revascularization is being offered to a growing number of patients. Because of its utility in peripheral and coronary arterial beds, the saphenous vein has become a valuable commodity that is often in short supply. It has been reported that in those patients needing primary revascularization of the lower extremity, as many as 30% lack suitable autogenous vein. This number increases to 50% in those patients requiring a secondary bypass procedure.[9] The use of duplex ultrasound has been increasingly implemented in these situations in order to locate acceptable vein that may not be readily apparent. However, there remains a significant number of patients in whom vein cannot be found. The most common reasons for this lack of vein include previous vein harvest for coronary revascularization or another peripheral bypass, excision of varicose veins, or vein that is unsuitable due to small size or postphlebitic changes.

ALTERNATIVE CONDUITS

Arm vein and lesser saphenous vein are alternative autogenous conduits when greater saphenous vein is not available. Holzenbien et al. of the Deaconess group[4] has championed the use of arm vein by demonstrating that there is an improved patency rate for arm vein bypasses as compared to PTFE alone. However, Calligaro et al.[3] demonstrated that arm vein may be only slightly better than PTFE for bypass to infrapopliteal arteries, and lesser saphenous vein may not function any better than PTFE material alone. Our experience with arm vein and lesser saphenous vein has been limited by the problem of sufficient conduit length. Arm veins and lesser saphenous segments may not be long enough to reach a distal tibial artery, especially when the proximal anastomosis must begin from the external iliac artery to avoid the presence of a heavily scarred groin from previous bypass attempts. Arm vein is also problematic in the diabetic patient with renal failure and a history of upper extremity arteriovenous fistulas for hemodialysis access. However, arm vein and lesser saphenous segments remain particularly good choices for autogenous reconstructions for younger patients in whom the vein is long enough to reach the appropriate recipient artery.

Cryopreserved vein and human umbilical vein are alternative conduits that are biologic in their properties and therefore have an intrinsic appeal for distal reconstruction. However, these grafts have been met with limited success when used for tibial bypass.[10] Farber et al.[11] reported a 30% patency rate, at 12 months, for cryopreserved veins used in infrapopliteal bypass procedures, with the presence of diabetes having a particularly adverse impact on graft patency in this study. Anticoagulation with warfarin sodium and aspirin did not improve durability of the cryopreserved vein graft function. The best use of cryopreserved vein may be limited to bypasses that must traverse infected fields in the absence of any autogenous conduit. The use of human umbilical vein grafts was impeded by aneurismal degeneration of the graft material. This complication has been addressed in recent modifications of the graft design. Dardik et al.[12] have reported experience using human umbilical vein grafts adding a concomitant anastomotic arteriovenous fistula. This alternative configuration resulted in 61% patency at 36 months, and may represent a nonprosthetic alternative in the absence of autogenous saphenous vein.

The alternative graft with the most inherent appeal is a prosthetic graft that could be readily available and easy to use. PTFE grafts have certain advantages in terms of ease of use and familiarity for most vascular surgeons.

This represents a significant difference as compared to the human umbilical vein graft. Unfortunately, PTFE used directly to a tibial artery has not led to consistently durable results. Some have argued that the results are so poor that primary amputation is a better choice than the effort and expense of putting a patient through a bypass using a PTFE graft to a tibial artery. Parsons et al.[13] reported poor primary patency rates for PTFE alone to infrapopliteal arteries. However, acceptable secondary patency and limb salvage rates supported their recommendation that a PTFE bypass should be attempted prior to primary amputation.

POLYTETRAFLUOROETHYLENE FOR TIBIAL ARTERY BYPASS GRAFTS

The use of PTFE as a lower extremity bypass conduit was originally reported by Campbell et al.[14] in 1976. This preliminary report described 15 patients undergoing lower extremity revascularization with PTFE grafts. Nine of the 15 bypass procedures were to infrapopliteal arteries. The authors reported 87% graft patency between 1 and 8 months, with a 75% patency rate at 28 months. Since that time, PTFE grafts have been used with greater frequency in the lower extremity, but primarily in the above-knee popliteal artery position. Several clinical series have questioned the use of PTFE for tibial bypass due to disappointing results.[1,15,16] Hobson et al.[15] reported on 547 lower extremity bypass procedures including 375 revascularizations performed over 5 years. Of the revascularization procedures, 91 were tibial bypasses, with saphenous vein used in 54% and PTFE in 46%. Limb salvage rates at 2 and 5 years were 53% and 47%, respectively, for tibial bypass with vein, versus 20% and 15% for tibial bypasses with PTFE. An additional observation of note in this series concerned perioperative mortality rates, with a 3% mortality rate in those patients undergoing revascularization compared to 13% for those patients undergoing primary amputation. This experience demonstrated that revascularization is preferable to primary amputation when feasible. However, one could also argue, based on this experience, that those patients requiring distal vascular reconstruction without the presence of adequate saphenous vein should be considered for primary amputation due to the poor long-term results of PTFE alone. Other clinical work lends support to this conclusion. As previously cited, clinical series involving PTFE bypasses to tibial arteries report 1-year patency rates between 20% and 50%, with 3-year patency rates between 12% and 37% for infrapopliteal bypasses using PTFE.

In an attempt to address this issue, a prospective, multicenter, randomized trial was conducted comparing autologous saphenous vein and PTFE for infrainguinal arterial revascularization.[2] A total of 845 patients were enrolled, with 485 undergoing popliteal bypasses and 360 undergoing tibial bypasses. Patients who had adequate ipsilateral saphenous vein were randomized to vein bypass or PTFE bypass for the vascular reconstruction. Patency differences became apparent within 1 month of operation and the difference increased progressively thereafter. At the 4-year interval, primary patency for vein bypasses was 49% as compared to a 12% patency rate for those randomized to PTFE. However, the difference in limb salvage rates at 3.5 years did not reach statistical significance (57% for saphenous vein and 61% for PTFE). The lack of a significant difference in limb salvage was due to the fact that PTFE graft failure was not always associated with limb loss due to ischemia. Additionally, secondary bypass procedures with vein were often performed after primary graft failure resulting in limb salvage. This well-recognized study supported previous suspicions of the inferior results for PTFE bypass grafts to tibial arteries, but seemed to argue against the issue of primary amputation in the population of patients without adequate autogenous conduit.

VEIN CUFFS, PATCHES, AND BOOTS

Several different configurations have been described in an attempt to improve PTFE bypass results by the interposition of venous tissue between the prosthetic graft and the recipient tibial artery. Each configuration has certain advantages and disadvantages, both real and potential. In 1979, Siegman[17] proposed using a vein cuff to ease the technical challenges of a difficult anastomosis to heavily calcified small arteries. However, he did not hypothesize any possible effects on intimal hyperplasia or graft patency. Subsequently, Miller et al.[6] proposed a variant of a vein cuff to overcome the technical difficulties of the anastomosis between a PTFE graft and a small artery, but also to attempt to improve graft patency by influencing the different elastic properties of the prosthetic graft and the target artery. The Miller vein cuff involved the longitudinal opening of a small piece of

vein and a running suture to secure the edge of the vein to the arteriotomy. The two cut ends of the vein were then sutured together in order to construct an oval venous cuff. The prosthetic graft was then sutured directly to the oval vein cuff (Fig. 24-1). Miller et al.[6] reported on 114 infrainguinal procedures using this cuff technique. The patient cohort included only 21 tibial artery bypass grafts. A patency rate of 72% was noted at 18 months. Since that initial report, other authors have reported on their experience with the Miller cuff configuration. Kansal et al.[18] obtained improved patency rates for prosthetic bypasses to popliteal and tibial arteries as compared to historical controls without the addition of a vein cuff.

However, several potential disadvantages have been recognized in association with the Miller vein cuff technique. Significant turbulence has been noted due to the deep anastomotic reservoir and the difficulty of achieving a narrow angle between the graft and recipient artery. This results in increased turbulence and shear stress at the distal anastomosis. These hemodynamic factors may help to explain the immediate and early graft failures reported in Miller's initial series.[1] Additionally, the oval formation of the Miller cuff is difficult to maintain in tight anatomic spaces such as those involved in very distal bypasses to the dorsalis pedis artery of the forefoot and the plantaris pedis branches of the posterior tibial artery.

Taylor et al.[8] have described a vein patch technique at the distal anastomosis in an effort to address several of these concerns. This experience began with a group of patients presenting for thrombectomy after graft failure. Taylor's technique required a long arteriotomy (3 to 4 cm) so that the patch could be constructed at least four to five times longer than the diameter of the PTFE conduit. A U-shaped slit approximately 1 cm in length was made on the underside of the graft with minimal angulation to ensure that the PTFE lay almost parallel to the artery. The heel of the graft was then sutured directly to the proximal portion of the arteriotomy with the suture line continued along each side of the arteriotomy. The anterior surface of the PTFE was then incised parallel to the arteriotomy to a point 2 cm proximal to the heel of the anastomosis. A vein patch varying from 5 to 6 cm was harvested to close this elliptical defect. The patch was begun distally

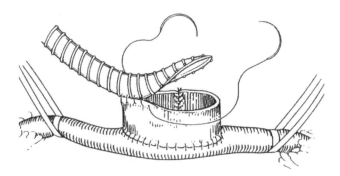

Figure 24-1 The Miller vein cuff. Venous tissue is opened longitudinally and sutured in an oval configuration to the artery with the polytetrafluoroethylene (PTFE), then sutured to the vein. (From Tyrrell MR, Chester JF, Vipond MN, et al. Experimental evidence to support the use of interposition vein collars/patches in distal PTFE anastomoses. *Eur J Vasc Surg.* 1990 Feb;4(1):95–101, with permission.)

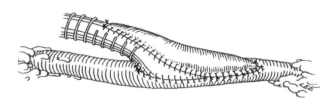

Figure 24-2 The Taylor patch. Polytetrafluoroethylene (PTFE) graft material is sutured to the proximal artery with a vein patch placed on the anterior surface of the graft extending onto the distal artery. Note the direct contact between PTFE and the artery for much of the anastomosis. (From Tyrrell MR, Chester JF, Vipond MN, et al. Experimental evidence to support the use of interposition vein collars/patches in distal PTFE anastomoses. *Eur J Vasc Surg.* 1990 Feb;4(1):95–101, with permission.)

on the tibial artery with interrupted sutures and completed proximally onto the PTFE with a running suture (Fig. 24-2). In his patients, Taylor used a vein patch at the proximal as well as the distal anastomosis. The proximal anastomosis was described as a conventional end-to-side anastomosis with a subsequent 3-cm, longitudinal incision across the inlet of the graft that was closed with a vein patch. Using this technique, Taylor reported on 256 grafts (only 83 to tibial arteries) with 1-, 3-, and 5-year patency rates of 74%, 58%, and 54%, respectively.

Taylor hypothesized that the improved graft patency noted with this patch technique was secondary to a reduction in the compliance mismatch between the PTFE graft material and the tibial artery wall, or, to the inherent properties of the vein endothelium located across the anastomosis. Recognizing that the anastomotic reservoir of the Miller cuff theoretically increased turbulence and shear stress at the distal anastomosis, Taylor felt this vein patch led to a more tapered funnel shape and theoretically decreased turbulence. However, there continue to be theoretical and practical disadvantages to the Taylor patch technique. The tibial artery intima is directly exposed to PTFE graft material for the proximal half of the distal anastomosis thereby losing the advantage of the venous endothelium for half the anastomosis. Additionally, a significant length of vein must be available to accomplish the anastomosis using the Taylor patch technique.

Recognizing the encouraging patency rates of the various vein cuff techniques, Tyrell and Wolfe[7] tried to reproduce these results. The group reported a 1-year patency rate of 74% (72 bypasses) with use of PTFE and the Taylor patch as compared to 47% (27 bypasses) with use of the PTFE with the Miller cuff technique. This experience confirmed some of the theoretical disadvantages of both techniques, most notably, the large anastomotic reservoir of the Miller cuff that increased turbulence, and the need for direct suturing of the PTFE graft to the tibial artery with the Taylor patch technique. This led to the development of the St. Mary's boot as described by Tyrell and Wolfe.[7] The St. Mary's boot technique utilizes a similar arteriotomy and venous harvest as the Miller cuff; however, the corner of the venous sheet is sutured to the

apex of the arteriotomy to form the anastomotic toe. The remainder of the venous-arterial anastomosis is formed in a similar fashion to the Miller cuff; however, the redundant vein is excised obliquely and sutured to the longitudinal edge. Next, a segment of the posterior collar is incised to increase the size of the anastomosis between the graft and vein collar (Fig. 24-3). Overall, the St. Mary's boot maintains a fully compliant venous collar, avoids any direct contact between artery and PTFE, and maintains the hemodynamic advantages of the Taylor patch. Its main drawback is the technical difficulty of its construction.

WHY DOES THE INTERPOSED VEIN SEGMENT HELP?

Bypass graft failure occurs for several reasons. In the early postoperative period, technical difficulty is the most common cause of graft failure. This includes a poor choice of the inflow or outflow artery, difficulty performing the anastomosis, and lack of appropriate conduit for the bypass. Graft stenosis due to myointimal hyperplasia becomes the leading cause of graft failure 6 to 24 months after the perioperative period. Beyond the 2-year postoperative period, progression of atherosclerosis proximal or distal to the graft is the most likely cause of graft failure. Myointimal hyperplasia at the anastomosis is particularly important in the failure of prosthetic bypass grafts.[19] The hyperplastic lesion is thought to originate from the proliferation of vascular smooth muscle cells in the arterial media, with subsequent cellular migration into the "injured" intimal layer of the arterial wall at the anastomotic site (Fig. 24-4). Possible stimuli for the cascade of events that result in this hyperplastic response include endothelial injury, abnormal hemodynamic patterns, and a stimulation of a variety of peptide growth factors.[20] The study of this hyperplastic response remains an area of active clinical interest as well as basic research, and is beyond the scope of this chapter.

The interposition of venous tissue between a PTFE graft and the recipient tibial artery may improve results in several ways. These bypasses are technically demanding, requiring an anastomosis between a small, diseased tibial artery and fairly noncompliant prosthetic material. The interposed venous tissue may simply make the bypass less technically demanding by suturing vein to the tibial artery. There may also be an effect on the thrombogenicity that may play a role at the interface between the high-resistance outflow artery and larger prosthetic graft.[21] Last, the venous tissue may reduce the hyperplastic myointimal response and thereby improve graft patency.

Several possible explanations have been proposed for the decreased hyperplastic reaction associated with vein cuffs, patches, and boots added to PTFE grafts. One

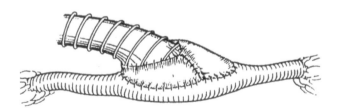

Figure 24-3 The St. Mary's boot. Venous tissue is sutured to the artery in an elliptical fashion with the polytetrafluoroethylene (PTFE), then sutured to the vein. Note the similarity to the Miller cuff. (From Tyrrell MR, Chester JF, Vipond MN, et al. Experimental evidence to support the use of interposition vein collars/patches in distal PTFE anastomoses. *Eur J Vasc Surg.* 1990 Feb;4(1):95–101, with permission.)

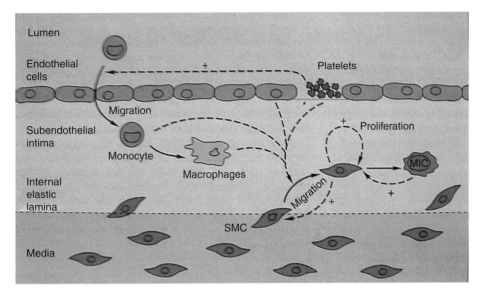

Figure 24-4 Myointimal hyperplasia. Vascular smooth muscle chemotactic and mitogenic stimulation after endothelial injury and platelet activation. SMC, smooth muscle cell. (From Neville RF, Sidawy AN, Foegh ML. The molecular biology of vein graft atherosclerosis and myointimal hyperplasia. *Curr Cardiol.* 1992;7: 930–938, with permission.)

possibility is the creation of a biologic "buffer zone" by the endothelium of the venous segment. Other benefits of the venous segment include a beneficial alteration of hemodynamic factors such as compliance and shear stress. Additionally, mechanical considerations, such as anastomotic surface area and the angle of the cuffed anastomosis, are altered by the venous tissue, possibly contributing to improved graft function and patency.

In an experimental animal model, the inhibition of myointimal hyperplasia by the use of a vein cuff with PTFE bypasses was demonstrated by Suggs et al.[22] Using a canine model, PTFE bypass grafts were placed bilaterally in the carotid artery with and without a vein cuff. Subsequent graft patency was assessed and luminal diameters were measured at three sites along the distal anastomosis and 1 mm beyond the anastomosis. Graft patency in the surviving animals was 36% for PTFE grafts and 64% for PTFE grafts with a vein cuff. Histologic analysis demonstrated that antibody positive cellular proliferation occurred predominantly at the PTFE anastomosis not using a vein cuff. Luminal encroachment was predominantly by cells highly reactive to smooth muscle–derived antibody. The area most affected by the myointimal hyperplastic response was the site 1 mm beyond the toe of the distal anastomosis, which is not usually seen with PTFE alone.

This redistribution of myointimal hyperplasia at the anastomotic site due to the interposed vein at the distal anastomosis has been noted by other authors as well. Kissin et al.[23] compared PTFE bypasses in Yorkshire pigs using a distal cuff of vein and a cuff made of PTFE material; several interesting observations were made. The vein cuff bypasses developed less myointimal hyperplasia with an actual regression of the hyperplastic response over 4 weeks. This result was attributed to compensatory vessel wall remodeling due to the presence of the vein cuff. Additionally, there was a redistribution

of the hyperplastic response away from the arterial portion of the anastomosis to the interface between the PTFE material and the vein segment, thus decreasing obstruction of the recipient artery by the hyperplastic tissue. The bypasses involving the PTFE cuff did not demonstrate these beneficial effects. This suggests that the favorable results noted in the presence of interposed vein are due to the biologic properties of the venous tissue, and not the geometric configuration that results due to the cuff.

Particle hemodynamic analysis has also been used to study the redistribution of myointimal hyperplasia due to venous tissue at the anastomosis. Archie et al.[24] performed a fluid dynamics analysis using computational models of distal anastomotic sites with and without a vein cuff. They were able to study near-wall residence time and shear stress factors that affect both platelet-wall activation and surface reactivity. These studies of particle hemodynamics demonstrated that the presence of a vein cuff significantly reduced the potentially detrimental changes in residence time and shear stress, as the hemodynamic abnormalities at the arterial portion of the suture line are shifted to the suture line between the PTFE and the vein. This supports the results noted in the animal model noted by Kissin et al.[23] Archie et al.[24] also noted a reduction in particle-wall interaction at the toe of the arterial anastomosis incorporating an interposed cuff. This would support the earlier observations described from the animal laboratory.

Other investigators have studied the contribution of mechanical factors to the effect on the hyperplastic response due to the vein cuff. Norberto et al.[25] used a canine carotid model and implanted bilateral PTFE grafts with a vein cuff at the distal anastomosis. On one side, the vein cuff was encircled with a PTFE jacket to decrease expansibility of the venous segment and minimize compliance as a significant factor. A second group had a PTFE segment without vein constructed between the graft and the carotid artery to create a fixed perpendicular angle at the anastomosis. At harvest, there was no significant difference between the hyperplastic reaction on the two sides in either group of dogs. This indicated that neither compliance nor the anastomotic angle seemed to play a prominent role in the reduction of hyperplasia. Another mechanical factor thought to play a role in the hyperplastic response at the anastomotic site is low wall shear stress. The effect of this wall shear stress was studied by How et al.[26] Flow velocity was assessed in graft models with and without a vein cuff under pulsatile flow conditions. Near-wall velocity vector measurements were used to determine wall shear stress. The addition of a vein cuff altered the wall shear stress at the anastomosis by decreasing areas of low shear stress in the recipient artery. This type of work on flow mechanics suggests that the beneficial effect of the vein cuff may not be mechanical in origin, thus emphasizing the concept of a venous endothelial "buffer zone" that is responsible for diminishing the hyperplastic response at the distal anastomosis.

VEIN CUFFS, PATCHES, AND BOOTS IN CURRENT PRACTICE

Several reports have examined the results of PTFE bypasses with vein cuffs and patches in clinical practice. Hobson et al.[23] reported a benefit for tibial bypass using the Miller vein cuff technique. In 30 grafts, they noted 54% patency with the vein cuffed grafts versus 12% patency for the noncuffed grafts at 24 months. A prospective, randomized trial utilizing PTFE grafts with and without a vein cuff was reported by Stonebridge et al.[27] This series did not demonstrate a statistically significant benefit for the vein cuff technique in tibial bypasses, although the patency was seemingly improved at 24 months, 52% versus 29%. The lack of statistical significance reflected the fact that the report randomized 246 femoral popliteal bypasses with only 15 tibial bypass grafts included in the analysis. Kreienberg et al.[28] compared grafts using PTFE with a vein cuff and composite saphenous vein grafts. Primary patency was similar at a 2-year interval: 49% cuff versus 44% composite vein. Secondary patency rates were somewhat better for the composite vein group, but there was no difference in limb salvage, and the composite vein group had a significantly higher number of wound complications. In the presence of adequate lengths of saphenous vein, a composite configuration should certainly be considered in order to establish an all autogenous reconstruction. However, composite grafts of poor quality vein may not function any better than PTFE with a vein cuff or patch.

After a suboptimal experience with the Miller and Tyrell configurations, and stimulated by a larger volume of patients without autogenous options to avoid limb loss, we developed our own vein cuff configuration. This configuration combined a standard vascular technique (the Linton patch) with a PTFE bypass. This distal vein patch (DVP) bypass utilizes a technique familiar to all vascular surgeons and requires a shorter arteriotomy, thereby decreasing the amount of venous tissue required for the procedure. A 2- to 3-cm segment of tissue for the patch is suitable and can include saphenous vein remnants, arm vein harvested under local anesthesia, superficial femoral vein, or a segment of occluded superficial femoral artery that is opened and endarterectomized. However, a segment of vein can usually be located. The segment is gently irrigated with prepared vein solution and opened longitudinally in preparation for the patch. Valves are excised and the vein segment is briefly stored in the vein solution. A 2- to 3-cm arteriotomy is then performed in the artery chosen for the distal anastomosis. The venous segment is cut to the appropriate length and width in preparation for the patch. In most cases, the width is left unaltered to allow for a generous patch, in order to permit bulging of the patch under arterial flow and to have a functional result similar to that of a vein cuff. After the patch is sewn in place, a longitudinal venotomy is made in the proximal two thirds of the patch (Fig. 24-5). An externally reinforced, 6-mm, thin-walled *e*-PTFE graft is then sutured

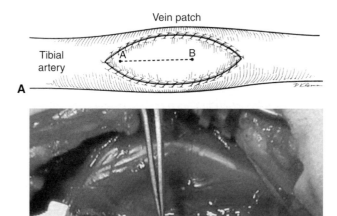

Figure 24-5 Distal vein patch. **A:** The vein patch is sutured to the artery and a proximal venotomy is cut from point A to B. **B:** Intraoperative photograph of the venotomy during construction of the distal vein patch (DVP) anastomosis. (From Neville RF, Attinger C, Sidawy AN. Prosthetic bypass with a distal vein patch for limb salvage. *Am J Surg.* 1997;174:173–176, with permission from Excerpta Medica, Inc.)

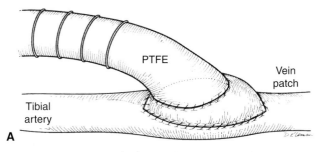

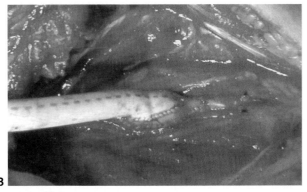

Figure 24-6 Distal vein patch. The polytetrafluoroethylene (PTFE) material is sutured to the proximal venous tissue. **A:** Schematic picture. **B:** Intraoperative photograph. (From Neville RF, Attinger C, Sidawy AN. Prosthetic bypass with a distal vein patch for limb salvage. *Am J Surg.* 1997;174:173–176, with permission from Excerpta Medica, Inc.)

to the vein patch using 6-0 Prolene monofilament suture (Fig. 24-6). The anastomosis is constructed in order to maintain a rim of venous tissue interposed between the PTFE graft and the entire circumference of the arterial wall. Because the venotomy is made in the proximal two thirds of the patch, more venous tissue is left interposed at the toe of the anastomosis than at the heel of the anastomosis. A heparin infusion is started 4 to 6 hours postoperatively, with coumadin administered on the first postoperative day. Long-term anticoagulation with coumadin is continued with an international normalized ratio (INR) of 2.0 as the goal.[29]

The initial data using this DVP technique included 79 patients with no autogenous vein available as conduit for a bypass.[30] In each patient who received a DVP graft, the ipsilateral and contralateral greater saphenous veins were either not present, having been used for previous revascularization procedures, or were unsuitable due to inadequate length or quality. In the 79 patients, 80 bypasses were performed. Follow-up ranged from 30 days to 4 years. During this time interval, the DVP group represented 16% of the total tibial bypass experience (500 cases). Patient demographics were similar to other series with 39 men, 40 women, and a mean age of 67 years. Risk factor analysis revealed 53% of patients with diabetes mellitus, 20% of patients with renal failure, and 60% of patients with increased perioperative cardiac risk as assessed by Eagle's criteria. The indication for revascularization was limb-threatening ischemia in all

patients, with rest pain in 49% of limbs and gangrene or nonhealing ulceration present in 51%. Reasons for the lack of adequate saphenous vein included previous failed lower extremity bypass at an outside institution in 47 patients (59%), previous coronary bypass in 21 (26%), unsuitable vein quality due to size or thrombosis in eight (10%), and absence of vein due to varicose vein stripping in four (5%). A fairly high percentage of grafts originated from the external iliac artery (43%) in order to avoid hostile, scarred groins from previous bypass attempts at outside institutions. Occasionally, the superficial femoral artery was a suitable source of inflow (8%), with the remainder of the grafts originating at the common femoral artery. Recipient arteries included the peroneal artery in 35 cases (44%), the posterior tibial artery in 28 cases (35%), and the anterior tibial artery in 17 cases (21%). Two of the posterior tibial bypasses were to inframalleolar plantar branches. Primary graft patency was 90% at 6 months, and 82%, 78%, 69%, and 62% at respective 12-month intervals up to 48 months. At the time of this analysis, six grafts remained patent beyond 48 months. Since that report, the DVP technique has been used to perform an additional 149 cases for a total of 229 DVP bypass grafts. This number represents 27% of the total tibial experience (841 cases) at our institution during that time.

SHOULD WE ADD A DISTAL ARTERIOVENOUS FISTULA AS WELL?

The addition of an arteriovenous fistula at the distal anastomosis has been attempted as another measure to improve graft patency, even with the use of saphenous vein as the conduit. As an alternative to PTFE when autogenous conduit is not available, Dardik et al.[12] have used human umbilical vein grafts and added a common ostium distal arteriovenous fistula in an attempt to decrease the thrombosis rate by reduction of outflow resistance. Ascer et al.[31] has described a technique involving construction of an arteriovenous fistula between the target tibial artery and corresponding tibial vein with a PTFE bypass to the involved vein as a type of vein cuff. Reported patency rates with this technique are 62% patency at 36 months, despite a fistula thrombosis rate of 37% within 2 years. Kreienberg et al. of the Albany group[28] have also reported a series using vein cuffs and arteriovenous fistulas. This retrospective series of popliteal and tibial bypasses compared PTFE grafts using the Tyrell/Wolfe vein boot technique to grafts performed with an arteriovenous fistula distal to the actual anastomosis. They noted similar graft patency rates between the two techniques at 12 months (96% boot vs. 86% dAVF) and 36 months (38% boot vs. 48% dAVF). Based on this work, the authors indicated a preference for the Tyrell/Wolfe boot technique due

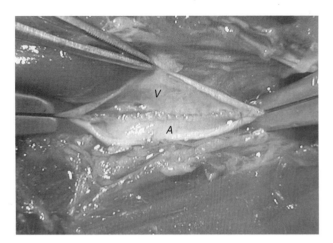

Figure 24-7 "Patchula." Distal vein patch (DVP) bypass with an arteriovenous fistula added at the distal anastomosis. A common ostium fistula is created between the recipient tibial artery *(A)* and its corresponding vein *(V)*.

to technical ease and other logistic considerations involving graft salvage and secondary patency. A prospective randomized trial by Hamsho et al.[32] compared distal prosthetic bypasses using PTFE with a Miller vein cuff both with and without a concomitant arteriovenous fistula. This series indicated that the fistula conferred no benefit, but did not stratify patients based on arterial runoff.

Based on the above experience, we have added an arteriovenous fistula to the distal anastomosis of a distal vein patch bypass ("patchula"). This modification has been performed in patients with no vein available and severely disadvantaged arterial runoff on the preoperative arteriogram. The target tibial artery is opened longitudinally with a venotomy in the corresponding tibial vein (Fig. 24-7). The vein patch is then sutured to the common ostium created by this fistulous connection. An anastomosis is then constructed between the vein patch and the PTFE, as described in the DVP bypass configuration (Fig. 24-8).

The initial group of patients has included several who would not have been offered an attempt at a bypass, due to the lack of a target artery with suitable runoff that would support a reasonable chance of success. The

arteriovenous fistula was added to the DVP in the hopes of decreasing outflow resistance in those patients with a severely diseased arterial runoff bed. This initial patient series includes 15 patients with tissue loss and/or gangrene as the indication for revascularization. The "patchula" was performed due to the appearance of the preoperative arteriogram that showed an isolated tibial segment or a diminutive tibial artery as the recipient artery for the bypass. These patients are at various stages of follow-up from 1 to 18 months, with one graft thrombosis and subsequent amputation in this patient cohort (author's unpublished data). Additional patient numbers and more complete follow-up are needed prior to any conclusions, but the initial results are promising in this very challenging group of patients with threatened limbs and the combination of lack of autogenous conduit and severely diseased distal runoff.

SUMMARY

In those patients requiring tibial bypass for revascularization in an attempt at limb salvage despite the lack of autogenous conduit, acceptable long-term patency can be achieved using PTFE with the interposition of venous tissue at the distal anastomosis. The results presented above suggest that the addition of venous tissue at the outflow anastomosis somehow alters the thrombotic and hyperplastic response, thereby improving patency of prosthetic bypasses to tibial arteries. However, this issue would best be answered by a randomized prospective trial of obligatory prosthetic bypasses in patients with unavailable autogenous vein requiring infrapopliteal bypass.

At this point in time, patients in danger of limb loss who lack adequate saphenous vein should be considered for tibial bypass with PTFE and a vein patch or cuff as the conduit. As the population ages and policies towards limb salvage become more aggressive, vascular surgeons will require alternative conduits to autogenous saphenous vein in a growing subset of patients. In our practice, PTFE with a DVP is preferred to both PTFE bypass alone or composite grafts constructed with PTFE and longer segments of saphenous vein. A multicenter, prospective, randomized trial may be of benefit to address the question of the best alternative for the patient without suitable autogenous saphenous vein for limb salvage. Until then, we will offer the patient without adequate vein PTFE bypasses to tibial arteries for limb salvage with the addition of a distal vein patch.

REFERENCES

1. Bergan JJ, Veith FJ, Bernhard VM, et al. Randomization of autogenous vein and polytetrafluoroethylene grafts in femoral-distal reconstruction. *Surgery.* 1982;92:921–930.

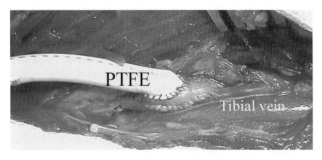

Figure 24-8 "Patchula." Distal anastomosis involving polytetrafluoroethylene (PTFE), a vein patch, and tibial vein/artery fistula.

2. Veith FJ, Gupta SK, Ascer E, et al. Six-year prospective multicenter randomized comparison of autologous saphenous vein and expanded polytetrafluoroethylene grafts in infrainguinal arterial reconstructions. *J Vasc Surg.* 1986;3:104–114.

3. Calligaro KD, Syrek JR, Dougherty MJ, et al. Use of arm and lesser saphenous vein compared with prosthetic grafts for infrapopliteal bypass: are they worth the effort? *J Vasc Surg.* 1997;26:919–927.

4. Holzenbien TJ, Pomposelli FB II, Miller A, et al. Results of a policy with arm veins used as the first alternative to an unavailable ipsilateral greater saphenous vein for infrainguinal bypass. *J Vasc Surg.* 1996;23:130–140.

5. Bell PR. Are distal vascular procedures worthwhile? *Br J Surg.* 1985;72:335.

6. Miller JH, Foreman RK, Ferguson L, et al. Interposition vein cuff for anastomosis of prosthesis to small artery. *Aust N Z J Surg.* 1984;54:283–285.

7. Tyrell MR, Wolfe JH. New prosthetic venous collar anastomotic technique: combining the best of other procedures. *Br J Surg.* 1991;78:1016–1017.

8. Taylor RS, Loh A, McFarland RJ, et al. Improved technique for polytetrafluoroethylene bypass grafting: long-term results using anastomotic vein patches. *Br J Surg.* 1992;79:348–354.

9. Brewster DC. Composite grafts. In: Rutherford RB, ed. *Vascular surgery.* Philadelphia, Pa: WB Saunders; 1989:481–486.

10. Anderson LI, Nielsen OM, Buchardt Hansen HJB. Umbilical vein bypass in patients with severe lower limb ischemia: a report of 121 consecutive cases. *Surgery.* 1985;97:294–298.

11. Farber A, Major K, Wagner WH, et al. Cryopreserved saphenous vein allografts in infrainguinal revascularization: analysis of 240 grafts. *J Vasc Surg.* 2003;38:15–21.

12. Dardik H, Silvestri F, Alasio T, et al. Improved method to create the common ostium variant of the distal arteriovenous fistula for enhancing crural prosthetic graft patency. *J Vasc Surg.* 1996;24: 240–248.

13. Parsons RE, Suggs WD, Veith FJ, et al. Polytetrafluioroethylene bypasses to infrapopliteal arteries without cuffs or patches: a better option than amputation in patients without autologous vein. *J Vasc Surg.* 1996;23:347–356.

14. Campbell CD, Brooks DH, Webster MW, et al. The use of expanded microporous polytetrafluoroethylene for limb salvage: a preliminary report. *Surgery.* 1976;79:485–491.

15. Hobson RW II, Lynch TG, Jamil Z, et al. Results of revascularization and amputation in severe lower extremity ischemia: a five-year clinical experience. *J Vasc Surg.* 1985;2:174–185.

16. Whittemore AD, Kent KC, Donaldson MC, et al. What is the proper role of polytetrafluoroethylene grafts in infrainguinal reconstruction? *J Vasc Surg.* 1989;10:299–305.

17. Siegman FA. Use of the venous cuff for graft anastomosis. *Surg Gynecol Obstet.* 1979;148:930.

18. Kansal N, Pappas PJ, Gwertzman GA, et al. Patency and limb salvage for polytetrafluoroethylene bypasses with vein interposition cuffs. *Ann Vasc Surg.* 1999;13:386–332.

19. DeWeese JA. Anastomotic intimal hyperplasia. In: Sawyer PN Kaplutt NJ, eds. *Vascular Grafts.* New York, NY: Appleton-Century-Crofts; 1978:147–152.

20. Neville RF, Sidawy AN, Foegh ML. The molecular biology of vein graft atherosclerosis and myointimal hyperplasia. *Curr Cardiol.* 1992;7:930–938.

21. Wolfe J, Tyrell M. Venous patches, collars, and boots improve the patency rates of polytetrafluoroethylene grafts. *Adv Vasc Surg.* 1995;3:134–143.

22. Suggs WD, Henriques HF, DePalma RG. Vein cuff interposition prevents juxta-anastomotic hyperplasia. *Ann Surg.* 1988;207: 717–723.

23. Kissin M, Kansal N, Pappas PJ, et al. Vein interposition cuffs decrease the intimal hyperplastic response of PTFE bypass grafts. *J Vasc Surg.* 2000;31:69–83.

24. Longest PW, Kleinstreuer C, Archie JP. Particle hemodynamics analysis of Miller cuff arterial anastomosis. *J Vasc Surg.* 2003;38: 1353–1362.

25. Norberto JJ, Sidawy AN, Trad KS, et al. The protective effect of vein cuffed anastomoses is not mechanical in origin. *J Vasc Surg.* 1995;21:558–566.

26. How TV, Rowe CS, Gilling-Smith GL, et al. Interposition vein cuff anastomosis alters wall shear stress distribution in the recipient artery. *J Vasc Surg.* 2000;31:1008–1017.

27. Stonebridge PA, Prescott RJ, Ruckley CL. Randomized trial comparing infrainguinal polytetrafluoroethylene bypass grafting with and without interposition vein cuff at the distal anastomosis. *J Vasc Surg.* 1997;26:543–550.

28. Kreienberg PB, Darling CR III, Chang BB, et al. Adjunctive techniques to improve patency of distal prosthetic bypass grafts: polytetrafluoroethylene with remote arteriovenous fistulae versus vein cuffs. *J Vasc Surg.* 2000;31:696–701.

29. Neville RF, Attinger C, Sidawy AN. Prosthetic bypass with a distal vein patch for limb salvage. *Am J Surg.* 1997;174:173–176.

30. Neville RF, Tempesta B, Sidawy AN. Tibial bypass for limb salvage using polytetrafluoroethylene and a distal vein patch. *J Vasc Surg.* 2001;33:266–272.

31. Ascer E, Gennaro M, Pollina RM, et al. Complementary distal arteriovenous fistula and deep vein interposition: a five-year experience with a technique to improve infrapopliteal prosthetic bypass patency. *J Vasc Surg.* 1996;24:134–143.

32. Hamsho A, Nott D, Harris PL. Prospective randomised trial of distal arteriovenous fistula as an adjunct to femoro-infrapopliteal PTFE bypass. *Eur J Vasc Endovasc Surg.* 1999;17:197–201.

25

Adjuvant Medical Therapy to Improve Patency of Infrainguinal Bypasses

William Andrew Tierney   *Samuel R. Money*

There is a wide range of patency rates for various vascular reconstructions depending on the vessels involved and the choice of conduit. Aortobifemoral bypasses have 5-year patency rates as high as 92%.[1] In these high-flow, lower-resistance grafts, aggressive antithrombotic therapy is not necessary to improve graft patency. At the other extreme are bypasses to infrapopliteal vessels using polytetrafluoroethylene (PTFE), where 4-year patency rates as low as 12% can be expected.[2] In these grafts using a thrombogenic prosthetic conduit and a small target vessel, antithrombotic medications are an important adjuvant therapy. The choice of antithrombotic therapy must be tailored to each vascular reconstruction to provide optimal graft patency in balance with the risk of the adjuvant therapy.

PLATELET INHIBITORS

Aspirin

Aspirin plays an important role in both maintaining patency of vascular reconstructions and reducing the incidence of cardiovascular complications in patients with peripheral arterial occlusive disease. Aspirin is by far the most studied antithrombotic agent used in vascular surgery.

Indium[111]-labled platelets show increased uptake on femoropopliteal bypasses composed of PTFE or Dacron. A combination of aspirin and dipyridamole significantly reduces platelet uptake on prosthetic grafts.[3] Although there are some conflicting data, the improvement in bypass patency with antiplatelet therapy which this would predict, is found in most studies. Of the seven trials evaluating the effect of aspirin and/or aspirin and dipyridamole on arterial bypasses, five demonstrated a significant improvement in patency in the treatment group[4–8] (Table 25-1). Three of these were well-constructed, randomized, controlled trials involving PTFE or Dacron bypasses.[4–6] In all of these, aspirin or aspirin and dipyridamole were started preoperatively. Although most studies used a combination of aspirin and dipyridamole, the study by Green et al.[4] showed no difference in benefit between aspirin and dipyridamole or aspirin alone. A trial of 148 patients with a mix of autogenous and prosthetic graft material found a significant increase in patency of prosthetic bypasses with aspirin and dipyridamole, but no difference in the patency of vein grafts.[7] Possible explanations for the lack of benefit in vein grafts

TABLE 25-1

TRIALS WITH ASPIRIN AND DIPYRIDAMOLE

Author, Year	Graft Material	Rx Start	No. of Pts	Limb Salvage	Follow-up	Patency in Treatment	Patency in Controls
Green, 1982[4]	PTFE	Preop	49	82%	1 y	100%[a]	50%
Goldman, 1983[5]	PTFE Dacron	Preop	67	76%	1 y	67%[a]	36%
Kohler, 1984[9]	PTFE Vein	Postop	102	67%	2 y	54% PTFE 58% vein	58% PTFE 73% vein
Donaldson, 1985[6]	Dacron	Preop	73	0%	1 y	85%[a]	59%
Clyne, 1987[7]	PTFE Vein	Preop	148	73%	1 y	85% PTFE[a] 81% vein	53% PTFE 72% vein
McCollum, 1991[10]	Vein	Preop	549	60%	3 y	61%	60%
Franks, 1992[8]	Vein	Preop	145	60%	3 y	83%[a]	66%

PTFE, polytetrafluoroethylene.
[a]$p < 0.05$.

are that only dipyridamole was given preoperatively while aspirin and dipyridamole were given postoperatively, and the length of treatment was unusually short, lasting only 6 weeks. Given the expected higher patency of vein grafts, any improvements in patency with this regimen may have been too small to reach statistical significance; a type II error may have occurred.

Two trials of aspirin and dipyridamole failed to show a benefit on patency.[9,10] The first involved 102 patients with PTFE and vein bypasses. The most striking difference between this study and those that clearly showed a benefit to therapy is that the aspirin and dipyridamole were started postoperatively.[9] The second is a large, randomized, controlled trial from Britain that involved 549 patients with vein grafts who were treated with aspirin and dipyridamole.[10] In addition to finding no effect on graft patency, the treated patients were twice as likely to require reoperation for bleeding. The only proven benefit of treatment was a significant reduction in the risk of myocardial infarction (MI) and stroke in the treatment group. The greatest weakness of this trial was poor patient compliance. A separate analysis of a subset of 145 patients in whom salicylate levels were measured revealed a significant improvement in patency in patients with detectable salicylate levels.[8] These results suggest that patients who are compliant with taking their aspirin will obtain a better patency.

Two meta-analyses have evaluated the effect of aspirin and dipyridamole on peripheral arterial bypasses. Tangelder et al.[11] analyzed five randomized, controlled trials including 816 patients and found a relative risk (RR) of graft occlusion of 0.78% in treated patients. The most extensive meta-analysis was done by the Antiplatelet Trialists' Collaboration.[12] This trial involved 3,000 patients, and showed a significant increase in the patency of vascular grafts as well as a significant reduction in the

risk of MI, stroke, and vascular death in patients taking aspirin or aspirin and dipyridamole. Clearly, aspirin should be used, not only to improve patency, but also to reduce major cardiovascular risk. This medication is overwhelmingly cost-effective, with proven results.

Ticlopidine, Dextran-40, and Clopidogrel

In a single well-designed, randomized, controlled trial involving 243 patients with femoropopliteal or femorotibial vein grafts, ticlopidine was shown to significantly improve bypass graft patency. After 2 years of follow-up, primary patency in the ticlopidine group was 66.4% compared to 51.2% in the placebo group. There was no difference in the occurrence of major adverse events between the two groups. The study also evaluated the rates of MI and stroke and found no risk reduction with ticlopidine.[13]

Dextran-40 was also evaluated in a single well-designed study in which 156 patients with autogenous and prosthetic bypasses were treated for 3 days. After 1 week, 93.1% of treated grafts were patent versus 79.5% of controls. This difference was even more significant for the subset of patients with prosthetic grafts. However, at 1-month follow-up, the improvement in patency was no longer significant.[14]

Clopidogrel is an adenosine diphosphate (ADP)-receptor antagonist and a potent inhibitor of platelet function. The CAPRIE trial[15] showed a significant reduction in nonfatal MI, nonfatal stroke, and vascular death among high-risk patients taking clopidogrel compared to those taking aspirin. Furthermore, this benefit was even more pronounced in patients with lower extremity ischemia. Analysis of a subset of the CAPRIE population with a history of aortocoronary bypass also revealed a 42.8% RR reduction in vascular death in patients treated with clopidogrel versus aspirin.[16] This would seem to suggest improved patency of aorto-coronary bypass grafts with clopidogrel. However, despite good evidence for its use in cardiovascular protection of patients with peripheral arterial occlusive disease, there has been very little investigation into its role in improving the patency of vascular bypass grafts. Only a single poorly designed Turkish study has addressed the effect of clopidogrel on peripheral bypasses. In the Turkish study, 76 bypasses were performed on 54 patients, with 28 patients receiving aspirin and 26 patients receiving clopidogrel. Follow-up was short, 11 months and 7 months for aspirin and clopidogrel, respectively. The patency was 81% in the aspirin group versus 84% in the clopidogrel group.[17] This study included a significant number of aortofemoral, aortoiliac, and aortobifemoral bypasses. Due to the high-flow, low-resistance nature of these grafts, they are far less likely to benefit from antithrombotic therapy. Therefore, we feel that no significant conclusions can be gleaned from this paper.

ORAL ANTICOAGULANTS

Compared to antiplatelet therapy, oral anticoagulation (OAC) is clearly more inconvenient for the patient. Another concern is the potential for hemorrhagic complications. However, due to its potential to provide a greater level of protection against graft thrombosis, it has been evaluated in several trials involving peripheral arterial reconstruction (Table 25-2). As with studies of platelet inhibitors, several of these trials provide conflicting results. However, the data still provide a basis for rational recommendations regarding oral anticoagulation in certain types of vascular reconstructions.

Kretschmer et al.[21] followed 130 patients with femoropopliteal vein grafts for 10 years using phenprocoumon with a target international normalized ratio (INR) of 2.5 to 3.5, and compared them to controls with no anticoagulation. They reported a significant improvement in graft patency, limb salvage, and survival. The only reported bleeding complication was a fatal gastrointestinal hemorrhage in a patient in the treatment group. In contrast, Arfvidsson et al.[22] found no increase in patency, and reported a 4% to 5% incidence of major bleeding complications. This study included patients with prosthetic and vein grafts. It also used a lower target INR (1.8 to 2.8).

The Veterans Affairs Cooperative study[23] was a large, multicenter, prospective, randomized trial comparing warfarin plus aspirin (WASA) therapy to aspirin alone in patients with vein and prosthetic bypasses. With a total of 831 patients followed for up to 5 years, they found no improvement in the patency of vein bypasses in patients treated with WASA. Subgroup analysis of the patients with prosthetic bypasses revealed a significant improvement in patency in patients with 6-mm PTFE grafts. However, they also found a significant increase in overall mortality and both minor and major hemorrhagic complications in the WASA group. The patency data in this study are difficult to interpret because 40% of the patients in the warfarin group were no longer taking the drug at the time of graft thrombosis, and an additional 33% had an INR <1.4. Still, the increase in hemorrhagic complications is concerning.

The largest trial examining the effect of oral anticoagulants on arterial bypass grafts is the Dutch Bypass Oral Anticoagulants or Aspirin study.[20] In this multicenter, randomized trial, 2,690 patients with either autogenous or prosthetic infrainguinal bypass grafts were treated with either aspirin or phenprocoumon

TABLE 25-2
TRIALS WITH ORAL ANTICOAGULANTS

Author, Year	INR	No. of Pts (Material)	Limb Salvage	Follow-up	Patency in Treatment	Patency in Controls
Flinn, 1988[18]	2–3	75 (PTFE)	97%	4 yr	50%[a]	12% (historical)
Arfvidsson, 1990[22]	1.8–2.8	116 (total) 49 (vein)	79%	3 yr	46%	42%
Kretschmer, 1992[21]	2.5–3.5	130 (vein)	52%	10 yr	71%[a]	44%
Sarac, 1998[19]	2–3	56 (vein)	95%	3 yr	74%[a]	51%
Dutch BOA, 2000[20]	3–4.5	858 (prosthetic) 1496 (vein)	49%	21 mo	RR 1.32 RR 0.71	– –
VA Study, 2002[23]	1.4–2.8	373 (PTFE) 458 (vein)	Unknown	5 yr	71.4% 75.3%	57.9% 74.9%

INR, international normalized ratio; PTFE, polytetrafluoroethylene; RR, risk reduction.
[a]p <0.05.

and aspirin with a target INR of 3.0 to 4.5. Although there was no significant difference between the overall patency in the OAC group versus the aspirin group, subgroup analysis showed a significant increase in patency in patients with vein grafts in the OAC group. Conversely, patients with prosthetic grafts had better patency when treated with aspirin alone. Although anticoagulation also provided a reduction in the rate of vascular death, MI, stroke, and amputation, it came at the cost of an almost twofold increase in bleeding complications.

Using coumadin with a target INR of 2 to 3 to treat patients with limb-threatening ischemia, Flinn et al.[18] found an increase in the patency of PTFE bypasses. In patients with a therapeutic INR, the graft patency at 4 years was 50% compared to 12% in historical controls. In another paper, Sarac et al.[19] compared coumadin and aspirin versus aspirin alone in patients with infrainguinal vein grafts deemed to be at high risk for failure. In this study, 95% of patients were operated on for limb-threatening ischemia. The OAC group had a significantly higher patency rate and a higher rate of limb salvage. However, OAC was also associated with a higher rate of postoperative hematoma.

An additional benefit of oral anticoagulation is a reduction in the ischemic consequences of prosthetic graft thrombosis. It has been shown that thrombosis of a PTFE graft leads to more severe ischemia than thrombosis of vein grafts.[24] In a multicenter clinical trial, 402 patients with femoropopliteal bypass grafts using PTFE or autogenous vein were randomized to coumadin plus aspirin or aspirin alone. Patients with PTFE and subsequent graft occlusion had significantly less severe ischemia if treated with coumadin and aspirin compared to aspirin alone.[25]

Although three trials with OAC in vascular bypasses reported significant increases in bleeding complications, other large studies of chronically anticoagulated patients have provided conflicting results. In five randomized trials of OAC with a target INR of 2 to 3 for atrial fibrillation, the risk of major bleeding was 1.3% in treated patients versus 1% in placebo-treated controls.[26] In practice, it is quite difficult to keep many patients in this range. Several risk factors have been identified that convey a higher risk for hemorrhagic complications with anticoagulation. These risks are age >65, history of gastrointestinal bleeding, history of stroke, or the presence of one of four comorbid conditions (recent MI, anemia, renal insufficiency, or diabetes). Using this model, the cumulative incidence of major bleeding at 48 months was 3%, 12%, and 53% in low-, intermediate-, and high-risk patients, respectively.[27] This allows more accurate risk/benefit analysis of patients with vascular reconstructions who have an indication for anticoagulation.

HEPARIN

Standard unfractionated heparin (UFH) has long been used intraoperatively around the time of arterial cross-clamping. There is little good scientific data to support this, but it seems intuitive to provide anticoagulation to protect against thrombosis in areas of stagnant flow and in the presence of denuded endothelium or prosthetic material. Furthermore, the consequences of thrombosis in the setting of a fresh vascular reconstruction would make performing such a randomized, controlled study difficult.

There are, however, several studies relating to the use of UFH and low-molecular-weight heparin (LMWH) in the postoperative period. In the most intriguing of these, Edmondson et al.[28] followed 200 patients for 1 year after femoropopliteal bypass with vein, Dacron, or PTFE. Patients were randomized to receive either LMWH (Fragmin, Pharmacia, Stockholm, Sweden) or aspirin and dipyridamole for 3 months. Although there was no benefit to patients operated on for claudication, there was a significant increase in graft patency among the patients in the LMWH group with limb-threatening ischemia. In a similar study, Samama et al.[29] compared postoperative LMWH (Lovenox, Aventis, Kansas City, Missouri) to UFH for the prevention of graft thrombosis. There was a significant improvement in patency in the LMWH group. Although the treatment was discontinued after 10 days, the difference in patency remained significant after 1 month. A third study compared LMWH (Fragmin) and UFH when used intraoperatively at the time of arterial cross-clamping. There was no difference in the rate of graft thrombosis. However, due to an extremely small sample size, it is difficult to draw meaningful conclusions from this trial.[30]

OTHER TREATMENTS

There are strong data in the cardiology literature to suggest that the use of statins to treat hyperlipidemia increases the patency of aortocoronary bypass grafts. A meta-analysis of 14 angiographic trials evaluating the effect of lipid-lowering medications on coronary anatomy found a 49% reduction in the odds for disease progression and a 219% increase in the odds for disease regression.[31] Although there are no studies to confirm that this benefit also applies to peripheral arterial bypasses, all vascular patients with hyperlipidemia should be aggressively treated to lower their risk of cardiovascular complications.

One of the most interesting treatments on the horizon is the use of gene therapy to modify autogenous bypass grafts. The most promising target is the pivotal cell-cycle transcription factor E2F. Animal studies using oligodeoxynucleotides as E2F factor decoys have shown a reduction in intimal hyperplasia and susceptibility to atherosclerosis.[32] One randomized, controlled trial used E2F factor decoys in human vein grafts for infrainguinal arterial bypasses. The study, involving 41 patients, used *ex vivo* pressure-mediated transfection to deliver the decoy to vein grafts. The transfection efficiency was 89%, and at 12-month follow-up, treated patients had significantly fewer graft occlusions, revisions, and critical stenoses. Furthermore, there was no difference in complications between the groups.[33] It has also been shown that while neointimal hyperplasia is inhibited, E2F factor decoys do not suppress normal endothelial proliferation in response to vessel injury and bypass grafting.[34] This form of adjuvant therapy is extremely promising, but more research is required before widespread clinical application is possible.

New anticoagulants are on the horizon. There are numerous new agents that are presently in clinical testing. Many of these will work on different parts of the clotting cascade. Some of these may reduce bleeding, improve patency, and not require frequent monitoring. It is hopeful that one or more of these agents will serve to reduce bypass failures.

RECOMMENDATIONS

Although some of the data conflict and newer treatments such as clopidogrel and gene therapy must be investigated further, several recommendations can be made given the available evidence.

- Aspirin has been proven to increase the patency of infrainguinal bypasses and decrease cardiovascular morbidity and mortality. Given the high association of peripheral arterial occlusive disease with coronary and cerebrovascular disease, it is prudent to treat all patients having lower extremity revascularization with aspirin.
- The necessity of adding dipyridamole to an aspirin regimen is questionable. Although most studies used a combination of aspirin and dipyridamole, there is evidence that aspirin alone is equally effective. Animal experiments in which dipyridamole was found to increase the antithrombotic effect of aspirin on prosthetic surfaces may favor the combination of aspirin and dipyridamole in the treatment of patients with prosthetic grafts, but most practicing vascular surgeons simply use aspirin.[35]
- The effect of clopidogrel on the patency of infrainguinal bypasses has not been sufficiently studied. Therefore, it is not possible to recommend its use for this indication based on clear evidence-based research. In our practice, we frequently use this drug

in patients with bypasses at high risk for failure. These include below-knee prosthetic bypasses and composite below-knee or tibial bypasses.

- Dextran-40 is beneficial in preventing thrombosis of vascular grafts in the early postoperative period. However, this benefit was lost on 1-month follow-up. Due to its limited benefit and the cumbersome nature of a continuous intravenous infusion, Dextran-40 has a very limited role in antithrombotic therapy of infrainguinal bypasses.
- Ticlopidine also has proven benefit in preventing thrombosis of vein grafts. However, aspirin has a better effect on cardiovascular morbidity. Ticlopidine may be used as an alternative in patients with vein grafts who are intolerant of aspirin. However, the problems with bone marrow suppression and hepatotoxicity have severely limited ticlopidine's use.
- Oral anticoagulation combined with aspirin should be used to improve patency of bypasses at high risk for failure. Grafts considered at high risk for failure include those with poor arterial runoff, suboptimal venous conduit, redo infrainguinal bypasses, and PTFE grafts to infrageniculate vessels.
- Routine use of OAC in all infrainguinal bypasses is not recommended.

REFERENCES

1. McDaniel MD, Macdonald PD, Haver RA, et al. Published results of surgery for aortoiliac occlusive disease. *Ann Vasc Surg.* 1997;11:425–441.
2. Vieth FJ, Gupta SK, Ascer E, et al. Six-year prospective multicenter randomized comparison of autologous saphenous vein and expanded polytetrafluoroethylene grafts in infrainguinal arterial reconstructions. *J Vasc Surg.* 1986;3:104–113.
3. Pumphrey CW, Chesebro JH, Dewanjee MK, et al. *In vivo* quantitation of platelet deposition on human peripheral arterial bypass grafts using Indium-111-labled platelets: effect of dipyridamole and aspirin. *Am J Cardiol.* 1983;51:796–801.
4. Green RM, Roedersheimer R, DeWeese JA. Effects of aspirin and dipyridamole on expanded polytetrafluoroethylene graft patency. *Surgery.* 1982;92:1016–1026.
5. Goldman M, Hall C, Dykes J, et al. Does [111]Indium-platelet deposition predict patency in prosthetic arterial grafts? *Br J Surg.* 1983;70:635–638.
6. Donaldson DR, Salter MCP, Kester RC, et al. The influence of platelet inhibition on the patency of femoro-popliteal Dacron bypass grafts. *Vasc Surg.* 1985;19:224–230.
7. Clyne CA, Archer TJ, Atuhaire LK, et al. Random control trial of a short course of aspirin and dipyridamole (Persantin) for femorodistal grafts. *Br J Surg.* 1987;74:246–248.
8. Franks PJ, Sian M, Kenchington GF, et al. Aspirin usage and its influence on femoro-popliteal vein graft patency. The Femoropopliteal Bypass Trial Participants. *Eur J Vasc Surg.* 1992;6:185–188.
9. Kohler TR, Kaufman JL, Kacoyanis G, et al. Effect of aspirin and dipyridamole on the patency of lower extremity bypass grafts. *Surgery.* 1984;96:462–466.
10. McCollum C, Alexander C, Kenchington G, et al. Antiplatelet drugs in femoropopliteal vein bypasses: a multicenter trial. *J Vasc Surg.* 1991;13:150–162.

11. Tangelder M, Lawson JA, Algra A, et al. Systematic review of randomized controlled trials of aspirin and oral anticoagulants in the prevention of graft occlusion and ischemic events after infrainguinal bypass surgery. *J Vasc Surg.* 1999;30:701–709.

12. Antiplatelet Trialists' Collaboration. Collaborative overview of randomized trials of antiplatelet therapy-II: maintenance of vascular graft or arterial patency by antiplatelet therapy. *Br Med J.* 1994;308:159–168.

13. Becquemin J. Effect of ticlodipine on the long-term patency of saphenous-vein bypass grafts in the legs. *N Engl J Med.* 1997;337:1726–1731.

14. Rutherford RB, Jones DN, Bergentz S, et al. The efficacy of dextran 40 in preventing early postoperative thrombosis following difficult lower extremity bypass. *J Vasc Surg.* 1984;1:765–772.

15. CAPRIE Steering Committee. A randomized, blinded, trial of clopidogrel versus aspirin in patients at risk of ischemic events (CAPRIE). *Lancet.* 1996;348:1329–1339.

16. Bhatt DL, Chew DP, Hirsch AT, et al. Superiority of clopidogrel versus aspirin in patients with prior cardiac surgery. *Circulation.* 2001;103:363–368.

17. Duran E, Canbaz S, Ege T, et al. Aspirin versus clopidogrel for synthetic graft patency after peripheral arterial bypass grafting. *Platelets.* 2001;12:503–504.

18. Flinn WR, Rohrer MJ, Yao JST, et al. Improved long-term patency of infragenicular polytetrafluoroethylene grafts. *J Vasc Surg.* 1988;7:685–690.

19. Sarac TP, Huber TS, Back MR, et al. Warfarin improves the outcome of infrainguinal vein bypass grafting at high risk for failure. *J Vasc Surg.* 1998;28:446–457.

20. Dutch Bypass Oral Anticoagulants or Aspirin (BOA) Study Group. Efficacy of oral anticoagulants compared with aspirin after infrainguinal bypass surgery (The Dutch Bypass Oral Anticoagulants or Aspirin study): a randomized trial. *Lancet.* 2000;355:346–351.

21. Kretschmer G, Herbst F, Prager M, et al. A decade of oral anticoagulant treatment to maintain autologous vein grafts for femoropopliteal atherosclerosis. *Arch Surg.* 1992;127:1112–1115.

22. Arfvidsson B, Lundgren F, Drott C, et al. Influence of coumarin treatment on patency and limb salvage after peripheral arterial reconstructive surgery. *Am J Surg.* 1990;159:556–560.

23. Johnson WC, Williford WO. Benefits, morbidity, and mortality associated with long-term administration of oral anticoagulant therapy to patients with peripheral arterial bypass procedures: a prospective randomized study. *J Vasc Surg.* 2002;35:413–421.

24. Jackson MR, Belott TP, Dickason T, et al. The consequences of a failed femoropopliteal bypass: comparison of saphenous vein and PTFE grafts. *J Vasc Surg.* 2000;32:498–505.

25. Jackson MR, Johnson WC, Williford WO, et al. The effect of anticoagulation therapy and graft selection on the ischemic consequences of femoropopliteal bypass graft occlusion: results from a multicenter randomized clinical trial. *J Vasc Surg.* 2002;35:292–298.

26. Atrial Fibrillation Investigators. Risk factors for stroke and efficacy of antithrombotic therapy in atrial fibrillation: analysis of pooled data from five randomized controlled trials. *Arch Intern Med.* 1994;154:1449–1457.

27. Beyth RJ. Management of haemorrhagic complications associated with oral anticoagulant treatment. *Expert Opin Drug Saf.* 2002;1:129–136.

28. Edmondson RA, Cohen AT, Das SK, et al. Low-molecular weight heparin versus aspirin and dipyridamole after femoropopliteal bypass grafting. *Lancet.* 1994;344:914–918.

29. Samama CM, Gigou F, Ill P. Low-molecular-weight heparin vs. unfractionated heparin in femorodistal reconstructive surgery: a multicenter open randomized study. *Ann Vasc Surg.* 1995;9(Suppl):S45–S53.

30. Swedenborg J, Nydahl S, Egberg N. Low molecular mass heparin instead of unfractionated heparin during infrainguinal bypass surgery. *Eur J Vasc Endovasc Surg.* 1996;11:59–64.

31. Rossouw JE. Lipid-lowering interventions in angiographic trials. *Am J Cardiol.* 1995;76:86c–92c.

32. Ehsan A, Mann MJ, Dell'Acqua G, et al. Long-term stabilization of vein graft wall architecture and prolonged resistance to experimental atherosclerosis after E2F decoy oligonucleotide gene therapy. *J Thorac Cardiovasc Surg.* 2001;121:714–722.

33. Mann MJ, Whittemore AD, Donaldson MC, et al. Ex-vivo gene therapy of human vascular bypass grafts with E2F decoy: the PREVENT single center, randomized, controlled trial. *Lancet.* 1999;354:1493–1498.

34. Ehsan A, Mann MJ, Dell'Acqua G, et al. Endothelial healing in vein grafts: proliferative burst unimpaired by genetic therapy of neointimal disease. *Circulation.* 2002;105:1686–1692.

35. Hanson SR, Harker LA. Effects of platelet-modifying drugs on arterial thromboembolism in baboons. *J Clin Invest.* 1985;75:1591–1599.

Infrainguinal Bypass in Patients with Renal Failure

26

John C. Lantis, II   Michael S. Conte

End-stage renal disease (ESRD), defined as a lack of native renal function that requires renal replacement therapy (hemodialysis, peritoneal dialysis, or renal transplantation), is undergoing a dramatic increase in prevalence. Critical limb ischemia (CLI) secondary to the severe arteriopathy that accompanies ESRD has therefore become a growing problem for the vascular surgeon. As evidence of this trend, the proportion of ESRD patients among all infrainguinal bypass grafts (IBG) performed at one tertiary care institution rose dramatically from 2% (1978 through 1992) to 14% (1993 through 1997) over the last 2 decades.[1] Historically, ESRD patients with CLI have presented a major surgical challenge manifested by increased perioperative mortality, reduced long-term survival, diminished graft patency, and inferior limb salvage following arterial reconstruction. In this review, we will summarize the contemporary results of lower extremity bypass in this challenging patient group, outline our management strategy, and explore the evolving role of endovascular interventions.

EPIDEMIOLOGY

In 2001, the number of ESRD patients in the United States was 398,553, of whom 94,905 patients required renal replacement therapy for the first time.[2] This population, of whom approximately one third are diabetic,

is expected to roughly double by 2010.[3] With ongoing improvements in the treatment of hypertension and coronary artery disease, more diabetic patients are developing ESRD as a late complication.[4] Furthermore, since the atherosclerotic burden in patients with type 2 diabetes mellitus (DM) is high at the outset, it may be expected that the growing diabetic fraction of the ESRD population will have a high incidence of peripheral vascular complications.[5]

The population of patients with type 2 DM and ESRD continues to exhibit a markedly reduced life expectancy, with a reported 5-year survival rate of 25% in all age categories as of 1999. The 5-year survival rate ranges from 51% for the group that begins renal replacement therapy secondary to diabetes at ages 40 to 49, and drops to 8% for those beginning renal replacement therapy after 80 years of age.[2] These sobering statistics provide an important framework for clinical decision making.

ETIOLOGY

There is a consensus among physicians specializing in vascular disease that lower extremity atherosclerosis associated with chronic renal failure is unique in its pattern and poor response to standard therapy. While some of the distribution of this disease mimics the lower leg arterial pathology seen in DM, the occlusive disease in ESRD

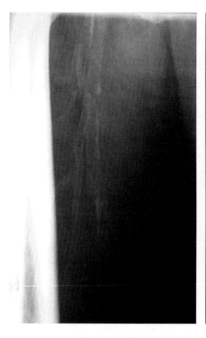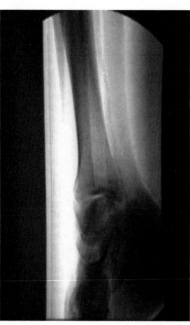

Figure 26-1 Lower extremity radiographs in patients with limb ischemia and end-stage renal disease (ESRD) demonstrate extensive calcification of the deep and superficial femoral (**left panel**) as well as the posterior tibial (**right panel**) arteries.

appears to involve the pedal vasculature more extensively and does not respond to revascularization as successfully. The arteriopathy of ESRD is accompanied by calcification of the media of arteries of all sizes, with a marked predilection for the infrageniculate vessels (Fig. 26-1).

This incredibly problematic form of arteriosclerosis may exist for several interrelated reasons. These include DM, uremia, hyperlipidemia, hypertension, and elevated homocystine levels, among other reasons. The well-defined arteriosclerotic risk factors of DM and hypertension are present in nearly 100% of the patients with ESRD requiring IBG. These atherogenic factors are augmented by the expression of uremic dyslipidemia: Elevated cholesterol, lipoprotein A, and triglycerides, with lowered high density lipoprotein (HDL) levels. The increased oxidation of low density lipoprotein (LDL) in uremia further adds to this process.[6,7] In addition to this profile, homocysteine, an independent risk factor for atherosclerosis, is consistently elevated in patients with ESRD, especially while on hemodialysis.[8,9] The medial calcinosis may be accelerated by secondary hyperparathyroidism, and chronic endothelial activation and dysfunction have been described in ESRD.[10]

OUTCOMES OF LOWER EXTREMITY REVASCULARIZATION IN END-STAGE RENAL DISEASE PATIENTS

Perioperative Mortality, Morbidity, and Long-term Survival

The aggressive atherosclerotic pathology observed in ESRD affects not only the distal arterial tree but the coronary vasculature as well. Approximately half of all deaths in patients with ESRD are cardiac related.[2,11] The significant prevalence of cardiac disease weighs heavily in clinical decision making in ESRD patients with critical limb ischemia, elevating the surgical risk and reducing the potential long-term benefits of limb salvage. A recent large, single-institution study of IBG in ESRD patients reported the following perioperative complication rates: Congestive heart failure, 2%; myocardial infarction, 3%; arrhythmia, 5%; and wound infection, 10%.[12] Historically, operative mortality and 2-year survival rates reported in the literature ranged from 0% to 27% (mean 9%) and 32% to 62% (mean 49%), respectively, for ESRD patients undergoing IBG.[13] One author reported no ESRD patients being alive with a salvaged limb 4 months after revascularization.[11] In a review of data from the Department of Veterans Affairs' National Surgical Quality Improvement Program (NSQIP), O'Hare et al.[14] noted a significantly increased perioperative mortality (10%) and incidence of cardiovascular complications in dialysis patients following IBG. ESRD has also been identified as an independent predictor of long-term mortality following IBG in patients with tissue loss.[15] While these statistics have led some authors to propose primary amputation as a safer alternative to arterial reconstruction in the ESRD patient, others have shown similar operative mortality figures for major amputation in this cohort.[16]

In our most recent reported experience,[13] the perioperative mortality for ESRD patients ($n = 60$) who underwent IBG was 1.3%, not significantly different from that observed in patients without renal failure. In addition, the 2- and 4-year survival rates in the ESRD group were 65% and 51%, respectively, consistent with the best outcomes reported by others[17] and markedly improved in comparison to a historical series from our institution.[18] In another recent study comparing a similar group of patients with large lower extremity tissue defects that underwent revascularization versus those with adequate blood supply, the 3-year survival for the group was 49%; 79% of wounds healed, and an 89% limb salvage rate was reported when adequate blood supply was combined with the aggressive use of amputations and soft-tissue transfers.[19] These results suggest that the risk-to-benefit ratio for performing arterial reconstruction in the ESRD patient may be somewhat more favorable than it has generally been portrayed to be.

Graft Patency and Limb Salvage

Modern techniques of arterial reconstruction have resulted in improved outcomes for patients with critical limb ischemia. However, the subset of patients with dialysis-dependent ESRD continues to represent one of the more difficult vascular surgical challenges. A recent review of published reports noted an early graft thrombosis rate of 14% and a >14% amputation rate with a functioning graft.[11] It has long been recognized that ESRD patients are unique among the population of patients who undergo IBG, consistently experiencing a long-term limb salvage rate that is inferior to graft patency.[16,20,21] In recent years, there have been several reports regarding the use of IBG for limb salvage in patients with ESRD (Table 26-1).[12-16,21-25] A recent meta-analysis reviewing 16 studies of IBG in patients with ESRD from 1987 to 2000 showed promising, if not ideal, outcomes. The pooled results demonstrated an average graft patency rate of 74%, limb salvage rate of 73%, and patient survival of 42% at 2 years.[26]

Recently, we reported on a series of 60 patients with ESRD undergoing IBG ($n = 78$ procedures) for limb salvage at our institution.[13] These revascularizations were performed for rest pain (15%), ulceration (54%), or gangrene (31%), and the majority (94%) were primary bypasses. All reconstructions were performed exclusively with autogenous vein, including nonreversed greater saphenous vein (NRGSV) (51%), in situ greater saphenous vein (GSV) (18%), reversed GSV (16%), spliced vein (9%), arm (4%), and lesser saphenous vein (2%) conduits. Distal inflow sites, including the proximal superficial femoral artery (26% vs. 12%) and the above-knee popliteal artery (23% vs. 13%), were used more frequently in patients with ESRD, as compared to a contemporaneous control group with normal renal function. Distal anastomoses were to tibial or pedal arteries in 90%, with the anterior tibial (27% vs. 15%) and the dorsalis pedis (24% vs. 9%) arteries more commonly employed in ESRD patients versus controls. This pattern of graft configurations has been observed by other authors.[24]

In our experience, primary (60%) and secondary (86%) graft patency in the ESRD cohort at 4 years was not significantly different from controls (Figs. 26-2 and 26-3). Unfortunately, 13% of patients with patent grafts still went on to undergo a major (transtibial or above) amputation, resulting in a 77% limb salvage rate at 4 years, which, while quite encouraging, was significantly less than that observed in the control population (92%) (Fig. 26-4).

More recently, a larger single institution experience in ESRD patients was published from the Beth Israel Deaconess Medical Center.[12] In a cohort of 146 ESRD patients (171 limbs), 92% had diabetes and 91% presented with tissue loss; secondary patency rates were 85% at 1 year and 68% at 3 years. The 3-year limb salvage rate was 80%. However, the overall patient survival

TABLE 26-1

RESULTS FROM SELECTED SERIES OF INFRAINGUINAL BYPASS GRAFTS IN END-STAGE RENAL DISEASE PATIENTS

Author, Year	Limbs/ Patients	Periop. Mortality	Follow-up Duration	Patency	Limb Salvage	Patient Survival
Korn, 2000[22]	31/23	—	5 y	79% secondary	59% (2 y)	47% (2 y)
Lantis, 2001[13]	78/60	1.3%	4 y	86% secondary	77%	51%
Cox, 2001[23]	78/63	—	3 y	48% secondary	62%	55% (5 y)
Myerson, 2001[24]	82/64	4.9%	3 y	67% secondary	59%	60%
Biancari, 2002[25]	25/21	—	2 y	74%	85%	23%
Ramdev, 2002[12]	177/146	3%	3 y	68% secondary	80%	18%
Kimura, 2003[27]	33/22	18%	2 y	85% secondary	83%	45%

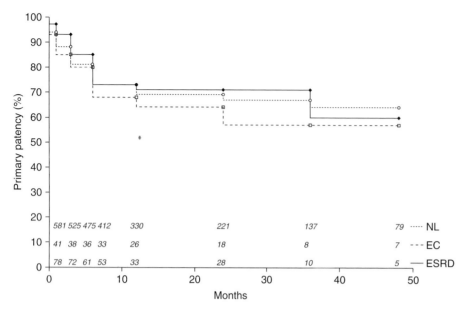

Figure 26-2 Primary graft patency for autogenous infrainguinal bypass grafts (IBG) performed at a single institution (1993 to 1999) by life table method. Patency of three contemporaneous groups are illustrated: Normal renal function (*NL*; serum creatinine ≤1.2 mg per dL; n = 581), elevated creatinine (*EC*; serum creatinine >1.2 mg per dL; n = 41), and end-stage renal disease (ESRD; n = 78). (From Lantis JC II, Conte MS, Belkin M, et al. Infrainguinal bypass grafting in patients with end-stage renal disease: improving outcomes? *J Vasc Surg*. 2001;33:

rate was 60% at 1 year, 18% at 3 years, and only 5% of the entire cohort was alive at 5 years.

Predictors of Poor Outcome

As noted, diminished graft patency and a disturbing incidence of limb loss despite a functioning graft (hemodynamic failure) have been repeatedly observed in ESRD patients.[20] Other investigators have identified several predictors of adverse outcome in this population, including preoperative foot infection,[28] poor functional status,[29] tobacco abuse,[28] >2 cm ischemic ulceration,[30] heel necrosis >4 cm,[28] forefoot gangrene,[29] preoperative toe pressures <20 mm HG,

pedal angiographic resistance score of >2.5 (3.0 representing no named pedal arteries), peritoneal dialysis,[22] number of years on dialysis, age,[12] and distal vessels with only collateral outflow (Society for Vascular Surgery and International Society for Cardiovascular Surgery [SVS/ISCVS] runoff score = 10).[25]

In reviewing our recent experience, we also attempted to identify clinical variables associated with poor outcome following IBG in ESRD patients.[13] Although other investigators have found that amputation despite a patent bypass was more common in patients with poor runoff scores,[31] runoff scores were not predictive of adverse outcomes in our series. Furthermore, age, tobacco use, type of conduit used, or use of an isolated

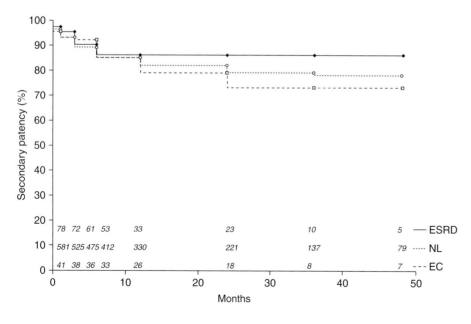

Figure 26-3 Cumulative secondary patency for autogenous infrainguinal bypass grafts (IBG) performed at a single institution (1993 to 1999), grouped by renal functional status. Patency of three contemporaneous groups are illustrated: Normal renal function (*NL*; serum creatinine ≤1.2 mg per dL; n = 581), elevated creatinine (*EC*; serum creatinine >1.2 mg per dL; n = 41), and end-stage renal disease (ESRD; n = 78). (From Lantis JC II, Conte MS, Belkin M, et al. Infrainguinal bypass grafting in patients with end-stage renal disease: improving outcomes? *J Vasc Surg*. 2001;33:1171–1178, with permission.)

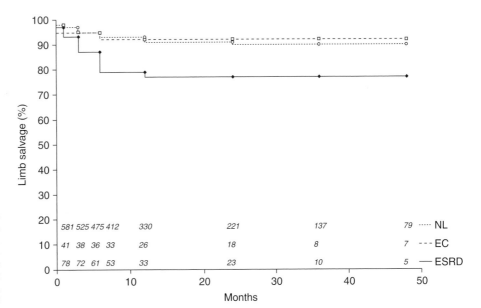

Figure 26-4 Cumulative limb salvage for a consecutive series of autogenous infrainguinal bypass grafts (IBG) at a single institution (1993 to 1999), grouped by renal functional status. Patency of three contemporaneous groups are illustrated: Normal renal function (*NL*; serum creatinine ≤1.2 mg per dL; *n* = 581), elevated creatinine (*EC*; serum creatinine >1.2 mg per dL; *n* = 41), and end-stage renal disease (*ESRD*; *n* = 78). (From Lantis JC II, Conte MS, Belkin M, et al. Infrainguinal bypass grafting in patients with end-stage renal disease: improving outcomes? *J Vasc Surg.* 2001;33:1171–1178, with permission.)

anterior tibial target vessel were also not predictive of graft failure or limb loss.

In our analysis, the only significant predictor of limb loss despite a patent graft in ESRD patients was the presence of extensive heel necrosis (>4-cm diameter). Notably, the majority of patients with smaller heel lesions went on to complete healing following IBG, even those with grafts that did not provide direct outflow to the posterior circulation. This observation is supported by previous studies demonstrating that non-direct flow bypasses in patients without ESRD will heal tissue loss.[32]

Renal Transplantation

The improvement in the quality of life that is conveyed to the ESRD patient that undergoes renal transplantation is extended to the area of limb salvage. Patients who undergo renal transplantation have better outcomes when undergoing IBG than patients with ESRD who have not been transplanted. In one series, the major complication rate in kidney transplant recipients who underwent IBG was 12%, with a 30-day mortality rate of 1.3%.[33] Most impressively, the 1-year survival was 93% and the 5-year survival was 67% for this group. Limb salvage was 78% at 5 years, with a primary patency of 44%. These results were obtained in a group that had working renal grafts in place at the time of bypass.

Quality of Life

The likelihood of preserving independent function and quality of life with successful limb salvage surgery is a critical aspect of the preoperative clinical assessment. A report assessing Quality of Life scores in 57 patients

with ESRD who underwent IBG noted that these patients had significantly lower scores at both 30 days and 1 year than normal (NL) patients undergoing IBG.[34] Other recently published series have indicated that only 31% to 21% of patients with ESRD who underwent IBG were ambulating at 1 year.[34,35] In one series, this number has been noted to decrease to 6% walking independently at 2 years. Others have noted a 1.72-year median survival in ESRD patients undergoing IBG; 50% of the group experienced limb loss at 1.24 years from the time of IBG.[36] However, a more optimistic study documented that of the patients who were alive at 1-year follow-up, 73% were independently ambulating and 27% were bound to a wheelchair or bed. Of this group, 82% of the patients were very satisfied with the salvage attempt, and this included a cohort that underwent extensive tissue reconstruction.[19] One investigator using Markov decision analysis has shown a measurable increase in the expected quality-adjusted life years for ESRD patients with tissue loss who undergo IBG.[23] The average hospital cost of this intervention has been estimated to be $44,000 per year of limb salvage.[22]

The question remains, is revascularization in the ESRD patient with CLI worthwhile? Clearly the approach must be individualized to each patient's comorbidities and expectations. In addition, the quality of life and cost of revascularization must be compared with the very limited rehabilitation potential for those undergoing major limb amputation among this severely debilitated population. Given that perioperative mortality rates for IBG appear no greater than those associated with major amputation, it appears reasonable to attempt revascularization as a primary approach in the majority of patients who feel strongly about limb preservation.

CURRENT APPROACH TO CRITICAL LIMB ISCHEMIA IN END-STAGE RENAL DISEASE

Patient Evaluation

On the basis of our most recent experience, we have taken a moderately aggressive approach to offering IBG for limb salvage in patients with ESRD. The clinical decision making in this setting requires a careful, individualized evaluation of the potential risks and benefits. Knowledge of their current quality of life and expectations weighs heavily into the treatment decisions. For those who are more debilitated and inactive, or when tissue necrosis is extensive, primary amputation is recommended. Conversely, motivated functional patients on chronic dialysis therapy should be offered attempts at limb salvage if they are otherwise stable medically and there are good anatomic options for revascularization.

Our preoperative evaluation includes a cardiac risk assessment focusing on careful clinical review, with selective application of stress testing or cardiac catheterization. Pharmacotherapy with β-adrenergic blocking agents for control of heart rate in the perioperative period is the cornerstone of medical management. Antiplatelet therapy, generally using aspirin, is also standard. In order to minimize hemodynamic or electrolyte derangement, we attempt to coordinate hemodialysis treatments so that preoperative and postoperative dialysis sessions are both within 24 hours of surgery.

Perhaps more than any other subgroup of patients with peripheral vascular disease, diabetics with ESRD tolerate infection poorly and are prone to rapid acceleration of local sepsis in the foot. Even seemingly minor ulcerations or skin infections require aggressive treatment with surgical debridement, antibiotics, and close surveillance of wounds. When extensive debridement or multiple toe amputations are required to control infection, an assessment of the viability of remaining tissue and the likelihood of salvage of a functional foot is critical before proceeding with further attempts at vascular reconstruction.

For imaging of the vascular anatomy in these patients, we continue to prefer digital subtraction angiography, which facilitates our ability to choose the best distal outflow tract. If more than one infrageniculate vessel is visualized, then we try to determine the vessel that appears to fill the pedal arch. If presented with two equal-appearing target vessels, the one with the better runoff to the foot should be chosen.

When no adequate vessel is visualized on angiography, other imaging techniques may be of value. We have used magnetic resonance angiography (MRA) with gadolinium or time-of-flight techniques, as well as duplex ultrasound to help visualize target vessels in the distal calf or foot. On occasion, surgical exploration of the distal vessel is undertaken in the absence of a definable target on imaging, especially when a pedal Doppler signal is present. It is not unreasonable to take the patient with tissue loss of the foot to the operating room for exploration with an understanding that if the target vessel is unusable, then a primary major amputation will be performed.

Techniques of Revascularization

In performing infrainguinal bypass grafts in patients with ESRD, conduit usage, vessel handling, and wound management are issues requiring particular attention. For all IBG, standard surgical techniques, including loupe magnification and completion arteriography, are employed. We employ Duplex ultrasound for vein mapping and intraoperative completion imaging as well. The patients undergo general or regional anesthesia. Using a two-team approach, vein harvesting and arterial exposures can be performed simultaneously, and complex operations, including those requiring spliced vein grafts, can be executed more expeditiously.

Our preference for all infrainguinal revascularizations, particularly in the context of limb salvage, is to complete the bypass graft entirely with autogenous vein conduit. The use of prosthetic grafts for IBG in the ESRD patient appears to be of little utility due to high rates of early occlusion. Although our group has not had to resort to this technique, other surgeons report a 2-year patency of 27% with prosthetic versus a 3-year patency rate of 67% with autogenous vein in these patients.[24] A study reviewing 33 IBGs in 28 limbs demonstrated that significantly poorer outcomes were related to attempts at limb salvage with nonautogenous conduit.[27]

Venous conduit of a minimum diameter of 3.5 mm, without discernible areas of phlebosclerosis, is utilized even if this means excising segments and performing a spliced vein graft. More than any other single factor, the quality of the venous conduit is of primary import in achieving a successful outcome with distal bypass in these challenging patients. In our experience, the use of contralateral saphenous vein or spliced vein grafts in patients without adequate ipsilateral GSV has been associated with excellent outcomes.[37,38] We believe that a flexible approach is important to make optimal use of available vein sources, particularly in the absence of ipsilateral GSV. Our preference has been to optimize the size-match between the graft and the native vessels at both the proximal and distal anastomoses, and in spliced-vein bypass, to create a gradual taper of the composite graft. To prepare nonreversed segments, valves are lysed under distension using a Mills valvulotome. Venovenostomies are performed using beveled, end-to-end anastomoses with fine polypropylene suture. Obviously, the patient undergoing hemodialysis is less likely to have an available arm vein. In the face of a well-functioning arteriovenous fistula (AVF), the use of contralateral arm vein may be cautiously considered, but we have generally avoided it to preserve alternative sites for dialysis access in the future.

Proximal and distal arterial exposures are performed via standard approaches. In the diabetic population in particular, we have found great utility in so-called distal origin grafts (DOGs), where the superficial femoral or popliteal artery serves as the inflow site.[39] In our experience, the long-term performance of DOGs is excellent when the proximal femoral segment is minimally diseased. We will often employ the proximal GSV, harvested from the groin down and oriented in a nonreversed fashion, to complete these grafts. The advantage of translocating the proximal vein down the leg for a DOG is that it avoids a long harvest incision in the more ischemic distal calf, allowing the bypass to be tunneled under intact skin and soft tissue. This helps to avoid difficult wound complications in this high-risk population. We generally prefer subcutaneous positioning of grafts to facilitate ultrasound surveillance

and revisions, but deeper tunnels are not infrequently employed in this patient group to avoid areas of potential skin breakdown or infection.

In the patient with ESRD, hemostatic control and suturing of the distal vessel can be difficult secondary to medial calcinosis. In addition, choosing the best site for the anastomosis can be troublesome. We correlate the digital subtraction angiogram with the vessel and try to avoid areas of extensive calcification where possible. The vessel can also be palpated with a finger or a forcep against a right angle to find the softest spot at which to create the distal anastomosis. Techniques to facilitate the clamping and suturing of calcified vessels, such as gentle crushing of circumferential calcium or limited endarterectomy, are occasionally employed and usually technically successful. Fine metal spring clamps (Yasergil or Bulldog) may be employed for hemostatic control of the distal vessel. Pneumatic tourniquets may be quite useful, depending on the extensiveness of the proximal artery calcification; often they must be supplemented by one of the other techniques to obtain a clear field (Fig. 26-5). We

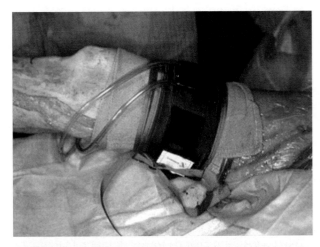
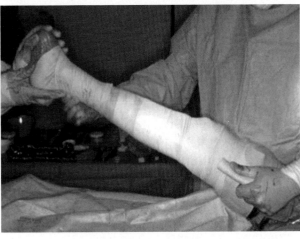
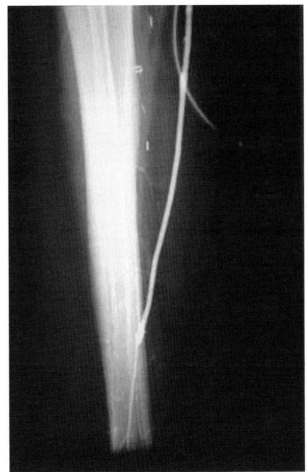

Figure 26-5 Tibial bypass in the end-stage renal disease (ESRD) patient. Use of pneumatic tourniquet and Esmarch bandage to achieve vascular control is illustrated on the **left**. Intraoperative angiogram (**right**) demonstrates a patent saphenous vein bypass to the posterior tibial artery.

have also used Fogarty embolectomy balloons inflated within the lumen of the vessel. Proximal anastomoses are completed first, and after the graft is carefully passed through any tunnels, it is allowed to fill under arterial pressure, and antegrade flow is checked. At this point, the conduit is cut to length on a bevel appropriate for the target vessel. The heel of the vein is then parachuted into place and, in vessels <2 mm, the toe is often parachuted into place. Prior to completion of the anastomosis, the distal outflow tract is checked for patency with a fine olive-tipped coronary probe. If necessary, hemostasis is augmented with topical thrombin and Gel-foam.

Endovascular Therapy

Owing to the anatomic pattern of disease, percutaneous interventions have a limited role in ESRD patients with advanced peripheral atherosclerosis. Angioplasty or stenting of inflow disease at the aortoiliac level is employed when suitable lesions with a significant pressure gradient are identified. In addition, angioplasty of focal stenoses within the superficial femoral or even popliteal segments is sometimes employed to allow for a more distal inflow site for bypass, particularly in patients who have limited autogenous conduit. Rarely, a patient with rest pain or limited tissue loss will have diseased but continuous single vessel runoff, with a series of focal lesions that are potentially amenable to angioplasty. This approach may be considered in patients with high surgical risk or lacking adequate vein, but the success rates and durability appear limited in our anecdotal experience.

Evolving catheter technology has spawned a growing interest in percutaneous transluminal angioplasty (PTA) as a treatment modality for CLI.[40] In many cases, the high-risk nature of ESRD patients with tissue loss makes them attractive candidates for less invasive approaches to revascularization. However, the pathophysiology of the disease process in this population may severely limit the applicability of endovascular therapies for the ESRD patient with possible limb loss. These adverse factors include the volume and infrageniculate location of disease, the high penetrance of diabetes, the highly calcified vessels, the poor runoff, and the degree of tissue loss associated with the arteriopathy of renal failure. Each of these factors has been independently identified as indicators of poor outcome for attempted endovascular revascularization of the lower limb.[41] At the present time, we would consider an endovascular approach as a primary option in patients with favorable anatomy, but our feeling is that extensive occlusions of the popliteal and tibial arteries are most effectively treated with surgical bypass to a suitable outflow vessel.

To date, there are relatively few reports looking at the treatment of CLI with an endovascular approach, and none specifically at limb salvage in ESRD.[25] Limb salvage at early end points, <1 year, has been reported in a small series using endovascular interventions.[42] Technical success can be achieved as frequently as 90% of the time, with an 8-month limb salvage rate of 75%. Infragenicular subintimal angioplasty has been associated with an 86% technical success rate and an 80% clinical success rate, with 3-year limb salvage rates of 84%.[43] However, this study did not subdivide patients with ESRD, but patients with DM had a significantly higher failure rate than those without DM. Other retrospective studies of infrainguinal PTA for limb salvage have demonstrated that the need for repeat procedures is high at 1.9 invasive procedures per critically ischemic limb.[44] The same review exhibited a 5-year limb salvage rate of 60%, but a corresponding life with limb rate of 18%. Reports of combination endovascular therapy, including debulking procedures, have looked at long limb revascularization for gangrene, fair results have been noted when bypass is added for those who fail PTA alone.[45] However, these have not included ESRD patients in any analyzable numbers.

In our limited experience with PTA for limb salvage, the anatomic distribution and volume of disease appear to be more important than the presence of ESRD, as we have salvaged several limbs in the ESRD population when the intervention was limited to the superficial femoral artery or above-knee popliteal artery. Similar efficacy has been noted in the non-ESRD population when there are fewer diseased distal vessels. These therapies should be viewed as complementary, and not necessarily competitive, to surgical revascularization. Further developments in minimally invasive debulking technology may augment endovascular approaches in this very difficult population.

Wound Management

When closing incisions in the diabetic ESRD patient, extreme care must be exercised due to their impaired wound-healing capacity. Meticulous hemostasis and careful layered closures of subcutaneous tissue are performed. Incisions in the lower calf and foot, particularly those overlying the graft, are generally closed using vertical mattress nylon sutures for skin. When necessary, concomitant foot debridement or toe amputations should be carried out at the completion of the bypass operation, which in this population is necessary 50% of the time. Tissue should be cut back to healthy, bleeding tissue. For the heel ulcer, this may require partial or near complete calcanectomy, or open transmetatarsal amputation for the forefoot. For large or complex wounds that are clean but not readily closable, we have often employed the Vacuum Assisted Closure device (KCI, Inc.) on the wound in the operating room.[46] For lesser wounds and amputations, in the absence of surrounding sepsis, primary closure should be explored as open wounds generally heal quite slowly in the ESRD patient. Attempts at local rotational and advancement flaps are warranted and can facilitate primary closure. In one review of 71 wounds in this population, the average time to wound healing among a group that required revascularization was 79 days. The overall complication rate in this population was 43%.[19]

CONCLUSION

It is clear from epidemiologic evidence that a growing proportion of the patients requiring IBG for limb salvage will suffer from ESRD and DM. Recent surgical series demonstrate that good to excellent perioperative mortality, graft patency, and limb salvage are possible in carefully selected patients with ESRD. However, overall survival remains limited, and careful clinical decision making is required to maximize the opportunity for functional benefit. Certain technical aspects, such as the manipulation of calcified arteries and wound management, are uniquely difficult in ESRD. Nonetheless, the available evidence suggests that the postimplantation biology of the vein graft per se is similar to that of a non-ESRD population. The role for endovascular therapy in this population remains to be defined, though at present, the limited data available concerning infragenicular PTA would indicate that it has very limited application in the ESRD patient. Continued improvements in technology may make these techniques more widely applicable.

Novel methods to promote wound healing in the ESRD patient need to be developed to improve the chances for successful limb preservation. Such approaches may include innovative methods of antibiotic delivery, tissue debridement, tissue coverage, and modulation of growth factors. The use of antibiotic beads, pulse irrigation at the bedside, artificial skin substitutes, and anabolic steroids are all methods already being investigated. Although the technical success in this population is high, the overall outcome analysis remains poor with a median survival of approximately 2 years.

In conclusion, our experience continues to support an attempt at IBG for limb salvage in carefully selected ESRD patients presenting with CLI that is not complicated by one of the following: Unsalvageable wet or dry gangrene of the foot, overwhelming patient comorbidity, fixed contracture of the knee, or a level of advanced debility such that the patient would be unlikely to benefit from limb preservation.

REFERENCES

1. Conte MS, Belkin M, Upchurch GR, et al. Impact of increasing comorbidity on infrainguinal reconstruction: a 20 year perspective. *Ann Surg.* 2001;233:445–452.

2. Renal Data System. *USRDS 2003 annual data report.* Bethesda, Md: National Institute of Diabetes and Digestive and Kidney Diseases; 2003.

3. Abt Associates, Ad Hoc Committee on Nephrology Manpower Needs. Estimated workforce and training requirements for nephrologists through the year 2010. *J Am Soc Nephrol.* 1997;8:S1–32.

4. Ritz E, Stefanski A. Diabetic nephropathy in type II diabetes. *Am J Kidney Dis.* 1996;27:167–194.

5. Luke RG. Chronic renal failure—a vasculopathic state. *N Engl J Med.* 1998;339:841–843.

6. Maggi E, Bellazzi R, Falaschi F, et al. Enhanced LDL oxidation in uremic patients: an additional mechanism for accelerated atherosclerosis? *Kidney Int.* 1994;45:876–883.

7. Becker BN, Himmelfarb J, Henrich WL, et al. Reassessing the cardiac risk profile in chronic hemodialysis patients: a hypothesis on the role of oxidant stress and other non-traditional cardiac risk factors. *J Am Soc Nephrol.* 1997;8:475–486.

8. Jungers P, Chauveau P, Bandin O, et al. Hyperhomocysteinemia in association with atherosclerotic occlusive arterial accidents in predialysis chronic renal failure patients. *Miner Electrolyte Metab.* 1997;23:170–173.

9. Bachmann J, Tepel M, Raidt H, et al. Hyperhomocysteinemia and the risk for vascular disease in hemodialysis patients. *J Am Soc Nephrol.* 1995;6:121–125.

10. Gris JC, Branger B, Vecina F, et al. Increased cardiovascular risk factors and features of endothelial activation and dysfunction in dialyzed uremic patients. *Kidney Int.* 1994;46:807–813.

11. Dovgan PS, Shepard AD, Nypaver TJ. Critical limb ischemia in patients with end-stage renal disease: do long-term results justify an aggressive surgical approach? In: Gloviczki P, ed. *Perspectives in vascular surgery,* Vol 12:1. New York, NY: Thieme; 2000.

12. Ramdev P, Rayan SS, Sheahan M, et al. A decade experience with infrainguinal revascularization in a dialysis-dependent patient population. *J Vasc Surg.* 2002;36:969–974.

13. Lantis JC, Conte MS, Belkin M, et al. Infrainguinal bypass in patients with end stage renal disease: improving outcomes? *J Vasc Surg.* 2001;33:1171–1178.

14. O'Hare AM, Feinglass J, Sidawy AN, et al. Impact of renal insufficiency on short term morbidity and mortality after lower extremity revascularization: data from the Department of Veterans Affairs' National Surgical Quality Improvement Program. *J Am Soc Nephrol.* 2003;14:1287–1295.

15. Peltonen S, Biancari F, Lindgen L, et al. Outcome of infrainguinal bypass surgery for critical limb ischemia in patients with chronic renal failure. *Eur J Vasc Endovasc Surg.* 1998;15:122–127.

16. Seeger JM, Pretus HA, Carlton LC, et al. Potential predictors of outcome in patients with tissue loss who undergo infrainguinal vein bypass grafting. *J Vasc Surg.* 1999;30:427–435.

17. Dossa CD, Shepard AD, Amos AM, et al. Results of lower extremity amputation in patients with end stage renal disease. *J Vasc Surg.* 1994;20:14–19.

18. Whittemore AD, Donaldson MC, Mannick JA. Infrainguinal reconstruction for patients with chronic renal insufficiency. *J Vasc Surg.* 1993;17:32–41.

19. Attinger CE, Ducic I, Neville RF, et al. The relative roles of aggressive wound care versus revascularization in salvage of the threatened lower extremity in the renal failure diabetic patient. *Plast Reconstr Surg.* 2002;109:1281–1290.

20. Edwards JM, Taylor LM, Porter JM. Limb salvage in end-stage renal disease (ESRD). *Arch Surg.* 1988;123:1164–1168.

21. O'Hare Am, Sidawy AN, Feinglass J, et al. Influence of renal insufficiency on limb loss and mortality after initial lower extremity surgical revascularization. *J Vasc Surg.* 2004;39:709–716.

22. Korn P, Hoenig SJ, Skillman JJ, et al. Is lower extremity revascularization worthwhile in patients with end-stage renal disease? *Surgery.* 2000;128:472–479.

23. Cox MH, Robinson JG, Brothers TE, et al. Contemporary analysis of outcomes following lower extremity bypass in patients with end-stage renal disease. *Ann Vasc Surg.* 2001;15:374–382.

24. Myerson SL, Skelly CL, Curi MA, et al. Long term results justify autogenous infrainguinal bypass grafting in patients with end-stage renal failure. *J Vasc Surg.* 2001;34:27–33.

25. Biancari F, Kantonen I, Matzke S, et al. Infrainguinal endovascular and bypass surgery for critical leg ischemia in patients on long-term dialysis. *Ann Vasc Surg.* 2002;16:210–214.

26. Albers M, Romiti M, Braganca Pereira CA, et al. A meta-analysis of infrainguinal arterial reconstruction in patients with end-stage renal disease. *Eur J Vasc Surg.* 2001;22:294–300.

27. Kimura H, Miyata T, Sato O, et al. Infrainguinal arterial reconstruction for limb salvage in patients with end-stage renal disease. *Eur J Vasc Endovasc Surg.* 2003;25:29–34.

28. Baele HR, Piotrowski JJ, Yuhus J, et al. Infrainguinal bypass in patients with end-stage renal disease. *Surgery.* 1995;117:319–324.

29. Simsir SA, Cabellon A, Kohlman-Trigoboff D, et al. Factors influencing limb salvage and survival after amputation and revascularization in patients with end-stage renal disease. *Am J Surg.* 1995;170:113–117.

30. Leers SA, Reifsnyder T, Delmonte R, et al. Realistic expectations for pedal bypass grafts in patients with end stage renal disease. *J Vasc Surg.* 1998;28:976–983.

31. Desai TR, Meyerson SL, Skelly CL, et al. Patency and limb salvage after infrainguinal bypass with severely compromised ("blind") outflow. *Arch Surg.* 2001;136:635–642.

32. Raftery KB, Belkin M, Mackey WC, et al. Are peroneal artery bypass grafts hemodynamically inferior to other tibial artery bypass grafts? *J Vasc Surg.* 1994;19:964–968.

33. McArthur CS, Sheahan MG, Pomposelli FB Jr, et al. Infrainguinal revascularization after renal transplantation. *J Vasc Surg.* 2003;37:1181–1185.

34. Nicholas GG, Bozorgnia M, Nastasee SA, et al. Infrainguinal bypass in patients with end-stage renal disease: survival and ambulation. *Vasc Surg.* 2000;34:147–155.

35. Albers M, Fratezi A, DeLuccia N. Assessment of quality of life of patients with severe ischemia as a result of infrainguinal arterial occlusive disease. *J Vasc Surg.* 1992;16:54–59.

36. Reddan DN, Marcus RJ, Owen WF Jr, et al. Long-term outcomes of revascularization for peripheral vascular disease in end-stage renal disease patients. *Am J Kidney Dis.* 2001;38:57–63.

37. Chew D, Conte MS, Donaldson MC, et al. Autogenous composite vein bypass for infrainguinal arterial reconstruction. *J Vasc Surg.* 2001;33:259–265.

38. Chew DKW, Owens CD, Belkin M, et al. Bypass in the absence of ipsilateral greater saphenous vein-safety and superiority of the contralateral greater saphenous vein. *J Vasc Surg.* 2002;35:1085–1092.

39. Reed AB, Conte MS, Belkin M, et al. Usefulness of autogenous bypass grafts originating distal to the groin. *J Vasc Surg.* 2002;35:48–55.

40. Nasr MK, McCarthy RJ, Hardman J, et al. The increasing role of percutaneous transluminal angioplasty in the primary management of critical limb ischaemia. *Eur J Vasc Endovasc Surg.* 2002;23:398–403.

41. Clark TW, Groffsky JL, Soulen MC. Predictors of long-term patency after femoropopliteal angioplasty: results from the STAR registry. *J Vasc Interv Radiol.* 2001;12:923–933.

42. Tefera G, Turnipseed W, Tanke T. Limb salvage angioplasty in poor surgical candidates. *Vasc Endovascular Surg.* 2003;37:99–104.

43. Ingle H, Nasim A, Bolia A, et al. Subintimal angioplasty of isolated infragenicular vessels in lower limb ischemia: long term results. *J Endovasc Ther.* 2002;9:411–416.

44. Jamsen T, Manninen H, Tulla H, et al. The final outcome of primary infrainguinal percutaneous transluminal angioplasty in 100 consecutive patients with chronic critical limb ischemia. *J Vasc Interv Radiol.* 2002;13:455–463.

45. Gray BH, Laird JR, Ansel GM, et al. Complex endovascular treatment for critical limb ischemia in poor surgical candidates: a pilot study. *J Endovasc Ther.* 2002;9:599–604.

46. Argenta LC, Morykwas MJ. Vacuum-assisted closure: a new method for wound control and treatment-clinical experience. *Ann Plast Surg.* 1997;38:563–576.

Infrapopliteal Bypass Following Proximal Angioplasty

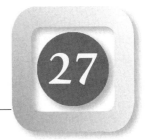

Christopher J. Abularrage   **Jonathan M. Weiswasser**
Paul W. White   **Subodh Arora**   **Anton N. Sidawy**

DeBakey et al.[1] described symptomatic arterial insufficiency as a general and time-dependent process that begins in the coronary circulation and extends to the peripheral and cerebrovascular beds. Further descriptions of peripheral vascular disease patterns divide location of disease into proximal aortoiliac (type I) and distal infrainguinal disease (type II). Typical patients suffering from lower extremity peripheral vascular disease will present with one of these patterns, the former being more frequent in smokers and the latter more common in people with diabetes. Type I disease has been shown to progress to multilevel, or type III, disease in 13% to 42% of patients.[2,3] Patients with multilevel disease tend to be older and more morbid and symptomatic than patients with single-level disease.[4] Sixty-five percent of patients requiring lower extremity revascularization will have multilevel disease.[5] This is especially true of the diabetic population who, along with the typical infragenicular distribution of atherosclerotic disease, will frequently have inflow disease as well.

In the setting of often severe comorbidity, simultaneous revascularization of both the inflow and outflow circulation has been viewed with caution given the magnitude of the procedure. Recent advances in endovascular therapy and minimally invasive techniques have allowed for safe revascularization and reduced morbidity in the patient with multilevel disease. Herein, we outline the debate over the need for combined procedures in patients with multilevel disease with an emphasis on the importance of inflow on distal revascularization, alternatives to open aortoiliac surgery, and results of tibial bypass after proximal angioplasty.

MULTILEVEL DISEASE AND THE IMPORTANCE OF INFLOW ON DISTAL BYPASSES

Disease involving multiple levels of the lower extremity arterial tree is challenging to identify, manage, and treat. Furthermore, adequate inflow, outflow, and runoff are all essential to the success of a distal revascularization. In the era of open inflow revascularization, many surgeons attempted to identify those patients with multilevel disease who would need a combined procedure.

Brewster et al.[5] used multivariate analysis to identify five independent predictors of a poor result after inflow operation alone in patients with multilevel occlusive disease. These included lack of a femoral pulse, inflow disease with >75% stenosis, poor outflow circulation determined by digital subtraction angiography (DSA), and abnormal noninvasive vascular indices after the successful performance of the inflow procedure. They recommended staged inflow and outflow procedures for patients with any of these findings.

Others argued that identification of multilevel disease might be difficult based on clinical evidence alone. Charlesworth et al.[6] retrospectively reviewed 29 femoropopliteal bypasses with no clinical or angiographic evidence of aortoiliac insufficiency, and showed that there was a highly significant decrease in the infrainguinal arterial revascularization (IAR) patency in patients who had a low preoperative femoral pulsatility index. Some have found that hemodynamically significant inflow stenoses might escape detection until after the IAR has been performed. Gupta et al.[7] measured the gradient between the femoral and radial artery pressures after completion of lower extremity bypass. Unexpected postbypass gradients >15 mm Hg developed in 8% of the patients undergoing femoropopliteal and femorotibial bypass, most likely due to undetected proximal disease. Many were treated immediately by either percutaneous transluminal angioplasty or proximal extension of the inflow. Treatment of the inflow pressure gradient did not increase bypass patency, although the study was not designed to answer this question.

Approximately 75% of symptomatic patients will improve with an inflow procedure alone, avoiding the morbidity of a combined procedure. While this is true for many patients, singular success decreases to 50% in the presence of an ulcerated foot lesion, suggesting that not all distal procedures can be avoided with the correction of proximal disease.[8] In patients with tissue loss, a combined inflow and outflow procedure is more likely necessary to provide robust blood flow to the ischemic tissue bed and result in successful healing.

Adequate inflow is an important factor in the success of a distal bypass. In one large series examining the importance of inflow on distal revascularization graft patency, Eagleton et al.[9] reviewed 551 infrainguinal bypasses in 495 patients and compared the patency rates of those with normal inflow and those requiring an inflow procedure prior to IAR. In this study group, 62 patients had a vein IAR combined with an inflow procedure (27 below-knee popliteal and 35 tibial) and 218 had an IAR alone (88 below-knee popliteal and 130 tibial). Inflow procedures included aorto-iliofemoral bypass, iliofemoral endarterectomy, iliac artery angioplasty (15% overall), and extra-anatomic bypass. The 4-year primary patency was significantly less in patients with combined inflow procedures and autogenous bypasses compared to autogenous bypass alone (41% vs. 54%; $p = 0.006$). There were no differences in the assisted primary and secondary patency rates, the limb salvage rate, or the patient survival rate. Patency rates did not significantly differ when stratified by the type of inflow procedure; however, this determination was limited by the small patient populations in each inflow procedure group. The most common cause of IAR failure in the combined group was inflow failure, while the most common cause in the autogenous bypass alone group was the bypass itself. The authors concluded that normal inflow is critical to the success of lower extremity revascularization and that bypasses dependent upon intrinsically normal inflow fared significantly better in overall success compared to their diseased counterparts.

Last, timing of a combined procedure is another crucial aspect in the treatment of multilevel disease. Combined procedures are considered more morbid given the extent of dissection and the duration of anesthesia, and it is for this reason that procedures are often staged. While most surgeons perform staged inflow and outflow procedures for these reasons, others have reported similar limb salvage rates in patients undergoing synchronous procedures and argue that distal disease may worsen during the period between surgeries.[10]

METHODS OF INFLOW RESTORATION

Open aorto(bi)femoral anatomic bypass (AFB) has traditionally been considered the gold standard for the treatment of iliac occlusive disease. This procedure has excellent primary patency rates, but the magnitude of the procedure and duration of anesthesia are associated with a 1% to 5% operative mortality, a 5% to 10% major complication rate, and an 11% to 33% late morbidity rate, including graft infection, impotence, and sexual dysfunction.[11] In patients considered to be high-risk, extra-anatomic methods, such as the axillobifemoral and femorofemoral bypasses, can be used to treat iliac occlusive disease. These procedures may avoid the risks of an anatomic intracavitary bypass, but primary patency and overall success are significantly less.

Endovascular treatment of arterial occlusive disease can be traced back to 1964 when Dotter and Judkins[12] first performed arterial dilation using a coaxial catheter. The creation of the balloon angioplasty catheter by Gruntzig in 1974 made percutaneous transluminal angioplasty (PTA) more practical, and first permitted dilation of vessels >4 mm.[13] By the 1980s, success and short-term primary patency rates increased, and PTA was applied to different regions of the vascular system that were susceptible to atherosclerosis. Although PTA was considered an effective alternative to standard open surgical revascularization, it could not match the long-term success rates of open bypass. While morbidity rates were less than AFB,[14] the 5-year primary patency rates remained between 34% and 85%.[15,16] Furthermore, with this new technique came unforeseen complications. Complications secondary to angiography include contrast nephropathy, arterial dissection, thromboembolism, and pseudoaneurysm formation. Additional complications of primary PTA include arterial perforation, dissection, arterial recoil, acute thrombosis requiring emergent surgery, and inadequate angiographic result secondary to arterial calcification.

With the introduction of intra-arterial stents in the mid-1980s, many of the complications seen with primary PTA could be safely treated and the long-term patency of iliac artery PTA increased. Bosch et al.[17] performed a meta-analysis of six iliac artery PTA studies (1,300 patients) and eight iliac artery PTA with stent studies (816 patients). Four-year patency rates increased from 65% to 77% after stent placement in patients treated for claudication. Results were slightly lower when patients were treated for limb-threatening ischemia, with an increase from 53% to 67% after stent placement. The incidence of complications was the same between the PTA and the PTA with stent groups, but the risk of long-term failure was reduced by 39% after stent placement.

Short-term complications unique to stenting compared to PTA alone include inadequate or incorrect deployment, in-stent restenosis secondary to intimal hyperplasia, and stent infection requiring removal of the foreign body. Long-term complications include migration, erosion through the vessel wall, and fracture, especially when stents are placed across a joint.

Noninvasive techniques, such as intravascular ultrasound, have been developed for the treatment of inadequate stent deployment. Stemming from their observation that 40% of stent deployments were inadequate, Buckley et al.[18] found that 6-year patency could be increased from 69% to 100% with the use of adjunctive intravascular ultrasound. This was attributed to the ability of intravascular ultrasound to more accurately estimate complete stent–vessel wall apposition compared to DSA alone.

Stents generally become incorporated in the arterial wall after 3 weeks and therefore do not prevent subsequent intimal hyperplasia.[19] The development of in-stent restenosis in the form of neointimal hyperplasia or primary disease progression has been addressed more recently by the development of peripheral arterial brachytherapy (radioactive stents) and drug eluting stents. Vascular brachytherapy may improve the short-term patency rate of peripheral endovascular applications, although the effects on long-term patency rates remain indeterminate compared to conventional therapy.[20]

INDICATIONS FOR ENDOVASCULAR INFLOW RESTORATION

Initially, the surgeon must determine the hemodynamic significance of a detected proximal stenosis prior to instituting treatment. The mere presence of a stenosis does not necessarily indicate the need for treatment, as the impact of that lesion on distal arterial blood flow may be negligible. Hemodynamically significant lesions can be identified by DSA, and correspond to 80% to 85% stenosis of the artery (or 50% to 60% reduction in transluminal diameter). Measurements of translesional pressure gradients with and without vasodilators, reactive hyperemia, or pedal exercise improve the sensitivity of DSA for treatment evaluation. A systolic gradient of 10 to 15 mm Hg or a mean gradient 5 mm Hg across a lesion is considered hemodynamically significant.[21]

Iliac Artery

The classification of iliac artery occlusive disease has recently been revised to better represent available endovascular means of therapy. Originally classified by the Society of Interventional Radiology (SIR) according to lesion length (Table 27-1), the TransAtlantic InterSociety Consensus (TASC) working group stratified iliac disease based on complexity in 2000 (Table 27-2).[22] This more detailed classification system was better suited to newer endovascular techniques.

According to the TASC working group, endovascular treatments are the procedure of choice for focal, short, type A iliac artery lesions (Table 27-2). Type D lesions, on the other hand, are more diffuse and complex, requiring open surgical reconstruction. The TASC did not specify the preferred treatment for type B and C lesions due to a lack of sufficient data.

Timaran et al.[23] compared iliac artery stenting versus open surgical reconstruction in patients with type B and C lesions. They found that iliac artery PTA and stenting had a statistically significant decrease in 5-year primary patency (64%) compared to surgical reconstruction (86%), although there were more systemic complications in the surgical group. Multivariate analysis identified poor infrainguinal runoff, external iliac artery (EIA) disease, and female gender as independent risk factors for poor outcome after iliac stenting in this group. After accounting for these risk factors, there were no statistically significant differences in primary patency rates.

TABLE 27-1

MODIFIED SOCIETY OF INTERVENTIONAL RADIOLOGY GUIDELINES FOR GRADING ILIAC ARTERY LESIONS

Grade	Morphologic Description
0	No lesion
1	Symmetric lesion <3 cm
2	Lesion 3–5 cm
3	Lesion >5 cm
4	Occlusion

From Guidelines for percutaneous transluminal angioplasty. Standards of Practice Committee of the Society of Cardiovascular and Interventional Radiology. *Radiology*. 1990;177:619–626, with permission.

TABLE 27-2

TRANSATLANTIC INTERSOCIETY CONSENSUS MORPHOLOGIC STRATIFICATION OF ILIAC LESIONS

Type	Definition
A	Single stenosis of CIA or EIA <3 cm long (unilateral or bilateral)
B	Single stenosis 3–10 cm long, not extending into CFA
	Two stenoses of CIA or EIA not involving CFA <5 cm
	Unilateral CIA occlusion
C	Bilateral stenoses of CIA and/or EIA not involving CFA 5–10 cm long
	Unilateral EIA occlusion not involving CFA
	Unilateral EIA stenosis extending into CFA
	Bilateral CIA occlusion
D	Diffuse stenosis of entire CIA, EIA, and CFA of >10 cm
	Unilateral occlusion of CIA and EIA
	Bilateral EIA occlusions
	Iliac stenosis adjacent to aortic or iliac aneurysms

CIA, common iliac artery; EIA, external iliac artery; CFA, common femoral artery.
From Timaran CH, Prault TL, Stevens SL, et al. Iliac artery stenting versus surgical reconstruction for TASC (TransAtlantic InterSociety Consensus) type B and type C iliac lesions. *J Vasc Surg.* 2003;38(2):272–278, with permission.

Other studies have confirmed these findings, demonstrating decreased patency rates in women, patients with renal insufficiency,[24] and patients undergoing EIA PTA.[25]

Femoropopliteal Segment

Femoropopliteal disease has been classified by the TASC in much the same way as iliac lesions (Table 27-3). The

TABLE 27-3

TRANSATLANTIC INTERSOCIETY CONSENSUS MORPHOLOGIC STRATIFICATION OF FEMOROPOPLITEAL LESIONS

Type	Definition
A	Single stenosis of up to 3 cm long, not at origin of superficial femoral artery or distal popliteal artery
B	Single stenosis or occlusion 3–5 cm long, not involving distal popliteal artery
	Multiple stenoses or occlusions, each <3 cm long
C	Single stenosis or occlusion >5 cm
	Multiple stenoses or occlusions, each 3–5 cm long
D	Complete common femoral artery or superficial femoral artery occlusion or complete popliteal and proximal trifurcation occlusions

From Costanza MJ, Queral LA, Lilly MP, et al. Hemodynamic outcome of endovascular therapy for TransAtlantic InterSociety Consensus type B femoropopliteal arterial occlusive lesions. *J Vasc Surg.* 2004;39(2):343–350, with permission.

categories are descriptive of morphologic complexity and are more applicable to endovascular therapeutics. As in their recommendations for the treatment of iliac arterial disease, the TASC working group has advocated endovascular treatment of type A lesions, and surgical bypass for type D lesions.

The treatment of femoropopliteal stenoses with endovascular techniques has been plagued by poor long-term results. Five-year patency ranges from 38% to 58% overall, while 5-year patency of lesions <1 to 2 cm increases to approximately 75%.[26] This has led many to perform femoropopliteal PTA only for these short, focal lesions. Unlike the iliac system, uncomplicated femoropopliteal PTA patency does not increase with the use of stents. Vroegindeweij et al.[27] compared femoropopliteal PTA to primary stent balloon angioplasty (SBA) and found a primary patency at 1 year to be 62% for the stent group compared to 74% for the PTA group (p = NS).

Becquemin et al.[28] examined 103 consecutive PTA of the femoropopliteal segment and found that the probability of angiographic success at 2 years was 80% in patients with a stenosis of <2 cm, and 62% in patients with a stenosis of >2 cm. Success, defined as restenosis <70%, was <50% in those patients with an occluded segment regardless of length, and cumulative 2-year patency was only 51.3%. Also, secondary stent placement failed to improve patency. They concluded that femoropopliteal angioplasty is a safe alternative in a select group of patients.

As in the iliac system, a lack of outcome data of the endovascular treatment of intermediate (type B and type C) lesions has made the indications for treatment more vague. Costanza et al.[29] studied the outcome of endovascular treatment of type B femoropopliteal lesions in patients with claudication. They found that the 1-year primary patency was 58% for patients who underwent primary PTA, and 51% for patients who underwent primary PTA with secondary stenting.

RESULTS OF TIBIAL BYPASS FOLLOWING ILIAC ANGIOPLASTY

As success of endovascular treatment of significant iliac artery disease approached that of its open counterpart, vascular surgeons began to rely on these interventions to provide inflow for tibial bypasses. Moreover, it became clear that the additional runoff provided by the bypass contributed positively to the success of the bypass. Combined procedures increased the iliac patency in the presence of poor runoff from 30% to 73%, making the inflow procedure itself more durable.[30]

Combined iliac PTA and IAR was first performed in the 1980s. Peterkin et al.[31] found a 76% 3-year primary patency in patients who underwent iliac PTA and ipsilateral femoropopliteal or femoroinfrageniculate bypass. These short-term results were comparable to that of open iliac artery repair combined with distal revascularization. Corey et al.[32] reported on 15 high-risk patients who underwent combined iliac PTA and IAR, six of whom had a bypass to the distal popliteal or tibial arteries. Life table analysis showed a 3-year iliac patency of 86% and distal bypass patency of 76%. They also had a 3-year limb salvage rate of 86%. Katz et al.[33] reported on iliac PTA prior to distal revascularization, with a total of 37 IAR, of which two were tibial bypasses, and 18 were below-knee popliteal bypasses. Patients who had an unsuccessful iliac PTA were excluded from the study. They reported an iliac patency of 76%, a primary graft patency of 75% for all popliteal and distal tibial bypasses, and an overall limb salvage rate of 78% at 5 years. There were six patients who had early iliac PTA failure, four of whom had recurrent symptoms. They concluded that iliac PTA prior to IAR is feasible in patients with multilevel disease with a low morbidity. Siskin et al.[34] reported on 85 patients who underwent staged iliac PTA and IAR. They found 4-year primary and secondary patency rates of 63% and 71%, respectively. When the analysis was performed only on patients who had a saphenous vein conduit, these patencies increased to 78% and 86%, allowing them to conclude that combined iliac PTA and IAR is durable.

One of the largest reported series was by Brewster et al.,[35] and included iliac PTA performed in 79 patients who needed IAR, with 96% of the iliac procedures completed prior to the surgical procedure. Patients who had an unsuccessful iliac PTA were excluded from the study. There were nine PTA complications, with five (6%) major complications classified as thrombosis, embolization, and pseudoaneurysm. Four of these required immediate conversion to an open groin approach and infrainguinal surgical bypass procedure. The IAR included 45 femoropopliteal and 10 tibial bypasses. Five-year primary patency of these bypasses was 68% overall (75% for autogenous vein and 54% for prosthetic grafts). There were 12 bypass failures, three due to failed EIA PTA, and one due to a new common iliac artery (CIA) stenosis. The other eight failures were not due to the inflow disease. The 5-year cumulative limb salvage rate was 90%. They concluded that combined iliac PTA and IAR reduces the extent of surgical intervention while increasing the comprehensiveness of the revascularization.

Perhaps the only published series comparing PTA, PTA with selective stent placement, and aortobifemoral bypass in patients who required multilevel revascularizations was performed by Timaran et al.[36] They examined the effect of an inflow procedure on infrainguinal arterial bypass patency. Forty-two percent of these patients had a tibial bypass, and 36% underwent above-knee popliteal bypass. Five-year primary patency of the

IAR was 68% in the stent group, 61% in the AFB group, and 46% in the PTA group. Stratified analysis revealed that the presence of EIA lesions decreased the primary patency of the IAR compared to those patients with only CIA lesions. This study was limited in that it did not specifically look at tibial bypasses. Last, there were no statistically significant differences in limb salvage rates between all three groups.

Last, early studies found that iliac PTA was less successful in patients with diabetes, suggesting that this group of patients would require an open inflow procedure in order to increase patency rates of the IAR.[37,38] Faries et al.[14] performed a retrospective study to compare the results of combined iliac angioplasty and IAR in diabetics and nondiabetics with multilevel disease and limb-threatening ischemia. They evaluated 45 femoropopliteal bypasses and 54 infragenicular bypasses in diabetic patients, and 11 femoropopliteal bypasses and 16 infragenicular bypasses in nondiabetic patients. There were no statistical differences in 3-year patency rates of the diabetic (73%) and nondiabetic (70%) patients. They concluded that iliac PTA combined with IAR is a safe and durable technique for revascularization of multilevel disease in the diabetic patient. Spence et al.[39] found similar results in their comparison of diabetic and nondiabetic patients undergoing iliac PTA and IAR. There were no statistically significant differences in iliac patency, IAR patency, and 4-year limb salvage rates between groups.

While iliac artery PTA with or without stenting combined with IAR produces similar results to aortobifemoral bypass, what may not be clear is whether treatment should be staged or performed successively during one sitting. Simultaneous PTA and IAR may be more cost-efficient and may reduce complications by allowing immediate identification and repair in the same sitting. With staging, however, the iliac PTA can be done at the time of preoperative arteriography, usually with better imaging equipment. This also allows for evaluation of the results of initial treatment and helps to determine if an outflow procedure is necessary to accomplish the desired treatment goals.[40]

RESULTS OF TIBIAL BYPASS FOLLOWING FEMOROPOPLITEAL ANGIOPLASTY

In the early days of proximal angioplasty, Wengerter et al.[41] evaluated 19 cases of femoropopliteal PTA and subsequent popliteal-to-distal bypass, a subgroup of 153 nonsequential popliteal-to-distal artery bypasses. In order to optimize the results of PTA, only nonoccluded lesions <3 cm long with >35% stenosis were included in the study. The femoropopliteal lesions were then followed for an average of 2.4 months, during which failures were excluded from the study. Two-year primary graft patency was 68%. They did not find any statistically significant differences in primary graft patency and limb salvage between those patients with >35% stenosis who underwent PTA and those with <35% stenosis who did not. Limb salvage was improved over those patients who had >35% stenosis but either did not undergo angioplasty or had a PTA failure (55% vs. 82%, $p < 0.01$). They concluded that femoropopliteal PTA of properly selected lesions prior to popliteal-to-distal bypass was associated with adequate results, although these results were not directly compared to more proximal surgical bypass.

Schneider et al.[26] compared a group of 12 diabetic patients undergoing combined intraoperative superficial femoral artery angioplasty and popliteal-to-distal bypass to 46 patients undergoing femorodistal bypass, and 52 patients without proximal occlusive disease undergoing popliteal-to-distal bypass. The surgical indication for all patients was distal gangrene. All patients with a single lesion <3 cm causing >50% stenosis were included in the angioplasty group. They found no statistical difference in 5-year primary or secondary patency rates between the groups. Two of the 12 patients required subsequent PTA for recurrent stenosis. They argued in favor of endovascular balloon angioplasty when the saphenous vein is not of adequate length to permit a longer bypass. Furthermore, the additional runoff provided by the bypass may contribute to patency of the angioplasty. These findings agree with Clark et al.[42] who found that poor tibial runoff was an independent risk factor for poor long-term patency of femoropopliteal PTA. Stent design may also affect outcome, as some authors have reported a 1-year femoropopliteal primary patency of 86% in patients treated with a nitinol stent,[43] and 6-month patency of 93% in patients treated with a sirolimus-eluting stent.[44]

CONCLUSION

In conclusion, tibial artery bypass following proximal angioplasty produces results comparable to traditional, open methods of multilevel revascularization with decreased morbidity. Currently, proximal PTA should be performed on TASC type A lesions, and surgical bypass for type D lesions. There is not enough current evidence to advocate proximal PTA of type B or C lesions. Further advances in stent technology may lead to better long-term patency rates, and the ability to base a distal bypass on PTA of type B and C lesions.

REFERENCES

1. DeBakey ME, Lawrie GM, Glaeser DH. Patterns of atherosclerosis and their surgical significance. *Ann Surg.* 1985;201:115–131.

2. Mozersky DJ, Sumner DS, Strandness DE. Long-term results of reconstructive aortoiliac surgery. *Am J Surg.* 1972;123:503–509.

3. Dickinson PH, McNeil IF, Morrison JM. Aortoiliac occlusion, a review of 100 cases treated by direct arterial surgery. *Br J Surg.* 1967; 54:764–770.

4. Laborde JC, Palmaz JC, Rivera FJ, et al. Influence of anatomic distribution of atherosclerosis on the outcome of revascularization with iliac stent placement. *J Vasc Interv Radiol.* 1995;6:513–521.

5. Brewster DC, Perler BA, Robison JG, et al. Aortofemoral graft for multilevel occlusive disease: predictors of success and need for distal bypass. *Arch Surg.* 1982;117:1593–1600.

6. Charlesworth D, Harris PL, Cave FD, et al. Undetected aorto-iliac insufficiency: a reason for early failure of saphenous vein bypass grafts for obstruction of the superficial femoral artery. *Br J Surg.* 1975;62:567–570.

7. Gupta SK, Veith FJ, Kram HB, et al. Significance and management of inflow gradients unexpectedly generated after femorofemoral, femoropopliteal, and femoroinfrapopliteal bypass grafting. *J Vasc Surg.* 1990;12:278–283.

8. Imparato AM, Sanoudos G, Epstein HY, et al. Results in 96 aortoiliac reconstructive procedures: preoperative angiographic and functional classifications used as prognostic guides. *Surgery.* 1970; 68:610–616.

9. Eagleton MJ, Illig KA, Green RM, et al. Impact of inflow reconstruction on infrainguinal bypass. *J Vasc Surg.* 1997;26:928–938.

10. Nypaver TJ, Ellenby MI, Mendoza O, et al. A comparison of operative approaches and parameters predictive of success in multilevel arterial occlusive disease. *J Am Coll Surg.* 1994;179:449–456.

11. Elkouri S, Hudon G, Demers P, et al. Early and long-term results of percutaneous transluminal angioplasty of the lower abdominal aorta. *J Vasc Surg.* 1999;30:679–692.

12. Dotter CT, Judkins MP. Transluminal treatment of arteriosclerotic obstruction: description of a new technique and a preliminary report of its application. *Circulation.* 1964;30:654–670.

13. Gruntzig A, Hopff H. Percutaneous recanalization after chronic arterial occlusion with a new dilator-catheter (modification of the Dotter technique). *Dtsch Med Wochenschr.* 1974;99:2502–2511.

14. Faries PL, Brophy D, LoGerfo FW, et al. Combined iliac angioplasty and infrainguinal revascularization surgery are effective in diabetic patients with multilevel arterial disease. *Ann Vasc Surg.* 2001;15:67–72.

15. Stokes KR, Strunk HM, Campbell DR, et al. Five-year results of iliac and femoropopliteal angioplasty in diabetic patients. *Radiology.* 1990;174:977–982.

16. Tegtmeyer CJ, Hartwell GD, Selby JB, et al. Results and complications of angioplasty in aortoiliac disease. *Circulation.* 1991;83 (Suppl 2):I53–160.

17. Bosch JL, Hunink MG. Meta-analysis of the results of percutaneous transluminal angioplasty and stent placement for aortoiliac occlusive disease. *Radiology.* 1997;204:87–96.

18. Buckley CJ, Arko FR, Lee S, et al. Intravascular ultrasound scanning improves long-term patency of iliac lesions treated with balloon angioplasty and primary stenting. *J Vasc Surg.* 2002;35:316–323.

19. Lau H, Cheng SWK. Intraoperative endovascular angioplasty and stenting of iliac artery: an adjunct to femoro-popliteal bypass. *J Am Coll Surg.* 1998;186:408–415.

20. Sidawy AN, Weiswasser JM, Waksman R. Peripheral vascular brachytherapy. *J Vasc Surg.* 2002;35:1041–1047.

21. Bonn J. Percutaneous vascular intervention: value of hemodynamic measurements. *Radiology.* 1996;201:18–20.

22. Dormandy JA, Rutherford RB. Management of peripheral arterial disease (PAD). TASC Working Group. TransAtlantic Inter-Society Consensus (TASC). *J Vasc Surg.* 2000;31(1 Pt 2):S1–S296.

23. Timaran CH, Prault TL, Stevens SL, et al. Iliac artery stenting versus surgical reconstruction for TASC (TransAtlantic Inter-Society Consensus) type B and type C iliac lesions. *J Vasc Surg.* 2003;38: 272–278.

24. Timaran CH, Stevens SL, Freeman MB, et al. Predictors for adverse outcome after iliac angioplasty and stenting for limb-threatening ischemia. *J Vasc Surg.* 2002;36:507–513.

25. Parsons RE, Suggs WD, Lee JJ, et al. Percutaneous transluminal angioplasty for the treatment of limb threatening ischemia: do the results justify an attempt before bypass grafting? *J Vasc Surg.* 1998;28:1066–1071.

26. Schneider PA, Caps MT, Ogawa DY, et al. Intraoperative superficial femoral artery balloon angioplasty and popliteal to distal bypass graft: an option for combined open and endovascular treatment of diabetic gangrene. *J Vasc Surg.* 2001;33:955–962.

27. Vroegindeweij D, Vos LD, Tielbeek AV, et al. Balloon angioplasty combined with primary stenting versus balloon angioplasty alone in femoropopliteal obstructions: a comparative randomized study. *Cardiovasc Intervent Radiol.* 1997;20:420–425.

28. Becquemin JP, Cavillon A, Haiduc F. Surgical transluminal femoropopliteal angioplasty: multivariate analysis outcome. *J Vasc Surg.* 1994;19:495–502.

29. Costanza MJ, Queral LA, Lilly MP, et al. Hemodynamic outcome of endovascular therapy for TransAtlantic InterSociety Consensus type B femoropopliteal arterial occlusive lesions. *J Vasc Surg.* 2004;39:343–350.

30. Johnston KW. Iliac arteries: reanalysis of results of balloon angioplasty. *Radiology.* 1993;186:207–212.

31. Peterkin GA, Belkin M, Cantelmo NL, et al. Combined transluminal angioplasty and infrainguinal reconstruction in multilevel atherosclerotic disease. *Am J Surg.* 1990;160:277–279.

32. Corey CJ, Bush HL, Widrich WC, et al. Combined operative angiodilation and arterial reconstruction for limb salvage. *Arch Surg.* 1983;118:1289–1292.

33. Katz SG, Kohl RD, Yellin A. Iliac angioplasty as a prelude to distal arterial bypass. *J Am Coll Surg.* 1994;179:577–582.

34. Siskin G, Darling RC 3rd, Stainken B, et al. Combined use of iliac artery angioplasty and infrainguinal revascularization for treatment of multilevel atherosclerotic disease. *Ann Vasc Surg.* 1999;13:45–51.

35. Brewster DC, Cambria RP, Darling RC, et al. Long-term results of combined iliac balloon angioplasty and distal surgical revascularization. *Ann Surg.* 1989;210:324–330.

36. Timaran CH, Stevens SL, Freeman MB, et al. Infrainguinal arterial reconstructions in patients with aortoiliac occlusive disease: the influence of iliac stenting. *J Vasc Surg.* 2001;34:971–978.

37. Cambria RP, Faust G, Gusberg R, et al. Percutaneous angioplasty for peripheral arterial occlusive disease. Correlates of clinical success. *Arch Surg.* 1987;122:283–287.

38. Kwasnik EM, Siouffi SY, Jay ME, et al. Comparative results of angioplasty and aortofemoral bypass in patients with symptomatic iliac disease. *Arch Surg.* 1987;122:288–291.

39. Spence LD, Hartnell GG, Reinking G, et al. Diabetic versus nondiabetic limb-threatening ischemia: outcome of percutaneous iliac intervention. *AJR Am J Roentgenol.* 1999;172:1335–1341.

40. Melliere D, Cron J, Allaire E, et al. Indications and benefits of simultaneous endoluminal balloon angioplasty and open surgery during elective lower limb revascularization. *Cardiovasc Surg.* 1999;7:242–246.

41. Wengerter KR, Yang PM, Veith FJ, et al. A twelve-year experience with the popliteal-to-distal artery bypass: the significance and management of proximal disease. *J Vasc Surg.* 1992;15:143–149.

42. Clark TW, Groffsky JL, Soulen MC. Predictors of long-term patency after femoropopliteal angioplasty: results from the STAR registry. *J Vasc Interv Radiol.* 2001;12:923–933.

43. Jahnke T, Voshage G, Muller-Hulsbeck S, et al. Endovascular placement of self-expanding nitinol coil stents for the treatment of femoropopliteal obstructive disease. *J Vasc Interv Radiol.* 2002; 13:257–266.

44. Duda SH, Pusich B, Richter G, et al. Sirolimus-eluting stents for the treatment of obstructive superficial femoral artery disease: six-month results. *Circulation.* 2002;106:1505–1509.

45. Guidelines for percutaneous transluminal angioplasty. Standards of Practice Committee of the Society of Cardiovascular and Interventional Radiology. *Radiology.* 1990;177:619–626.

Surveillance of Distal Bypasses

28

Gabor A. Winkler   Keith D. Calligaro   Kevin Doerr
Sandy McAffee-Bennett   Matthew J. Dougherty

It is estimated that 20% to 40% of all infrainguinal bypass grafts will develop stenosis.[1] Meaningful long-term graft salvage is seldom possible once thrombosis occurs. Therefore, it is crucial to identify failing bypass grafts during the postoperative follow-up. Over the last 2 decades, there has been growing support for the post-operative surveillance of arterial bypass grafts to improve long-term patency. This is particularly the case for infrainguinal revascularizations. Early methods of graft surveillance included clinical examination and segmental pressures with pulse volume recordings. Over time this was supplemented with duplex ultrasonography monitoring. Initial surveillance protocols were developed for autogenous grafts only, but later prosthetic bypass grafts were also included and suggested to be candidates for surveillance.[2] At our institution, patients are currently undergoing routine postoperative surveillance of all infrainguinal bypass grafts at regular intervals.

NATURAL HISTORY

Primary patency is defined as uninterrupted patency without any further procedures performed on the graft. Procedures on adjacent native vessels are included in this definition, as long as they serve to treat progression of disease. Any procedures performed on the graft itself, including either anastomosis, and even if these are only percutaneous interventions, contribute to assisted primary patency. These interventions are intended to prevent impending graft failure. Secondary patency is achieved by restoring patency to a thrombosed graft.[3] It is well established that the outcome of procedures to prevent graft failure is better than that of procedures to restore patency to an occluded graft.[4]

Veith et al.[5] reported patency rates in a large, prospective, randomized, multicenter study. The authors performed infrainguinal bypasses using autologous vein grafts and compared them with prosthetic polytetrafluoroethylene (PTFE) grafts. For infrainguinal bypasses to the above-knee popliteal artery, primary patency rates at 48 months were 76% and 54% for vein grafts and PTFE grafts, respectively. For infrainguinal bypasses to the infrapopliteal arteries, primary patency rates at 48 months were 49% and 12% for vein grafts and PTFE grafts, respectively. This study demonstrated the "true" natural history of these revascularization efforts, since graft failure was recorded when graft thrombosis occurred or when any secondary intervention became necessary to treat graft thrombosis. Subsequent reports have demonstrated some improvement in patency rates for prosthetic grafts when adjunctive techniques, such as vein patch,[6] vein cuff,[7] or distal arteriovenous fistula[8] were used.

Other series compared primary, assisted primary, and secondary patency rates. A retrospective review of infrapopliteal arterial bypasses performed at our institution with PTFE analyzed if distal arteriovenous fistulae improved graft patency rates.[9] In this study, a total of 43 bypasses were included. Six-mm ringed PTFE grafts were used. Twenty-one were created with a distal arteriovenous fistula and 22 without. Postoperatively, all patients were anticoagulated with intravenous heparin, which was converted to life-long oral warfarin therapy with a goal international normalized ratio (INR) ≥2.0. The primary patency rate for grafts constructed with distal arteriovenous fistulae was 22% at 2 years, compared to 5% without this adjunct ($p < 0.05$). Assisted primary patency rates at 3 years were 34% with distal arteriovenous fistulae and 15% without ($p > 0.05$). Secondary patency rates were 61% with this adjunct and 45% without ($p > 0.05$). Limb salvage rates were not affected by this adjunct (74% vs. 71%).

The natural history of bypass grafts showing duplex abnormalities that are not treated is less clear. Approximately 100 total grafts reported in the literature were followed without revision. Idu et al.[10] reported high occlusion rates in a small group of bypass grafts with reduction in diameter exceeding 50% on arteriogram if left unrevised. In a subsequent prospective, randomized study, superior patency rates were found in grafts that were revised based on duplex ultrasonographic abnormalities.[11] However, only 18 grafts were treated. Mattos et al.[12] followed 38 grafts with duplex ultrasonographic abnormalities and found similarly inferior patency rates in failing grafts that were left unrevised when compared with failing grafts that were revised. In contrast, Ho et al.[13] followed 15 grafts with duplex abnormalities and found no occlusions over 2 years. We followed 46 failing arterial bypass grafts over a median of 10 months that were not treated for a variety of reasons (scarred redo groins, patient refusal, etc.).[14] Only five (10.9%) showed progression of abnormal findings. Only three of the 46 failing grafts (6.5%) occluded during the follow-up period.

DUPLEX ULTRASONOGRAPHY

Clinical parameters, including return of ischemic symptoms, and reduction in ankle-brachial indices (ABI) and pulse volume recordings lack sufficient sensitivity to detect early failing grafts and often suggest a problem only after graft occlusion. Two European studies relying on clinical symptoms to diagnose >50% reduction in graft diameter missed 62% to 89% of these lesions.[15,16] Even by adding the measurement of ABI, only 46% of grafts with >50% reduction in diameter were diagnosed.[16] In contrast, duplex ultrasonography detected 100% of grafts with the same diameter reduction.[15] There was some disagreement in earlier publications about the value of ABI to detect failing grafts, and the ABI appears to be insensitive for predicting graft failure.[17,18]

In 1985, Bandyk et al.[19] published one of the earliest reports about the use of duplex ultrasonography–derived blood flow velocity measurements to predict failing

grafts. The two most important predictors in this series were low peak systolic velocities (<45 cm per second) throughout the graft and the absence of diastolic forward flow, indicating high outflow resistance. The authors also noted that all grafts experienced some degree of increased outflow resistance in the early postoperative period, as evidenced by a generalized drop in peak systolic velocities during follow-up studies. These results were later confirmed by Mills et al.[20] on a much larger patient cohort. Once again, a peak systolic velocity of 45 cm per second was determined as the cutoff to predict early graft failure. If the peak systolic velocity was >45 cm per second in this series, the chance for graft failure was 2.1% compared with a 12.6% graft failure rate if the peak systolic velocity was <45 cm per second. Only 29% of failing grafts, as diagnosed by duplex ultrasonography, showed a reduction in ABI measurement >0.15, clearly indicating the higher sensitivity of duplex ultrasonography surveillance. These parameters were used in three positions: Proximal anastomosis, midgraft, and distal anastomosis. This sampling method is prone to miss focal stenoses in the body of the graft, therefore current technique includes an investigation of the graft with segmental peak systolic velocity measurements along its entire length. In our noninvasive laboratory, velocities are measured every 10 cm along the graft.

Surveillance of prosthetic bypass grafts in the infrainguinal position has been received with more skepticism. Regional vascular societies and several authors have suggested that surveillance protocols are not beneficial for prosthetic grafts.[10,21-26] We and others experienced significant benefits in following subsets of prosthetic grafts according to a similar surveillance protocol as with autologous vein grafts.[2,4,27,28] Lesions causing prosthetic graft failure, similar to those causing autologous vein graft failure, can be located at an anastomosis, in adjacent inflow or outflow arteries or, much less frequently, within the body of the graft. If these stenoses are identified prior to graft thrombosis, interventions can be relatively straightforward. One report demonstrated 90% of lesions present in inflow or outflow arteries, 5% within the body of the graft, and 5% at either anastomosis.[28] In contrast, our institution demonstrated 50% of stenoses to be perianastomotic in nature, supporting findings indicating intimal hyperplasia, particularly at the distal anastomosis, to be a common cause of prosthetic graft failure.

As has been demonstrated for vein grafts, secondary patency rates of previously thrombosed grafts are superior to assisted primary patency rates for failing prosthetic grafts.[4] An occluded prosthetic graft that has undergone thrombolysis or surgical thrombectomy may be more prone to rethrombosis than a graft that has never been lined with thrombus. Endovascular and surgical intervention to salvage patent but failing grafts is more straightforward than when the graft has already thrombosed. When a patient presents with a thrombosed graft, options include thrombolysis or surgery, either of which have a high failure rate. Thrombolysis is expensive, associated with a higher incidence of hemorrhage than surgery, and frequently requires subsequent surgery for definitive treatment of the causative lesion. Operating on a thrombosed graft, without knowing the cause of the thrombosis, is generally more time consuming and requires possibly larger or extra incisions than to correct a known focal problem. Balloon thrombectomy catheter passage through a thrombosed graft may be unsuccessful due to angulation at an anastomosis, may lead to residual thrombus retention, and may cause damage in the native artery distal to the distal anastomosis. Often thrombosed grafts present emergently in the middle of the night, thus precluding potential endovascular interventional or combined therapeutic options at some hospitals.

Prosthetic grafts are much more sensitive to low-flow states and resulting thrombosis than autologous vein grafts. When reviewing duplex surveillance data on 89 infrainguinal prosthetic bypass grafts at our institution, we found that the sensitivity of abnormal duplex ultrasonographic findings that correctly diagnosed a failing graft was 88% for femorotibial bypasses but only 57% for femoropopliteal bypasses.[2] The positive predictive value (correct abnormal studies/total abnormal studies) was 95% for femorotibial grafts and 65% for femoropopliteal grafts. Therefore, we concluded that duplex surveillance is indicated and probably worthwhile for femorotibial grafts, while utility for femoropopliteal grafts remains unproven.

According to our protocol, both vein and prosthetic bypass grafts are routinely evaluated by duplex sonography in the early postdischarge period.[14] After that, the graft is followed every 3 months for the first year after bypass operation, every 6 months for the second year, and annually thereafter. A graft surveillance study typically uses transmitting frequencies from 4.0 to 7.5 MHz. It is essential that the examiner is aware of the origin of the graft and its course. Due to their more superficial location, in situ vein grafts are much easier to follow than anatomically tunneled grafts. The entire graft is scanned, beginning at the inflow artery, crossing the proximal anastomosis, moving along the body of the graft every 10 cm, and beyond the distal anastomosis. Liberal use of color flow enhancement may expedite studies. Peak systolic and diastolic velocities are recorded at these sites. Any focal increase in flow velocities is more precisely investigated with measurements performed proximal and distal to the focus. At the distal anastomosis, the Doppler angle must be carefully adjusted, due to the relatively steep angle of the graft. If consistently low peak systolic velocities are detected throughout the graft, a more detailed examination of the

inflow and outflow vessels is necessary. These findings, however, could be consistent with normal flow through a relatively large diameter graft.

ABNORMAL FINDINGS

Although duplex findings have been compared with arteriography, there is no firm consensus on strict criteria for abnormal findings on duplex ultrasonography, especially when to perform revision of a failing graft.[12,29,30] Some reports focused on uniform low peak systolic flow velocities,[26,31,32] whereas others considered focal increases in peak systolic flow velocities with reference to adjacent areas more important.[10,11,27,30,33–35] A combination of both findings has also been recommended.[36] There has also been considerable variation in the definition of abnormal peak systolic velocity values between the different studies. The current criteria used to determine failing grafts at our institution are illustrated in Table 28-1.

INDICATIONS FOR INTERVENTIONS

The optimal threshold of intervention for arterial bypass grafts is still controversial. Most authorities would agree that impending failure of a graft is suggested by lack of diastolic forward flow throughout the graft, as evidenced by monophasic Doppler signals, decreased peak systolic velocities <45 cm per second throughout the graft, focal elevations of peak systolic velocities >250 to 350 cm per second, and elevated peak systolic velocity ratios between two adjacent segments. Suggested abnormal elevated ratios range between 1.5 and 4.0.[10,12,37–42] Gupta et al.[40] recommended peak systolic velocity ratios >3.4 and focal peak systolic velocities >300 cm per second. Similar values were also confirmed by Mills et al.[41]

In 1993, two reports described results in grafts surveyed by duplex ultrasonography that underwent subsequent revision.[10,12] It was concluded in both studies that duplex ultrasonography surveillance was very effective in detecting graft-threatening stenotic lesions. If early intervention was performed based on surveillance

TABLE 28-1

CRITERIA TO IDENTIFY FAILING ARTERIAL BYPASS GRAFTS AT PENNSYLVANIA HOSPITAL

Monophasic signal throughout the graft
Uniform peak systolic velocities <45 cm/sec
Any focal peak systolic velocity >300 cm/sec
Peak systolic velocity ratio between two adjacent segments >3.5

results, the secondary patency rate was improved by 20% over 3 to 5 years compared with grafts that were not revised when stenotic lesions were identified, as well as with grafts undergoing clinical follow-up alone. However, these were not prospective randomized studies.

Conversely, a prospective, randomized study from Finland found no benefits of routine duplex ultrasound surveillance compared to clinical surveillance supplanted with Doppler-based pressure measurements for primary assisted patency rates, secondary patency rates, or limb salvage rates.[43] This study is in contrast with a large body of evidence in favor of routine surveillance using duplex ultrasonography.

We reviewed the results of 572 infrainguinal revascularizations performed at our institution between 1991 and 1995. Eighty-five bypass grafts showed duplex ultrasonographic signs of pending graft failure.[44] The mean time from initial surgery to the first abnormal duplex study was 4.5 months. Three subgroups were identified based on the timing of the revision: Early (<2 months after first abnormal duplex), late (>2 months after first abnormal duplex), and those not revised at all, despite abnormal duplex findings. Primary patency rates at 12 months were 78.9% in the unrevised group, 43.1% in the early revision group, and 63.8% in the late revision group (p <0.05). Assisted primary patency rates were 78.9%, 69.8%, and 67.2%, respectively (p >0.1). Secondary patency rates were 89.6%, 87.6%, and 85.7% (p >0.1). Last, limb salvage rates were 94.8%, 91.6%, and 95.2%, respectively (p >0.1). Although this study apparently does not support routine duplex surveillance of infrainguinal bypass grafts, we cannot explain why the unrevised group contained mostly lesions that did not progress over time. Also, peak systolic velocity ratio of 3.0 was selected as the cutoff, which may be too liberal as a value to predict graft failure.

In another study by our group examining the natural history of failing grafts, seven bypasses were followed without intervention for various reasons that had peak systolic velocity ratios >7.0.[14] Only three of the seven bypasses occluded during follow-up, and two of the three bypasses that occluded had both focal abnormalities (peak systolic velocity ratios >7.0 in this case) and uniform peak systolic velocities <45 cm per second throughout the graft. It is interesting that unless both focal and diffuse abnormalities were present, occlusion was significantly less likely.

As suggested by the previous study from our group, abnormal duplex findings do not always mandate further therapy. This is especially true if abnormal findings are encountered at the proximal anastomosis.[1] It is speculated that the hemodynamics at vessel bifurcations, which occurs at the typical end-to-side proximal anastomosis, is not strictly comparable to flow dynamics within the graft because of size discrepancies between the graft and native artery. Possibly, this turbulence and the resulting abnormalities in peak systolic velocity ratios at the proximal anastomosis are less predictive of graft thrombosis than the same abnormalities at other locations.

Controversy surrounds whether short stenoses detected in failing grafts are better treated with operative revision or percutaneous balloon angioplasty.[45] Many believe that balloon angioplasty approximates the patency rate of surgical therapy and should be used as a primary therapy for vein graft stenoses. This is supported further by the fact that balloon angioplasty is less invasive than surgery.[46] When Sanchez et al.[47] performed balloon angioplasty for simple lesions (nonrecurrent single lesions <1.5 cm in a vein graft at least 3 mm in diameter), graft patency rates were 66% at 2 years. The same procedure yielded only a 17% 2-year patency rate for more complex lesions (>1.5 cm long, recurrent, multiple, or within grafts <3 mm in diameter). Berkowitz et al.[48] observed the relevance of location of the lesion. This group advocated surgical revision for midgraft and distal anastomotic lesions due to inferior results with balloon angioplasty when compared with proximal graft lesions. It was further recommended to revise recurrent lesions operatively. Perler et al.[49] reported a very disappointing 2-year patency rate of 22% for balloon angioplasty in contrast with a 62% 5-year patency rate for surgically revised vein graft stenoses. Similarly, <30% 3-year patency rates with balloon angioplasty were noted by Whittemore et al.[50,51] compared with a 5-year patency of 86% for surgically revised grafts. The results of our institution of balloon angioplasty for failing vein grafts are in line with those of others, and showed high initial success rates with disappointingly low long-term patency rates.[45] Overall, some reports have shown that balloon angioplasty of short lesions tends to have better results than those of longer lesions. We recommend that balloon angioplasty should be reserved for "short" stenotic lesions (<2 cm) when surgical revision is associated with an inordinate risk or difficulty, such as a scarred groin wound in an obese patient.

As previously mentioned, routine graft surveillance of prosthetic grafts is controversial and not widely accepted. We have previously analyzed these grafts and made the following recommendations. Graft surveillance may not be worthwhile for femoropopliteal prosthetic grafts, but was shown to have excellent sensitivity and positive predictive values for femorotibial grafts.[2] We also believe duplex may be worthwhile for axillofemoral and aortobifemoral prosthetic grafts, perhaps at less frequent intervals than for vein grafts, specifically to identify stenosis at the femoral anastomosis. If duplex ultrasonographic examination reveals peak systolic velocities of <45 cm per second, or monophasic signals throughout an infrainguinal prosthetic graft and arteriogram does not confirm a lesion, we recommend anticoagulation for these patients. In these cases, it is our belief that duplex ultrasonography may detect unfavorable prosthetic graft–blood interactions that are not due to a specific lesion, but may lead to low flow and early graft thrombosis.[27]

SUMMARY

Duplex ultrasonography is the method of choice for surveillance of infrainguinal bypass grafts. It is every vascular laboratory's duty to continuously correlate their interpretations with arteriographic findings and clinical outcomes. A peak systolic velocity ratio >3.5 between two adjacent segments is generally accepted as a strong indicator for a focal stenosis. Also low peak systolic velocities throughout the graft (<45 cm per second), as well as lack of diastolic forward flow, as evidenced by loss of biphasic Doppler signals throughout the graft, are indicators of either inflow or outflow problems and should be further investigated. Judicious use of arteriographic follow-up and appropriate endovascular or open surgical revision of failing grafts requires careful thought and expertise on the part of the vascular surgeon.

REFERENCES

1. Ryan SV, Dougherty MJ, Chang M, et al. Abnormal duplex findings at the proximal anastomosis of infrainguinal bypass grafts: does revision enhance patency? *Ann Vasc Surg.* 2001;15: 98–103.
2. Calligaro KD, Doerr K, McAffee-Bennett S, et al. Should duplex ultrasonography be performed for surveillance of femoropopliteal and femorotibial arterial prosthetic bypasses? *Ann Vasc Surg.* 2001; 15:520–524.
3. Rutherford RB, Baker JD, Ernst C, et al. Recommended standards for reports dealing with lower extremity ischemia: revised version. *J Vasc Surg.* 1997;26:517.
4. Sanchez LA, Suggs WD, Veith FJ, et al. Is surveillance to detect failing polytetrafluoroethylene bypasses worthwhile? *Am J Surg.* 1993;18:981–990.
5. Veith FJ, Gupta SK, Ascer E, et al. Six-year prospective multicenter randomized comparison of autologous saphenous vein and expanded polytetrafluoroethylene grafts in infrainguinal arterial reconstructions. *J Vasc Surg.* 1986;3:104–114.
6. Taylor RS, McFarland RJ, Cox MI, et al. An investigation into the causes of failure of PTFE grafts. *Eur J Vasc Surg.* 1987;1:335.
7. Miller JH, Foreman RK, Ferguson L, et al. Interposition vein cuff for anastomosis of prosthesis to small artery. *Aust N Z J Surg.* 1984;54:283.
8. Ascer E, Gennaro M, Pollina R, et al. Complementary distal arteriovenous fistula and deep vein interposition: a five-year experience with a new technique to improve infrapopliteal prosthetic bypass patency. *J Vasc Surg.* 1996;24:134–143.
9. Syrek JR, Calligaro KD, Dougherty MJ, et al. Do distal arteriovenous fistulae improve patency rates of prosthetic infrapopliteal bypasses? *Ann Vasc Surg.* 1998;12:148–152.
10. Idu MM, Blankenstein JD, de Gier P, et al. Impact of color-flow duplex surveillance program on infrainguinal vein graft patency: a five-year experience. *J Vasc Surg.* 1993;17:42–53.

11. Lundell A, Lindblad B, Bergqvist D, et al. Femoropopliteal-crural graft patency is improved by an intensive surveillance program: a prospective randomized study. *J Vasc Surg.* 1995;21:26–34.
12. Mattos MA, van Bemmelen PS, Hodgson KJ, et al. Does correction of stenoses identified with color duplex scanning improve infrainguinal graft patency? *J Vasc Surg.* 1993;17:54–66.
13. Ho GW, MpII FI, Kuipers MM, et al. Long-term surveillance by duplex scanning of non revised infra genicular graft stenosis. *Ann Vasc Surg.* 1993;18:981–990.
14. Dougherty MJ, Calligaro KD, DeLaurentis DA. The natural history of "failing" arterial bypass grafts in a duplex surveillance protocol. *Ann Vasc Surg.* 1998;12:255–259.
15. Moody P, Gould DA, Harris PL. Vein graft surveillance improves patency in femoropopliteal bypass. *Eur J Vasc Surg.* 1990;4:117–121.
16. Disselhoff B, Bluth J, Jakimowicz J. Early detection of stenosis of femoral-distal grafts: a surveillance study using color-duplex scanning. *Eur J Vasc Surg.* 1989;3:43–48.
17. Barnes RW, Thompson BW, MacDonald CM, et al. Serial noninvasive studies do not herald postoperative failure of femoropopliteal or femorotibial bypass grafts. *Ann Surg.* 1989;210:486–492.
18. Berkowitz J, Hobbs C, Roberts B, et al. Value of routine vascular laboratory studies to identify vein graft stenoses. *Surgery.* 1981; 90:971–979.
19. Bandyk DF, Cato RF, Towne JB. A low flow velocity predicts failure of femoropopliteal and femorotibial bypass grafts. *Surgery.* 1985;98:799–809.
20. Mills JL, Harris EJ, Taylor LM Jr, et al. The importance of routine surveillance of distal bypass grafts with duplex scanning: a study of 379 reversed vein grafts. *J Vasc Surg.* 1990;12:379–386, discussion 387–389.
21. Strandness DE, Andros G, Bake D, et al. Vascular laboratory utilization and payment report of the Ad Hoc Committee of the Western Vascular Society. *J Vasc Surg.* 1992;16:163–168.
22. Lalak NJ, Hanel KC, Junt J, et al. Duplex scan surveillance of infrainguinal prosthetic bypass grafts. *J Vasc Surg.* 1994;20:637–641.
23. TASC Working Group. Management of peripheral arterial disease. *J Vasc Surg.* 2000;31:234–258.
24. Baker JD. The vascular laboratory: regulations and other challenges. *J Vasc Surg.* 1994;19:901–904.
25. TASC Working Group. Management of peripheral arterial disease Recommendations. *J Vasc Surg.* 2000;31:1.
26. Hobollah JJ, Nassal MM, Ryan SM, et al. Is color duplex surveillance of infrainguinal polytetrafluoroethylene grafts worthwhile? *Am J Surg.* 1997;174:131–135.
27. Calligaro KD, Musser DJ, Chen AY, et al. Duplex ultrasonography to diagnose arterial prosthetic grafts. *Surgery.* 1996;120:455–459.
28. Sanchez LA, Gupta SK, Veith FJ, et al. A ten-year experience with one hundred fifty failing or threatened vein and polytetrafluoroethylene arterial bypass grafts. *J Vasc Surg.* 1991;14:729–738.
29. Buth J, Disselhoff B, Sommeling C, et al. Color-flow duplex criteria for grading stenosis in infrainguinal vein grafts. *J Vasc Surg.* 1991;14:716–728.
30. Grigg MJ, Nicolaides AN, Wolfe JHN. Detection and grading of femorodistal vein graft stenoses: duplex velocity measurements compared with angiography. *J Vasc Surg.* 1988;8:661–666.
31. Bandyk DR, Schmitt DD, Seabrook GR, et al. Monitoring functional patency of *in situ* saphenous vein bypasses: the impact of a surveillance protocol and elective revision. *J Vasc Surg.* 1989;9:286–296.
32. Bandyk DF, Cates RF, Towne JB. A low flow velocity predicts failure of femoropopliteal and femorotibial bypass grafts. *Surgery.* 1985;98:799–809.
33. Bergamini TM, George SM, Massey HT, et al. Intensive surveillance of femoropopliteal-tibial autogenous vein bypasses improves long-term graft patency and limb salvage. *Ann Surg.* 1995;221:507–516.
34. Gahtan V, Payne LP, Roper LD, et al. Duplex criteria for predicting progression of vein graft lesions: which stenoses can be followed? *J Vasc Tech.* 1995;19:211–215.

35. Belkin M, Schwartz LB, Donaldson MC, et al. Hemodynamic impact of vein graft stenoses and their prediction in the vascular laboratory. *J Vasc Surg.* 1997;25:1016–1022.

36. Sladen JG, Reid JDS, Cooperberg PL, et al. Color-flow duplex screening of infrainguinal grafts combining low and high velocity criteria. *Am J Surg.* 1989;158:107–112.

37. Bandyk DF, Johnson BL, Gupta AK, et al. Nature and management of duplex abnormalities encountered during infrainguinal vein bypass grafting. *J Vasc Surg.* 1996;24:430–438.

38. Caps MT, Cantwell-Gab K, Bergelin RO, et al. Vein graft lesions: time of onset and rate of progression. *J Vasc Surg.* 1995;22:466–474, discussion 475.

39. Chalmers RT, Hoballah JJ, Kresowik TF, et al. The impact of color duplex surveillance on the outcome of lower limb bypass with segments of arm veins. *J Vasc Surg.* 1994;19:279–286, discussion 286–288.

40. Gupta AK, Bandyk DF, Cheanvechai D, et al. Natural history of infrainguinal vein graft stenosis relative to bypass grafting technique. *J Vasc Surg.* 1997;25:211–220, discussion 220–225.

41. Westerband A, Mills JL, Kistler S, et al. Prospective validation of threshold criteria for intervention in infrainguinal vein grafts undergoing duplex surveillance. *Ann Vasc Surg.* 1997;11:44–48.

42. Idu MM, Buth J, Hop WC, et al. Vein graft surveillance: is graft revision without angiography justified and what criteria should be used? *J Vasc Surg.* 1998;27:399–411, discussion 412–413.

43. Ihlberg L, Luther M, Alback A, et al. Does a completely accomplished duplex-based surveillance prevent vein-graft failure? *Eur J Vasc Endovasc Surg.* 1999;18:395–400.

44. Dougherty MJ, Calligaro KD, DeLaurentis DA. Revision of failing lower extremity bypass grafts. *Am J Surg.* 1998;176:126–130.

45. Rua I, Calligaro KD, Dougherty MJ, et al. Is balloon angioplasty indicated for "short" stenoses of failing vein grafts? *Ann Vasc Surg.* 1998;12:134–137.

46. Alpert JR, Ring EJ, Berkowitz HD, et al. Treatment of vein graft stenosis by balloon catheter dilatation. *JAMA.* 1979;242:2769–2771.

47. Sanchez LA, Suggs WD, Marin MD, et al. Is percutaneous balloon angioplasty appropriate in the treatment of graft and anastomotic lesions responsible for failing vein bypass? *Am J Surg.* 1994;168:97–101.

48. Berkowitz HD, Fox AD, Deaton DH. Reversed vein graft stenosis: early diagnosis and management. *J Vasc Surg.* 1992;15:130–142.

49. Perler BA, Osterman FA, Mitchell SE, et al. Balloon dilatation versus surgical revision of infrainguinal autogenous vein graft stenoses: long-term follow-up. *J Cardiovasc Surg.* 1990;31:656–661.

50. Whittemore AD, Donaldson MD, Polak JF, et al. Limitations of balloon angioplasty for vein graft stenosis. *J Vasc Surg.* 1991;14:340–345.

51. Whittemore AD, Clowes AW, Couch NP, et al. Secondary femoropopliteal reconstruction. *Ann Surg.* 1981;193:35–42.

Infrainguinal Catheter-based Endovascular Interventions

29

Glenn M. LaMuraglia   **Giuseppe R. Nigri**

Though angioplasty can trace its roots to the pioneering work of Dotter and Judkins,[1] it was not until the work of Gruntzig in 1974,[2] with the introduction of nonelastomeric balloons, that the application of angioplasty became a viable therapeutic option. Since its introduction, transluminal angioplasty has evolved into a safe and effective method for the treatment of obstructive vascular stenoses. There have been technological advances, driven primarily for coronary applications, in materials and engineering, such as the development of new dependable, low-profile, high-pressure balloon catheters; hydrophilic-coated guidewires; and catheters that facilitate the safe manipulation across vascular stenoses or occlusions. Stents have been introduced as an adjunct for the treatment of stenoses that develop elastic recoil or flow-limiting flaps.[3] Improvements in high-definition, digital-imaging technology with software adjuncts, such as road-mapping, have permitted improved visualization of stenoses and enabled the conservation of iodinated contrast administration to patients with renal failure for these procedures. Progress in antiplatelet therapy, though not proven in peripheral applications, may also lead to better results as seen in the coronary literature.[4] These have all led to a wider acceptance and application of balloon angioplasty in the treatment armamentarium for atherosclerotic stenoses.

The mechanism of action of balloon angioplasty was originally thought to be a compression and remodeling of atherosclerotic plaque. It is now known that fracture with localized, "controlled" dissection of the intima of the plaque is the major mechanism.[5] Overdistension of the vessel wall with medial and adventitial dissection or rupture is clearly undesirable; however, medial stretching represents an important part of the therapy. This may be occasionally accompanied by transient, localized pressure or discomfort related to balloon inflation, attributed to stretching of the media. Unremitting, sustained pain, even after deflation of the balloon is, however, an unfavorable sign that may indicate vessel rupture or bleeding into adjacent tissue.

INDICATIONS

In the infrainguinal arterial system, percutaneous balloon angioplasty (PTA) can provide definitive therapy for patients presenting with disabling claudication or limb-threatening ischemia.[6–8] On the basis clinical criteria with vascular laboratory confirmation, one should decide the need for intervention to improve lower extremity circulation. Once that decision is made, then the anatomic detail of the limb needs to be characterized either with a contrast arteriogram or, if possible, in patients with significant renal insufficiency, a magnetic resonance angiogram (MRA). This information is considered with the patient's comorbidities, functional status, and expected survival before the selection of the therapeutic options can be considered.

PTA is less invasive than open surgical reconstruction for lower extremity ischemia and is therefore better tolerated. However, the natural tendency to broaden the application and become less stringent with the therapeutic indications when considering a percutaneous approach should be resisted. A technical misadventure or a poor clinical result with a percutaneous route can result in an inferior long-term outcome than the natural history of mild-moderate chronic lower extremity ischemia and, therefore, the algorithm used for determining patient indications for an intervention should be based on the clinical presentation and not the method of treatment.[6,9] Another factor that should be considered is the extent and anatomy of the disease process. The intention to treat extensive infrainguinal occlusive disease, or its location in the distal popliteal or crural vessels, should result from more stringent clinical indications.[7]

This is not to mean that therapy should be withheld for those patients requiring treatment. It just means that patients should have their risk factors modified as best as possible and other conservative measures, such as a walking program for the mild-moderate claudication patient, before proceeding with a reconstruction procedure.

PATIENT SELECTION

Catheter-based infrainguinal reconstruction can be used as a stand-alone method or in combination with surgical reconstruction. The scenarios for joint procedures can be varied and are dependant on anatomic considerations and the clinical necessity for completeness of the revascularization.[10] Commonly, these include inflow procedures that are not amenable to endovascular reconstruction, but require surgery, such as extensive common femoral lesions, long occlusions, or diminutive inflow vessels. This can be approached by a surgical endarterectomy or bypass with ensuing distal outflow vessel angioplasty, if clinically indicated at the time by hemodynamic assessment.

Alternatively, there may be limited venous conduit and extensive distal small-vessel disease or occlusion with concomitant proximal stenosis where the combination of surgery and endoluminal revascularization may be in the reverse configuration. In this instance, the proximal lesion can undergo PTA to provide adequate inflow. If the distal disease was not readily amenable to percutaneous intervention or is too extensive, and the clinical and hemodynamic assessments indicate that a more complete revascularization is needed, a more distal surgical bypass may be required to supplement the more proximal angioplasty procedure. The various combinations and permutations are not limited to the described scenarios, but these combined technique reconstructions can be devised for any particular set of clinical circumstances. However, these patient-specific treatment algorithms appear to be best determined by those very skilled in both interventional and open surgical skills. This is true not only during formulation of the plan, by judging the possible limitations and benefits of each available approach such as PTA or surgery, but during the interventional procedure as well. The decision when to continue and persist with a catheter-based intervention or when to back out and alter the plan and proceed with another option during a complex case is best made by a single individual. This includes a good understanding of the patient's comorbidities and surgical risks, all of which should be factored in to make the best possible decision for the patient's ultimate outcome.

TECHNICAL CONSIDERATIONS

The percutaneous infrainguinal artery reconstructions using balloon angioplasty or plaque excision devices are most easily accessed under local anesthesia from either the left brachial, the contralateral femoral artery in a retrograde fashion, or the ipsilateral femoral artery in an antegrade fashion. Although a retrograde popliteal artery access has been described and can be used in specific circumstances, it is of limited benefit since the majority of patients do not tolerate remaining prone on a hard angiogram table for an extended period of time, and sheath pulling can be challenging if the patient needs to be supine.

The left brachial approach is indicated when there is concern for groin access due to complicated anatomy, multiple or tenuous surgical reconstructions, or anastomotic aneurysms that preclude femoral access. This approach can be used when there is a strong, brisk pulse present. Although the right brachial approach has been used for access to the coronary arteries, it is not ideal for the lower extremities, and by traversing across the aortic arch, there is a higher expected incidence of stroke than left brachial access.

A retrograde femoral approach should be undertaken from the contralateral side of the anatomy of principal clinical interest when the anatomic detail of the patient is not known. This approach facilitates angiography of the aorta, pelvis, and bilateral runoff. Although the ipsilateral runoff can be performed through the sheath, the arteriogram of the contralateral side, which is the side of interest, can be undertaken after selecting the common femoral artery after traversing over the aortic bifurcation. In this fashion, an antegrade angiogram is performed for full diagnostic imaging of the contralateral ischemic extremity. This provides the best delineation of the lower extremity anatomy with the use of less iodinated contrast, and provides the ability of further selective cannulation and repeat arteriogram with or without intervention of infrainguinal lesions. The theoretical argument that this increased manipulation of the arteries can cause injury holds little merit when considering its very low incidence with trained interventionalists, and the significantly better anatomic detail obtained by this approach. It is the author's preferred approach in routine cases when the specifics of the patient's vascular anatomy are not known (Fig. 29-1). This is significantly different than trying to convert a retrograde femoral access into an antegrade femoral access, since the manipulations with the wire to undertake this maneuver, which can only be done well in very thin individuals, can result in arterial dissection.

In patients with preprocedure imaging (such as computertized tomography angiography [CTA] or MRA) without need for a proximal intervention, an ipsilateral, antegrade common femoral artery approach can be used. This approach is best undertaken in nonobese patients. The location and angle of the skin and artery puncture need to be carefully planned with periodic fluoroscopic visualization of the femoral head of the femur. This helps avoid too low of a stick in the superficial femoral artery, and with attention to technique, can be very safe without complications. Generally, if the occlusive disease is within 5 cm of the origin of the superficial femoral artery or if an intervention is considered for the profunda femoral artery, a remote approach (brachial or contralateral femoral artery) is preferable. If the lesions requiring treatment are infrageniculate, it is preferable, when the anatomy is amenable, to approach them with this antegrade approach from the ipsilateral femoral artery. This is not to say that a combination of access sites cannot be used for a particular case; it is not uncommon that after the diagnostic procedure is undertaken, for intervention, a separate puncture is performed on the affected extremity with an antegrade femoral approach (Fig. 29-2). This ipsilateral femoral access provides the best ability to accurately manipulate guidewires across stenoses or through occlusions. Although this may not be a consideration in straightforward cases, another consideration is the distances that wires, catheters, and balloons can travel. In normal-height people, it is generally difficult to access the below-knee popliteal artery from the arm, but one can generally get to the proximal calf from the contralateral femoral approach. The longest balloon catheters available commercially are 150 cm in length.

Iodinated contrast is utilized at full strength for aortography and bolus-chase nonsubtracted runoff arteriography. To keep contrast at a minimum, hand injections with half-strength contrast and subtraction angiography can be utilized with selective catheterization at the area of interest. In patients with severe chronic renal insufficiency, a mixture of Gadolinium, nonionic-iodinated contrast, and saline (1:1:1), with selective catheterization and subtraction angiography can further minimize

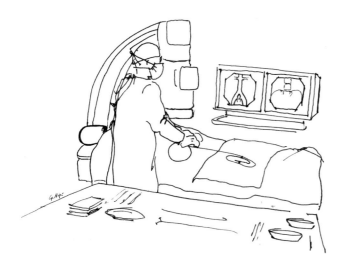

Figure 29-1 The position of operator and working table when a retrograde femoral access is obtained. It is easiest to access and work in the groin closest to the operator, and the table with the equipment and devices is best positioned behind the operator.

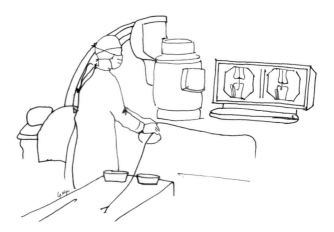

Figure 29-2 The position of operator and working table when an antegrade femoral access is obtained. It is easiest to access and work in the groin closest to the operator, and the table with the equipment and devices is best positioned perpendicular to the patient and in front of the operator. The placement of two basins at the corners assist the operator to keep the wires and catheters from falling off the table and getting contaminated.

the use of iodinated contrast.[11] The use of CO_2 digital subtraction arteriography below the femoral artery does not generally provide enough detail to be useful for diagnostic or therapeutic endeavors as it is for the aorta and iliac arteries.[12] Preadministration of 200 μg of intra-arterial nitroglycerin before contrast administration for the arteriogram is hemodynamically well tolerated in properly hydrated patients, and helps open the collaterals and improve distal visualization during arteriography. It should be emphasized that nonselective placement of a catheter in the distal aorta and using step-table technique to obtain runoff arteriography, even in the subtraction mode, is generally effective only to the level of the proximal tibial vessels, requires significantly more contrast administration than selective arteriography, and does not provide the anatomic detail obtained with selective angiography.

When performing a diagnostic arteriogram, it is important to adequately visualize the arteries by opacifying them with contrast. When further characterization of the iliac arteries is indicated, oblique arteriograms of the iliac systems or runoff vessels may identify otherwise poorly defined stenoses. It is a good technique to well visualize the origin of the profunda femoral artery. A steep ipsilateral oblique view of the groin should be routinely used to delineate the posterior wall of the common femoral artery and the profunda origin, which is commonly diseased and may factor importantly into the treatment algorithm.

It should be again emphasized that selective catheter placement proximal to the anatomic area of interest with local contrast injections provide better anatomic delineation of the arteries and minimizes the quantity of contrast administered, an important factor for diabetic patients who generally suffer from renal insufficiency. This antegrade injection of contrast can be performed either as a bolus chase or just proximal to the area of interest with digital subtraction. When performed with subtraction, it is the ideal method to perform the diagnostic angiogram and set up "road-mapping" of the site for possible intervention. In fact, when using this technique of an antegrade femoral puncture with a focused angiogram, and intervention, the whole procedure can sometimes be completed with only a total of 30 to 40 cc of iodinated contrast.

The smaller the sheath size compared to the size of the artery, the lower the complication rate.[13] Accessing the brachial artery or an antegrade femoral puncture with a 4F micropuncture kit provides the added safety of using a small needle to localize and gain access to the artery before placing a larger wire and sheath. Micropuncture kits should be used when difficult access is expected, and are useful for antegrade femoral puncture. Fluoroscopically visualizing the femoral head helps determine the needle versus targeted access site, especially if a previous arteriogram has been conducted

of the area and the location of the femoral artery is known. The 4F is readily converted to a 5F sheath through which a full diagnostic and most therapeutic balloon angioplasty procedures can be undertaken, with upsizing sheath size only needed if a stent is required. For antegrade femoral punctures, a 5F sheath with a radio-opaque marker on the tip of the sheath can be helpful, especially if there are lesions in the proximal superficial femoral artery that require treatment. From the brachial approach a long (90-cm), flexible, reinforced 5F sheath is helpful since it can be left in the iliac system during distal catheterization, and from the contralateral groin access, a long (35-cm to 55-cm) 5F or 6F flexible, reinforced sheath is useful to position in the common or superficial femoral artery prior to a distal therapeutic procedure.

Anticoagulation with heparin or other intravenous-appropriate anticoagulant is routinely used in small doses during the diagnostic studies and therapeutic doses for interventions. For longer procedures, the activating clotting time (ACT) measurements are used to help regulate the dosing of the anticoagulant during the procedure.

When performing an intervention on the lower extremity, it is always advantageous to have a radio-opaque ruler or other radio-opaque markers (needles or similar devices) adjacent to the patient's leg within the radiographic image. This is especially true in the thigh, where the femur does not have unique bony landmarks in the diaphysis, and the ruler provides a frame of reference for the lesion location for directed therapy (Fig. 29-3A). This is particularly useful when changing magnifications for improved visualization at the time of traversing a lesion, or when undertaking an intervention of multiple lesions in different radiographic fields, so that arteriography does not need to be repeated each time the image intensifier is moved.

A directed floppy-tipped wire (platinum) with a torque device is the safest method to cross an obstructing stenosis. These guidewire tips are very soft and cannot dissect or traverse occlusions, thereby minimizing the possibility of endoluminal trauma. A guidewire should never fold over itself, and if there is a stenosis and not an occlusion, one can achieve a visual-tactile feel for the endoluminal irregular anatomy. In fact, there is the contention that blood flow channeling into a stenosis can help direct the smaller (0.014-in.) wires through the obstruction. Glide-tipped wires are very useful to traverse vascular total occlusions, but their very low coefficient of friction also predisposes them to injury, by creating false channels, and occasionally perforate the vessel. These types of injuries can result in a dissection and other problems that, occasionally, cannot be easily remedied by an endovascular approach. For this reason, although a glide-tipped wire may occasionally be required to achieve access beyond obstructions, reasonable attempts

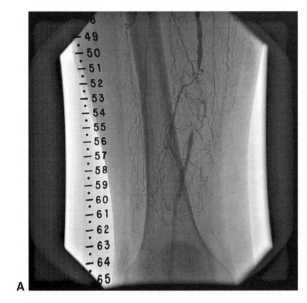
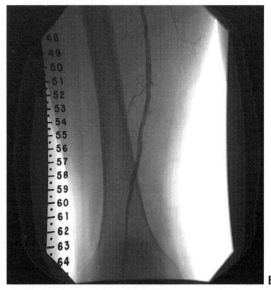

A   **B**

Figure 29-3   A: Angiogram of an occluded superficial femoral artery, with the ruler marker indicating the occlusion is between 52 and 56 cm markers. The ruler provides a frame of reference that is useful for intervention and remains constant between different magnifications. Notice the collaterals present. Post angioplasty **(B)** demonstrates a successful result. Notice the small dissection at the site of intervention. With excellent flow across the lesion there is no need to treat the lesion with a stent.

should be made to exchange them through a catheter for the less traumatic floppy-tipped wire before an intervention. If that is not possible, the location of the tip should be kept under constant observation to avoid its downstream migration and possible artery injury or perforation.

Prior to an intervention, the location of the wire should always be verified by an angiogram, since its inadvertent passage into a side branch (especially a geniculate at the knee) with subsequent intervention into the small vessel can be disconcerting (Fig. 29-4). For antegrade puncture, a 0.014-in. platform and rapid exchange balloons are readily used. They can also be used with a contralateral retrograde access over the top of the aortic bifurcation only after the placement of a flexible, reinforced sheath to facilitate passage of balloons over the aortic bifurcation.

Arterial occlusions are best crossed with a straight 0.035-in. glide wire with an angled or, occasionally, a straight 4F glide catheter. For long or chronic occlusions, the administration of a small amount of thrombolytic agent (1 mg tissue plasminogen activator [tPA] or 5,000 U urokinase) into or at the origin of the occlusion (not above the occlusion) can help facilitate recanalization of the occluded artery. Once beginning the traversion of an extended occlusion (>10 to 15 cm), a small dose of thrombolytic drug into the occlusion may further assist in recanalization. After the glide catheter is placed beyond the recanalized segment, the wire is removed and an angiogram is performed to verify its intraluminal location. A floppy-tipped wire is then advanced into the distal artery prior to retrieval of the catheter and undertaking the intervention.

For occlusions, it is always advisable to start the PTA with smaller balloons and work up to larger diameters, always inflating them slowly. Very rapid inflations can result in unnecessary injury, and there is evidence that keeping the balloon inflated for at least 1 to 2 minutes (at the given atm of pressure, with no decrease in the pressure value) provides superior results. Although the choice of balloon length is determined by the radio-opaque ruler placed adjacent to the artery, the ultimate

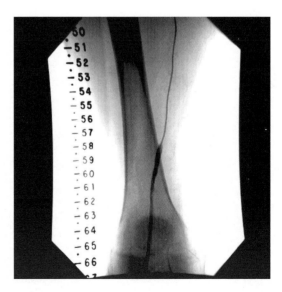

Figure 29-4 Angiogram through the recanalized segment of superficial femoral artery (Fig. 29-3A) by injecting through a catheter that tracked along with the wire during the recanalization. This verifies that the position of the catheter is in the popliteal artery and not subintimal or in a geniculate sidebranch.

balloon diameter is best judged by comparing an angiogram of the distal vessel and the radiographic image of inflated PTA balloon just utilized. Using too large a balloon diameter or inflation pressure can lead to a distal intimal tear, dissection, and a flow-limiting flap. Having the patient awake to disclose pain or pressure at the site of the PTA during the procedure is also valuable information. Higher balloon pressures or larger balloon sizes should not be used to avoid vessel rupture or perforation. If the patient has discomfort with a balloon diameter that appears to be small when compared to the adjacent artery, the PTA procedure can always be repeated at a later date, as long as the vessel is not found on a computed tomography (CT) scan to be severely calcified. When multiple tandem lesions are to be treated, there should be an overlap by 3 to 5 mm between inflations, and the author generally permits a period of blood flow between successive balloon inflations to prevent stagnation of blood and clot formation. The length of time of balloon inflation should approach 1 minute and should always be longer than when the balloon pressure has stabilized without further drift. Between inflations, intra-arterial nitroglycerin (200 μg) can also be administered to help open up the outflow vessels and increase blood flow across the lesions. Completion angiography should be undertaken to verify the anatomic outcome of the intervention (Fig. 29-3B). An important thing to remember is to be gentle to the arteries. They will generally treat you as well as you treat them.

All of the infrainguinal arteries can be treated with success using PTA. Coronary balloons of small diameters, as small as 1.5 mm, can be used for tibial artery PTA, while balloon diameters of >6 mm are rarely needed in the superficial femoral artery. While balloon lengths of 10 to 40 mm are the most frequently used, there are balloons that measure up to 100 mm. The most commonly treated arteries are the superficial femoral and popliteal arteries (Fig. 29-3), keeping in mind that treating behind the knee joint has a higher risk, and the use of a stent in this location should be avoided whenever possible. Tibial lesions can be readily treated for patients with limb-threatening ischemia (Fig. 29-5). Bifurcation lesions can also be addressed using the "buddy wire" technique, with wire access across both lesions at the bifurcation while they are being treated (Fig. 29-6A and D). Angioplasty for these lesions is preferentially undertaken sequentially (Fig. 29-6C and D), but can be done simultaneously in the "kissing balloon" technique.

In restenosis and in plaques involving the origin of the vessels, the use of a focal plaque excision or atherectomy device could be considered.[14,15] These are undergoing constant development and are quite safe, but long-term data is not available. Another problem that can occasionally be encountered is the stenotic lesion that is resistant to PTA while using nominal pressures or pressures that are close to the limit of the balloon rating. During these cases, it is important to restrain from using balloon diameters that are too large since they can result in vessel rupture. Options that can be used to attempt to achieve a successful angioplasty include the use of as short a balloon length that will not result in "watermelon seeding" (inflation-related balloon-migration, either proximally or distally),

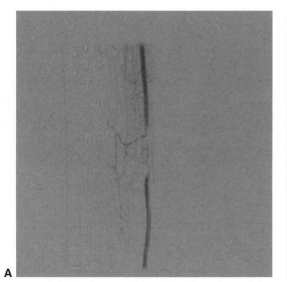
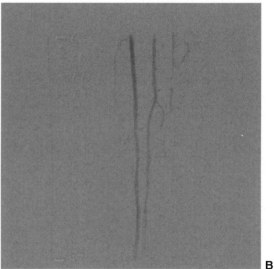

A **B**

Figure 29-5 **A:** Subtraction angiogram of an anterior tibial artery by selective injection that identifies the severe stenosis between the ruler markers of 79 through 82 cm. Although the markers are best seen on native imaging, minor movements during subtraction angiography help identify the markers through the movement in the mask, as seen in the arteriogram. **B:** Postprocedure subtraction angiogram demonstrates an excellent result.

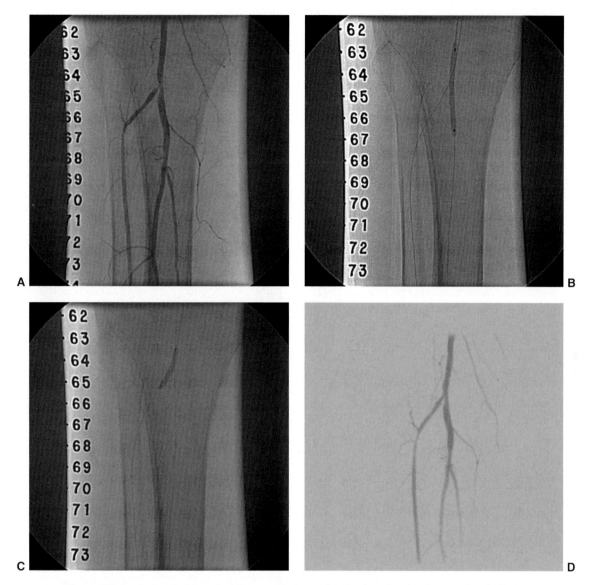

Figure 29-6 **A:** Arteriogram of a bifurcated lesion at the distal popliteal at the anterior tibial take-off, which was accessed by "buddy wires" from the same sheath into both the anterior tibial and the tibioperoneal arteries. Angioplasty was first undertaken for the larger tibioperoneal artery **(B)** and then the anterior tibial artery **(C)** before undertaking a completion arteriogram **(D)**, verifying adequate treatment of the obstructing lesion.

use of very noncompliant, high-pressure balloons, and also the use of "cutting balloons." The cutting balloons (available in sizes up to 6 mm) are most useful for very fibrotic lesions (as in vein graft stenoses), but have been useful for small-diameter, PTA-resistant stenoses, while maintaining a low insertion profile.[16] Although long-term data is not available in peripheral arteries, the short-term data available would suggest that it is a safe and feasible technique to use in these special circumstances.[17]

The use of stents as an adjuvant for infrainguinal PTA is controversial.[18–21] One indication where there is general agreement is the use of stents for a flow-limiting dissection, since they are likely to promote early patency in these circumstances. The stents are introduced into the area of interest after PTA and should cover the point of origin of the flap and the area of maximal lumen compromise. With the introduction of self-expanding nitinol stents, these flexible stents have been advocated to be superior to the balloon-expandable stents for infrainguinal applications. With the high range of motion of the hip and knee joints, placement of stents in these areas, when possible, should be particularly avoided.

The pharmacologic treatment of these patients post infrainguinal balloon angioplasty has not been well studied. Initial experience with the use of abciximab given intravenously at the time of infrainguinal PTA has been positive.[22] On the basis of data with coronary PTA, it is likely that the postprocedure administration of aspirin and clopidrogel for at least 6 to 8 weeks is likely to assist in maintaining early patency in arteries after PTA; this has become the practice of the author.[4]

RESULTS

The results of infrainguinal PTA have evolved over time with the technological advances and the improvement in medical therapy for peripheral vascular disease.[23] Although there is variability between reports of the immediate technical and interval success rates and parameters that affect durability of infrainguinal PTA, many of the observations of determinants of procedural outcome presented by Johnston et al.[24,25] almost 20 years ago remain relevant today. The patency data, low by present standards, for PTA of femoropopliteal artery in all patients was 89% at 1 month and 36% at 6 years, by Kaplan-Meier estimates. However, several factors could significantly predict success of PTA; these factors include the indication for the procedure (claudication > salvage), severity of lesion (stenosis > occlusion), good runoff vessels, fewer number of lesions, and absence of diabetes mellitus.

Angiographic findings at the time of PTA are often cited as the major determinants of procedural success. The TransAtlantic InterSociety Consensus (TASC) classification categorizes the complexity and lesion length of femoropopliteal disease to help reporting standards and predict outcomes. However, this has not been reliable or consistent in predictive value as demonstrated by the Society of Cardiovascular Interventional Radiology (SCVIR) Transluminal Angioplasty and Revascularization Registry (STAR) data of femoropopliteal angioplasty.[26] Other factors, such as patient selection, also have relevance to PTA durability. In a study of patients with critical ischemia, PTA of the superficial femoral artery occlusion >5 cm was found to have an inferior 5-year primary patency than those with occlusions <5 cm (12% vs. 32%).[27] More recent studies compared results of PTA between short or long occlusions and found no significant differences in long-term patency.[28,29] These data would not support the sole use of the TASC classification for the type of lesion to determine whether PTA would be an appropriate method of treatment for a patient.

The results of PTA in the infrageniculate arteries, which should be limited to patients with critical limb ischemia, have also been reported with varied success. It is important when reviewing reported results of crural artery PTA to consider the date of publication since technological advances in equipment have a high likelihood of effecting these results because of the small artery diameters. Reflecting this point, a prospective

study reported PTA procedural success in 84% of stenoses and 61% of occlusions while using 0.035-in. guidewire platform systems rather than the 0.014-in. generally used in coronary-sized arteries, which are similar in diameter to tibial arteries.[30] There are no prospective, randomized trials examining infrageniculate PTA, and most of the reports include patients that have had concomitant inflow procedures. A recent large, prospective series of consecutive patients having infrapopliteal PTA reported a 5-year clinical follow-up of 266 treated limbs in 215 patients.[31] This report of the subgroup of the 92% procedurally successful cases identified an 8% surgical crossover for limb salvage, and a 9% significant amputation rate in the 56% of patients who survived the 5-year duration of the study. As in other publications of infrageniculate PTA,[30,32,33] different endpoints (clinical vs. anatomic) and methods provide a spectrum of outcomes. The only predictors that correlated with poor long-term outcome were chronic renal insufficiency and lack of angiographic improvement after PTA.[30] However, PTA of the infrageniculate arteries should be considered a reasonable primary treatment for severe chronic limb ischemia because of its low complication rate; its very good clinical success rate in a generally elderly, infirm population with a limited life expectancy; and the fact that this treatment modality has not been shown to preclude eventual surgical reconstructions should they become necessary.

The use of intravascular stents as an adjuvant to PTA is considered by many to improve the immediate and long-term results of treatments. In a randomized, controlled trial of PTA treatment of the superficial femoral artery alone or supplemented with a stent, there were no significant hemodynamic or clinical differences (85% vs. 74%) or patency (74% vs. 62%) between the two groups at 1 year.[21] Another multicenter, prospective, randomized study between selective or systematic stenting with a Palmaz balloon-expandable stent with PTA for lesions in the superficial femoral artery did not identify any differences between the two groups. Stents were used in the selective stent group for a 30% or greater angiographic residual stenosis compared to the systematic stent group. At 1 year (32% vs. 35%) there were comparable rates of >50% stenosis, and at 4 years, both groups required an equivalent number of 45% of secondary interventions.[18]

Though routine primary treatment of infrainguinal lesions may have good outcomes with PTA alone, recurrent lesions after PTA may fare better with the use of an intravascular stent.[20] Restenosis after PTA is common and has been described as high as 60% of patients; however, the outcome of PTA alone of recurrent lesions versus primary lesions (33% vs. 61%) at 1 year is significantly different.[34] Therefore, this has led to the search for adjuvant techniques, such as brachytherapy and/or stenting,[35] to improve these results. Though brachytherapy has not been shown conclusively to have improved results in the periphery, the patency rate of PTA and stent for recurrent femoropopliteal lesions were superior to PTA alone.[34]

PTA is becoming more attractive as the primary treatment of critical limb ischemia.[36,37] Its minimally invasive features make it an appealing option for poor-risk patients, those lacking adequate autogenous bypass conduit, or those debilitated from lower extremity lesions. A shorter hospitalization and earlier rehabilitation to baseline activity can be of paramount importance to elderly patients with limited longevity. It is accepted that successful revascularization of patients with critical limb ischemia have improved survival and a better quality of life.[38,39] In the application of PTA as a first-line treatment for critical limb ischemia, Molloy et al.[37] identified a 1-year primary and secondary limb salvage rate (113, 67% vs. 88%), which included surgical bypass for limb salvage for the PTA failures (13 of 24, 54%). This study concluded that percutaneous techniques and surgical bypass can be complementary in the treatment of patients with critical lower limb ischemia.

There is no evidence that using PTA as a primary treatment modality for infrainguinal disease can result in a worse long-term outcome, either by resulting in accelerated atherosclerosis or loss of outflow during failure of the reconstruction. This is supported by Jamsen et al.,[29] who followed 233 consecutive patients with claudication treated with PTA, primarily for infrainguinal disease. Almost half of the treated extremities required repeated treatment (151 of 304 limbs, 49.7%), 47% of which were open surgical reconstructions. Despite the crossover to surgery, this combined treatment approach resulted in only 1.8% of patients per year progressing to critical ischemia. This compared favorably with the quoted natural history progression of claudication to critical ischemia rate of 4.5% in untreated patients.[6]

Diabetes mellitus has been associated with a less favorable outcome after PTA of the femoropopliteal arteries and may decrease the primary patency by as much as 50% when compared to nondiabetic patients.[26,40] Whether this is a result of the diabetes itself, the anatomic pattern of disease involving the crural vessels, or the higher incidence of renal insufficiency, is unclear. Since diabetes was not found to be a significant predictor of patency after distal arterial reconstruction and data have supported improved results of limb salvage after comprehensive revascularization,[41] careful assessment of the patient's vascular anatomy, extent of tissue loss, and general state of health need to be undertaken before determining the type of vascular reconstruction.

Renal failure and dialysis are powerful predictors of poor outcome after surgical revascularization.[42,43]

Although PTA has been advocated in this patient population due to their high surgical morbidity and limited life expectancy, the results suggest caution.[26,29,44] Despite this, since the goal is generally a positive short-term outcome with early return to a normal functional status, it is appropriate to aggressively pursue limb salvage in these patients with a percutaneous approach while considering surgical options as ultimately needed.

CONCLUSION

Although historical series have demonstrated inferior results with PTA compared to bypass surgery, recent results have demonstrated significant improvement in procedural success and long-term patency. As patients are living longer, and revascularization of the lower extremity becomes more of a necessity in a much older patient population that may be much more infirm and have a shorter life expectancy, returning to normal independent function within a short period of time is of prime importance. Early PTA has not been shown to compromise the options of secondary surgical procedures. Therefore, the time has come to re-evaluate the paradigm of patients with severe lower extremity vascular insufficiency and identify which patients should be treated initially with a percutaneous endovascular technique before considering an open bypass operative intervention.

REFERENCES

1. Dotter CT, Judkins MP. Transluminal treatment of arteriosclerotic obstruction. Description of a new technic and a preliminary report of its application. *Circulation*. 1964;30:654–670.
2. Gruntzig A, Hopff H. Percutaneous recanalization after chronic arterial occlusion with a new dilator-catheter (modification of the Dotter technique) (author's transl). *Dtsch Med Wochenschr*. 1974;99:2502–2510, 2511.
3. Palmaz JC, Richter GM, Noldge G, et al. Intraluminal Palmaz stent implantation. The first clinical case report on a balloon-expanded vascular prosthesis. *Radiologe*. 1987;27:560–563.
4. Calver AL, Blows LJ, Harmer S, et al. Clopidogrel for prevention of major cardiac events after coronary stent implantation: 30-day and 6-month results in patients with smaller stents. *Am Heart J*. 2000;140:483–491.
5. Block PC. Mechanism of transluminal angioplasty. *Am J Cardiol*. 1984;53:69C–71C.
6. Hertzer NR. The natural history of peripheral vascular disease. Implications for its management. *Circulation*. 1991;83(2 Suppl): I12–I19.
7. Atar E, Siegel Y, Avrahami R, et al. Balloon angioplasty of popliteal and crural arteries in elderly with critical chronic limb ischemia. *Eur J Radiol*. 2005;53:287–292.
8. Bostrom Ardin A, Lofberg AM, Hellberg A, et al. Selection of patients with infrainguinal arterial occlusive disease for percutaneous transluminal angioplasty with duplex scanning. *Acta Radiol*. 2002;43:391–395.
9. Karch LA, Mattos MA, Henretta JP, et al. Clinical failure after percutaneous transluminal angioplasty of the superficial femoral and popliteal arteries. *J Vasc Surg*. 2000;31:880–887.

10. Schneider PA, Caps MT, Ogawa DY, et al. Intraoperative superficial femoral artery balloon angioplasty and popliteal to distal bypass graft: an option for combined open and endovascular treatment of diabetic gangrene. *J Vasc Surg.* 2001;33:955–962.

11. Spinosa DJ, Angle JF, Hartwell GD, et al. Gadolinium-based contrast agents in angiography and interventional radiology. *Radiol Clin North Am.* 2002;40:693–710.

12. Bees NR, Beese RC, Belli AM, et al. Carbon dioxide angiography of the lower limbs: initial experience with an automated carbon dioxide injector. *Clin Radiol.* 1999;54:833–838.

13. Kaufman J, Moglia R, Lacy C, et al. Peripheral vascular complications from percutaneous transluminal coronary angioplasty: a comparison with transfemoral cardiac catheterization. *Am J Med Sci.* 1989;297:22–25.

14. Zeller T, Rastan A, Schwarzwalder U, et al. Midterm results after atherectomy-assisted angioplasty of below-knee arteries with use of the Silverhawk device. *J Vasc Interv Radiol.* 2004;15:1391–1397.

15. Gordon IL, Conroy RM, Tobis JM, et al. Determinants of patency after percutaneous angioplasty and atherectomy of occluded superficial femoral arteries. *Am J Surg.* 1994;168:115–119.

16. Engelke C, Sandhu C, Morgan RA, et al. Using 6-mm Cutting Balloon angioplasty in patients with resistant peripheral artery stenosis: preliminary results. *AJR Am J Roentgenol.* 2002;179:619–623.

17. Rabbi JF, Kiran RP, Gersten G, et al. Early results with infrainguinal cutting balloon angioplasty limits distal dissection. *Ann Vasc Surg.* 2004;18:640–643.

18. Becquemin JP, Favre JP, Marzelle J, et al. Systematic versus selective stent placement after superficial femoral artery balloon angioplasty: a multicenter prospective randomized study. *J Vasc Surg.* 2003;37:487–494.

19. Chatelard P, Guibourt C. Long-term results with a Palmaz stent in the femoropopliteal arteries. *J Cardiovasc Surg (Torino).* 1996;37(3 Suppl. 1):67–72.

20. Conroy RM, Gordon IL, Tobis JM, et al. Angioplasty and stent placement in chronic occlusion of the superficial femoral artery: technique and results. *J Vasc Interv Radiol.* 2000;11:1009–1020.

21. Vroegindeweij D, Vos LD, Tielbeek AV, et al. Balloon angioplasty combined with primary stenting versus balloon angioplasty alone in femoropopliteal obstructions: a comparative randomized study. *Cardiovasc Intervent Radiol.* 1997;20:420–425.

22. Stavropoulos SW, Solomon JA, Soulen MC, et al. Use of abciximab during infrainguinal peripheral vascular interventions: initial experience. *Radiology.* 2003;227:657–661.

23. Ruef J, Hofmann M, Haase J. Endovascular interventions in iliac and infrainguinal occlusive artery disease. *J Interv Cardiol.* 2004;17:427–435.

24. Johnston KW. Femoral and popliteal arteries: reanalysis of results of balloon angioplasty. *Radiology.* 1992;183:767–771.

25. Johnston KW, Rae M, Hogg-Johnston SA, et al. 5-year results of a prospective study of percutaneous transluminal angioplasty. *Ann Surg.* 1987;206:403–413.

26. Clark TW, Groffsky JL, Soulen MC. Predictors of long-term patency after femoropopliteal angioplasty: results from the STAR registry. *J Vasc Interv Radiol.* 2001;12:923–933.

27. Lofberg AM, Karacagil S, Ljungman C, et al. Percutaneous transluminal angioplasty of the femoropopliteal arteries in limbs with chronic critical lower limb ischemia. *J Vasc Surg.* 2001;34:114–121.

28. Murray JG, Apthorp LA, Wilkins RA. Long-segment (> or = 10 cm) femoropopliteal angioplasty: improved technical success and long-term patency. *Radiology.* 1995;195:158–162.

29. Jamsen TS, Manninen HI, Tulla HE, et al. Infrainguinal revascularization because of claudication: total long-term outcome of endovascular and surgical treatment. *J Vasc Surg.* 2003;37:808–815.

30. Soder HK, Manninen HI, Jaakkola P, et al. Prospective trial of infrapopliteal artery balloon angioplasty for critical limb ischemia: angiographic and clinical results. *J Vasc Interv Radiol.* 2000;11:1021–1031.

31. Dorros G, Jaff MR, Dorros AM, et al. Tibioperoneal (outflow lesion) angioplasty can be used as primary treatment in 235 patients with critical limb ischemia: five-year follow-up. *Circulation.* 2001;104:2057–2062.

32. Boyer L, Therre T, Garcier JM, et al. Infrapopliteal percutaneous transluminal angioplasty for limb salvage. *Acta Radiol.* 2000;41:73–77.

33. Tsetis D, Belli AM. The role of infrapopliteal angioplasty. *Br J Radiol.* 2004;77:1007–1015.

34. Schillinger M, Mlekusch W, Haumer M, et al. Angioplasty and elective stenting of de novo versus recurrent femoropopliteal lesions: 1-year follow-up. *J Endovasc Ther.* 2003;10:288–297.

35. Minar E, Pokrajac B, Ahmadi R, et al. Brachytherapy for prophylaxis of restenosis after long-segment femoropopliteal angioplasty: pilot study. *Radiology.* 1998;208:173–179.

36. Parsons RE, Suggs WD, Lee JJ, et al. Percutaneous transluminal angioplasty for the treatment of limb threatening ischemia: do the results justify an attempt before bypass grafting? *J Vasc Surg.* 1998;28:1066–1071.

37. Molloy KJ, Nasim A, London NJ, et al. Percutaneous transluminal angioplasty in the treatment of critical limb ischemia. *J Endovasc Ther.* 2003;10:298–303.

38. Klevsgard R, Risberg BO, Thomsen MB, et al. A 1-year follow-up quality of life study after hemodynamically successful or unsuccessful surgical revascularization of lower limb ischemia. *J Vasc Surg.* 2001;33:114–122.

39. Kalra M, Gloviczki P, Bower TC, et al. Limb salvage after successful pedal bypass grafting is associated with improved long-term survival. *J Vasc Surg.* 2001;33:6–16.

40. Hewes RC, White RI Jr, Murray RR, et al. Long-term results of superficial femoral artery angioplasty. *AJR Am J Roentgenol.* 1986;146:1025–1029.

41. Pomposelli FB, Kansal N, Hamdan AD, et al. A decade of experience with dorsalis pedis artery bypass: analysis of outcome in more than 1000 cases. *J Vasc Surg.* 2003;37:307–315.

42. Korn P, Hoenig SJ, Skillman JJ, et al. Is lower extremity revascularization worthwhile in patients with end-stage renal disease? *Surgery.* 2000;128:472–479.

43. Seeger JM, Pretus HA, Carlton LC, et al. Potential predictors of outcome in patients with tissue loss who undergo infrainguinal vein bypass grafting. *J Vasc Surg.* 1999;30:427–435.

44. Ramdev P, Rayan SS, Sheahan M, et al. A decade experience with infrainguinal revascularization in a dialysis-dependent patient population. *J Vasc Surg.* 2002;36:969–974.

Surgical Repair of Vein Graft Stenoses

Michael L. Miller   *Joseph L. Mills, Sr.*

In 1973, Szilagyi et al.[1] published a landmark study that addressed, for the first time, the development, frequency, and natural history of intrinsic vein graft stenoses. This report analyzed 377 patients who had been studied by means of serial postoperative arteriography following infrainguinal bypass with autogenous vein conduit; an intrinsic graft stenosis developed over time in one third of these vein bypass grafts. These arteriographic defects were categorized and attributed to a variety of causes including, in decreasing order of importance, intimal thickening, atherosclerosis, fibrotic valve leaflets, fibrotic vein stenosis, aneurysmal dilation, and suture (anastomotic) stenosis.

Since the seminal contribution by Dr. Szilagyi and his group at Henry Ford Hospital, numerous investigators have confirmed that at least 25% to 30% of infrainguinal autogenous grafts placed for occlusive disease ultimately develop intrinsic stenosis.[2-4] This problem has been most commonly attributed to myointimal hyperplasia and is the persistent Achilles' heel of arterial reconstructive surgery. A significant proportion of such stenotic lesions are progressive and lead to vein graft occlusion and its associated morbidity. A subset of lesions exhibit a more benign natural history and thus may be safely observed. Since the mid-1980s, duplex ultrasound has replaced conventional arteriography as the surveillance tool of choice for infrainguinal vein bypass grafts because it is noninvasive, safer, cheaper, and provides useful hemodynamic information of prognostic and clinical importance. Specific hemodynamic parameters have been developed that permit detection and grading of vein graft stenosis.[3,5-8] These parameters correlate with the relative risk of subsequent graft occlusion and are useful in appropriately selecting graft-threatening lesions for targeted intervention to prevent untimely graft occlusion. The vascular surgeon, therefore, must not only possess the technical expertise to repair selected graft-threatening lesions, but also must offer duplex-based graft surveillance to all his infrainguinal vein graft patients, and be able to interpret the available data to determine which grafts require intervention.

Despite the tidal wave of enthusiasm for numerous less invasive, catheter-based interventions for peripheral vascular disease, the primary and most effective treatment method for lower extremity vein graft stenosis remains open repair. Although selected, focal, late-appearing vein graft lesions may respond favorably to percutaneous transluminal angioplasty (PTA) (Table 30-1), in general, the results of conventional PTA for vein graft stenosis are distinctly inferior to those of open repair.[9-13] There are two reports detailing the use of cutting balloon angioplasty for infrainguinal vein graft lesions, but long-term durability is unproven.[14,15] At the present time, the best treatment option for the majority of primary vein graft stenotic lesions is open surgical revision (Table 30-2) because it yields 5-year assisted-primary patency rates of 75% to 85%, compared to 50% assisted-primary patencies at 2 to 3 years following PTA.[9,11,12]

GRAFT SURVEILLANCE: TECHNIQUE AND ALGORITHM

Graft failures can be categorized as early, intermediate, or late. Early graft failures are those that occur in the

TABLE 30-1

PATENCY RATE FOLLOWING PERCUTANEOUS TRANSLUMINAL ANGIOPLASTY FOR GRAFT STENOSIS

Reference	6 mo	12 mo	24 mo	36 mo	48 mo	60 mo
Perler[9]	69%	29%	—	22%	—	—
Sanchez[11]	60.2%	52%	—	—	—	—
Gahtan[10]	86.4%	67.5%	60.8%	—	—	—
Avino[13]	82%	75%	63%	53%	—	—
Whittemore[12]	59%	42%	36%	25%	18%	18%
Carlson[16]	74.2%	62.7%	58.2%	—	—	—
Mean	**71.8%**	**54.7%**	**54.5%**	**33.3%**	**18%**	**18%**

first 30 postoperative days, and are usually due to poor conduit selection, judgmental errors, or technical imperfections made during the bypass procedure. Late failures are those that occur 3 or more years after the procedure, the vast majority of which are due to progressive atherosclerotic disease in the inflow and outflow tracts. Graft failures most frequently occur between 30 days and 3 years postoperatively, and such failures are termed intermediate. Intermediate vein graft failure is due primarily to focal intrinsic graft stenosis, and it is the outcome of this subset that is most strongly influenced by an aggressive duplex surveillance program. Idu et al.[19,20] found that virtually all unrevised >70% diameter-reducing graft stenoses progressed to total occlusion and subsequent graft failure. Wixon et al.[21] from our own group at the University of Arizona confirmed the malignant natural history of high-grade vein graft stenoses. Revision following graft thrombosis has been conclusively shown to be inferior to revision prior to thrombosis.[18,22–25] The identification of critical vein graft stenosis prior to graft occlusion is therefore the implicit goal of graft surveillance.

Prior to the advances in duplex ultrasound (DUS) technology over the last 2 decades, graft surveillance relying only upon history, clinical examination, and ankle-brachial index (ABI) determination was not sufficiently sensitive to reliably detect the failing graft prior to occlusion; serial arteriography proved to be prohibitively expensive and excessively invasive. The efficacy of DUS surveillance in identifying and grading hemodynamically significant lesions within the vein graft has been verified by numerous investigators and has made it the gold standard in graft surveillance.[5,26,27] Duplex-based surveillance programs have increased 5-year assisted-primary patency rates to 78% to 85% compared to 60% to 70% patency rates for those grafts followed by clinical observation alone.[8] Graft surveillance studies include serial color flow duplex surveillance of the entire graft and its anastomoses as well as the adjacent inflow and outflow arteries and ABI pressure determinations. These studies should begin within the first 4 weeks following the procedure, be repeated at 3-month intervals for the first year, every 6 months for the second and third postoperative years, and annually thereafter. Such intensive early surveillance is warranted because

TABLE 30-2

PATENCY RATE FOLLOWING OPEN SURGICAL REVISION FOR GRAFT STENOSIS

Reference	6 mo	12 mo	24 mo	36 mo	48 mo
Perler[9]	75%	62%	—	62%	62%
Sanchez[11]	91.4%	86.4%	—	—	—
Avino[13]	92%	79%	66%	63%	63%
Landry[17]	98.8%	95.7%	93.1%	90.6%	87.4%
Sullivan[18]	98%	98%	98%	95%	79%
Mean	**91.04%**	**84.22%**	**85.7%**	**82.87%**	**76.47%**

the vast majority of graft-threatening lesions develop within the first 3 postoperative years; 70% to 80% of all significant intrinsic graft lesions are detected within the first year after graft implantation.[2,3,28,29] Continued life-long surveillance, albeit less intense, is likewise warranted due to the persistent, ongoing rate of late graft failure. Threshold criteria for intervention have been validated via prospective studies and include the following: (a) High-velocity criteria (HVC) defined as peak systolic velocity (PSV) >300 cm per second and velocity ratio (VR) >3.5; and (b) low-velocity criteria (LVC) defined as PSV <45 cm per second ± an ABI decrease >0.15.[7,29]

Duplex vein graft surveillance can be justified not only on clinical but also on economic grounds. Wixon et al.[21] found that the total cost of the initial bypass procedure along with 5 years of surveillance was slightly less than the cost of a major limb amputation ($35,649 vs. $36,273). Additionally, the expenses incurred in the care of patients with grafts revised for stenosis detected by duplex were significantly less than costs for those patients in whom grafts were revised after thrombosis ($17,677 vs. $45,252 for 1 year). Visser et al.[30] have also confirmed the economic superiority of duplex vein graft surveillance compared to clinical observation alone.

TECHNIQUES OF REPAIR

In general, there are three options whenever a vein graft stenosis is identified: Continued observation, percutaneous endovascular repair, or open surgical revision. The first option, continued observation without intervention, is inappropriate for grafts harboring a severe stenosis. Failure to intervene for vein graft stenoses exceeding 70% diameter reduction inevitably leads to graft thrombosis. Several studies have shown that revision after thrombosis results in 1- and 2-year patency rates of 20% to 50%.[17,28,31] This outcome stands in mark contrast to 5-year assisted-patency rates exceeding 80% for those grafts revised prior to failure[23,32]; such patency is nearly equivalent to those grafts in which no stenosis was ever detected. A recent report by Landry et al.[17,33] from Oregon has even documented 10-year assisted-primary patency rates of 80% in revised grafts and 5-year patency rates of 91% for grafts requiring multiple revisions. These findings strongly support expeditious, elective, open revision of severe vein graft stenoses detected by duplex surveillance.

Once a hemodynamically significant graft stenosis has been confirmed and treatment deemed necessary, the decision then becomes one of selection of the most efficacious technique. Revision technique remains somewhat controversial since there is no consensus on which procedure provides the best outcome. The two basic options are endovascular repair (PTA) or open surgical revision. When first introduced, many clinicians were of the opinion that PTA would be an effective means of treating vein graft stenosis and would yield results comparable to open surgical repair. Although no randomized, prospective trials have been performed, available data suggest that PTA is generally inferior to open repair.[9,11,12] Additionally, the indiscriminate use of PTA frequently results in an increased requirement for multiple reinterventions. One recent study suggested that PTA is efficacious when selectively and judiciously applied. Avino et al.[13] noted that results of PTA were nearly equivalent to surgical revision when specifically applied to focal lesions (<2 cm in length), developing after 4 months following the original bypass procedure, in good-caliber veins (>3.5 mm). Thus, the use of PTA as the primary intervention for vein graft stenosis remains controversial and is of limited clinical applicability. There is insufficient clinical data to determine whether cutting balloon technology will improve the results of standard PTA. Such less invasive techniques are, however, an option when the patient refuses surgery or is at excessively high risk for open surgery due to medical comorbidities.

From the previous discussion, one can conclude that open surgical revision is still the procedure of choice for severe vein graft stenosis. The precise technique of open repair is dictated by the location and etiology of the lesion. Sixty percent to 70% of vein graft failures in the first 5 postoperative years are due to focal intrinsic graft stenosis.[1,2] Midgraft lesions are often the result of retained or sclerotic valve leaflets; many of these can be corrected by partial excision of the valve leaflets and vein patch angioplasty. Circumferential fibrotic lesions, however, will require total, segmental excision with interposition vein graft replacement. Stenoses occurring near the anastomosis are termed juxta-anastomotic lesions. Whether at the proximal or distal anastomosis, these lesions usually occur on the venous side of the anastomosis and are the result of focal intimal hyperplasia. Such lesions can sometimes be repaired by excision of the stenotic portion of the vein graft and translocation of the anastomosis to an adjacent arterial site, thus obviating the need to harvest additional conduit. Proximal graft lesions may often be treated in this manner if the original anastomosis was to the common femoral artery, and the origin and proximal deep femoral artery is widely patent and relatively free of obstruction. If there is insufficient length to allow relocation of the vein graft, an interposition vein graft can be used.

Graft-threatening lesions can also develop in the inflow or outflow tracts. Although 80% of intrinsic vein graft lesions are solitary, it should be noted that in approximately 20% of cases there will either be synchronous or metachronous lesions elsewhere in the graft, the inflow vessels, or the outflow vessels. Therefore, it is imperative that at some point, the entire conduit and its inflow and outflow be evaluated arteriographically to ensure that no other lesions are present.

SURGICAL TREATMENT STRATEGIES

In the remainder of this chapter, specific graft-threatening lesions will be discussed, and the surgical interventions designed to correct them will be reviewed in some detail. Lesions of importance include preexisting vein conduit defects, postoperative intrinsic vein graft stenosis, and progressive disease of inflow and outflow vessels.

Preexisting Vein Conduit Defects

The best strategy for treatment of stenoses due to conduit defects is to discover and repair them at the time of initial graft implantation. With attention to detail, many such defects can be identified during conduit preparation. The vein should be carefully palpated and flushed. Sclerotic areas within the vein are suggested by the findings of firmness or hardness to palpation, and nondistensibility during gentle graft irrigation with manual compression. These lesions should be excised and the conduit repaired prior to implantation. Upgrading the conduit by the identification of a significant intrinsic focal defect can prevent the development of an early graft occlusion. Angioscopy is useful in identifying such lesions, especially when the surgeon is employing arm vein conduits that are prone to contain intraluminal webs and synechiae.

It is essential in the early postoperative period to detect any evidence of a suboptimal, hemodynamic result. If missed, valvular lesions or other technical defects can result in platelet deposition and resultant graft thrombosis. The presence of such lesions almost invariably leads to graft failure within the first 3 months. Careful, serial clinical examinations in conjunction with early duplex studies will salvage many such at-risk grafts.

Postoperative Intrinsic Vein Graft Stenosis

Approximately 80% of intrinsic vein graft lesions will be solitary, focal stenoses. These lesions may occur in the juxta-anastomotic area or midgraft. Juxta-anastomotic lesions are almost exclusively found on the vein side of the arterial to vein graft anastomosis, and are found with nearly equal frequency at the proximal and distal ends of the graft. Proximal lesions may occur more frequently following reversed vein graft placement, while distal lesions may be more common after *in situ* grafting. Figure 30-1A demonstrates a typical, focal, proximal, juxta-anastomotic graft stenosis. The primary etiology of these stenoses is likely myointimal hyperplasia. What causes intimal hyperplasia to develop in some grafts and not others is presently an area of intense research investigation. Potential causes being studied include genetic predisposition, operative trauma, or flow and shear stress abnormalities.

A variety of procedures, such as interposition vein grafting, vein patch angioplasty, or anastomotic translocation can be employed to repair focal juxta-anastomotic stenoses. The technique of anastomotic translocation, as illustrated in Figure 30-1B and C, is especially useful when the stenosis is at the proximal anastomosis and there is limited additional vein conduit. By excising the stenosis and relocating the anastomosis to a more distal origin (often the deep femoral artery), no additional conduit will be required. Figure 30-1D is an intraoperative arteriogram performed following a proximal anastomotic translocation for a focal high-grade proximal graft stenosis.

Occasionally, juxta-anastomotic stenoses may be more diffuse and therefore not amenable to angioplasty or translocation. In such cases, vein graft interposition can be used to correct the abnormality. Almost equal in frequency to proximal juxta-anastomotic stenoses are distal juxta-anastomotic lesions. These are most easily repaired either by vein patch angioplasty or by resection and interposition vein grafting.

Midgraft stenoses (Fig. 30-2A) are most often the result of fibrosis at valve sites or idiopathic, fibrotic intimal hyperplasia.[34] These lesions can usually be addressed either by vein patch angioplasty or by interposition vein grafting (Fig. 30-2B).

No matter which technique of open repair is undertaken, it is essential that the intervention minimize potential additional injury to the arterialized vein conduit. The graft is especially subject to injury during dissection in a scarred field or by traumatic clamp placement directly on the vein. These injuries can be prevented through the use of distal exsanguination with an Esmarch bandage and proximal tourniquet control, obviating the need for clamp placement (Fig. 30-3). Revision of focal graft stenosis can often be performed under local anesthesia, especially if the graft has been subcutaneously tunneled. Since redo vein grafts and those employing alternate conduits, such as arm vein, are associated with an increased requirement for subsequent revision,[35] we frequently tunnel such grafts subcutaneously. This approach renders graft surveillance studies easy and greatly simplifies open graft repair should the need arise.

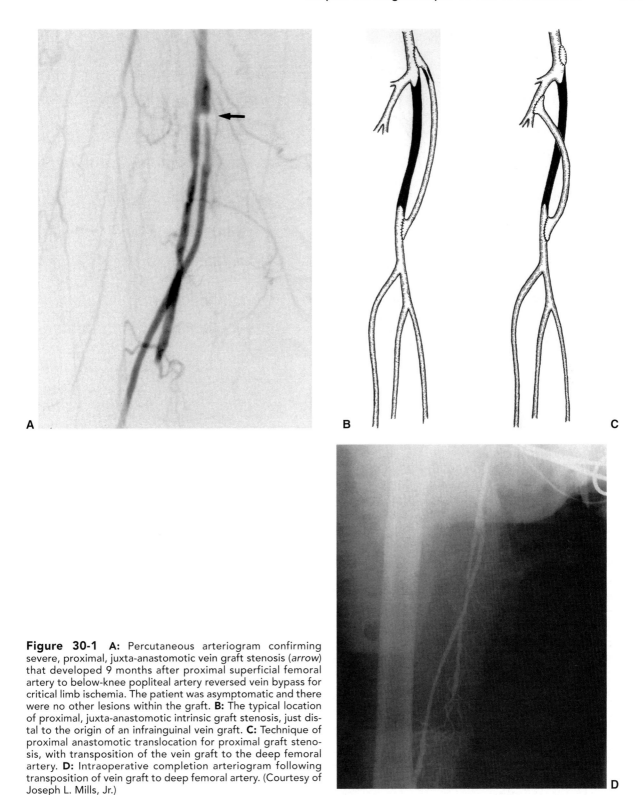

Figure 30-1 A: Percutaneous arteriogram confirming severe, proximal, juxta-anastomotic vein graft stenosis (*arrow*) that developed 9 months after proximal superficial femoral artery to below-knee popliteal artery reversed vein bypass for critical limb ischemia. The patient was asymptomatic and there were no other lesions within the graft. **B:** The typical location of proximal, juxta-anastomotic intrinsic graft stenosis, just distal to the origin of an infrainguinal vein graft. **C:** Technique of proximal anastomotic translocation for proximal graft stenosis, with transposition of the vein graft to the deep femoral artery. **D:** Intraoperative completion arteriogram following transposition of vein graft to deep femoral artery. (Courtesy of Joseph L. Mills, Jr.)

Arterial Disease Progression

Graft failures after 3 years following implantation are frequently the result of progressive arterial occlusive disease in either the inflow or outflow tract.[34] These lesions may be isolated to the native arterial tree or may develop in conjunction with juxta-anastomotic graft stenosis; all such lesions are readily identifiable by duplex surveillance. Figure 30-4A demonstrates a distal

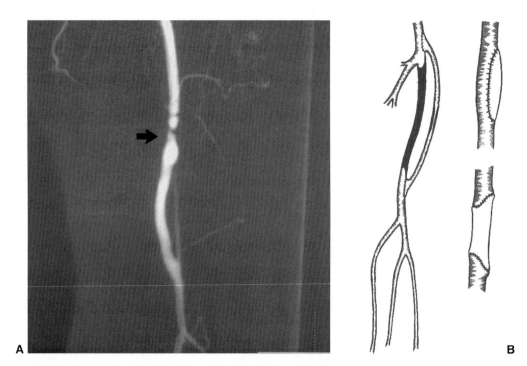

Figure 30-2 **A:** Arteriogram of complex, midgraft vein graft lesion (*arrow*) that was detected by surveillance 14 months following femoropopliteal graft implantation. At exploration, two focal valve lesions were excised and vein patch angioplasty was performed. **B:** Midgraft lesions may be corrected by vein patch angioplasty or short vein graft interposition. The latter method is more appropriate for circumferential, fibrous, napkin ring–like stenoses and for lesions exceeding 1 to 2 cm in length. (Courtesy of Joseph L. Mills, Jr.)

juxta-anastomotic stenosis in conjunction with progressive arterial outflow disease. Such tandem lesions are best repaired using an extension or jump graft originating from patent graft just proximal to the intrinsic stenosis, with insertion distal to the native arterial stenosis (Fig. 30-4B). Figure 30-5 shows preoperative (Fig. 30-5A) and completion (Fig. 30-5B) arteriograms showing the treatment of a severe popliteal artery stenosis just distal to an *in situ* vein graft that was detected by duplex and ABI measurement in the fourth year following graft implantation. In this case, the jump graft was tunneled through the interosseous membrane to allow its insertion into the dominant runoff vessel, the anterior tibial artery.

Less frequently seen are high-grade stenoses or occlusive lesions in outflow arteries below patent functioning

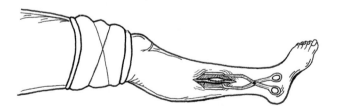

Figure 30-3 Distal exsanguination with an Esmarch bandage followed by tourniquet application is a useful technique for repair of many vein graft lesions. This approach minimizes dissection and obviates the need for placement of silastic vessel loops or traumatic clamps. (Courtesy of Joseph L. Mills, Jr.)

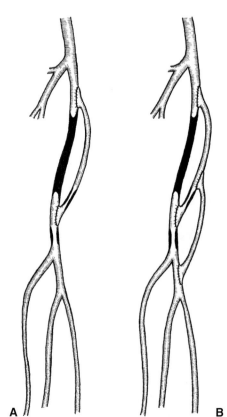

Figure 30-4 **A:** Illustration of distal juxta-anastomotic graft stenosis in conjunction with native popliteal artery stenosis distal to the graft insertion site. **B:** A sequential graft or graft extension addresses both lesions. (Courtesy of Joseph L. Mills, Jr.)

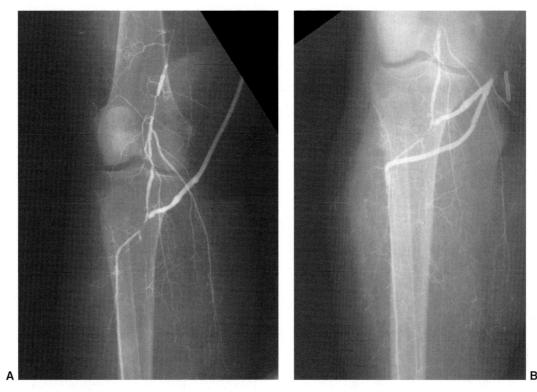

Figure 30-5 **A:** Arteriogram demonstrating nearly occlusive arterial stenosis distal to an *in situ* femoral to below-knee popliteal artery bypass 3 $^1/_2$ years following graft placement. **B:** Completion arteriogram after extension graft to anterior tibial artery, tunneled through the interosseous membrane. (Courtesy of Joseph L. Mills, Jr.)

grafts. When such lesions result in low graft flow velocities, there is an increased risk of graft thrombosis and recurrent foot ischemia. An example of such a lesion is depicted in Figure 30-6A. Occasionally, lesions of this type may be treated by translocating the distal anastomosis to an alternate runoff artery, if available (Fig. 30-6B), or by extending the bypass to a more distal target artery.

Progressive atherosclerotic occlusive disease may also develop over time in the inflow arteries leading to stenosis or even occlusion of the inflow artery, while the graft itself remains patent but in a low-flow state. The patient may be asymptomatic or may notice return of claudication or rest pain; a key finding is that diminished or absent femoral pulses will be noted on physical examination. In addition, DUS will reveal low flow velocities within the graft (<45 cm per second, usually <30 cm per second). While mature, arterialized vein grafts without intrinsic defects are remarkably tolerant to low-flow states, such a situation will put the graft at increased risk for eventual failure, making it essential that the responsible lesion be corrected. Procedures commonly used to restore adequate inflow include percutaneous transluminal iliac angioplasty or local endarterectomy for focal lesions, and aortofemoral bypass, axillofemoral bypass, or femorofemoral bypass for more diffuse

disease. The appropriate procedure must be based upon the anatomic distribution of disease and the patient's medical condition.

SUMMARY

While peripheral bypass procedures can be formidable undertakings in and of themselves, the major challenge in the management of patients requiring such interventions lies in attempting to optimize long-term outcome. A patent infrainguinal bypass graft reduces the incidence of recurrent limb ischemia and major limb amputation and is most readily provided by a thorough program of routine postoperative surveillance with timely intervention for severe or progressive vein graft lesions. Although the majority of autogenous vein bypasses remain patent for many years, significant stenosis develops with sufficient frequency to warrant lifelong surveillance. All grafts found to have severe stenoses should be expeditiously repaired. If repair is performed before the onset of thrombosis, subsequent graft patency will rival that of nonstenotic grafts. Grafts which thrombose, however, exhibit dismal patency rates following repair. The type of revision needed is dictated by the location and extent of the responsible lesion and the ingenuity of

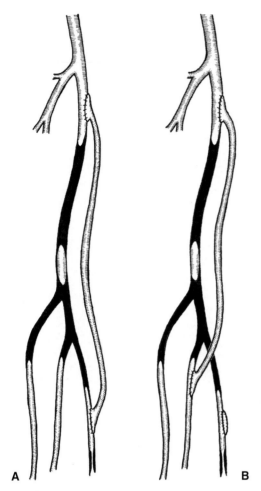

Figure 30-6 A: Illustration of outflow tract atherosclerotic disease progression in posterior tibial artery distal to graft insertion site. These lesions typically occur 3 or more years after the initial reconstruction, and may result in low graft flow velocities with high resistance patterns on duplex surveillance. **B:** If a suitable, patent, parallel outflow artery is available (in this illustration, the peroneal vessel) the graft may be salvaged by distal anastomotic translocation. (Courtesy of Joseph L. Mills, Jr.)

the surgeon, as outlined in the preceding sections. Routine duplex graft surveillance and judicious surgical repair of graft-threatening lesions unquestionably reduces the significant morbidity associated with vein graft thrombosis.

REFERENCES

1. Szilagyi DE, Elliot JP, Hageman JH, et al. Biologic fate of autogenous vein implants as arterial substitutes: clinical, angiographic and histopathologic observations in femoro-popliteal operations for atherosclerosis. *Ann Surg.* 1973;178:232–246.
2. Mills JL, Fujitani RM, Taylor SM. The characteristics and anatomic distribution of lesions that cause reversed vein graft failure: a five-year prospective study. *J Vasc Surg.* 1993;17:195–206.
3. Mills JL, Wixon CL, James DC, et al. The natural history of intermediate and critical vein graft stenosis: recommendations for continued surveillance or repair. *J Vasc Surg.* 2001;33:273–280.
4. Mills JL, Bandyk DF, Gahtan V. The origin of infrainguinal vein graft stenosis: a prospective study based on duplex surveillance. *J Vasc Surg.* 1995;21:16–25.
5. Mills JL, Harris EJ, Taylor LM, et al. The importance of routine surveillance of distal bypass grafts with duplex scanning: a study of 379 reversed vein grafts. *J Vasc Surg.* 1990;12:379–389.
6. Idu MM, Buth J, Hop WC, et al. Vein graft surveillance: is graft revision without angiography justified and what criteria should be used? *J Vasc Surg.* 1998;27:399–413.
7. Westerband A, Mills JL, Kistler S, et al. Prospective validation of threshold criteria for intervention in infrainguinal vein grafts undergoing duplex surveillance. *Ann Vasc Surg.* 1997;11:44–48.
8. Bandyk DF. Infrainguinal vein bypass graft surveillance: how to do it, when to intervene, and is it cost effective? *J Am Coll Surg.* 2002;194(S1):40–52.
9. Perler BA, Osterman FA, Mitchell SE, et al. Balloon dilation versus surgical revision of infrainguinal autogenous vein graft stenosis: long-term follow-up. *J Cardiovasc Surg.* 1990;31:656–661.
10. Gahtan V, Weiss JP, Kerstein MD, et al. Percutaneous transluminal angioplasty in the treatment of vein graft stenosis. *Vasc Surg.* 1997;31:721–726.
11. Sanchez LA, Suggs WD, Marin ML, et al. Is percutaneous balloon angioplasty appropriate in the treatment of graft and anastomotic lesions responsible for failing vein bypasses? *Am J Surg.* 1994;168:97–101.
12. Whittemore AD, Donaldson MC, Polak JF, et al. Limitations of balloon angioplasty for vein graft stenosis. *J Vasc Surg.* 1991;14: 340–345.
13. Avino AJ, Bandyk DF, Gonsalves AJ, et al. Surgical and endovascular intervention for infrainguinal vein graft stenosis. *J Vasc Surg.* 1999;29:60–71.
14. Mauri L, Bonan R, Weiner BH, et al. Cutting balloon angioplasty for the prevention of restenosis: results of the cutting balloon global randomized trial. *Am J Cardiol.* 2002;90:1079–1083.
15. Engelke C, Morgan RA, Belli AM. Cutting balloon percutaneous angioplasty for salvage of lower limb arterial bypass grafts: feasibility. *Radiology.* 2002;223:106–114.
16. Carlson GA, Hoballah JJ, Sharp WJ, et al. Balloon angioplasty as a treatment of failing infrainguinal autologous vein bypass grafts. *J Vasc Surg.* 2004;39(2):421–426.
17. Landry GJ, Moneta GL, Taylor LM. et al. Long-term outcome of revised lower-extremity bypass grafts. *J Vasc Surg.* 2002;35:56–63.
18. Sullivan TR Jr, Welch HJ, Iafrati MD, et al. Clinical results of common strategies used to revise infrainguinal vein grafts. *J Vasc Surg.* 1996;24:909–919.
19. Idu MM, Blankenstein JD, DeGier P, et al. Impact of colour-flow duplex surveillance program on infrainguinal vein graft patency: a five year experience. *J Vasc Surg.* 1993;17:42–53.
20. Idu MM, Truyen E, Buth J. Surveillance of lower vein grafts. *Eur J Vasc Endovasc Surg.* 1992;6:456–462.
21. Wixon CL, Mills JL, Westerband A, et al. An economic appraisal of lower extremity bypass graft maintenance. *J Vasc Surg.* 2000; 32:1–12.
22. Donaldson MC, Mannick JA, Whittemore AD. Causes of primary graft failure after *in situ* saphenous vein bypass grafting. *J Vasc Surg.* 1992;15:113–120.
23. Bandyk DF, Bergamini TM, Towne JB, et al. Durability of vein graft revision: the outcome of secondary procedures. *J Vasc Surg.* 1991;13:200–210.
24. Nielsen TG, Jensen LP, Schroeder TV. Early vein bypass thrombectomy is associated with an increased risk of graft related stenosis. *Eur J Vasc Endovasc Surg.* 1997;13:134–138.
25. Bergamini TM, Towne JB, Bandyk DF, et al. Experience with *in situ* vein bypasses during 1981 to 1989: determinant factors of long-term patency. *J Vasc Surg.* 1991;13:137–149.
26. Golledge J, Beattie DK, Greenlaugh RM, et al. Have the results of infrainguinal bypass improved with the widespread utilization

of postoperative surveillance? *Eur J Vasc Endovasc Surg.* 1996;11: 388–392.

27. Lundell A, Lindblad B, Bergqvist D. Femoropopliteal-crural graft patency is improved by an intensive surveillance program: a prospective randomized study. *J Vasc Surg.* 1995;21:26–34.

28. Mattos MA, Bemmelen PS, Hodgson KJ, et al. Does correction of stenosis identified with color duplex scanning infrainguinal graft patency? *J Vasc Surg.* 1993;17:54–66.

29. Mills JL, Wixon CL. Pathobiology, detection and treatment of vein graft stenosis. In: Mills JL, ed. *Management of chronic lower limb ischemia.* London: Arnold; 2000:113–129.

30. Visser K, Idu MM, Buth J, et al. Duplex scan surveillance during the first year after infrainguinal autologous vein bypass grafting surgery: Costs and clinical outcomes compared with other surveillance programs. *J Vasc Surg.* 2001;33:23–30.

31. Belkin M, Donaldson MC, Whittemore Ad, et al. Observations on the use of thrombolytic agents for thrombotic occlusion of infrainguinal vein grafts. *J Vasc Surg.* 1990;11:289–296.

32. Nehler MR, Moneta GL, Yeager RA, et al. Surgical treatment of threatened reversed infrainguinal vein grafts. *J Vasc Surg.* 1994; 20:558–565.

33. Landry GJ, Moneta GL, Taylor LM, et al. Patency and characteristics of lower extremity vein grafts requiring multiple revisions. *J Vasc Surg.* 2000;32:23–31.

34. Mills JL. Mechanisms of vein graft failure: the location, distribution and characteristics of lesions that predispose to graft failure. *Semin Vasc Surg.* 1993;6:78–91.

35. Landry GJ, Moneta GL, Taylor LM, et al. Choice of autogenous conduit for lower extremity vein graft revisions. *J Vasc Surg.* 2002; 36:238–244.

Secondary Surgical Procedures for Failed Bypasses

Gautam Shrikhande   **Bernadette Aulivola**   **Frank Pomposelli**

As the population ages, the frequency of limb-threatening ischemia secondary to atherosclerotic peripheral vascular disease increases. Despite the excellent patency rates associated with primary lower extremity revascularization procedures, vascular surgeons will inevitably encounter patients with recurrent limb-threatening ischemia after failed bypasses. Many surgeons maintain an aggressive policy of repeated limb revascularization, even in the face of multiple previous graft failures. A unique set of challenges is associated with the performance of repeat leg bypass, including progressively distal bypass target locations and shortage of autogenous vein conduit. In general, two types of secondary revascularization are used in the setting of graft failure. One approach aims at salvage of part or all of the previous bypass graft utilizing thrombectomy techniques, vein patching, and jump grafting. The second approach involves performing an entirely new bypass graft. The choice of which option is most appropriate in a given situation depends on multiple factors, including conduit type, location of the primary bypass, etiology of graft failure, and available inflow and outflow target vessels. This chapter focuses on the management of the lower extremity with a failed bypass graft, with an emphasis on the technical aspects unique to secondary bypass procedures.

INDICATIONS

Secondary arterial reconstruction is indicated in the presence of ischemic rest pain, nonhealing ischemic ulcer, and gangrene. The threshold for performing redo bypass procedures for claudication is generally higher and should be considered mainly in patients with truly disabling claudication. In general, immediate limb salvage is the main indication for secondary arterial reconstructions. The presence of diabetes does not preclude aggressive therapy; however, careful selection and judgment should be used with end-stage renal disease patients, given their decreased long-term survival.[1,2]

ETIOLOGY OF GRAFT FAILURE

Graft failure occurs by markedly different mechanisms in autogenous versus prosthetic bypass conduit. Whereas the most common cause of graft failure in bypasses constructed with autogenous vein is disease intrinsic to the vein conduit, prosthetic bypass grafts tend to fail as a result of lesions at the anastomoses.[3]

Factors that may contribute to early graft failure (<30 days) are technical error, poor inflow or outflow target vessel selection, poor distal runoff, multisegment disease, poor conduit quality, and low-flow states. The etiology of early graft failure is unknown in up to half of cases. A study investigating the incidence of early graft failure associated with technical failure in femorodistal bypass grafts noted that early graft failure occurred in a total of 7.3% of bypasses. Causes of graft failure were determined to be coagulation disorders in 16.1%, technical defects in 14.5%, inadequate runoff in 11.3%, and embolization in 9.7% of cases. No identifiable cause of graft thrombosis was identified in 48% of cases; however, 83% of these grafts were salvaged with surgical thrombectomy and anticoagulation.[4] Early graft failure has also been described in the setting of vascular clamp injury to the native vessel above the proximal anastomosis causing thrombosis of the native vessel as well as the bypass graft. In this setting, resulting ischemic symptoms may be more severe than those noted preoperatively, given proximal extension of thrombus and extension into the profunda femoris artery.[5] Furthermore, occurrences of transient, low-flow states may be to blame for graft thrombosis in some cases. Interestingly, despite the potential for differing degrees of anesthesia-related hypotension, type of anesthetic administered (spinal, epidural, general) has not been noted to significantly impact upon early graft thrombosis rate.[6]

Late graft failure (>30 days) may result from similar causes as early failure. However, late graft failure is most commonly the result of intimal hyperplasia and progression of native arterial atherosclerotic disease. Intimal hyperplasia usually occurs between 2 and 18 months after revascularization, and can involve any portion of the vein graft, although the distal anastomosis is most commonly affected. After 18 months, the most common cause of graft failure is thought to be progression of native vessel atherosclerotic disease. In a series of 450 infrainguinal revascularization procedures where native inflow occlusion was noted to occur in 16 limbs, no cases of associated bypass graft failure were noted. This series brings to question the implication that native inflow disease contributes to the failure of infrainguinal bypass grafts.[7] One series of 227 infrainguinal revascularizations noted the cause of late reversed vein graft failure to be intrinsic graft stenosis in 59.6%, inflow failure in 12.8%, outflow failure in 8.5%, muscle entrapment in 4.3%, and hypercoagulable state in 4.3% of cases.[8] Other series have found progression of outflow vessel disease to account for a higher proportion of graft failures, as much as 67.6%.[9]

The extent of arterial calcification has been implicated as a factor associated with increased susceptibility to graft failure. However, comparable graft patency rates have been observed in cases of clampable and unclampable calcified vessels. This suggests that the finding of severe, circumferential calcification of outflow target arteries should not preclude their use as bypass targets.[10]

DIAGNOSIS OF GRAFT FAILURE

Patients with graft failure often present with recurrence of prebypass symptoms such as rest pain, claudication, or a notable deceleration in wound healing. Graft surveillance with ultrasound or physical examination can aid in the identification of both the failing and the failed bypass graft. A documented change in the quality of palpable pulses or Doppler signals may be the only indicator of graft failure. Graft failure is usually categorized as early or late, as detailed above; the timing of failure may impact treatment decisions.

MANAGEMENT OF EARLY GRAFT FAILURE

In cases of initial infrainguinal reconstruction for limb salvage, early graft failure is commonly associated with recurrent limb threat. Given that angiography was likely performed prior to the initial operation, additional angiographic study is usually unnecessary prior to reoperation (Fig. 31-1). Once graft failure is identified,

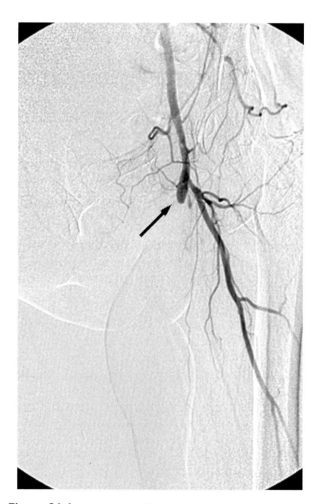

Figure 31-1 Angiogram of the failed graft. The *arrow* shows the stump of a polytetrafluoroethylene (PTFE) graft.

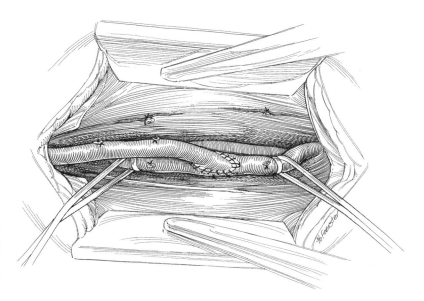

Figure 31-2 Operative exposure of the distal bypass anastomosis. The hood of the graft is incised within 1 mm of its distal end. (From Ouriel K, Rutherford RB, eds. *Atlas of vascular surgery-operative procedures.* New York, NY: WB Saunders Company; 1998, with permission.)

immediate systemic heparinization should begin and arrangements should be made for return to the operating room.

Vein Graft Failure

Prompt reoperation is especially important in vein graft bypass given the risk of graft ischemia and injury secondary to the presence of thrombus within the vein. The prior incision is opened or reincised and the vein graft is inspected to confirm thrombosis. Exploration of the vein is begun at the distal anastomosis. Dissection of the distal portion of the graft is usually relatively straightforward due to the absence of scar tissue early after initial bypass. Additional systemic heparin should be administered after proximal and distal control of the native artery around the distal anastomosis is obtained. The hood of the graft is longitudinally incised to within approximately 1 mm of its distal end (Fig. 31-2). The anastomosis should be carefully inspected and the presence of lesions, such as intimal flaps, should prompt redo of the anastomosis. Thrombotic material is then extracted from the graft and adjacent artery by gentle passage of a thrombectomy balloon catheter (Fig. 31-3). Care must be taken when inflating the balloon as disturbances to the endothelial surface can incite an inflammatory response. If normal inflow is not restored, the same series of events should be performed at the proximal anastomosis. In addition, if reversed positioning of the vein graft with intact valves prevents passage of the balloon catheter from the distal anastomosis, exploration from the proximal anastomosis should be pursued. Doppler examination, intraoperative angiography, or direct arterial pressure measurements may be performed if necessary to aid in identification of causative lesions.

Identification of an intrinsic vein conduit lesion likely to have caused graft thrombosis should prompt graft replacement with the most suitable available

alternative conduit. If a retained valve is identified in a nonreversed vein conduit, valve lysis should be performed and angioscopy considered for vein inspection to document adequate valve lysis. If adequate inflow and outflow are achieved, vein graft incisions are closed with fine monofilament suture and intraoperative angiography may then be performed to document graft patency and detect other lesions.

When the vein graft is nonsalvageable, replacement with the best available conduit should be performed. The options for vein conduit should include contralateral leg and arm vein; therefore, the appropriate area should be prepped into the surgical field if the need of additional conduit is suspected. When no vein conduit is available, prosthetic graft may be used.

Identification of an inflow lesion in the setting of a failed graft should be addressed with inflow procedures such as axillofemoral, femorofemoral, or aortofemoral bypasses or balloon angioplasty prior to attempting secondary infrainguinal bypass. If vein graft failure is thought to be due to a lesion in the outflow tract, a

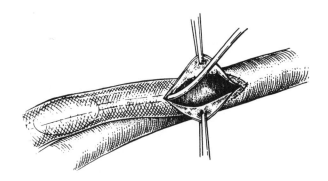

Figure 31-3 Balloon catheter thrombectomy through the distal end of the graft. (From Veith FJ, Quintos RT II, Ascher E, et al. Secondary arterial reconstructions in the lower extremity. In: Rutherford RB, ed. *Vascular surgery.* New York, NY: WB Saunders Company; 2000:1025–1035, with permission.)

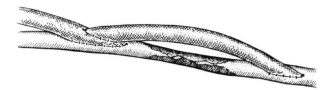

Figure 31-4 Graft extension for a distal anastomotic lesion. (From Veith FJ, Quintos RT II, Ascher E, et al. Secondary arterial reconstructions in the lower extremity. In: Rutherford RB, ed. *Vascular surgery.* New York, NY: WB Saunders Company; 2000: 1025–1035, with permission.)

more distal outflow bypass should be performed. For focal stenoses, patch angioplasty of the region is an excellent option. Longer areas of stenosis may be addressed by performing a jump graft originating from the preexisting bypass or a composite extension of the distal end of the previous bypass (Fig. 31-4).

Prosthetic Graft Failure

Early failure of the prosthetic graft is managed in a similar fashion to vein graft failure. The distal anastomosis is exposed, a longitudinal incision in the hood of the graft over the anastomosis is made, and proximal thrombectomy of the graft is performed. In >50% of early prosthetic graft failures, a cause is not determined and thrombectomy alone is sufficient for restoring graft patency. In one series, failed above-knee prosthetic grafts with no identifiable cause of thrombosis achieved a 50% 3-year patency rate after thrombectomy alone.[11] Unlike the case of vein graft failure, the prosthetic conduit itself is virtually never the cause of early graft failure. If upon inspection, however, the graft is noted to be malpositioned, causing kinking or twisting, redo of an anastomosis is warranted. This situation emphasizes the importance of initial correct positioning of the graft close to and parallel to the artery (Fig. 31-5).

As is the case with early vein graft failure, identification of inflow disease should be addressed with an inflow enhancing procedure. Outflow disease is treated with either extension of the graft to a more distal, nondiseased target or patch angioplasty of the distal anastomosis assuming the lesion is within this area.

MANAGEMENT OF LATE GRAFT FAILURE

Several key differences in the management of late versus early graft failure exist. In contrast to early thrombosis, patients with late (>30 days) graft thrombosis should only be considered for reoperation if recurrent limb threat is present. Although some patients with late graft occlusion may present with acute limb ischemia, others may not demonstrate signs of recurrent limb threat at the time of thrombosis. Approximately 10% to 25% of patients can tolerate occlusion of a limb salvage bypass

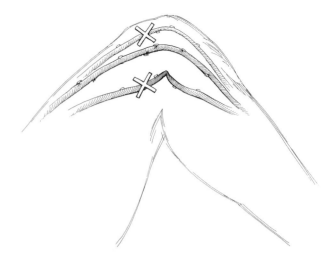

Figure 31-5 Kinking of the bypass graft: a potential cause of graft failure. (From Ouriel K, Rutherford RB, eds. *Atlas of vascular surgery-operative procedures.* New York, NY: WB Saunders Company; 1998, with permission.)

presumably because of collateral formation and healing of previously ischemic tissue.[12] Critically threatened limbs require aggressive intervention. All symptomatic patients with late graft failure should undergo complete arteriography of the abdominal aorta and lower extremity, unless absolutely contraindicated. In some cases, where a delay in operative intervention might place the limb in further jeopardy, intraoperative arteriography may be performed if needed.[13] In these cases, the availability of intraoperative fluoroscopy is especially helpful in the complete angiographic evaluation of inflow, conduit, and outflow.

In reoperation for late graft failure, alternative surgical approaches to the proximal and distal target vessels may be considered in order to avoid dissection through areas of dense scar tissue. These approaches are also useful in the setting of graft infection where a remote site for redo bypass is sought. These approaches include a direct posteromedial or lateral approach to the profunda femoris artery,[14–16] lateral approach to the popliteal artery,[17] and lateral or medial approaches to the infrapopliteal arteries. The lateral approach to the arteries in the calf may involve resection of a segment of fibula, but provides excellent exposure to the distal peroneal and tibial arteries.[18] Often, these alternative approaches may shorten the length of conduit required for bypass, an important factor in patients with limited autogenous conduit.

Vein Graft Failure

Late vein graft failure is usually due to intimal hyperplasia or progression of native vessel atherosclerotic disease. As mentioned above, preoperative arteriography should routinely be obtained in the setting of late graft failure for complete evaluation of the inflow and runoff vessels. Specifically, arteriography should evaluate possible causes of graft failure and potential inflow and outflow target vessels for redo revascularization. If renal function is of concern, magnetic resonance arteriography (MRA) can be obtained with adjunctive use of limited arteriography, if needed. If time allows, preoperative upper and lower extremity vein mapping via duplex ultrasonography should be performed to identify available vein conduit. This may reveal the presence of unsuspected accessory greater saphenous vein in patients otherwise thought to lack saphenous conduit due to a history of prior harvest.

Thrombectomy alone of an occluded vein graft is generally not attempted in the late period, as success in achieving long-term patency in this setting is limited. Graft revision or extension may be performed in conjunction with thrombectomy or endarterectomy. In some instances, focal lesions may be bypassed with a jump graft using autogenous vein conduit. Due to the short nature of these grafts, autogenous vein can be preserved for future revascularization procedures.[19] In many cases of late vein graft failure, redo revascularization is required and should be performed when and if recurrent limb-threatening ischemia occurs.

Although ultrasound vein mapping is useful in the identification of available conduit, there is no substitute to surgical exploration for investigation of the suitability of vein for use. In the absence of an adequate ipsilateral greater saphenous vein, a situation commonly encountered when performing secondary bypass, various alternative conduits exist (Table 31-1). Contralateral greater saphenous vein may be used and has been demonstrated to yield superior results to other conduits.[20] Alternatively, lesser saphenous vein may be used, although its harvesting is most easily performed in the prone position, and this may be inconvenient in the setting of emergent reoperation. The use of arm vein, specifically basilic and cephalic, has been shown to be associated with increased patency and limb salvage rates when compared with prosthetic grafts in femoral–below-knee-popliteal and femorotibial bypasses.[21] Furthermore, multisegment composite arm vein conduit has been shown to result in superior long-term patency and limb salvage rates when compared to composite prosthetic-autogenous grafts.[22] In evaluating vein conduit, employment of routine angioscopy is quite helpful in assessing adequate luminal diameter and valve lysis.

Prosthetic graft material is an acceptable alternative to autogenous conduit in the femoral–above-knee-popliteal bypass; however, its use in more distal locations should be reserved for cases in which absolutely no autogenous vein conduit is available.[23] If some vein is available, composites of vein and polytetrafluoroethylene (PTFE) have been shown to achieve long-term limb salvage in threatened extremities, although patency rates do not significantly differ from the use of prosthetic conduit alone.[24] Cryopreserved vein has patency rates that approach those of PTFE,[25] demonstrating no advantage over PTFE. We limit our use of nonautogenous vein conduit to ring-reinforced PTFE when performing infrainguinal bypass.

Prosthetic Graft Failure

In the setting of late failure of the prosthetic graft, thrombectomy can be performed from the distal anastomosis in a fashion similar to that described previously. This approach is generally accepted for femoral–above-knee-popliteal bypass grafts. In the treatment of failed PTFE femoral–above-knee-popliteal grafts with anastomotic stenoses, thrombectomy combined with open surgical repair (patch angioplasty) has been shown to result in superior patency rates than thrombolysis combined with balloon angioplasty. Given these findings, balloon angioplasty should be reserved for patients who are at high risk for surgery.[26] Given that intimal hyperplasia is often the cause of late prosthetic graft failure, the ideal treatment for some lesions may be patch angioplasty at the affected anastomosis (Fig. 31-6). After thrombectomy, if good inflow is achieved, arteriography may reveal progression of disease distal to the bypass. The best method for addressing this is to extend the graft to a distal patent artery. This may be performed as a jump graft from the old bypass conduit to a distal patent artery. In cases of infrapopliteal distal anastomosis of a PTFE graft, our recommendations are to redo the bypass graft without use of the thrombosed primary bypass. Preoperative arteriography is especially helpful in these cases, as there may be thrombosis of the native vessels proximal and distal to the graft itself, affecting plans for the secondary procedure. Surprisingly, many patients presenting with thrombosed below-knee prosthetic grafts have available vein for use in secondary bypass. This point emphasizes the importance of preoperative ultrasound vein mapping of all extremities.

TABLE 31-1

OPTIONS FOR BYPASS CONDUIT

Arm vein (basilic or cephalic)
Lesser saphenous vein
Contralateral greater saphenous vein
Prosthetic graft

FAILED SECONDARY BYPASS

Secondary infrainguinal bypasses are associated with an increased rate of graft failure and limb loss. Particularly susceptible to secondary graft failure are patients with tissue loss and rest pain, and who are women.[27] Also at increased risk of secondary graft failure are those with a history of early primary graft failure.[28]

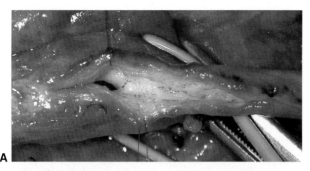

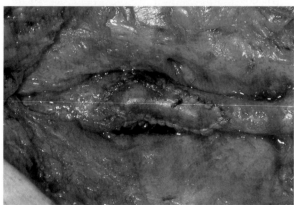

Figure 31-6 A: Anastomotic stenosis due to intimal hyperplasia. **B:** Vein patch angioplasty.

One series examined patients with lower extremity ischemia after failure of two or more prior infrainguinal bypasses in the ipsilateral leg, and demonstrated 4-year patency and limb salvage rates of 79.8% and 69.6%, respectively. Such series justify an aggressive policy of limb revascularization after multiple failed prior bypasses.[29]

An important principle in primary as well as secondary bypasses is to construct the shortest bypass graft necessary to bypass the lesion present. It is essential to realize that all infrapopliteal bypasses need not originate from the femoral artery. This principle serves to minimize the use of autogenous vein graft, preserving vein for future revascularization procedures. With careful selection of bypass inflow and outflow sites, the use of prosthetic graft material for secondary bypass procedures can be avoided. In fact, short vein grafts have been shown to have superior patency rates when compared to longer grafts.[19]

SUMMARY

Secondary arterial procedures play a critical role in limb salvage. When faced with the failed secondary bypass, some surgeons may be reluctant to make further attempts at revascularization. However, an overwhelming amount of data exists in support of the benefits of secondary lower extremity revascularization.

Vascular surgeons should welcome the unique challenge of lower extremity arterial reconstruction in the setting of multiple failed prior bypasses. Results in this setting demonstrate that patients can benefit from repeated limb salvage procedures. Moreover, the benefits of redo revascularization outweigh the potential risks of infection and limb loss. By employing the strategies detailed in this chapter, the patient is afforded an opportunity for continued limb salvage.

REFERENCES

1. Akbari CM, Pomposelli FB, Gibbons GW, et al. Lower extremity revascularization in diabetes: late observations. *Arch Surg.* 2000;133:452–456.
2. Korn P, Hoenig SJ, Skillman JJ, et al. Is lower extremity revascularization worthwhile in patients with end-stage renal disease? *Surgery.* 2000;128:472–479.
3. Ouriel K, Shortell CK, Green RM, et al. Differential mechanisms of failure of autogenous and non-autogenous bypass conduits: An assessment following successful graft thrombolysis. *J Vasc Surg.* 1995;3:469–473.
4. Stept LL, Flinn WR, McCarthy WJ, et al. Technical defects as a cause of early graft failure after femorodistal bypass. *Arch Surg.* 1987;122:599–604.
5. Archie JP. Early postoperative femoral-distal bypass graft failure due to vascular clamp injury induced common femoral artery thrombosis. *Am Surg.* 1988;54:167–168.
6. Pierce ET, Pomposelli FB, Stanley GD, et al. Anesthesia does not influence early graft patency or limb salvage rates of lower extremity arterial bypass. *J Vasc Surg.* 1997;25:226–232.
7. Taylor SM, Mills JL, Fujitani RM, et al. Does arterial inflow failure cause distal vein graft thrombosis? A prospective analysis of 450 infrainguinal vascular reconstructions. *J Vasc Surg.* 1994;8:92–98.
8. Mills JL, Fujitani RM, Taylor SM. The characteristics and anatomic distribution of lesions that cause reversed vein graft failure: A five-year prospective study. *J Vasc Surg.* 1993;17:195–206.
9. Gutierrez IZ, Barone DL, Makula P. Progression of arteriosclerotic disease in the failed infrainguinal bypass. *Am Surg.* 1987;53:482–484.
10. Misare BD, Pomposelli FB, Gibbons GW, et al. Infrapopliteal bypasses to severely calcified, unclampable outflow arteries: two-year results. *J Vasc Surg.* 1996;24:6–15.
11. Ascer E, Collier P, Gupta SK, et al. Reoperation for polytetrafluoroethylene bypass failure: the importance of distal outflow and the operative technique in determining outcome. *J Vasc Surg.* 1987;5:298–310.
12. Veith FJ, Quintos RT II, Ascher E, et al. Secondary arterial reconstructions in the lower extremity. In: Rutherford RB. ed. *Vascular surgery.* New York, NY: WB Saunders Company; 2000:1025–1035.
13. Veith FJ, Gupta SK, Daly V. Management of early and late thrombosis of expanded polytetrafluoroethylene (PTFE) femoropopliteal bypass grafts: favorable prognosis with appropriate reoperation. *Surgery.* 1980;87:581–587.
14. Mills JL, Taylor SM, Fujitani RM. The role of the deep femoral artery as an inflow site for infrainguinal revascularization. *J Vasc Surg.* 1993;18:416–423.
15. Nunez A, Veith FJ, Collier P, et al. Direct approach to the distal portions of the deep femoral artery for limb salvage bypasses. *J Vasc Surg.* 1988;8:576–581.
16. Bertucci WR, Marin MD, Veith FJ. Posterior approach to the deep femoral artery. *J Vasc Surg.* 1999;29:741–744.
17. Veith FJ, Ascer E, Gupta SK, et al. Lateral approach to the popliteal artery. *J Vasc Surg.* 1987;6:119–123.

18. Dardick H, Dardick I, Veith FJ. Exposure of the tibial-peroneal arteries by a single lateral approach. *Surgery.* 1974;75:377–382.

19. Ascer E, Veith FJ, Gupta SK, et al. Short vein grafts: a superior option for arterial reconstructions to poor or compromised outflow tracts? *J Vasc Surg.* 1988;7:370–378.

20. Chew DK, Owens CD, Belkin M, et al. Bypass in the absence of ipsilateral greater saphenous vein: safety and superiority of the contralateral greater saphenous vein. *J Vasc Surg.* 2002;35:1085–1092.

21. Faries PL, LoGerfo FW, Arora S, et al. A comparative study of alternative conduits for lower extremity revascularization: all-autogenous conduit versus prosthetic grafts. *J Vasc Surg.* 2000;32:1080–1090.

22. Faries PL, LoGerfo FW, Arora S, et al. Arm vein conduit is superior to composite prosthetic-autogenous grafts in lower extremity revascularization. *J Vasc Surg.* 2000;31:1119–1127.

23. Veith FJ, Gupta SK, Ascer E, et al. Six-year prospective multicenter randomized comparison of autologous saphenous vein and expanded polytetrafluoroethylene grafts in infrainguinal arterial reconstructions. *J Vasc Surg.* 1986;3:104–114.

24. Chang JB, Stein TA. The long-term value of composite grafts for limb salvage. *J Vasc Surg.* 1995;22:25–31.

25. Harris L, O'Brien-Irr M, Ricotta JJ. Long-term assessment of cryopreserved vein bypass grafting success. *J Vasc Surg.* 2001;33:528–532.

26. AbuRahma AF, Hopkins ES, Wulu JT, et al. Lysis/balloon angioplasty versus thrombectomy/open patch angioplasty of failed femoropopliteal polytetrafluoroethylene bypass grafts. *J Vasc Surg.* 2002;35:307–315.

27. Henke PK, Proctor MC, Zajowski PJ, et al. Tissue loss, early primary graft occlusion, female gender and a prohibitive failure rate of secondary infrainguinal graft failure. *J Vasc Surg.* 2002;35:902–909.

28. Robinson KD, Sato DT, Gregory RT, et al. Long-term outcome after early infrainguinal graft failure. *J Vasc Surg.* 1997;26:425–437.

29. De Frang RD, Edwards JM, Moneta GL, et al. Repeat leg bypass after multiple prior bypass failures. *J Vasc Surg.* 1994;19:268–277.

Thrombolytic Therapy for Failed Bypass Grafts

Kenneth Ouriel

Acute limb ischemia develops when a peripheral arterial occlusion occurs abruptly and in the absence of adequate collateral circulation. The underlying etiology may be the thrombosis of a native artery, occlusion of a bypass graft, or an embolic event to a lower extremity vessel. With the increase in the performance of peripheral bypass grafting over the last 2 decades, occlusion of an artificial or autogenous bypass graft has become the most common cause of lower extremity arterial occlusion in most centers.[1]

Irrespective of etiology, the acute occlusive event may be catastrophic for the patient, with great risk to the patient's limb and life (Table 32-1). In a classic study by Blaisdell et al.[2] published over 25 years ago, amputation and mortality rates in excess of 25% were documented following open surgical repair for acute leg ischemia. Despite improvements in operative technique and postoperative patient care, more recent series continue to verify unacceptably high rates of morbidity. Jivegård et al.[3] observed a 20% mortality rate in patients treated operatively. Even the more recent prospective studies of operatively treated patients document rates of limb loss and death that exceed desired targets.[4–7]

What factors explain the high morbidity and mortality following open surgical intervention? The baseline medical status of patients who present with acute limb ischemia may underlie this observation. Patients are frequently elderly and have a high rate of cardiac and other comorbidities that render them ill-equipped to tolerate the insult of ischemia of an extremity, let alone an invasive surgical intervention to relieve the obstruction. A multivariable analysis of the data from a single-center study of peripheral arterial thrombolysis uncovered several variables that were predictive of poor outcome, irrespective of the type of treatment instituted.[8] A summary of available literature would appear to confirm that patients who present with acute, limb-threatening ischemia comprise one of the sickest subgroup of patients that the peripheral vascular practitioner is asked to treat.[1]

There is some evidence to confirm the impression that a less invasive intervention is better tolerated in patients who develop acute limb ischemia. That said, poor technique, inadequate devices, and inferior agents colored the initial experiences with catheter-directed thrombolytic therapy decades ago. For instance, the now well-accepted principle of ensuring infusion of the thrombolytic agent directly into the substance of the occluding thrombus was not always ardently adhered to. End-hole catheters were employed; it was not until the late 1980s that multisided-hole catheters were available. Last, streptokinase was the most frequently used agent until the landmark article of McNamara and Fischer in 1985[9] documented improved results with locally administered high-dose urokinase.

PHARMACOLOGY OF THROMBOLYTIC AGENTS

In 1933, Tillett and Garner[10] at the Johns Hopkins Medical School discovered that filtrates of broth cultures of certain strains of hemolytic *Streptococcus* bacteria had fibrinolytic properties. This streptococcal

TABLE 32-1

EARLY (IN-HOSPITAL OR 30-DAY) RATES OF AMPUTATION AND DEATH IN SELECTED SERIES OF PATIENTS WITH RECENT PERIPHERAL ARTERIAL OCCLUSION, TREATED WITH PRIMARY OPEN SURGICAL INTERVENTION

Study	Year	Amputation Rate	Mortality Rate
Blaisdell[2]	1978	25%	30%
Jivegård[3]	1988	—	20%
Rochester[4]	1994	14%	18%
STILE[6]	1994	5%	6%
TOPAS[5]	1998	2%	5%

byproduct was originally termed *Streptococcal fibrinolysin*. The purity of this agent was poor, however. Clinical use, of necessity, awaited adequate purification. Tillett and Sherry[11] administered streptokinase intrapleurally to dissolve loculated hemothoraces in the late 1940s, but intravascular administration was not attempted until the following decade. Tillett et al.[12] first reported intravascular administration of a thrombolytic agent in an article published in 1955. A concentrated and partially purified streptokinase (SK) (Varidase, Lederle Laboratories) was injected into 11 patients. This investigation was performed with the intent to gain data on the safety of the agent in volunteers; in no case was the SK administered to dissolve pathologic thrombi. Fever and hypotension developed as the amount of SK approached therapeutic levels. Whereas fever was generally mild and controllable with antipyretics, hypotension was sometimes prominent. The mean fall in systolic pressure was 31 mm Hg, and three of the patients manifested systolic pressures <80 mm Hg. These untoward reactions were more likely a result of contaminants in the preparation rather than the SK itself. Despite these reactions, systemic proteolysis was observed, with a decrease in fibrinogen and plasminogen, concurrent with a mild increase in the prothrombin time.

These early studies were followed by reports on the use of SK in patients with occluding vascular thrombi. In 1956, E. E. Cliffton[13] at the Cornell University Medical College in New York was responsible for the first brief description of the clinical effectiveness of intravascular thrombolytic administration. The following year, Cliffton published his results in 40 patients with occlusive thrombi treated with an SK-plasminogen combination.[14] The location of the thrombi was diverse, and included peripheral arterial thrombi, venous thrombi, pulmonary emboli, retinal occlusions, and (in two patients) occlusive carotid thrombi. Cliffton's clinical results were far from exemplary; recanalization was not uniform, and bleeding complications were frequent. Nevertheless, he must be credited with the first use of

thrombolytic agents for the treatment of pathologic thrombi, as well as with the first use of catheter-directed administration of a thrombolytic agent.

Several schemes may be used to classify thrombolytic agents. The agents may be grouped by their mechanism of action: Those that directly convert plasminogen to plasmin versus those that are inactive zymogens and require transformation to an active form before they can cleave plasminogen. Thrombolytic agents can be grouped by their mode of production: Those that are manufactured via recombinant techniques and those that are of bacterial origin. Of interest, recombinant agents harvested from a bacterial expression system such as *Escherichia coli* do not contain carbohydrates, while products of mammalian hybridoma (e.g., recombinant prourokinase from mouse hybridoma SP2/0 cells) are fully glycosylated. Thrombolytic agents can be classified by their pharmacologic actions: Those that are "fibrin-specific" (bind to fibrin but not fibrinogen) versus nonspecific, and those that have a great degree of "fibrin-affinity" (bind avidly to fibrin) versus those that do not. We have found it most useful to classify thrombolytic agents into groups based on the origin of the parent compound. It is most efficient to divide the agents into four groups: The streptokinase compounds, the urokinase compounds, the tissue plasminogen activators, and an additional, miscellaneous group consisting of novel agents that are distinct from agents in the three other groups.

Streptokinase Compounds

SK, originating from the *Streptococcus* bacteria, was the first thrombolytic agent to be described; 0.4 SK is a 50-kDa molecule with a biphasic half-life comprising a rapid $t1/2$ of 16 minutes and a second, slower $t1/2$ of 90 minutes.[15] Whereas the initial half-life is accounted for by complexing of the molecule with SK antibodies, the second half-life represents the actual biologic elimination of the protein. SK differs from other thrombolytic agents with respect to the stoichiometry of plasminogen binding. Whereas other agents directly convert plasminogen to plasmin, SK must form an equimolar stoichiometric complex with a plasmin or plasminogen molecule to gain activity. Only then can this SK-plasmin(ogen) complex activate a second plasminogen molecule to form active plasmin; thus, two plasminogen molecules are utilized in SK-mediated plasmin generation. Unfortunately, SK suffers from the limitation of antigenic potential. Preformed antibodies exist to a certain extent in all patients who have been infected with the *Streptococcus* bacterium. Similarly, patients with exposure to SK may have high antibody titers on repeat exposure. These neutralizing antibodies inactivate exogenously administered SK. SK antibodies may be overwhelmed through the use of a large initial bolus of drug, and a large initial SK loading dose may be employed in this regard. Some investigators have recommended measurement of antibody titers prior to beginning SK therapy, gauging the loading dose on the basis of this titer.[16] SK administration is complicated by allergic reactions in approximately 2% of patients treated, with the development of urticaria, periorbital edema, and bronchospasm. Pyrexia may also occur, but is usually adequately treated with acetaminophen. The major untoward effect associated with SK is hemorrhage. SK-associated hemorrhage may be no different than bleeding associated with any thrombolytic agent. The primary cause is likely the actions of systemic agent on the thrombi sealing the sites of vascular disintegrity. The generation of free plasmin, however, can contribute to the problem, with degradation of fibrinogen and other serum-clotting proteins, as well as the release of fibrin(ogen)-degradation products that are potent anticoagulants themselves and exacerbate the coagulopathy.

Recognizing potential limitations with SK, anisoylated plasminogen-streptokinase activator complex (APSAC) was developed by pharmacologists at Beecham Laboratories.[17,18] APSAC has a longer half-life than SK, since acylation rendered the complex less susceptible to degradation. Because of this property, it was anticipated that APSAC would be associated with a reduced risk of rethrombosis. Contrary to expectations, APSAC offered little clinical benefit over other agents, and, at present, is not used to treat thrombi in the peripheral vasculature.

Urokinase Compounds

Macfarlane and Pinot[19] first described the fibrinolytic potential of human urine in 1947. The active molecule was extracted, isolated, and named "urokinase" (UK) in 1952.[20] This urokinase-type plasminogen activator is a serine protease composed of two polypeptide chains, occurring in a low-molecular-weight (32-kDa) and high-molecular-weight (54-kDa) form. The high-molecular-weight form predominates in UK isolated from urine, while the low-molecular-weight form is found in UK obtained from tissue culture of kidney cells. Unlike SK, UK directly activates plasminogen to form plasmin; prior binding to plasminogen or plasmin is not necessary for activity. Also in contrast to SK, preformed antibodies to UK are not observed. The agent is nonantigenic and untoward reactions of fever or hypotension are rare. Presently, the most commonly employed UK in the United States is of tissue-culture origin, manufactured from human neonatal kidney cells (Abbokinase, Abbott Laboratories, North Chicago, IL). UK has been fully sequenced, and a recombinant form of UK (r-UK) was tested in a single trial of patients with acute myocardial infarction and in two multicenter trials of patients with peripheral arterial occlusion.[4,5] r-UK is fully glycosylated, since it is derived from a murine hybridoma cell line. r-UK differs from Abbokinase in several

respects. First, r-UK has a higher molecular weight than Abbokinase. Second, r-UK has a shorter half-life than its low-molecular-weight counterpart. Despite these differences, however, the clinical effects of the two agents have been quite similar.

A precursor of UK was discovered in urine in 1979.[21] Prourokinase was characterized and subsequently manufactured by recombinant technology using *E. coli* (nonglycosylated) or mammalian cells (fully glycosylated).[22] This single-chain form is an inactive zymogen, inert in plasma, but can be activated by kallikrein or plasmin to form active two-chain UK. This property accounts for amplification of the fibrinolytic process—as plasmin is generated, more prourokinase is converted to active urokinase, and the process is repeated. Prourokinase is relatively fibrin-specific, that is, its fibrin degrading (fibrinolytic) activity greatly outweighs its fibrinogen degrading (fibrinogenolytic) activity. This feature is explained by the preferential activation of fibrin-bound plasminogen found in a thrombus over free plasminogen found in flowing blood. Nonselective activators such as SK and UK activate free and bound plasminogen equally and induce systemic plasminemia with resultant fibrinogenolysis and degradation of factors V and VII. Given the potential advantages of prourokinase over urokinase, Abbott Laboratories produced a recombinant form of prourokinase (r-ProUK) from a murine hybridoma cell line. This recombinant agent, which was named Prolyse (Abbott Laboratories), is converted to active two-chain urokinase by plasmin and kallikrein. Prolyse has been studied in the settings of myocardial infarction, stroke, and peripheral arterial occlusion. To date, it appears that r-ProUK offers the advantages associated with an agent that does not originate from a human cell source. Fibrin specificity, however, may be lost at the higher dose levels necessary to effect more rapid thrombolysis than Abbokinase.

Tissue Plasminogen Activators

Tissue plasminogen activator, or tPA, is a naturally occurring fibrinolytic agent produced by endothelial cells and intimately involved in the balance between intravascular thrombogenesis and thrombolysis. Wild-type tPA is a single-chain (527 amino acid) serine protease with a molecular weight of approximately 65 kDa. Plasmin hydrolyses the Arg275-Ile276 peptide bond, converting the single-chain molecule into a two-chain moiety. In contrast to most serine proteases (e.g., urokinase), the single-chain form of tPA has significant activity. tPA has potential benefits over other thrombolytic agents. The agent exhibits significant fibrin specificity.[23] In plasma, the agent is associated with little plasminogen activation. At the site of the thrombus, however, the binding of tPA and plasminogen to the fibrin surface induces a conformational change in both molecules, greatly facilitating the conversion of plasminogen to plasmin, and dissolution of the clot. tPA also manifests the property of fibrin affinity, that is, it binds strongly to fibrin. Other fibrinolytic agents such as prourokinase do not share this property of fibrin affinity. Recombinant tPA (rt-PA [alteplase]) was produced in the 1980s after molecular cloning techniques were used to express human tPA deoxyribonucleic acid (DNA).[24] Activase (Genentech, South San Francisco, CA), a predominantly single-chain form of rt-PA, was eventually approved in the United States for the indications of acute myocardial infarction and massive pulmonary embolism. rt-PA has been studied extensively in the setting of coronary occlusion. In the Global Utilization of Streptokinase and tPA for Occluded Coronary Arteries (GUSTO-I) study of approximately 41,000 patients with acute myocardial infarction, rt-PA was more effective than SK in achieving vascular patency.[25] Despite a slightly greater risk of intracranial hemorrhage with rt-PA, overall mortality was significantly reduced. In an effort to lengthen the duration of bioavailability of tPA, the molecule was systematically bioengineered. Initial investigations identified regions in kringle 1 and the protease portion of tPA that mediated hepatic clearance, fibrin specificity, and resistance to plasminogen activator inhibitor. Three sites were modified to create TNK-tPA, a novel molecule with a greater half-life and fibrin specificity.[26] The longer half-life of TNK-tPA allowed successful administration as a single bolus, in contrast to the requirement for an infusion with rt-PA. In addition, TNK-tPA manifests greater fibrin specificity than rt-PA, resulting in less fibrinogen depletion. In studies of acute coronary occlusion, TNK-tPA performed at least as well as rt-PA, concurrent with greater ease of administration.[27]

Reteplase

Similar to TNK-tPA, the novel recombinant plasminogen activator reteplase comprises the kringle 2 and protease domains of tPA. Reteplase was developed with the goal of avoiding the necessity of a continuous intravenous infusion, thereby simplifying ease of administration.[28] Reteplase (Retavase, Centocor), produced in *E. coli* cells, is nonglycosylated, demonstrating a lower fibrin-binding activity and a diminished affinity to hepatocytes.[29] This latter property accounts for a longer half-life than rt-PA, potentially enabling bolus injection versus prolonged infusion. The fibrin affinity of reteplase was only 30% of that exhibited with tPA, similar to UK. The decrease in fibrin affinity was hypothesized to reduce the incidence of distant bleeding complications, in a manner similar to that of SK over rt-PA in the GUSTO trial. In fact, several properties of reteplase may account for a decreased risk of hemorrhage, including poor lysis of platelet-rich, older clots. Reteplase has demonstrated some benefit over rt-PA in the Reteplase Angiographic Phase II International Dose-Finding (RAPID 1 and RAPID 2) studies, as well as in

GUSTO III.[30] To date, peripheral arterial and venous studies remain few in number.[31]

Miscellaneous Agents

There exist a wide variety of novel thrombolytic agents, all of which have undergone extensive preclinical study, but few of which have been adequately evaluated in patients. Vampire bat plasminogen activator (bat PA) was cloned and expressed from the saliva of the vampire bat *Desmodus rotundus*.[32] This agent manifests extraordinary fibrin specificity; the plasminogenolytic activity is over 100,000 times greater in the presence of fibrin. The half-life of bat PA is five to nine times slower than that of rt-PA, offering some potential advantages with respect to ease of administration. To date, clinical trials have been limited to a phase I study with healthy volunteers.[33] Fibrolase is a metalloproteinase originating from venom of the southern copperhead snake.[34] Fibrolase is a unique fibrinolytic agent that does not require plasminogen for its activity. Rather, the agent directly degrades fibrin without the requirement of any other blood components. Staphylokinase is a byproduct of *Staphylococcus aureus* bacterium, and was originally mentioned in the classic streptococcal fibrinolysin paper of Tillett and Garner in 1933.[10] Staphylokinase has been produced by recombinant techniques and has been studied in the settings of myocardial infarction, peripheral arterial occlusion, and deep venous thrombosis.[35] Like SK, staphylokinase is inactive and must bind to plasminogen to activate other plasminogen molecules. Unlike SK, staphylokinase is relatively fibrin-specific and spares circulating plasminogen and fibrinogen. While staphylokinase is antigenic, antigenicity has been reduced with newer recombinant mutants and the initial clinical results have been quite acceptable.[36]

COMPARISON OF THE AGENTS IN STUDIES OF PERIPHERAL VASCULAR DISEASE

To date, there have been few well-designed clinical comparisons of various thrombolytic agents in the peripheral vasculature. There exist a variety of *in vitro* studies and retrospective clinical trials, most pointing to improved efficacy and safety of UK and rt-PA over SK. In an analysis of data collected in a prospective, single institution registry at the Cleveland Clinic Foundation, UK demonstrated a diminished rate of bleeding complications when compared with rt-PA.[37] Efficacy was not evaluated in this trial.

There have been two prospective, randomized comparisons of UK and rt-PA. Neither was blinded. Meyerovitz et al.[38] from the Brigham and Women's Hospital randomized 32 patients with peripheral arterial or bypass graft occlusions of <90 days' duration to rt-PA

(10 mg bolus, 5 mg per hour to a maximum of 24 hours) or UK (60,000 IU bolus, 4,000 IU per minute for 2 hours, 2,000 IU per minute for 2 hours, then 1,000 IU per minute to a maximum of 24 hours' total administration).[38] There was significantly greater systemic fibrinogen degradation in the rt-PA group ($p = 0.01$), indicating that the fibrin-specificity of rt-PA was lost at this dosing regimen. rt-PA patients achieved more rapid initial thrombolysis, but efficacy was identical in the two groups by 24 hours. The tradeoff to more rapid thrombolysis was a trend toward a higher rate of bleeding complications in the rt-PA–treated patients ($p = 0.39$). The second randomized comparison of UK and rt-PA was the Surgery or Thrombolysis for the Ischemic Lower Extremity (STILE) trial, a three-armed, multicenter comparison of UK (250,000 IU bolus, 4,000 IU per minute for 4 hours, then 2,000 IU per minute for up to 36 hours), rt-PA (0.05 to 0.1 mg/kg/hour for up to 12 hours), and primary operation.[6] There was one intracranial hemorrhage in the UK group (0.9%) and two in the rt-PA group (1.5%, no significant difference). Although actual rates of overall bleeding complications and efficacy were not reported for the two thrombolytic groups, the authors remarked that there were no significant differences detected in any of the outcome variables. In a subsequent reanalysis of the data, reported in 1999, the frequency of complete clot lysis was similar with UK and rt-PA at the time of the early arteriographic study.[39] These recent data suggest that the rate of thrombolysis may be quite similar, in direct contradistinction to the popularly held view that rt-PA is a much more rapidly acting agent. A multicenter, blinded trial compared the results of thrombolysis with UK versus r-UK in 300 patients with peripheral arterial occlusion. This data was never published. There were no significant differences noted between the two agents. A North American multicenter trial compared three different doses of r-ProUK to UK in 241 patients with lower extremity arterial occlusions of <14 days' duration.[40] While the higher r-ProUK dose was associated with slightly greater percentage of patients with complete (>95%) clot lysis at 8 hours, there was a mild increase in the rate of bleeding complications compared with either the UK or the lower-dose r-ProUK groups. The fibrinogen levels fell in the higher r-ProUK group, suggesting that fibrin specificity is lost at the higher dose regimens for this compound.

THROMBOLYSIS VERSUS SURGERY AS THE INITIAL INTERVENTION: OBJECTIVE DATA

There have been three well-controlled, randomized comparisons of thrombolytic therapy versus primary operation in patients with recent peripheral arterial occlusion. The first study, the Rochester series, compared UK to primary operation in 114 patients presenting with what

has subsequently been called "hyperacute ischemia."[4] Enrolled patients in this trial all had severely threatened limbs (Rutherford class IIb) with mean symptom duration of approximately 2 days. This was a single-center trial that was partially funded by the Thrombolysis and Thrombosis Program Project National Institutes of Health (NIH) grant at the University of Rochester. After 12 months of follow-up, 84% of patients randomized to UK were alive, compared to only 58% of patients randomized to primary operation (Fig. 32-1). By contrast, the rate of limb salvage was identical at 80%. A closer inspection of the raw data revealed that the defining variable for mortality differences was the development of cardiopulmonary complications during the periprocedural period. The rate of long-term mortality was high when such periprocedural complications occurred, but was relatively low when they did not occur. It was only the fact that such complications occurred more commonly in patients taken directly to the operating theatre that explained the greater long-term mortality rate in the operative group.

The second prospective, randomized analysis of thrombolysis versus surgery was the STILE trial.[6] Genentech (South San Francisco CA), the manufacturer of the Activase brand of rt-PA, funded the study. At its termination, 393 patients were randomized to one of three treatment groups, rt-PA, UK, or primary operation. Subsequently, the two thrombolytic groups were combined for purposes of data analysis when the outcome was found to be similar. While the rate of the composite endpoint of untoward events was higher in the thrombolytic patients, the rate of the more relevant and objective endpoints of amputation and death were equivalent (Fig. 32-2). Articles were written that comprised subgroup analyses of the STILE data, one relating to native artery occlusions[41] and one to bypass graft occlusions.[42]

In the STILE subgroup analysis of graft occlusions, thrombolysis appeared more effective than immediate

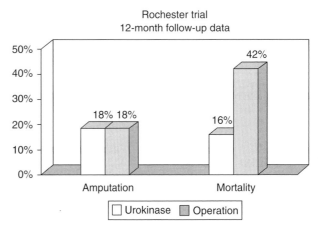

Figure 32-1 The rate of amputation was identical in the two treatment groups in the Rochester Trial, but the mortality rate was significantly lower in patients assigned to the thrombolytic arm.

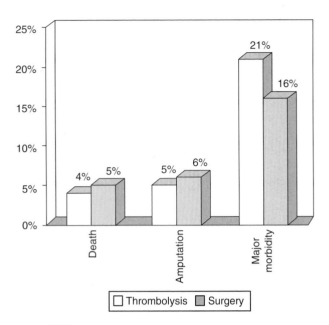

Figure 32-2 Outcome measures from the Surgery or Thrombolysis for the Ischemic Lower Extremity (STILE) data after 30 days of follow-up. Note that the rate of death and amputation are similar.

operation. The rate of major amputation was lower in patients with acute graft occlusions treated with thrombolysis ($p = 0.026$). In the study, 124 patients with lower limb bypass graft occlusion (46 autogenous and 78 prosthetic) were prospectively randomized to surgery ($n = 46$) or intra-arterial catheter-directed thrombolysis ($n = 78$) with rt-PA (0.1 mg/kg/hour, later modified to 0.05 mg/kg/hour for up to 12 hours), or UK (250,000 U bolus followed by 4,000 U per minute for 4 hours, then 2,000 U per minute for up to 36 hours). In this study, 39% of patients in the thrombolytic group failed attempts at catheter placement and crossed over to surgical revascularization. Overall, there was a better composite clinical outcome at 30 days ($p = 0.023$) and 1 year ($p = 0.04$) in the surgical group, predominately due to a reduction in ongoing or recurrent ischemia that was most prominent in autogenous grafts. However, following successful catheter placement, patency was restored by lysis in 84%, and 42% had a major reduction in their planned operation. Patients who presented within 14 days of symptoms demonstrated a trend toward a lower major amputation rate at 30 days when treated with thrombolysis ($p = 0.074$) and significantly at 1 year ($p = 0.026$). By contrast, those with a more chronic presentation demonstrated no difference in limb salvage, but had a higher rate of ongoing or recurrent ischemia when treated with thrombolysis ($p < 0.001$). In this trial, patients with occluded prosthetic grafts had greater major morbidity than did those with occluded autogenous grafts ($p < 0.02$).

The third and final randomized comparison of thrombolysis and surgery was the Thrombolysis or Peripheral Arterial Surgery (TOPAS) trial, funded by Abbott Laboratories (Abbott Park, IL). Following completion of a preliminary dose-ranging trial in 213 patients,[43] 544 patients were randomized to a recombinant form of UK or primary operative intervention.[5] After a mean follow-up period of 1 year, the rate of amputation-free survival was identical in the two treatment groups, 68.2% and 68.8% in the UK and surgical patients, respectively (Table 32-2).

TABLE 32-2

RESULTS OF THE THROMBOLYTIC OR PERIPHERAL ARTERIAL SURGERY TRIAL, DEMONSTRATING SIMILAR MORTALITY RATES AND AMPUTATION-FREE SURVIVAL RATES IN THE THROMBOLYTIC AND SURGERY GROUPS

Intervention	Native-Artery Occlusions ($n = 242$)			Bypass-Graft Occlusions ($n = 302$)		
	Urokinase ($n = 122$)	Surgery ($n = 120$)	p value	Urokinase ($n = 150$)	Surgery ($n = 152$)	p value
Complete dissolution of clot on final angiogram—no./total no. of patients (%)	67/112 (60%)	NA	—	100/134 (75%)	NA	—
Increase in ankle–brachial index[a]	0.44 ± 0.04	0.52 ± 0.04	0.15[b]	0.48 ± 0.03	0.50 ± 0.03	0.76[b]
Mortality (%)						
6 mo	20.8	15.9	0.33[c]	12.1	9.4	0.45[c]
1 y	24.6	19.6	0.36[c]	16.2	15.0	0.77[c]
Amputation-free survival (%)						
6 mo	67.6	76.1	0.15[c]	75.2	73.9	0.79[c]
1 y	61.2	71.4	0.10[c]	68.2	68.8	0.91[c]

NA, not applicable.
[a]Plus–minus values are means ± Standard Error (SE).
[b]The p value was based on one-way analysis of variance.
[c]The p value was based on Kaplan–Meier analysis.

While this trial failed to document improvement in survival or limb salvage with thrombolysis, fully 31.5% of the thrombolytic patients were alive without amputation with nothing more than a percutaneous procedure after 6 months of follow-up (Table 32-3). After 1 year, this number had decreased only slightly, with 25.7% alive without amputation and with only percutaneous interventions. Thus, the original goal of the TOPAS trial, to generate data on which regulatory approval of r-UK would be based, was not achieved. Nevertheless, the findings confirmed that acute limb ischemia could be managed with catheter-directed thrombolysis, achieving similar amputation and mortality rates, but avoiding the need for open surgical procedures in a significant percentage of patients.

TABLE 32-3
RESULTS OF THE THROMBOLYTIC OR PERIPHERAL ARTERIAL SURGERY (TOPAS) TRIAL

Intervention or Outcome	Urokinase Group (n = 272)		Surgery Group (n = 272)	
	6 mo	1 y	6 mo	1 y
	no. of interventions			
Operative intervention				
Amputation	48	58	41	51
Above the knee	22	25	19	26
Below the knee	26	33	22	25
Open surgical procedures	315	351	551	590
Major	102	116	177	193
Moderate	89	98	136	145
Minor	124	137	238	252
Percutaneous procedures	128	135	55	70
	% of patients			
Worst outcome				
Death	16.0	20.0	12.3	17.0
Amputation	12.2	15.0	12.9	13.1
Above the knee	5.6	6.5	6.1	7.5
Below the knee	6.6	8.5	6.8	5.6
Open surgical procedures	40.3	39.3	69.0	65.4
Major	23.6	24.3	39.3	39.3
Moderate	10.3	8.7	16.3	13.4
Minor	6.4	6.3	13.4	12.7
Endovascular procedures	16.9	15.4	2.1	1.7
Medical treatment alone	14.6	10.3	3.7	2.8

A significant number of patients in the thrombolytic group achieved similar rates of limb loss and mortality without the need for open surgical intervention.

PARADIGM FOR ACUTE OCCLUSION OF A BYPASS GRAFT TO THE TIBIAL ARTERIES

When a bypass graft to a tibial artery occludes, there are three basic options.

1. In some cases, the treating physician may conclude that further intervention would be futile and would place a substantial risk on the patient's life in efforts to save the limb. This scenario is rare, but revascularization in the form of open surgery or thrombolytic therapy may be inappropriate when it does arise. Some of these patients may be able to function with their symptoms for long periods of time; others may require amputation as a primary intervention. Of note, there is data to suggest that the long-term survival of many medically compromised patients is improved with revascularization compared with major amputation, attesting to the infrequency with which primary amputation is warranted.[44]

2. Patients who occlude a tibial bypass graft and who have a suitable length of autogenous conduit (e.g., contralateral saphenous vein) should undergo angiography and be offered a second revascularization procedure if:

    a. They are of acceptable medical risk

    b. A suitable outflow target vessel has been identified

3. In most cases, patients with occluded distal bypass grafts present with a long list of medical comorbidities, concurrent diseases that are severe enough that an urgent open surgical procedure is unwise. In other patients, the preprocedural imaging studies fail to demonstrate a suitable target vessel for an operative bypass. Thrombolysis should be considered as the most appropriate initial therapeutic option in these cases. In practice, most patients with occlusion of tibial bypass grafts fall into this group—a group where attempts at a percutaneous means of revascularization is justified.

It is important to discuss treatment options with the patient and the family prior to the diagnostic arteriogram. Open surgical and thrombolytic treatment options should be thoroughly discussed before the patient has been sedated, including the risk of complications associated with each modality. The diagnostic arteriogram should be performed through a site that will not be bathed in thrombolytic agent, if this option is eventually pursued. In most cases, the contralateral femoral artery is the best site for initial access. Once a thrombolytic treatment option has been elected, the catheter can be advanced over the aortic bifurcation, or, if the bypass graft originates distal to the proximal third of the superficial femoral artery, antegrade ipsilateral femoral access can be undertaken. In no case, however, should antegrade access be attempted in patients where the graft originates from the proximal superficial femoral artery.

The first step in pharmacologic thrombolysis of tibial grafts is the most important—access of the thrombosed conduit. Using oblique views to locate the proximal stump of the occluded graft, the presumed orifice is gently probed with an angled guidewire. The proximal cap of the thrombus is sometimes the toughest area to traverse, but the resistance drops significantly once the wire enters the body of the acutely occluded graft. Stenotic segments, usually at the distal anastomosis, represent challenges to guidewire negotiation, but the ultimate goal is to traverse the entire graft with the guidewire. Importantly, failure to access the graft should mandate the consideration of other, nonthrombolytic interventions. Upstream infusion of thrombolytic agent above an occluded graft rarely results in successful thrombolysis.

After guidewire access has been achieved, an infusion catheter must be advanced into the substance of the thrombus. In many cases, however, the stiff infusion catheters do not track well over the guidewire that has been used to gain access to the graft. Thus, consideration should be entertained for the use of a 4F or 5F hydrophilic catheter as an intermediate step. Once this catheter has been placed in the graft, the hydrophilic wire can be exchanged for a wire of a stiffer variety, facilitating placement of the infusion catheter.

Thrombolytic infusion catheters have small side-holes that promote the distribution of the lytic agent throughout the substance of the thrombus. Some catheters require the placement of a wire to occlude the larger distal end-hole so that the agent does not follow the path of least resistance and merely flow out the end of the catheter. In any event, one must be certain to place all of the side-holes within the thrombus; this is the most effective means of ensuring complete distribution of the agent into the thrombus. The infusion catheters have side-holes that are distributed in varying lengths along the catheter, and a catheter should be chosen such that the infusion length is just shorter than the length of the thrombus. When the occluded graft is long, an infusion wire can be used coaxially with the catheter to achieve a longer infusion length.

The thrombolytic infusion is begun with or without a "lacing" dose (bolus) of thrombolytic agent. Heparin is administered in small amounts through the sheath, usually <500 U per hour. One should ardently avoid mixing heparin with the thrombolytic agent in the same tubing, since the low pH of the heparin solution will result in precipitation of the agent into crystalline deposits with loss of fibrinolytic activity. The patient is returned to the angiography suite on a serial basis. The first return is usually at 8 to 12 hours, but the timing is variable and dependent on the clinical course of the patient. Thrombolytic infusion is discontinued when the bulk of the thrombus has been dissolved, when

dissolution has ceased in the absence of complete thrombolysis, or when a complication has occurred. Measuring fibrinogen levels is controversial; no study has ever demonstrated a correlation between fibrinogen level and bleeding. If fibrinogen is measured, however, a precipitous fall should prompt one to consider lowering the thrombolytic dose or to transiently terminate the infusion completely.

TREATMENT OF THE UNDERLYING LESION

Once successful recanalization of the arterial bypass graft has been achieved, any underlying culprit lesion must be addressed. Thrombolytic therapy alone is seldom sufficient therapy for acute arterial occlusion and must be followed by definitive therapy to address the underlying lesion that caused the occlusion (Fig. 32-3). In fact, when no such lesion can be found, the risk of early rethrombosis is unacceptably high.[45] As testimony

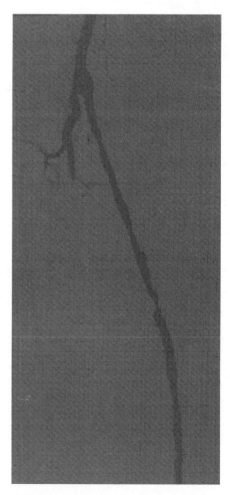

Figure 32-3 An occluded femoral-posterior tibial bypass graft that was successfully treated with catheter-directed urokinase. The conduit was diffusely diseased, but a focal, culprit stenosis was found in the proximal one third of the graft.

to this caveat, Sullivan et al.[45] observed postthrombolytic 2-year patency rates of 79% in bypass grafts with flow-limiting lesions identified and corrected by angioplasty or surgery, versus only 9.8% in those without such lesions. Multiple view arteriography, duplex ultrasound, and even intravascular ultrasound interrogation of a bypass graft should all be considered. Only after a wide array of diagnostic interrogations has been exhausted should one elect to merely treat the patient with long-term anticoagulation.

Surgical revascularization is unquestioned as appropriate therapy for addressing an underlying arterial lesion, and there exist three basic choices: Endarterectomy, patch angioplasty, and placement of a new bypass graft. Endarterectomy is an acceptable option when truly localized disease is present proximal to the bypass graft, for example, when upstream stenoses of the aorta or iliac arteries are found.[46] Presently, however, endarterectomy is infrequently utilized after successful thrombolytic recanalization; the same lesions appropriate for endarterectomy are suitable for percutaneous angioplasty or stenting procedures. Patch angioplasty continues to play an important role in the treatment of focal lesions uncovered after successful thrombolysis. This is particularly true for lesions within saphenous vein bypass conduits. While satisfactory results have been reported after balloon angioplasty of short vein graft lesions, many continue to advocate a localized operative approach. Patch angioplasty can be performed under local anesthesia with minimal morbidity. Lesions at anastomoses may be best treated with patch angioplasty as opposed to balloon dilatation, and long-term success can be anticipated.[47]

A localized procedure is not appropriate when thrombolysis uncovers a diffusely diseased bypass graft. Fortunately, the procedure can usually be delayed until the patient is adequately prepared for this major operative intervention. When adequate saphenous vein is available, the long-term patency rate of bypass to even the infrapopliteal (crural) vessels is quite satisfactory, approximating 70% to 80% at 5 years irrespective of whether the vein is reversed or left *in situ* with the valves disrupted.[48,49] Considering the quite dismal results of percutaneous angioplasty and stenting for disease in the crural arteries, autogenous vein bypass to the distal vessels should be considered as first-line therapy in patients with limb-threatening ischemia and distal disease.[50]

REFERENCES

1. Dormandy J, Heeck L, Vig S. Acute limb ischemia. *Semin Vasc Surg.* 1999;12:148–153.
2. Blaisdell FW, Steele M, Allen RE. Management of acute lower extremity arterial ischemia due to embolism and thrombosis. *Surgery.* 1978;84:822–834.
3. Jivegård L, Holm J, Scherstén T. Acute limb ischemia due to arterial embolism or thrombosis: Influence of limb ischemia versus pre-existing cardiac disease on postoperative mortality rate. *J Cardiovasc Surg.* 1988;29:32–36.
4. Ouriel K, Shortell CK, DeWeese JA, et al. A comparison of thrombolytic therapy with operative revascularization in the initial treatment of acute peripheral arterial ischemia. *J Vasc Surg.* 1994;19: 1021–1030.
5. Ouriel K, Veith FJ, Sasahara AA. A comparison of recombinant urokinase with vascular surgery as initial treatment for acute arterial occlusion of the legs. *N Engl J Med.* 1998;338:1105–1111.
6. Results of a prospective randomized trial evaluating surgery versus thrombolysis for ischemia of the lower extremity. The STILE trial. *Ann Surg.* 1994;220:251–266.
7. Ouriel K, Kandarpa K, Schuerr DM, et al. Prourokinase versus urokinase for recanalization of peripheral occlusions, safety and efficacy: the PURPOSE trial. *J Vasc Interv Radiol.* 1999;10: 1083–1091.
8. Ouriel K, Veith FJ. Acute lower limb ischemia: determinants of outcome. *Surgery.* 1998;124:336–342.
9. McNamara TO, Fischer JR. Thrombolysis of peripheral arterial and graft occlusions: improved results using high-dose urokinase. *AJR Am J Roentgenol.* 1985;144:769–775.
10. Tillett WS, Garner RL. The fibrinolytic activity of hemolytic streptococci. *J Exp Med.* 1933;58:485.
11. Tillett WS, Sherry S. The effect in patients of streptococcal fibrinolysin (streptokinase) and streptococcal desoxyribonuclease on fibrinous, purulent, and snaguinous pleural exudations. *J Clin Invest.* 1949;28:173.
12. Tillett WS, Johnson AJ, McCarty WR. The intravenous infusion of the streptococcal fibrinolytic principle (streptokinase) into patients. *J Clin Invest.* 1955;34:169–185.
13. Cliffton EE, Grunnet M. Investigations of intravenous plasmin (fibrinolysin) in humans. *Circulation.* 1956;14:919.
14. Cliffton EE. The use of plasmin in humans. *Ann N Y Acad Sci.* 1957;68:209–229.
15. Reddy DS. Newer thrombolytic drugs for acute myocardial infarction. *Indian J Exp Biol.* 1998;36:1–15.
16. Jostring H, Barth U, Naidu R. Changes of antistreptokinase titer following long-term streptokinase therapy. In: Martin M, Schoop W, Hirsh J, eds. *New concepts of streptokinase dosimetry.* Vienna: Hans Huber; 1978:110.
17. Smith RAG, Dupe RJ, English PD, et al. Fibrinolysis with acylenzymes: a new approach to thrombolytic therapy. *Nature.* 1981; 290:505.
18. Markland FS, Friedrichs GS, Pewitt SR, et al. Thrombolytic effects of recombinant fibrolase or APSAC in a canine model of carotid artery thrombosis. *Circulation.* 1994;90:2448–2456.
19. Macfarlane RG, Pinot JJ. Fibrinolytic activity of normal urine. *Nature.* 1947;159:779.
20. Sobel GW, Mohler SR, Jones NW, et al. Urokinase: an activator of plasma fibrinolysin extracted from urine. *Am J Physiol.* 1952;171: 768–769.
21. Husain S, Lipinski B, Gurewich V, inventors. Isolation of plasminogen activators useful as therapeutic and diagnostic agents. U.S. Patent No. 04381346.
22. Gurewich V. Pro-urokinase: history, mechanisms of action, and clinical development. In: Loscalzo J, Sasahara AA, eds. *New therapeutic agents in thrombosis and thrombolysis.* New York, NY: Marcel and Dekker; 1997:539–559.
23. Tanswell P, Tebbe U, Neuhaus KL, et al. Pharmacokinetics and fibrin specificity of alteplase during accelerated infusions in acute myocardial infarction. *J Am Coll Cardiol.* 1992;19:1071–1075.
24. Hoylaerts M, Rijken DC, Lijnen HR, et al. Kinetics of the activation of plasminogen by human tissue plasminogen activator: role of fibrin. *J Biol Chem.* 1982;257:2912.
25. The GUSTO Investigators. An angiographic study within the global randomized trial of aggressive versus standard thrombolytic strategies in patients with acute myocardial infarction. *N Engl J Med.* 1993;329:1615.

26. Cannon CP, McCabe CH, Gibson CM, et al. TNK-tissue plasminogen activator in acute myocardial infarction. Results of the Thrombolysis In Myocardial Infarction (TIMI) 10A dose-ranging trial. *Circulation.* 1997;95:351–356.

27. Cannon CP, Gibson CM, McCabe CH, et al., Thrombolysis in Myocardial Infarction (TIMI) 10B Investigators. TNK-tissue plasminogen activator compared with front-loaded alteplase in acute myocardial infarction: results of the TIMI 10B trial. *Circulation.* 1998;98:2805–2814.

28. Martin U. Clinical and preclinical profile of the novel recombinant plasmiogen activator retelplase. In: Sasahara AA, Loscalzo J, eds. *New therapeutic agents in thrombosis and thrombolysis.* New York, NY: Marcel Dekker; 1997:495–511.

29. Meierhenrich R, Carlsson J, Seifried E, et al. Effect of reteplase on hemostasis variables: analysis of fibrin specificity, relation to bleeding complications and coronary patency. *Int J Cardiol.* 1998;65:57–63.

30. The Global Use of Strategies to Open Occluded Coronary Arteries (GUSTO III) Investigators. A comparison of reteplase with alteplase for acute myocardial infarction [see comments]. *N Engl J Med.* 1997;337:1118–1123.

31. Ouriel K, Katzen B, Mewissen MW, et al. Initial experience with reteplase in the treatment of peripheral arterial and venous occlusion. *J Vasc Interv Radiol.* 2000;11:849–854.

32. Hawkey C. Plasminogen activator in the saliva of the vampire bat *Desmodus rotundus. Nature.* 1966;211:434–435.

33. Verstraete M, Lijnen HR, Collen D. Thrombolytic agents in development. *Drugs.* 1995;50:29–42.

34. Randolph A, Chamberlain SH, Chu HL, et al. Amino acid sequence of fibrolase, a direct-acting fibrinolytic enzyme from agkistrodon contortrix contortrix venom. *Protein Sci.* 1992;1:590–600.

35. Collen D. Staphylokinase: a potent, uniquely fibrin-selective thrombolytic agent. *Nat Med.* 1998;4:279–284.

36. Heymans S, Vanderschueren S, Verhaeghe R, et al. Outcome and one year follow-up of intra-arterial staphylokinase in 191 patients with peripheral arterial occlusion. *Thromb Haemost.* 2000;83:666–671.

37. Ouriel K, Gray BH, Clair DG, et al. Complications associated with the use of urokinase and recombinant tissue plasminogen activator for catheter-directed peripheral arterial and venous thrombolysis. *J Vasc Interv Radiol.* 2000;11:295–298.

38. Meyerovitz M, Goldhaber SZ, Reagan K, et al. Recombinant tissue-type plasminogen activator versus urokinase in peripheral arterial and graft occlusions: A randomized trial. *Radiology.* 1990;175:75–78.

39. Comerota AJ. A re-analysis of the STILE data. *Montefiore Vascular and Endovascular Symposium,* New York, NY, Nov 17th, 1999.

40. Ouriel K, Kandarpa K, Schuerr DM, et al. Prourokinase vs. urokinase for recanalization of peripheral occlusions, safety and efficacy: The PURPOSE Trial. *J Vasc Interv Radiol.* 1999;10:1083–1091.

41. Weaver FA, Comerota AJ, Youngblood M, et al., The STILE Investigators. Surgery versus Thrombolysis for Ischemia of the Lower Extremity. Surgical revascularization versus thrombolysis for nonembolic lower extremity native artery occlusions: results of a prospective randomized trial. *J Vasc Surg.* 1996;24:513–521.

42. Comerota AJ, Weaver FA, Hosking JD, et al. Results of a prospective, randomized trial of surgery versus thrombolysis for occluded lower extremity bypass grafts. *Am J Surg.* 1996;172:105–112.

43. Ouriel K, Veith FJ, Sasahara AA. TOPAS Investigators. Thrombolysis or peripheral arterial surgery: phase I results. *J Vasc Surg.* 1996;23:64–73.

44. Ouriel K, Fiore WM, Geary JE. Limb-threatening ischemia in the medically compromised patient: amputation or revascularization? *Surgery.* 1988;104:667–672.

45. Sullivan KL, Gardiner GAJ, Kandarpa K, et al. Efficacy of thrombolysis in infrainguinal bypass grafts. Circulation. 1991;83:(Suppl-105):99–105.

46. Brewster DC, Darling RC. Optimal methods of aortoiliac reconstruction. *Surgery.* 1978;84:739–748.

47. Whittemore AD, Donaldson MC, Polak JF, et al. Limitations of balloon angioplasty for vein graft stenosis. *J Vasc Surg.* 1991;14:340–345.

48. Veith FJ, Gupta SK, Ascer E, et al. Six-year prospective multicenter randomized comparison of autologous saphenous vein and expanded polytetrafluoroethylene grafts in infrainguinal arterial reconstructions. *J Vasc Surg.* 1986;3:104–114.

49. Taylor LM Jr, Edwards JM, Porter JM. Present status of reversed vein bypass grafting: five-year results of modern series. *J Vasc Surg.* 1990;11:193–206.

50. Belkin M, Knox J, Donaldson MC, et al. Infrainguinal arterial reconstruction with nonreversed greater saphenous vein. *J Vasc Surg.* 1996;24:957–962.

Percutaneous Transluminal Angioplasty for Infrainguinal Bypass Grafts

Sean D. O'Donnell   *Charles J. Fox*   *Todd E. Rasmussen*   *David L. Gillespie*

Infrainguinal bypass grafting has been used with increasing frequency, most predominantly for limb salvage. The preferred conduit remains autologous vein with postoperative graft surveillance being the standard for the maintenance of graft patency as noted in the prior chapter. With a rigorous graft surveillance program one can expect graft stenosis to be found in 16% to 27% of grafts. Once identified, options to manage graft stenosis include surgical patch angioplasty, interposition grafting, bypassing the stenosis, and percutaneous transluminal balloon angioplasty (PTA). Early results of angioplasty prior to the development of current catheter-based technologies were poor and led to a slow acceptance of percutaneous methods as a viable option for dealing with graft stenosis.[1-4] In recent years, more favorable reports of vein graft PTA compared with conventional open revisions have appeared.[5,6] Percutaneous methods have the advantage of complete angiographic evaluation of the inflow, graft, and outflow allowing treatment of multiple lesions at the same time. In addition, the percutaneous nature of the procedure allows it to be easily performed as an outpatient. This chapter will review the current status of PTA for infrainguinal vein graft stenosis and identify the setting in which it can be performed with successful results comparable to conventional open revisions.

LESION SELECTION

In general, any lesion that would appear suitable for open patch angioplasty is likely amenable to PTA. Objective criteria have been defined by Avino et al.[5] using clinical and duplex criteria to achieve results equivalent to surgical revision. They identified clinical and duplex criterion for optimal percutaneous intervention (Table 33-1). It is notable that in their series the site of the primary graft stenosis had no bearing on the development of a recurrent stenosis.

The clinical criterion was that of a graft stenosis identified >3 months following the primary bypass procedure. It has been demonstrated that graft stenosis occurring in the first few months following the primary procedure has signs of increased cellular activity and may not be well suited for PTA. Early graft stenosis is also often associated with technical abnormalities from the

TABLE 33-1

FACTORS ASSOCIATED WITH SUCCESSFUL VEIN GRAFT PERCUTANEOUS TRANSLUMINAL BALLOON ANGIOPLASTY

Factor	Favorable Parameter
Timing after initial procedure	>3 mo
Diameter of vein graft	>3.5 mm
Length of stenosis	<20 mm

primary procedure.[5] These include retained valves, anastomotic abnormalities, and torsion of the graft. Lesions noted in this early time frame may also be due to primary defects in the vein prior to harvest.[7] In Figure 33-1 you can see the appearance of torsion of the graft at the distal anastomosis at 6 weeks postoperatively. In this particular case, an attempt at PTA left a residual stenosis that was managed with an interposition graft.

Duplex criteria for a significant vein graft stenosis include a peak systolic velocity (PSV) at the lesion of >300 cm per second, a ratio of PSV at the lesion to PSV proximal to the lesion of >3.5, or low flow in the normal-appearing graft <45 cm per second.[8] Favorable duplex findings for a durable vein graft PTA include a graft diameter of >3.5 mm and a total lesion length of <2 cm. Figures 33-2 to 33-4 are examples of these short isolated lesions that may frequently render a successful result.

Patients with suspected graft stenosis by duplex are studied as outpatients, maintained on aspirin, and loaded with 300 mg of clopidogrel (Plavix), which is then continued at 75 mg per day for 6 weeks if a PTA is performed. We prefer contralateral femoral artery access for these procedures. This allows for complete inflow, graft, and outflow assessment as well as treatment. A 5 French sheath is placed into the contralateral femoral artery over a 0.035 guidewire. A 5 French pigtail catheter is placed in the distal aorta and a pelvic arteriogram is performed with 10 cc per second for a total of 20 cc to visualize the iliac inflow. A 20- to 30-degree oblique view of the iliac artery ipsilateral to the graft is also performed to complete the inflow evaluation. The contralateral iliac artery is then selected with a SOS 1 catheter (Rim or Internal Mammary catheters may also be used) and a 0.035 angled hydrophilic wire. A 5 or 6 French braided sheath is then placed over the guidewire into the distal contralateral external iliac artery, which is now ipsilateral to the graft directed in an antegrade fashion (Fig. 33-5). The entire graft is now assessed angiographically starting with 3 cc per second for a total of 6 cc using digital subtraction angiography and adjusted for optimal visualization of the graft and outflow. Once the lesion is identified, the patient is heparinized with 75 to 100 U per kg to obtain an activated clotting time (ACT) of >250 seconds. The graft is selected with a 5 French angled glide catheter and a 0.035 angled glide wire. The glide catheter is advanced into the graft and the 0.035

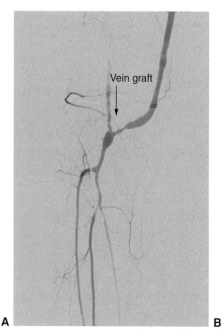
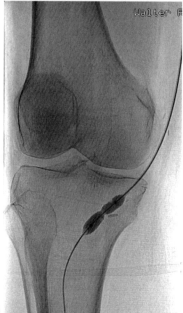
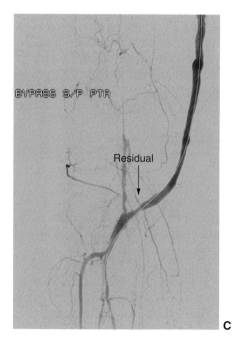

Figure 33-1 **A:** Right femoral–based vein bypass graft stenosis (*arrow*) identified by duplex sonography. **B:** Persistent waste due to residual twist in graft. **C:** Completion with residual stenosis (*arrow*).

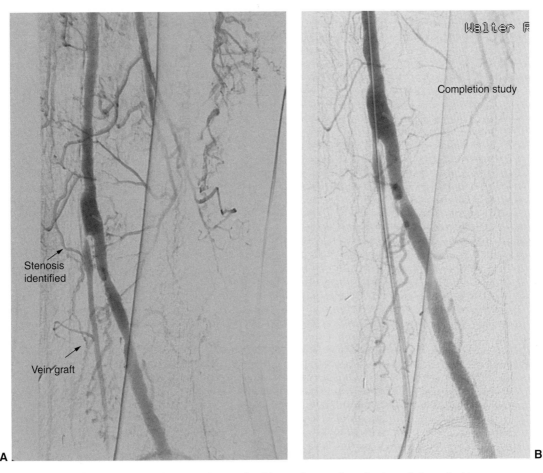

Figure 33-2   A: Arteriogram of left superficial femoral artery–based vein graft (*arrow*) with stenosis identified (*arrow*). **B:** Completion study after percutaneous transluminal balloon angioplasty.

hydrophilic wire is replaced with an exchange length (260 to 300 cm) 0.014 or 0.018 small-vessel wire, which is then used to cross the lesion and to perform the angioplasty. The angled glide catheter is then exchanged for a high-pressure (10 to 15 mm Hg), small-vessel or cardiac balloon. The balloon is sized to the normal adjacent graft for diameter and the length is sized to overlap the lesion but to avoid contact with as little as possible of the uninvolved graft. Inflation times were 30 to 60 seconds. The preoperative duplex can be useful in this regard to measure both the diameter of the normal adjacent graft and the length of the lesion.[9] A completion angiogram in at least two views is then performed. Inflow, outflow, and synchronous lesions are generally treated during the same procedure. The heparin is not reversed and the sheath is pulled when the ACT is <180 seconds and the patient discharged in 4 to 6 hours. The patient is then scheduled for a follow-up duplex in 4 to 6 weeks. Patients that predictably would not tolerate bed rest with limited motion of the access leg were liberally managed with a 6 French suture-mediated closure device and discharged in 2 hours.

Avino et al.[5] have advocated performing a completion duplex of the lesion at the site of the PTA. They referred to this as "duplex monitored" PTA. Their justification for this approach was a 35% incidence of unacceptable duplex velocities (PSV 150 to 300 cm per second or a Vr of >2.0) with completion angiogram that were otherwise acceptable. When a significant residual stenosis was identified by duplex, they retreated the lesion with either a 1- to 2-mm larger balloon or longer inflation time.

DISCUSSION OF THE RESULTS

When reviewing the results of vein graft stenosis, there can be confusion regarding number of patients, grafts, and stenoses treated. Also, the inclusion of various types of grafts makes definitive conclusions difficult. However, a trend toward more favorable results is apparent when PTA is applied to single, short, and primary lesions as opposed to less favorable results of multiple, long, or recurrent lesions.

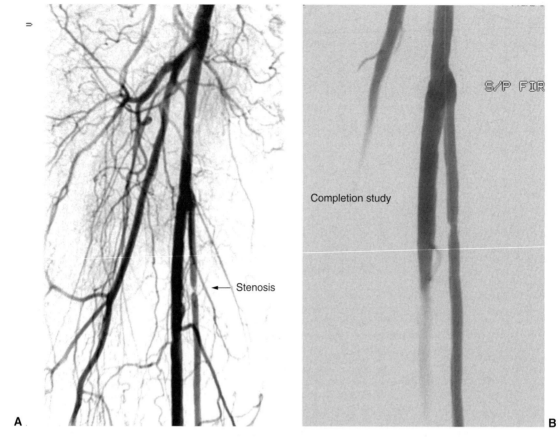

Figure 33-3 **A:** Arteriogram of right superficial femoral artery–based vein graft showing stenosis (*arrow*). **B:** Completion study after percutaneous transluminal balloon angioplasty.

Although early reports of PTA for graft stenosis were poor, more recent reports using improved catheter-based techniques and equipment have shown comparable results with conventional open revision (5). Results of recent series are listed in Table 33-2. Stenosis-free patencies of 59% to 89% and limb salvage of 88% can be expected with careful patient selection. It is notable that 75% of PTAs for graft stenosis are performed within 12 months of the primary graft procedure. In most series, PTA was performed for selected lesions

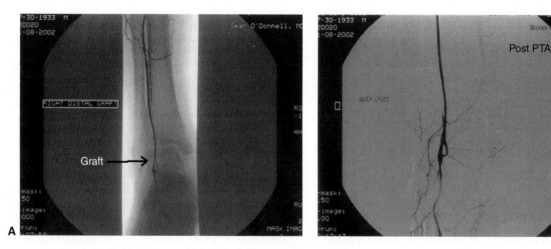

Figure 33-4 **A:** Arteriogram of right femoral–to–dorsalis pedis bypass with distal focal stenosis. **B:** Completion study after percutaneous transluminal balloon angioplasty.

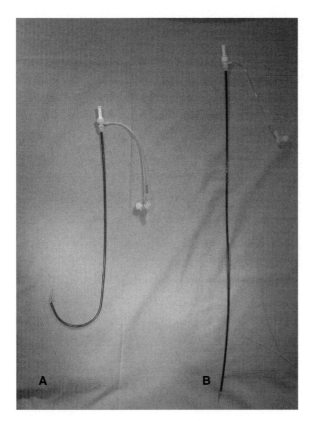

Figure 33-5   A: Balkin braided contralateral sheath. **B:** Straight braided sheath.

with similar criteria as identified earlier in this chapter. When all lesions were studied, as in the series by Whittemore et al.[1] or Sanchez et al.,[2] inferior results were seen, as noted in Table 33-2. Recurrent stenosis rates of 22% with a 2-year follow-up were reported by Avino et al.[5] and were similar to open revision. Others

have reported inferior results of PTA when applied to recurrent vein graft stenosis.[10]

Although conventional surgical revision has reproducible and durable results, there are still many challenges that confront this approach for all patients.[2,4,5,8,9,11] Many patients are significantly vein challenged, or have a lesion at a site of prior dissection or at a site that is anatomically difficult to access. In addition, many surgical interventions other than simple patch angioplasty for short midgraft lesions will require more than an overnight hospitalization.[4,6] Due to these challenges, PTA for graft stenosis has survived and a significant body of literature now supports its use in selected lesions which are <1.5 to 2 cm in length and in grafts >3 to 3.5 cm in diameter.[5,6,9,12]

Additional factors that may influence the use of PTA have also been suggested. Avino et al.[5] and Gonsalves et al.[13] have stated that graft stenosis that occurs within 30 days of the primary bypass procedure may not be well suited for angioplasty due to the biologic activity of the lesion at this stage. This notion was also supported in a study by Marin et al.[14] in which lesions with increased cellularity had a propensity to form intimal flaps. It has also been noted that proximal graft lesions may respond more favorably to PTA than distal graft lesions.[3] Certainly there is consistent data supporting less favorable results for PTA in the setting of recurrent stenosis and likely this is a testament to the varying biology of these lesions.[10,13] The complexity of the host biology can also be demonstrated by a patient in our experience who had an artery injury that occurred during the Vietnam War and underwent PTA for a graft stenosis. This recurred and was managed with an interposition saphenous vein. The excised vein graft stenosis demonstrated the typical smooth, white, firm, and

TABLE 33-2
RESULTS OF BALLOON ANGIOPLASTY FOR GRAFT STENOSIS

Author	Year	Number of Grafts	Assisted Patency Following PTA	Length of Follow-up
Whittemore[1]	1991	53	18%	5 y
			59% (lesions requiring single PTA)	3 y
Sanchez[2]	1994	41	44%	2 y
			66% (lesions <1.5 cm)	
Tonnesen[6]	1998	50	72% (included composite and PTFE)	0.75 y
Avino[5]	1999	67	63%	2 y
			89% (lesions <2 cm)	1 y

PTA, percutaneous transluminal balloon angioplasty; PTFE, polytetrafluoroethylene.

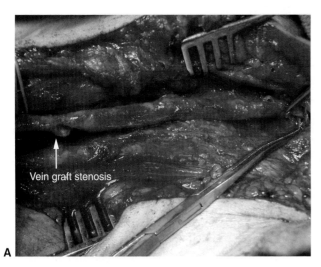 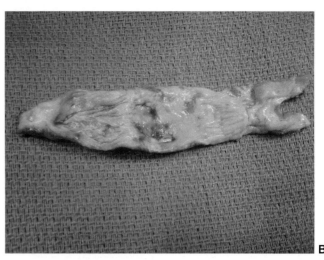

A

B

Figure 33-6 **A:** Operative photo showing gross external appearance of stenosis (*arrow*). **B:** Specimen showing the smooth, white, luminal stenosis.

fibrotic-appearing lesion (Fig. 33-6). He again developed a recurrent graft stenosis 6 months later, which was treated by PTA and has remained patent for the last 2 years.

Although not as well studied and beyond the scope of this discussion, it is worth noting that PTA has also been successfully utilized in polytetrafluoroethylene (PTFE) grafts and in graft stenosis detected following lytic therapy for graft thrombosis.[6,11,15,16] By the very nature of these series, the options of autologous vein revisions appear to have been limited, and, when available, conventional repairs with vein may be more favorable. Yet, in an established autologous vein graft, timely lysis and angioplasty of an inciting graft stenosis has the advantage of salvaging the best available conduit, that being the ipsilateral saphenous vein in most cases.[16]

Although most series of graft stenosis for PTA report no or minimal morbidity, arterial rupture has been reported.[6,12] The native artery beyond the distal anastomosis appears to be the region at risk. This is likely due to the fact that the graft and balloon diameter in most cases exceeds the diameter of the native tibial artery. It is therefore important to keep this in mind when treating a stenosis near the distal anastomosis.

There have been numerous factors identified that put grafts at risk for developing graft stenosis.[17–20] These factors include grafts with early flow disturbances, initial graft diameters <3.5 mm, composite or alternate vein grafts, smoking, hyperhomocysteinemia, and elevated levels of fibrinogen, lipoprotein (a), or 5-hydroxytryptamine. It would seem prudent to identify those factors that may be modulated in an effort to reduce the risk of recurrent graft stenosis following intervention.

TECHNICAL ADVANCES

Emerging angioplasty technologies may continue to improve on these reported results. Higher-pressure balloons exceeding 20 mm Hg and "cutting balloons" may be of use in treating the occasional short segment lesions that are unresponsive to standard angioplasty balloons. The use of a cutting balloon for fibrous lesions that resist dilatation even with high pressure angioplasty balloons is of particular interest. A recent report has demonstrated the successful use of these balloons with embedded cutting blades.[21] The cutting blades, called atherotomes, cause controlled longitudinal incisions in the neointimal lesion, allowing it to dilate (Fig. 33-7). Another technology is cryotherapy. When used in conjuction with angioplasty, cryotherapy may reduce the injury of the neointima and be advantageous for the fibrotic vein graft lesions.[22] The use of this technique has not yet been applied to vein graft stenosis. Drug-impregnated stents as well as brachiotherapy are additional technologies that may prove useful one day in managing these lesions.

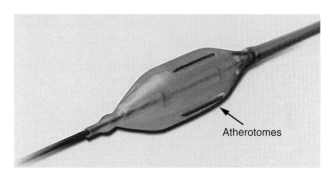

Atherotomes

Figure 33-7 Cutting balloon with atherotomes.

SUMMARY

Although conflicting results with percutaneous transluminal balloon angioplasty for vein graft stenosis are noted, it would appear that results comparable to conventional open revision can be achieved in selected patients. Favorable lesions can be identified by clinical, duplex, and angiographic criteria of lesions <2 cm in length, grafts >3.5 mm in diameter, and lesions occurring >3 months from the primary graft procedure (Table 33-1). Additional clinical considerations such as a difficult graft lesion to surgically access and the lack of available vein for a surgical revision may make vein graft PTA an attractive option. Open revision should be considered for recurrent lesions and those that do not meet the above criteria, multiple recurrences, and lesions detected during the first 3 months after the original bypass procedure.

REFERENCES

1. Whittemore AD, Donaldson MC, Polak JF, et al. Limitations of balloon angioplasty for vein graft stenosis. *J Vasc Surg.* 1991;14: 340–345.
2. Sanchez LA, Suggs WD, Marin ML, et al. Is percutaneous balloon angioplasty appropriate in the treatment of graft and anastomotic lesions responsible for failing vein bypasses? *Am J Surg.* 1994;168:97–101.
3. Dunlop P, Varty K, Hartshorne T, et al. Percutaneous transluminal angioplasty of infrainguinal vein graft stenosis: long-term outcome. *Br J Surg.* 1995;82:204–206.
4. Landry GJ, Moneta GL, Taylor LM Jr., et al. Comparison of procedural outcomes after lower extremity reversed vein grafting and secondary surgical revision. *J Vasc Surg.* 2003;38:22–28.
5. Avino AJ, Bandyk DF, Gonsalves AJ, et al. Surgical and endovascular intervention for infrainguinal vein graft stenosis. *J Vasc Surg.* 1999;29:60–70.
6. Tonnesen KH, Holstein P, Rordam L, et al. Early results of percutaneous transluminal angioplasty (PTA) of failing below-knee bypass grafts. *Eur J Vasc Endovasc Surg.* 1998;15:51–56.
7. Panetta TF, Marin ML, Veith FJ, et al. Unsuspected preexisting saphenous vein disease: an unrecognized cause of vein bypass failure. *J Vasc Surg.* 1992;15:102–110.
8. Sullivan TR Jr., Welch HJ, Iafrati MD, et al. Clinical results of common strategies used to revise infrainguinal vein grafts. *J Vasc Surg.* 1996;24:909–917.
9. Rua I, Calligaro KD, Dougherty MJ, et al. Is balloon angioplasty indicated for "short" stenoses of failing vein grafts? *Ann Vasc Surg.* 1998;12:134–137.
10. Tong Y, Matthews PG, Royle JP. Outcome of endovascular intervention for infrainguinal vein graft stenosis. *Cardiovasc Surg.* 2002;10:545–550.
11. Sanchez LA, Gupta SK, Veith FJ, et al. A ten-year experience with one hundred fifty failing or threatened vein and polytetrafluoroethylene arterial bypass grafts. *J Vasc Surg.* 1991;14:729–736.
12. Goh RH, Sniderman KW, Kalman PG. Long-term follow-up of management of failing *in situ* saphenous vein bypass grafts using endovascular intervention techniques. *J Vasc Interv Radiol.* 2000; 11:705–712.
13. Gonsalves C, Bandyk DF, Avino AJ, et al. Duplex features of vein graft stenosis and the success of percutaneous transluminal angioplasty. *J Endovasc Surg.* 1999;6:66–72.
14. Marin ML, Veith FJ, Gordon RE, et al. Analysis of balloon dilatation of human vein graft stenoses. *Ann Vasc Surg.* 1993;7:2–7.
15. Aburahma AF, Hopkins ES, Wulu JT Jr., et al. Lysis/balloon angioplasty versus thrombectomy/open patch angioplasty of failed femoropopliteal polytetrafluoroethylene bypass grafts. *J Vasc Surg.* 2002;35:307–315.
16. Berkowitz HD, Kee JC. Occluded infrainguinal grafts: when to choose lytic therapy versus a new bypass graft. *Am J Surg.* 1995; 170:136–139.
17. Cheshire NJ, Wolfe JH, Barradas MA, et al. Smoking and plasma fibrinogen, lipoprotein (a) and serotonin are markers for postoperative infrainguinal graft stenosis. *Eur J Vasc Endovasc Surg.* 1996; 11:479–486.
18. Irvine C, Wilson YG, Currie IC, et al. Hyperhomocysteinaemia is a risk factor for vein graft stenosis. *Eur J Vasc Endovasc Surg.* 1996; 12:304–309.
19. Gentile AT, Mills JL, Gooden MA, et al. Identification of predictors for lower extremity vein graft stenosis. *Am J Surg.* 1997;174: 218–221.
20. Idu MM, Buth J, Hop WC, et al. Factors influencing the development of vein-graft stenosis and their significance for clinical management. *Eur J Vasc Endovasc Surg.* 1999;17:15–21.
21. Kasirajan K, Schneider P. Early outcome of "cutting" balloon angioplasty for infrainguinal vein graft stenosis. *J Vasc Surg.* 2004;39:702–708.
22. Kataoka T, Honda Y, Bonneau HN, et al. New catheter-based technology for the treatment of restenosis. *J Interv Cardiol.* 2002; 15:371–379.

Lower Extremity Major Amputations

Marc E. Mitchell

Lower extremity amputation remains an important aspect of the practice of vascular surgery, with the vast majority of amputations resulting from complications of atherosclerosis. Unfortunately, for many vascular surgeons, amputations represent the primary manifestation of our limited ability to successfully treat peripheral arterial disease and prevent its complications. Amputations should instead be thought of as reconstructive procedures performed in patients with end-stage peripheral vascular disease. The initial objective of amputation is the removal of infected, ischemic, or gangrenous tissue and the relief of pain. The achievement of this objective is usually not difficult. The long-term goal is to create a stump that will successfully heal, and ultimately allow the patient to rehabilitate with a prosthesis and achieve independent ambulation. Patients undergoing amputation have severe arterial insufficency, frequently accompanied by multiple medical comorbidities, making the achievement of this objective one of the most challenging aspects of vascular surgery. The long-term success, measured by amputation mortality and morbidity, wound healing, and successful ambulation with a prosthesis, has not improved significantly over the last several decades.

Recent studies have determined the annual incidence of lower extremity amputation in the United States to be approximately 35 to 45 amputations per 100,000 people, the vast majority of which result from the complications of atherosclerotic peripheral arterial disease. Despite advances in techniques for limb salvage, the rate of major lower extremity amputations has remained relatively stable over the last 2 decades.

Approximately 30% to 50% of lower extremity amputations are performed at the above-knee level, 25% at the below-knee level, and the remainder at the level of the foot or toes.[1,2]

The risk factors for amputation are well known and mirror those for the development of atherosclerosis. Diabetes is one of the major risk factors, with 43% to 75% of patients undergoing amputation having diabetes.[1,3,4] It has been estimated that as many as 15% of diabetics will undergo a lower extremity amputation in their lifetime.[5] Men are more likely to undergo amputation than are women, with age-adjusted amputation rates 50% to 75% higher in men compared to women.[1,2] The incidence of amputation is directly related to age. Below-knee amputations are three times more frequent, and above-knee amputations six times more frequent in patients over 65 years of age compared to those younger than 65.[2] As the population ages, the number of amputations performed annually can be expected to increase, even if the amputation rate falls. There are racial differences in the amputation rate, with African Americans being two to three times more likely to undergo lower extremity amputation compared to other races, frequently at a higher level.[1,2,6] Native Americans and Hispanic Americans also have a markedly increased risk of amputation compared to other races.[6,7] These differences may be partially related to the incidence of diabetes and other risk factors in these populations.

Lower extremity amputation truly is one of the highest risk procedures performed by vascular surgeons. The 30-day operative mortality for major lower extremity amputation is 10% or higher.[3,4,8,9] Amputations done in the setting of acute limb ischemia are particularly high risk, with a mortality approaching 25%.[10,11] This extremely high operative mortality results from the associated ischemic heart disease and other comorbid conditions frequently seen in patients with end-stage vascular disease, and has not decreased significantly in recent years.[3] Similar to patients undergoing lower extremity revascularization, myocardial infarction is by far the leading cause of perioperative death in this group of patients. In addition, lower extremity amputation is associated with a dismal long-term outlook. The 1-year survival rate following major lower extremity amputation is approximately 50% to 60%, and is worse for patients undergoing above-knee compared to below-knee procedures.[3,4] Long-term mortality rates for amputees are more than double those of age-adjusted nonamputees with similar risk factors.[7]

Postoperative complications occur in approximately 40% of patients following major lower extremity amputation, the majority being wound-, cardiac-, or graft-related.[4,10] Failure of the amputated limb to heal is usually the result of progressive infection or ischemia. The resultant revision to a more proximal amputation subjects the patient to the potential morbidity and mortality of an additional operative procedure, and lessens the likelihood of successful rehabilitation and independent ambulation with a prosthesis. Selection of the proper amputation level is essential to avoid this complication, and is discussed in detail below.

In a recent series, 44% of lower extremity amputations were performed in the setting of a previous lower extremity bypass.[4] Failed previous lower extremity revascularization does not result in a higher amputation level or adversely affect wound healing.[4,8] Complications related to previous lower extremity bypass include graft infection, bleeding, and wound problems. Other common complications following major lower extremity amputation include deep venous thrombosis, decubitus ulcer formation, infections, and the development of flexion contractures.

The amputee's remaining limb is at risk for developing ischemic complications secondary to peripheral arterial disease, as well as long-term complications related to ambulation with a prosthesis. Seventeen percent to 20% of amputees eventually require amputation of the contralateral leg because of ischemia, and >5% undergo revascularization of the contralateral extremity for limb salvage.[3,4] Ambulating with a prosthesis produces an asymmetrical gait with abnormal forces and load applied to the contralateral leg. This results in accelerated degenerative disease of the leg. Amputees have a higher than normal incidence of osteoarthritis and degenerative joint disease in their remaining limb and back.[12,13]

For many patients, the most devastating consequence of major lower extremity amputation is the loss of independence. Recent studies indicate that only 25% of patients are discharged home following major lower extremity amputation, and that less than one third of patients are successfully fitted with a prosthesis and achieve independent ambulation.[3,4] Long-term care following lower extremity amputation places a significant financial and emotional burden on patients and their families. Much has been written regarding the cost of lower extremity amputation. There are several studies comparing the cost of primary amputation to the cost of lower extremity revascularization. This is a very difficult subject to study. The decision to perform a primary amputation or to attempt limb salvage is perhaps one of the more difficult ones a vascular surgeon must make, and it cannot be made solely on economic factors. It appears that the hospital costs for the two procedures are similar, but that the costs associated with failed lower extremity revascularization followed by amputation are significantly higher.[14-16] These findings underscore the importance of patient selection when deciding between primary amputation and revascularization. The long-term costs of amputation are high, with many patients requiring care in long-term nursing facilities. Perhaps one of the most frustrating aspects concerning lower extremity amputation is the fact that many can be avoided with appropriate patient education and preventive foot care. There is ample data to support the clinical and cost-effectiveness of these preventative programs.[17]

PREOPERATIVE EVALUATION

The extent of the preoperative workup required prior to lower extremity amputation is largely determined by the urgency of the procedure. For patients with an aggressive necrotizing lower extremity infection, an emergency open amputation is a life-saving procedure, and there is no time for an extensive preoperative evaluation. These patients should be rapidly resuscitated and taken to the operating room as quickly as possible. The majority of lower extremity amputations, however, are more elective in nature. Many patients will have already undergone a thorough preoperative evaluation prior to lower extremity revascularization. As previously discussed, lower extremity amputation is an extremely high-risk procedure with significant perioperative mortality and morbidity. Patients must undergo an appropriate preoperative evaluation in order to ensure the safest possible operation. The overall medical condition of the patient is one of the factors the vascular surgeon must consider when deciding between revascularization and primary amputation, or when selecting the appropriate level for amputation. This frequently entails a complete cardiac evaluation. For many patients, several days of medical management are required in order to optimize their overall medical condition. Many patients require invasive intraoperative monitoring as well as postoperative monitoring in an intensive care unit.

SELECTION OF AMPUTATION LEVELS

Once the decision to perform an amputation has been made, the appropriate level for the amputation must be determined. As a general rule, lower extremity amputations should be performed at the most distal level possible, in order to maintain maximal residual limb length and to allow the best chance for rehabilitation and successful ambulation with a prosthesis. Successful rehabilitation following digital or transmetatarsal foot amputation is common. Unfortunately the same cannot be said of below-knee or above-knee amputations. While more proximal above-knee amputations have an excellent chance of healing, the likelihood of successful ambulation with a prosthesis is small. Preservation of the knee joint is particularly important. A below-knee amputation preserves mobility and significantly increases the chances of successful rehabilitation compared to an above-knee amputation. The inability of patients to ambulate following lower extremity amputation is due in part to the increased energy required to ambulate with a prosthesis. Compared to normal walking, ambulation with a unilateral below-knee prosthesis requires a 40% increase in energy expenditure, and ambulation with a unilateral above-knee prosthesis, a 60% increase in energy expenditure.[18,19] In addition, ambulation with a prosthesis requires a degree of balance and motor coordination not possible for many patients. Consequently, <70% of below-knee amputees and <30% of above-knee amputees successfully rehabilitate to the point of independent ambulation with a prosthesis.[3,4,20,21] Because of the significantly higher rate of successful rehabilitation following below-knee amputations, they are usually preferred to above-knee amputations and should be performed more often.

There are exceptions to this rule. Patients who are not ambulatory prior to major amputation have little chance of ambulating following either a below-knee or above-knee amputation.[3,4] In these patients, the amputation should be performed at a level that is most assuredly going to heal—frequently above-knee. This avoids the risk of multiple procedures associated with a nonhealing wound. Additionally, nonambulatory patients frequently develop flexion contractures of the knee following below-knee amputations, leading to stump breakdown and eventual above-knee amputation. A primary through-knee or above-knee amputation avoids this complication and alleviates the need for an above-knee amputation in the future. Likewise, in patients that present an extremely high operative risk, a more proximal above-knee amputation is preferred. In these patients, it is important to perform a single procedure with a high probability of successful healing in order to avoid the risk associated with multiple operations.

Using clinical judgment alone, experienced surgeons can successfully predict healing in 80% of below-knee and 90% of above-knee amputations.[22–24] Clinicians are able to successfully predict the healing of amputations at the level of ankle or below only 40% of the time.[24] Physical examination alone does not offer any definitive signs that can assure successful wound healing. The presence of a palpable pulse just proximal to the amputation level is a good predictor of healing, but the absence of a pulse does not necessarily correlate with failure to heal.[25] Other clinical findings, such as skin temperature, dependent rubor, correlation with arteriographic findings, and bleeding during operation, have all been used with varying success to predict amputation wound healing.[24] Although clinicians are limited in their ability to predict wound healing, clinical judgment is better at predicting wounds that will not heal. Most experienced surgeons are successfully able to predict when a lower extremity amputation will not heal based on clinical findings alone.

Over the years, many techniques have been used by surgeons to improve their accuracy in predicting the most distal level at which an amputation will successfully heal. Segmental Doppler pressure measurements and pulse volume recordings are easily obtainable, inexpensive, noninvasive tests that have demonstrated usefulness in predicting the healing of amputation wounds. These tests are most useful when one is trying to decide between a below-knee and above-knee amputation. A significant pressure drop from the thigh to the calf or the absence of Doppler flow in the popliteal artery are reasonably good predictors of failure of a distal amputation to heal. Unfortunately, these techniques are not as accurate in predicting which amputations will heal. Doppler ankle pressures of <35 mm Hg are associated with nonhealing of foot amputations,[26] as are toe pressure measurements of <30 mm Hg.[27] There are limitations to the usefulness of segmental pressure measurements, especially in diabetic patients with noncompressible, calcified vessels. In such cases, pulse volume recordings are a valuable adjunct to segmental pressure measurements. Waveform analysis allows the surgeon to identify patients with falsely elevated pressure measurements due to arterial wall calcification.

The measurement of transcutaneous tissue oxygen tension ($TcPO_2$) has been used to predict the healing of specific amputation levels with good success.[24] An oxygen electrode is used to measure the oxygen tension of the skin after maximal dilation of the cutaneous vasculature by heating the skin to 43°C to 45°C. This measurement is believed to be an accurate representation of the actual PO_2 of the tissue. Like other methods used to predict amputation healing, $TcPO_2$ is more accurate at predicting wounds that will heal than wounds that will not heal. A $TcPO_2$ >40 mm Hg is predictive of successful wound healing. While a $TcPO_2$ <20 mm Hg is usually indicative of a wound that will not heal, there are reports of wounds with $TcPO_2$ measurements near zero healing.[28,29] Unfortunately, many patients fall into the indeterminate zone with a $TcPO_2$ measurement of between 20 and 40 mm Hg. The additional measurement of TcPo$_2$ with the leg elevated to 30 degrees for 3 minutes is useful in these patients. A decrease in the TcPo$_2$ of 15 mm Hg with elevation is predictive of failure to heal.[30] This technique is simple to perform and reproducible, and the equipment is relatively inexpensive, making it a commonly available test in many vascular laboratories. Many vascular surgeons have found TcPo$_2$ measurement to be a valuable adjunct to segmental pressure measurements and pulse volume recording when trying to determine the appropriate level for amputation.

The measurement of skin temperature has been reported to successfully predict amputation wound healing,[31] as has the use of ultraviolet Wood light fluorescence.[32] Cutaneous blood flow in response to hyperemia measured by laser Doppler velocimetry before and after skin heating is another technique that has been reported to accurately predict the healing of amputation wounds.[33] Laser Doppler velocimetry has also been used to measure skin perfusion pressure.[34] Radioactive isotopes can be used to measure both skin blood flow and skin perfusion pressure, and may be useful in predicting wound healing following amputation.[24] These techniques all require specialized equipment and are not widely used in clinical practice.

For the majority of patients, the clinical judgment of an experienced surgeon in conjunction with readily available noninvasive vascular testing will result in the selection of an amputation level that will heal. For more difficult cases, the measurement of TcPo$_2$ can provide valuable information. Using these techniques, vascular surgeons should be able to accurately predict amputation wound healing in well over 90% of cases. The overall clinical situation must also be taken into consideration when making the final decision regarding the level at which to perform an amputation. When considering young patients who are relatively healthy, highly motivated, and good candidates for successful rehabilitation with a prosthesis, one should err on the side of performing the most distal amputation and accept a higher rate of failure. Amputations below the ankle are frequently done under local or regional anesthesia and pose less operative risk to the patient. The long-term disability of these distal amputations is significantly less than that seen with below-knee or above-knee amputations, and it is sometimes in the best interest of the patient to attempt such a procedure even if the chance of success is relatively small. Similarly, below-knee amputations offer significant advantages over above-knee procedures. Surgical or endovascular revascularization is occasionally indicated to increase the probability of healing in order to preserve a below-knee amputation in good risk patients who have a high likelihood of successful rehabilitation. For older patients with multiple medical comorbidities and a

low likelihood of successful rehabilitation, the decision should be directed more towards initial operative success in order to avoid the risk of multiple procedures. In these patients, a more proximal amputation, often at the above-knee level, is indicated. Regardless of the level at which it is performed, a lower extremity amputation is a major, life-altering event, and the patient must be adequately informed of the likelihood of success and involved in the decision-making process.

TECHNICAL CONSIDERATION

Lower extremity amputations are frequently thought of as straightforward procedures assigned to junior members of the operating team. In reality, these procedures can be very challenging and require mature surgical skills and judgment. This is particularly true when one is trying to salvage a below-knee amputation in a patient with a failed lower extremity bypass and a gangrenous foot. The first step towards rehabilitation with a prosthesis following lower extremity amputation is successful healing of the amputation wound, resulting in a properly formed amputation stump that can accept a prosthesis. A successful amputation can significantly improve the quality of life for the patient, while the consequences of an improperly performed amputation requiring revision to a higher level can be devastating.

General Technical Principles

Perioperative antibiotics are indicated for all procedures, and may be required for an extended period in the presence of distal infection. Amputations at the foot or ankle level are usually performed under local or regional anesthesia. Diabetic patients with peripheral neuropathy often require little anesthesia for distal procedures. Below-knee or above-knee amputations can be done under regional or general anesthesia. Skin incisions must be carefully planned, taking into consideration previous surgical incisions, open wounds, and the presence of gangrenous tissue. Gentle handling of tissues and the use of proper surgical techniques are of paramount importance in order to avoid traumatizing relatively ischemic tissue that may be marginally viable. Forceps should be used sparingly, particularly on the skin. Skin incisions must be carefully placed in order to avoid the undermining of tissues, and to allow for a tension-free closure. Wounds closed under tension are a common error of the inexperienced surgeon and are destined for failure. The bones must be transected well above the level of the skin incision in order to avoid this complication. If the skin closure appears to be under tension, the bone must be resected more proximally. All nonviable tissue must be removed, and electrocautery used precisely and judiciously. Transected bones should be smooth and bone splinters removed. Nerves should be transected under tension and allowed to retract deep into the tissues in order to prevent the formation of painful neuromas that are irritated by pressure from the prosthesis. Hematoma or seroma formation can result in failure of the amputation wound to heal. Closed suction drains are used liberally in order to obliterate dead space and avoid these complications. Skin incisions are closed with monofilament sutures or stainless steel staples, and should be left in place for at least 3 weeks.

Single-stage closed amputations are generally preferred over open procedures. In the presence of wet gangrene or active infection, open procedures are performed. The open procedure should be done at a level that removes the infected and necrotic tissue, but allows for the construction of the most distal definitive amputation. If revascularization is contemplated, the open procedure should be planned with future surgical incisions in mind. Several days of antibiotics and local wound care are usually required before the definitive amputation is performed. If the extremity is severely edematous, the definitive procedure should be delayed until the edema has resolved.

Amputations done prior to or in conjunction with surgical revascularization or endovascular procedures deserve special consideration. Grossly infected and necrotic tissue should be removed at the time of the revascularization, but the wounds are usually left open. This approach allows for recovery of the chronically ischemic tissue following revascularization and the performance of a more distal definitive amputation at a later date. The amount of tissue recovery that occurs following revascularization of a chronically ischemic foot can be surprising. While it is important to remove necrotic tissue and drain infected areas, one should not commit a patient to a more proximal amputation by performing an overly aggressive procedure prior to revascularization. The postoperative edema frequently seen following revascularization can make the amputation more difficult and impair wound healing. Wound closure or definitive amputations should be delayed until the edema has subsided.

Toe Amputation

Toe amputation is indicated for gangrene involving the distal aspect of the toe, when there is adequate viable skin at the base of the digit to allow for a tension-free closure. The incision is slightly fish-mouthed, and the flaps are tailored based on the extent of the necrotic tissue. The phalynx is divided, leaving the proximal segment of bone covering the articular surface of the metatarsal head. The wound is closed in a single layer with 4-0 or 5-0 monofilament suture. Since the metatarsal head is the weight-bearing portion of the

foot, patients may ambulate within a few days of surgery following a toe amputation.

Ray Amputation

If the area of gangrene extends to the base of the toe, a ray amputation is required. A racquet-type incision is used. The circular head of the racquet encircles the base of the digit. The linear handle of the racquet is extended on the dorsum of the foot over the distal metatarsal. For first and fifth toe procedures, the handle is extended along the medial and lateral aspects of the foot, respectively. Care is taken to avoid injuring the neurovascular bundle or entering the metatarsal-phalyngeal joint of the adjacent toe. The tendons are divided as far proximally as possible. The metatarsal bone is divided in its midportion. The wound may be closed in layers or with a single layer of 4-0 monofilament suture encompassing the deeper tissue in addition to the skin. The patient should remain non–weight-bearing until complete healing, usually at least 3 weeks.

Transmetatarsal Amputation

Transmetatarsal amputation is indicated for gangrene involving several toes or metatarsal heads. When three or more digits require ray amputation, a transmetatarsal amputation is usually preferred. A long plantar flap is used for wound closure. Deep plantar space infections and gangrene involving the plantar surface of the foot are contraindications to transmetatarsal amputation. Open transmetatarsal amputation may be performed in the presence of infection, providing the infection does not extend proximally.

The dorsal incision is made across the foot at the midmetatarsal level (Fig. 34-1). The skin incision is made approximately 1 cm distal to the anticipated level of metatarsal transection. The incision is extended to the base of the toes medially and laterally along the foot, and then across the plantar aspect of the foot. The dorsal incision is carried down to bone. The metatarsals are divided with an oscillating saw proximal to the dorsal skin incision. The bones may be beveled slightly to facilitate closure. The shafts of the metatarsal bones are sharply excised from the plantar flap. The tendons are divided under tension and allowed to retract proximally. Excess tissue is removed from the plantar flap. The flap should be appropriately thinned to allow for easy dorsal rotation and a tension-free closure. The wound is closed in layers with 4-0 monofilament suture for the skin. The patient should not bear weight until the wound is completely healed. Patients have excellent functional results with minimal disability following transmetatarsal amputation. A short period of rehabilitation therapy is usually

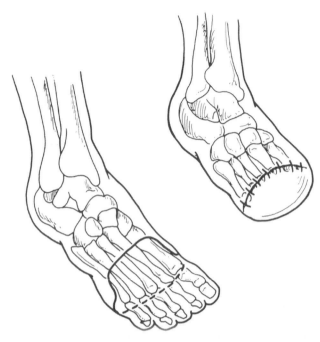

Figure 34-1 Transmetatarsal amputation plantar-based skin flap and completed amputation. (From Malone JM. Lower extremity amputation. In: Moore WS, ed. *Vascular surgery: a comprehensive review*. Philadelphia, Pa: WB Saunders Company; 1993, with permission.)

all that is required for ambulation following a midfoot amputation, and there is minimal increase in energy expenditure. Ankle-level amputees use a patellar tendon-bearing prosthesis attached to an artificial foot. Impaired wound healing is frequently a complication with these procedures because of the rather tenuous blood supply to the flap used for closure. Consequently, these amputations should not be attempted if the adequacy of arterial perfusion is in question. Stump breakdown is the most common long-term complication of these procedures, and results from the abnormal weight-bearing forces on the end of the stump. It is difficult to maintain functional ankle dorsiflexion with midfoot amputations, frequently resulting in a plantar flexion contracture and foot ulceration. This complication is most frequently seen in patients with peripheral neuropathy, making diabetes a relative contraindication. Syme amputations are sometimes complicated by a bulbous distal stump and posterior migration of the heel pad that is used to cover the end of the stump. This can lead to ulceration.

A disarticulation between the tarsal and metatarsal bones is known as a Lisfranc amputation. A Chopart amputation is a disarticulation of the talonavicular and calcaneocuboid joints. Both procedures are closed with a plantar flap, similar to a transmetatarsal amputation. The Syme amputation is the most commonly performed ankle-level amputation, and can be done in one or two stages. It is a technically difficult procedure, with a high rate of wound failure.[36] Most vascular surgeons have little experience with midfoot and ankle-level amputations, frequently referring these procedures to orthopedists or podiatrists.

necessary to return the gait to near normal. No specific prosthesis is required, but modifications to the shoe are necessary.

Failure of a transmetatarsal amputation usually results in a below-knee or above-knee amputation, with the concurrent functional disability. Because of the significant functional benefits of transmetatarsal amputation over below-knee amputation, it is sometimes in the best interest of the patient to make extraordinary efforts to preserve a transmetatarsal amputation. It is sometimes necessary to perform revascularization prior to or in conjunction with transmetatarsal amputation. Inadequate plantar flap for closure is one of the more common reasons for transmetatarsal amputation failure. Split-thickness skin grafting can be used to assist in the closure of a transmetatarsal amputation, providing the weight-bearing plantar surface of the foot is intact. The dorsum of the foot and the end of the stump can be covered with a skin graft. If the flap does not provide complete coverage and the open wound is small, it can be allowed to close by secondary intention.

Midfoot and Ankle Amputations

In cases of gangrene extending to the midportion of the foot, a transmetatarsal amputation may not be possible. In these cases, a midfoot or ankle amputation may be indicated. While technically more challenging, these procedures have excellent rehabilitation potential and are indicated in select patients.[35] A shoe prosthesis is

Below-knee Amputation

Below-knee amputation is indicated for the patient with severe lower extremity ischemia who is not a candidate for a more distal amputation. There are several techniques that can be used for this procedure. They vary in the type of flap used for closure. The creation of a long posterior myocutaneous flap based on the gastrocnemius and soleus muscles is the most commonly used technique (Fig. 34-2). Other techniques include a fishmouth incision with equal anterior and posterior flaps, or a sagittal incision with medial and lateral flaps. Traditional wisdom states that the blood supply to a posterior muscle flap is superior to that of an anterior flap, making this the technique of choice. Recent studies have challenged this belief,[37] and there are reports of excellent results using the other techniques for below-knee amputation. Since the pattern of distribution of the infection or gangrene and the presence of previous surgical incisions or scars may mandate the use of a particular technique, the vascular surgeon should be familiar with all the techniques for below-knee amputation.

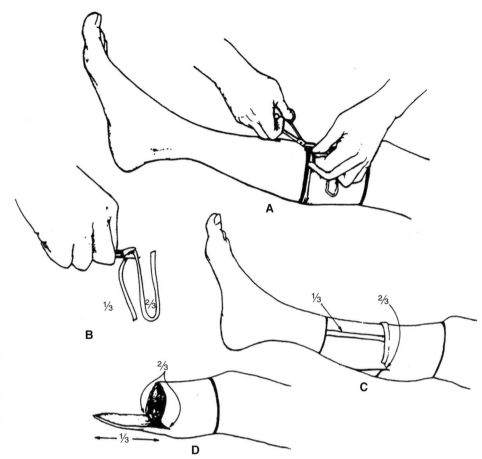

Figure 34-2 Technique for measuring the length of skin flaps in below-knee amputation. **A:** Umbilical tape or string is used to measure the circumference of the leg at the point of bone transection. **B:** Tape is divided in one-third and two-third lengths. **C:** The one-third piece measures the length of the posterior flap. The two-third piece measures the length of the anterior incision. Dog ears at each corner are avoided by cutting a curved triangle of skin from the anterior flap. **D:** The completed amputation before closure. (From Sanders RJ, Augspurger R. Skin flap measurement for below-knee amputation. *Surg Gynecol Obstet.* 1977;145:740, with permission.)

The tibia should be transected 10 to 12 cm below the tibial tuberosity for the best functional result. The tibial length may be shortened if the disease process extends proximally, but the insertion of the patellar tendon on the tibial tuberosity must be preserved in order to maintain knee extension. The skin incision should be made 1 cm distal to the level of tibial transection, or one hand's breath below the tibial tuberosity. The incision for creation of the skin flaps should be drawn on the leg as described by Sanders and Augspurger (Fig. 34-2). Dog ears at the corner of the anterior incision can be avoided by slightly curving the anterior portion of the incision proximally. The anterior compartment musculature and neurovascular bundle are divided. The periostium on the tibia is elevated proximally, and the bone transected proximal to the skin incision with an oscillating saw. The periostium should be elevated only to the level of bone transection. The tibia should be beveled at an angle of 45 degrees or more to avoid pressure of the anterior skin, which can lead to skin necrosis (Fig. 34-3). The fibula is transected at least 1 cm proximal to the tibia. The remaining neurovascular structures are divided, and the posterior flap created to complete the amputation. The muscle must be tailored to the appropriate thickness. The flap must be thick enough to provide adequate soft-tissue coverage over the tibia, but thin enough to rotate anteriorly for a tension-free closure. The fascia is approximated with absorbable 2-0 suture and the skin with monofilament suture or stainless steel staples. A close suction drain may be used. A rigid dressing is applied to protect the stump and maintain the knee in extension. A below-knee prosthesis can accommodate up to 25 degrees of flexion contracture at the knee, with more significant contractures causing disability. Sutures are left in place for at least 4 weeks. When the

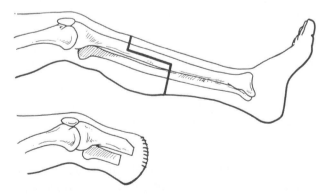

Figure 34-3 The standard posterior flap amputation. Note the beveled tibia and the proximal shortening of the fibula compared to the tibia. (From Malone JM. Lower extremity amputation. In: Moore WS. ed. *Vascular surgery: a comprehensive review.* Philadelphia, Pa: WB Saunders Company; 1993, with permission.)

wound is healed, a stump shrinker is applied. It takes several months for the stump to remodel and mature, at which time a permanent prosthesis is fitted.

Through-knee Amputation

Knee disarticulation or through-knee amputation is occasionally used in patients undergoing lower extremity amputation for ischemia. This procedure has several potential advantages compared to other lower extremity amputation including a high rate of primary wound healing; amputation at a level consisting primarily of tendons and ligaments, resulting in fewer bleedings; creation of a stump with a long lever arm resulting in better mobility, stability, and balance; and the avoidance of flexion contractures frequently seen in chronically bedridden patients following below-knee amputation.[38] The stump is durable and has good end weight-bearing capacity. Patients that would otherwise heal a below-knee amputation, but have a flexion contracture of the knee are well suited for a through-knee amputation.

Several techniques have been described for the procedure,[38–40] differing in the orientation of the skin flaps and management of the femoral condyles and patella. Anterior and posterior skin flaps are usually used, with a long anterior flap preferred. Sagittal orientation of the flaps is an acceptable alternative. Regardless of the orientation, the flaps should be of sufficient length to allow for a tension-free closure. The patellar tendon is taken off at its insertion on the tibial tuberosity. The lateral soft tissue structures, primarily tendons and ligaments, are divided at the level of the joint. The joint is entered, the knee disarticulated, and the neurovascular structures ligated. The patella may be left attached to its tendon or removed in a subperiosteal plane. The distal 1.5 to 2.0 cm of femur is transected. The patellar, semitendinous, and biceps femoris tendons are closed over the end of the femur. The fascia and skin are closed without tension. A drain may be used if necessary. A through-knee amputation can be performed quickly, with minimal blood loss, and may be preferable to above-knee amputation in many patients.

Above-knee Amputation

An above-knee amputation is indicated for patients with flexion contractures of the knee, when there is gangrene extending to the knee, or when severe ischemia prevents the healing of a below-knee amputation. Above-knee amputations have traditionally been classified as supracondylar, midfemur, and proximal femur. This classification is somewhat arbitrary, and the amputation should always be performed at the most distal level possible (Fig. 34-4). Longer femoral stumps have the benefit of better mobility, stability, and balance, making sitting in a wheelchair easier and more comfortable for the patient. A fished-mouth incision is usually used, with the

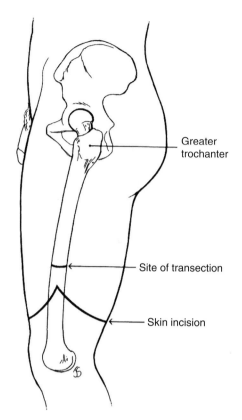

Figure 34-4 Above-knee amputation is carried out as caudad as possible, leaving a generous soft-tissue envelope for closure. (From Jacobs LA. Above-knee amputation and hip disarticulation. In: Ernst CB, Stanley JC, eds. *Current therapy in vascular surgery.* St Louis, Mo: Mosby; 2001, with permission.)

creation of equal anterior and posterior myocutaneous flaps. The soft tissue is divided with electocautery. The vessels are suture ligated, and the sciatic nerve is ligated under tension and allowed to retract proximally. The periostium of the femur is elevated proximally, and the bone divided well above the level of the skin incision. The periostium should be elevated just enough to allow division of the bone, and no more. If the femur is divided too far distally, the closure will be under tension and the wound will not heal. This technical error is one of the more common reasons for failure of an above-knee amputation to heal. The fascia is closed with interrupted absorbable sutures and the skin with staples or monofilament sutures. Drains may be used if needed.

Hip Disarticulation

Hip disarticulation is most commonly performed in the setting of trauma or malignancy, but occasionally may be indicated for severe ischemia, especially when there is extensive gangrene extending to the proximal thigh. Most patients, however, are able to heal a high above-knee amputation, including those with aortoiliac occlusions. Hip disarticulation is usually reserved for patients that fail to heal a proximal above-knee amputation. The operative mortality of hip disarticulation

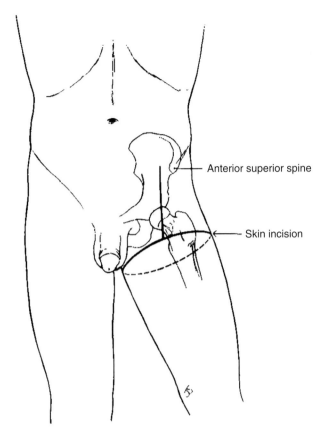

Figure 34-5 Simplified incision for hip disarticulation when done for ischemic gangrene. (From Jacobs LA. Above-knee amputation and hip disarticulation. In: Ernst CB, Stanley JC, eds. *Current therapy in vascular surgery.* St Louis, Mo: Mosby; 2001, with permission.)

physiatrist, and a number of support services. Ideally the physiatrist should see the patient prior to amputation. The early stages of rehabilitation consist of pain and edema control, strengthening and mobility, and the prevention of contractures. An elastic pressure dressing, known as a stump shrinker, is applied as soon as the wound is sufficiently healed. This helps to control the edema and shape the residual limb.

A temporary prosthesis is fitted approximately 6 weeks after surgery, at which time the patient begins to learn how to use the prosthesis. The temporary prosthesis can be easily modified as the patient's skill level increases and as the residual limb changes shape. Gait training begins with the temporary prosthesis. It is during this time that the physiatrist determines the most appropriate type of permanent prosthesis for the patient.

The permanent prosthesis is designed after the residual limb has stabilized in size and shape. The design of the socket is one of the most critical aspects of prosthetic design. The interface between the residual limb and socket of the prosthesis is one of the most critical aspects of rehabilitation. Difficulties in this area are the cause of many of the late complications seen with amputation wounds. The permanent prosthesis is very durable and can be expected to last at least 3 years.

is >50%, with a complication rate of nearly 80%.[41] Because of this extreme morbidity and mortality, aortoiliac revascularization may be indicated in order to avoid hip disarticulation and to facilitate healing of an above-knee amputation. The chances for successful rehabilitation following hip disarticulation are low in general, and are particularly dismal in patients with severe peripheral vascular disease.

A circumferential circular incision is made around the proximal thigh at the level of the gluteal crease, with extension onto the lower abdomen (Fig. 34-5). The retroperitoneal space is entered through the abdominal portion of the incision, by division of the muscles. The iliac vessels and femoral nerve are divided. The femoral head is exposed by dividing the posterior retroperitoneal musculature, creating side-to-side muscle flaps. The femur is transected, and then its head is disarticulated. The remainder of the muscles posterior to the femur are divided, and the wound closed in layers (Fig. 34-6).

REHABILITATION

Successful rehabilitation following lower extremity amputation requires the combined efforts of the surgeon,

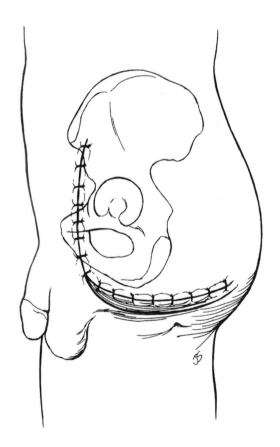

Figure 34-6 Closure of the hip disarticulation incision after trimming of "dog ears." (From Jacobs LA. Above-knee amputation and hip disarticulation. In: Ernst CB, Stanley JC, eds. *Current therapy in vascular surgery.* St Louis, Mo: Mosby; 2001, with permission.)

REFERENCES

1. Dillingham TR, Pezzin LE, MacKenzie EJ. Racial differences in the incidence of limb loss secondary to peripheral vascular disease: a population-based study. *Arch Phys Med Rehabil.* 2002;83: 1252–1257.

2. Feinglass J, Brown JL, LoSasso A, et al. Rates of lower-extremity amputation and arterial reconstruction in the United States, 1979 to 1996. *Am J Public Health.* 1999;89:1222–1227.

3. Fletcher DD, Andrews KL, Hallett JW Jr, et al. Trends in rehabilitation for geriatric patients with vascular disease: implications for future health resource allocation. *Arch Phys Med Rehabil.* 2002; 83:1389–1393.

4. Toursarakissian B, Shireman PK, Harrison A, et al. Major lower-amputation: contemporary experience in a single veterans affairs institution. *Am Surg.* 2002;68:606–610.

5. *Report of the national commission on diabetes.* Washington, DC: U.S. Government Printing Office; 1976. DHEW publication NIH 76-1002.

6. Lavery LA, Ashry HR, van Houtum W, et al. Variation in the incidence and proportion of diabetes-related amputation in minorities. *Diabetes Care.* 1996;19:48–52.

7. Chaturvedi N, Stevens LK, Fuller JH, et al. Risk factors, ethnic differences and mortality associated with lower-extremity gangrene and amputation in diabetes. The WHO multinational study of vascular disease in diabetes. *Diabetologia.* 2001;44: S65–S71.

8. Schina MJ Jr, Atnip RG, Healy DA, et al. The relative risk of limb revascularization and amputation in the modern era. *Cardiovasc Surg.* 1994;2:754–759.

9. Kazmers A, Perkins AJ, Jacobs LA. Major lower extremity amputation in Veterans Affairs Medical Centers. *Ann Vasc Surg.* 2000;14: 216–222.

10. Campbell WB, Marriott S, Eve R, et al. Amputation of acute ischaemia is associated with increased comorbidity and higher amputation level. *Cardiovasc Surg.* 2003;11:121–123.

11. Eliason JL, Wainess RM, Proctor MC, et al. A national and single institution experience in the contemporary treatment of acute lower extremity ischemia. *Ann Surg.* 2003;238:382–390.

12. Burke MJ, Roman V, Wright V. Bone and joint changes in lower limb amputees. *Ann Rheum Dis.* 1978;37:252–254.

13. Kulkarni J, Adams J, Thomas E. Association between amputation, arthritis and osteopenia in British male war veterans with major lower limb amputations. *Clin Rehabil.* 1998;12:348–353.

14. Gupta SK, Veith FJ, Samson RH, et al. Cost analysis of operations for infrainguinal atherosclerosis [Abstract]. *Circulation.* 1982; 66:II–I9.

15. Mackey WC, McCullough JL, Conlon TP, et al. The cost of surgery for limb-threatening ischemia. *Surgery.* 1986;99:26–35.

16. Raviola CA, Nichter LS, Baker JD. Cost of treating advanced leg ischemia: Bypass graft vs. primary amputation. *Arch Surg.* 1988; 123:495–496.

17. Tennvall GR, Apelqvist J. Prevention of diabetes-related foot ulcers and amputations: a cost-utility analysis based on Markov model simulations. *Diabetologia.* 2001;4:2077–2087.

18. Walters RL, Perry J, Antonelli D. Energy cost of walking amputees: the influence of level of amputation. *J Bone Joint Surg.* 1976;58: 42–46.

19. Pinzur MS. The metabolic cost of lower extremity amputation. *Clin Podiatr Med Surg.* 1997;14:599–602.

20. Couch NP, David JK, Tilney NL. Natural history of the leg amputee. *Am J Surg.* 1977;133:469–473.

21. Steinberg FU, Sunwoo I, Roettger RF, et al. Prosthetic rehabilitation of geriatric amputee patients: a follow-up study. *Arch Phys Med Rehabil.* 1985;66:742–745.

22. Keagy BA, Schwartz JA, Kotb M, et al. Lower extremity amputations: the control series. *J Vasc Surg.* 1986;4:321–326.

23. Robbs JV, Ray R. Clinical predictors of below-knee stump healing following amputation for ischaemia. *S Afr J Surg.* 1982; 20:305–310.

24. Durham JR. Lower extremity amputation levels: indications, determining the appropriate level, technique, and prognosis. In: Rutherford RB, ed. *Vascular surgery.* Philadelphia, Pa: WB Saunders; 2000.

25. Dwars BJ, van den Broek TA, Rauwerda JA. Criteria for reliable selection of the lowest level of amputation in peripheral vascular disease. *J Vasc Surg.* 1992;15:536–542.

26. Verta MJ, Gross WS, van Bellen B, et al. Forefoot perfusion pressure and minor amputation surgery. *Surgery.* 1976;80:729–734.

27. Bone GE, Pomajzl MJ. Toe blood pressure by photoplethysmography: an index of healing in forefoot amputations. *Surgery.* 1981;89:569–574.

28. Bunt TJ, Holloway GA. $TcPO_2$ as an accurate predictor of therapy in limb salvage. *Ann Vasc Surg.* 1996;10:224–227.

29. Ballard JL, Eke CC, Bunt TJ. A prospective evaluation of transcutaneous oxygen measurements in the management of diabetic foot problems. *J Vasc Surg.* 1995;22:485–490.

30. Bacharach JM, Rooke TW, Osmundson PJ, et al. Predictive value of transcutaneous oxygen pressure and amputation success by use of supine and elevation measurements. *J Vasc Surg.* 1992;15:558–563.

31. Wagner WH, Keagy BA, Kotb MM, et al. Noninvasive determination of healing of major lower extremity amputation: the continued role of clinical judgment. *J Vasc Surg.* 1988;8:703–710.

32. Bongard FS, Upton RA, Elings VB. Digital cutaneous fluorometry: Correlation between blood flow and fluorescence. *J Vasc Surg.* 1984;1:635–641.

33. Holloway GA Jr, Burgess EM. Preliminary experiences with laser Doppler velocimetry for the determination of amputation levels. *Prosthet Orthot Int.* 1983;7:63–66.

34. Black TL, Padberg FT, Thompson PN, et al. Probability of successful wound outcome determined by laser Doppler measurements using a heated probe (LDHP). *J Vasc Tech.* 1994;18:67–71.

35. Chang BB, Bock DE, Jacobs RL, et al. Increased limb salvage by the use of unconventional foot amputations. *J Vasc Surg.* 1994; 19:341–348.

36. Chang BB, Jacobs RL, Darling RC III, et al. Foot amputations. *Surg Clin North Am.* 1995;75:773–782.

37. Johnson WC, Watkins MT, Hamilton J. Transcutaneous partial oxygen pressure changes following skew flap and Burgess type below-knee amputations. *Arch Surg.* 1997;132:261–263.

38. Ayoub MM, Solis MM, Rogers JJ, et al. Thru-knee amputation: the operation of choice for non-ambulatory patients. *Am Surg.* 1993;59:619–623.

39. Nellis N, van de Water JM. Through-the-knee amputation: an improved technique. *Am Surg.* 2002;68:466–469.

40. Burgess EM. Disarticulation of the knee: a modified technique. *Arch Surg.* 1977;112:1250–1255.

41. Jacobs LA. Above-knee amputation and hip disarticulation. In: Ernst CB, Stanley JC, eds. *Current therapy in vascular surgery.* St. Louis, Mo: Mosby; 2001.